Genetic disorders among the Jewish people

A page from the Talmud (order Nashim, tractate Yevamot, 64b) giving the earliest account of hemophilia A

Richard M. Goodman, M.D.

Genetic disorders among the Jewish people

The Johns Hopkins University Press

BALTIMORE AND LONDON

The Johns Hopkins University Press, Baltimore, Maryland 21218
The Johns Hopkins Press Ltd., London

Library of Congress Catalog Card Number 78–21847
ISBN 0–8018–2120–7
Library of Congress Cataloging in Publication data will be found on the last printed page of this book.

To my dear parents
To my wife—my cherished companion—
and
To our sons, who bring us joy

Contents

Preface

THE SEEDS for the development of this text were planted in 1963 during my first visit to Israel when I came to study the problem of Buerger disease among Jews. As a by-product of the Buerger study I was introduced to a number of genetic disorders known to be common among the Jewish people. Through the years, as my knowledge and interest deepened concerning hereditary diseases in Jews, it became apparent that there was a need for a text to aid physicians, genetic counselors, and others who provide care for those individuals and families afflicted with these disorders.

Many questions, both medical and nonmedical in nature, arise when dealing with problems of genetic diseases in Jews. Although the answers are not always obvious or even known, knowledge of genetics, coupled with that of Jewish history, demography, and customs, has furthered our understanding of these disorders. However, much remains to be learned. The first chapters of this book serve as background material to introduce the reader to the historical and cultural development of the world's Jewish communities and to certain genetic principles applicable to the conditions discussed in later chapters. The disorders themselves are divided into the following categories: (1) genetic disorders among Ashkenazi Jews; (2) genetic disorders among Sephardi and Oriental Jews; (3) rare or isolated genetic syndromes; (4) disorders with complex or unproven inheritance; (5) nonpathological genetic traits and variants; and (6) misconceptions. This format was chosen as the one that would best represent the subject matter in terms of the number of conditions considered and their severity, mode of transmission, and distribution among the various Jewish ethnic groups.

In most instances the disorders are discussed according to *historical note, clinical features, diagnosis, basic defect, genetics, prognosis and treatment,* and *references.* At times, however, this format is not followed—for instance when the condition does not lend itself to such a presentation, or when only selected aspects of the disorder are being emphasized. Photographs permitting identification of patients have purposely been excluded. Introductory comments at the beginning of each chapter are meant to qualify or otherwise set the tone for the material discussed therein. References include supplemental readings as well as publications mentioned in the text.

It is hoped that this text will aid those responsible for bringing care and comfort to all who suffer from such disorders.

RICHARD M. GOODMAN, M.D.
Professor of Human Genetics
Tel Aviv University Sackler School of Medicine
The Chaim Sheba Medical Center, Tel Hashomer, Israel

xi

Acknowledgments

WERE IT NOT for the guidance and inspiration of three very special people, it is doubtful that this book would have been written.

Dr. Victor A. McKusick, who initially set the stage for my visit to Israel in 1963, not only helped me achieve this goal but also provided me with the opportunity to learn from him and others at The Johns Hopkins University Medical School about the evolving world of medical genetics.

The late Dr. Chaim Sheba opened avenues of thought regarding the Jewish people and their diseases that have served as fruitful sources for investigation and contemplation. In addition to intellectual stimulation, he offered warmth and understanding to all in his presence.

Through the years my dear friend and colleague Dr. Avinoam Adam and I have discussed many of the perplexing questions related to the subject of this text. He has always shared his thoughts and wealth of knowledge on genetic aspects of the Jewish communities.

I have indeed been fortunate to have these men as my mentors. To them and to the memory of Dr. Sheba I express my heartfelt thanks.

Numerous individuals at all levels of expertise have contributed enormously to the completion of this text, and to single out each person for his or her contribution would require several pages. Rather than offend those whose names might inadvertently be omitted, I would like to express my deep appreciation to all who have been so cooperative in sharing with me their scientific works, knowledge, advice, and varying talents. However, the efforts of some individuals have been of such magnitude that only through their guidance could certain topics be included in this text.

Professor Zvi Ankori has painstakingly and unselfishly guided me along the main roads and byways of Jewish history. For sharing with me his vast knowledge and expert advice, I express to him my deepest appreciation.

Under the tutelage of Rabbi Chaim Plato and Dr. Dov Erlich it has been possible for me to comment briefly on genetic disorders recorded or alluded to in the Bible and Talmud, and to both of these learned men I am grateful.

As in previous writings, I have been fortunate to have the assistance of two research associates, Dr. Beatrice Elian and Ms. Cheri Paper. Their tremendous efforts have made my work easier and to them I am grateful.

I would also like to thank Ms. Lesley Britles for typing the manuscript, Ms. Sara Asbel for her graphic work, and Mr. Mordecai Adato for his photographic assistance.

It has indeed been a pleasure to work with the staff of The Johns Hopkins University Press, and I am especially appreciative of the editorial efforts of Ms. Penny Moudrianakis.

Mr. George Crohn, Jr., president of the National Foundation for Jewish Genetic Diseases, deserves a special note of thanks for early support and encouragement. I would also like to thank the Lake Chemical Company (in memory of the late Dr. Lester Aronberg), the H. and E. Rosenberg Fund, and the Tel Aviv University Sackler School of Medicine for their support.

Perspective

GENETIC STUDIES on several ethnic and racial groups throughout the world show that many populations can be characterized by the high frequency or relative absence of certain genetic disorders common to each, and such is the situation with the Jewish people.

Although the ancient Hebrews during the Biblical and Talmudic periods were aware of a few genetic disorders, there is little evidence at present that these hereditary conditions can be traced to those now characteristically observed among the Jewish communities. It was not until the early 18th century that European physicians began to write about certain illnesses being more common in Ashkenazi Jews than in the surrounding non-Jewish population. Few of these conditions were thought to be of genetic etiology and much of this early medical reporting suffered from severe biases. However, by the end of the 19th century two genetic diseases (Tay-Sachs disease and Gaucher disease) were recognized as occurring more commonly in Ashkenazi Jews. By the beginning of the 20th century a voluminous amount of medical literature had been amassed purporting to show that Jews (Ashkenazim) were indeed afflicted more than other ethnic groups with a variety of illnesses, some of which were considered to be hereditary in nature. In 1911, in his book entitled *The Jews: A Study of Race and Environment*, Fishberg reviewed the status of a number of these disorders and for the most part concurred with the ongoing opinion that Jews have a special predilection for certain diseases. Many of the concepts acquired during this time concerning diseases in Jews were perpetuated and, unfortunately, some still exist today, despite the fact that they were based on poorly designed studies.

Very little was known about genetic diseases in the non-Ashkenazi Jewish communities until the immigration of Sephardi and Oriental Jews to Israel in the early 1950s. As Jews from all parts of the world began to settle in Israel, the country became an ideal laboratory for the investigation of a number of genetic disorders. This, coupled with the advances in medical genetics that occurred during the fifties, ushered in a new era of recognition of hereditary diseases among all populations. Over the past 20 years tremendous strides have been made in understanding a variety of genetic disorders, some of which are observed among the Jewish people. The existence of these more characteristic mutant genes in Jews is not due to some recent genetic or environmental happening, but rather is related to historical and cultural events that occurred centuries ago with the establishment of the different Jewish communities. It is precisely these past events that must be critically analyzed in the light of certain genetic principles in order that we may gain a perspective on why Jews suffer from these disorders today. Although a number of present-day medical services (genetic counseling, prenatal diagnosis, selective abortion, and screening programs), along with certain sociological changes in the Jewish communities themselves, will undoubtedly reduce the number of Jewish children born with these disorders, some of these mutant genes will continue to characterize certain specific Jewish ethnic groups.

Genetic disorders among the Jewish people

1

Comments on the origin and size of the world's Jewish communities

SOME OF THE REASONS why certain hereditary disorders occur among the Jewish people are intimately related to the historical development of the various Jewish communities. Thus, a rather detailed account of the origins and history of these communities is presented here along with information relating to their population size, past and present.

THE BEGINNING

According to the Scriptures the origin of the Jewish people began with Abraham, a native of Ur of the Chaldees, a city in Mesopotamia. Directed by G-d, Abraham left his country to settle in the Land of Canaan, where his divine mission was carried on by his son, Jacob. Jacob's wives, both Leah and Rachel, and their respective maids, Zilpah and Bilhah, bore him 12 sons. These 12 sons, with the exception of Joseph, became the "founding fathers" of the tribes of Israel. Joseph was not included, for he spent most of his life in Egypt, but his two sons, Ephraim and Manasseh, were given land rights in ancient Israel along with Joseph's brothers. Figure 1.1 traces the genetic origin of the 12 tribes of Israel.

The Jews' bondage in Egypt, the divine revelation of the Law, and the movement of the 12 tribes into the Land of Canaan all served as cohesive forces in the establishment of a nation, Israel. However, once established, it became difficult for the nation to maintain a sense of cohesion. Problems of diffusion, both geographical and biological, plagued the people, and in addition they had great difficulty defending themselves against the Philistines. The monarchy of Saul saved the Israelites from extinction and brought some degree of unity, but it was not until David became king that an entirely new concept was given to the Jewish people in terms of national identity and the establishment of new loyalties. David broke the tribal bonds and created a political and religious center, Jerusalem. The people became loyal to him, for his monarchy was the royal house chosen by G-d. Jerusalem, lying between the borders of Judah and Benjamin, was neutral with respect to the

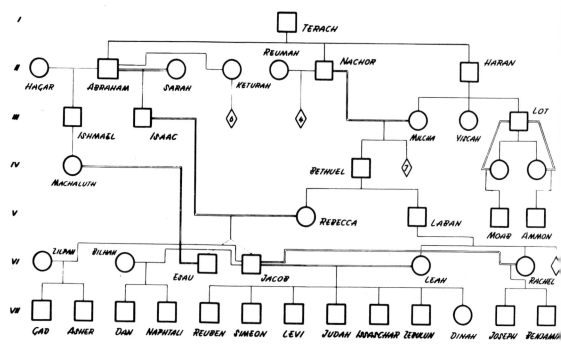

Figure 1.1. Origin of the 12 tribes of Israel beginning with Terach, the father of Abraham, and proceeding to Jacob and his 12 sons. Note the high degree of consanguinity indicated by the double lines.

tribal division of the land. The Ark of the Covenant was transferred to Jerusalem, making the city the center of religious allegiance. From this time on, the City of David and the Royal House of David became an integral part of the religious and cultural development of the Jewish people. The monumental task which David undertook was achieved in the face of the greatest difficulties. David's son, Solomon, went on to build the First Temple and greatly expanded the nation territorially. With this territorial expansion, however, came exposure to a number of diluting forces—religious, cultural, and biological. Moreover, the Jews' identity as a people was threatened by the forces of aggression as well as assimilation, for they found it increasingly difficult to defend the land.

The once unified nation of Israel was divided in 933 B.C.E.,* with 10 tribes forming the northern Kingdom of Israel, and Judah and Benjamin in the south making up the Kingdom of Judah. The northern Kingdom of Israel became cosmopolitan, with urban centers and commercial development reaching out to the sea. In addition, it interdigitated with various cultures, notably that of the Phoenicians. In contrast, the Kingdom of Judah was land-locked, backward, and poor, and as such became provincial. Nevertheless, the destiny of the Jewish people continued in Judah, while the broader policies of David and Solomon were carried on in Israel. The Kingdom of Israel faced the problem that has remained with the

* B.C.E., "before the Common Era," is the term used by Jews for the Christian era B.C.

Jewish people throughout their history—the conflicting forces arising from the desire to be open, with the resulting effects of dilution and assimilation, versus the desire for preservation, which leads to a degree of isolationism and inwardness.

In 722 B.C.E. the Kingdom of Israel fell. Although the legend of the "Ten Lost Tribes of Israel" has remained alive in Jewish history, not all the people of Israel were actually exiled. The rank and file of the population did not leave the land— only the upper classes (leaders, skilled workers, etc.) were exiled. In 587 B.C.E. the Kingdom of Judah fell, and again the upper eschelons of society were exiled to Babylonia while the common people remained. The 135 years in which Judah survived following the fall of Israel brought a tremendous change in the religious concepts of the Jewish people. What had happened in Israel was to serve as an example for Judah. Judah made Jerusalem the center of Judaism, and after Judah was captured it became entrenched in the minds of the people that Jerusalem could not be duplicated elsewhere and that a Jew could never forget Jerusalem. Following the destruction of the Jerusalem Temple, the Jewish people were without a spiritual center and thousands no longer lived in their homeland. How did they survive spiritually? Out of their Babylonian exile came a number of new concepts. Sacrifice gave way to prayer, the Temple was entrusted to synagogues, and collective responsibility before G-d gave way to individual retribution for sin and reward for good deeds. The Jewish religion remained institutionalized and state involvement in religion continued, but religious expression became personal rather than collective.

The Babylonian exile marked the beginning of Diaspora Jewry and the development of the various Jewish communities.

CLASSIFICATION OF JEWS

In a text dealing with genetic disorders among Jews, the classification of Jews becomes extremely important. If one is afflicted with a hereditary disease characteristically observed in Jews, in most cases that individual must be a Jew genetically. According to the *Halacha* (Jewish Law), however, one is a Jew if one's mother is Jewish or if one converts to Judaism according to the requirements of the Law. Those who convert to Judaism probably do not carry those mutant genes which account for the various disorders found among the Jewish people.

Leaving the question of religious classification to the rabbis, there is still some need to comment on a few terms that have been used in the past and that may also be found today with regard to the classification of Jews. Some authors have spoken of the Jews as a *race*. In terms of modern anthropology, however, the Jews cannot be considered a race, for physically they are a very heterogeneous group possessing no distinguishing racial features. This point will be discussed further in Chapter 2. Others have referred to the Jews as a *nation*—a nation in the tribal sense stemming from Biblical times. Such a broad definition is factual, in that it points to the early origin of Jews, but it is not sufficiently discriminating to be used when referring to genetic diseases among Jews. It is more acceptable to refer to the Jews as a *people*. They are a people composed of various groups, but they are one in that they share a common religion, culture, historical experience, and language (although Hebrew is not spoken by all Jews).

Unfortunately, Jewish historians, linguists, anthropologists, and population geneticists have not pooled their knowledge to produce a unified classification of Jews that is acceptable to all. The problem in classifying the Jewish communities pertains to the many dynamic events that have molded these groups. Their various migrations, with exposure to such forces as religious conversion, assimilation, and intermarriage, account for some of the difficulties in achieving a degree of uniformity in the classification of the various communities. Nevertheless, tenacious bonds have kept most of these groups together throughout their perilous history, thus maintaining their distinct identities. In addition, the various Jewish languages which developed in the Diaspora also aided in uniting the people both culturally and religiously. Common to these written languages were the Hebrew alphabet and elements of both Hebrew and Aramaic. Perhaps the best known of the Jewish languages are Yiddish (Judeo-German) and Ladino (Judeo-Spanish). Others include Judeo-French, Judeo-Italian, Judeo-Greek, Judeo-Arabic, Judeo-Persian, Judeo-Berber, and Tat (spoken by mountain Jews of the Caucasus), plus Gruzinic (the language of Jews of Georgia) and Crimchak (the language of Crimean Jews). For the linguist these languages provide an ideal means of classifying the various Jewish ethnic groups, since the linguistic history of the Jews accurately mirrors their dispersion throughout the world.

Certain Jewish historians, on the other hand, prefer to classify Jews according to the political regime or civilization under which they resided during a given period of time. One can therefore find broad divisions such as Jews under Islamic rule or Jews under Christian rule. Historians have also written about Jews under the Persian, Greek, Roman, Byzantine, and Ottoman empires. This method of classification is accurate in its depiction of a particular time period with its primary influencing factor, be it religious, political, or both.

From a genetic viewpoint, the Jewish people as a whole make up a heterogeneous population; however, more recent population studies using various genetic markers are beginning to show common threads reflecting the early Middle Eastern origin of the Jews (see Chapter 2). For various reasons, geneticists have not used the classifications put forth by historians or linguists, but rather have relied on such terms as *Ashkenazim*, *Sephardim*, and *Oriental*, or in some instances speak of the groups with reference to their present or former countries of origin. Essentially, this third method of classification will be used in the present text.

One problem with the terms *Sephardim* and *Oriental* is that they are too broad and therefore do not reflect the distinct features of particular subgroups. In such instances the country or place of origin also must be mentioned. For example, Yemenite and Persian Jews both come under the heading Oriental Jews, but the genetic traits and diseases of each are so different that it is essential to speak of them in terms of their place of origin. Such problems also exist among the Ashkenazim, and, when necessary, geographical regions will be noted.

Obviously, each authority views the classification of Jews through the eyes of his or her discipline. However, the geneticist must seek the advice of the Jewish historian and linguist, for the geneticist is examining the present, which can be seen in proper perspective only by understanding the past.

DEVELOPMENTAL FEATURES OF THE THREE MAJOR
JEWISH COMMUNITIES

The Jews are a Middle Eastern people. They originated in this region, and throughout their long history there has always been a segment of the population living in this part of Asia and North Africa. With the destruction of the First Temple, part of the community moved eastward and became the founders of Babylonian Jewry, which still exists today. Those Jews who remained in ancient Israel formed what may be called the Palestinian branch of Oriental Jewry.

Babylonian Jewry has gone through periods of expansion and contraction but has never disappeared. In times of great difficulty, segments of the community left Babylonia (modern-day Iraq) and established themselves in other parts of Asia— in countries and places known today as Iran, India, Kurdistan, Afghanistan, Bukhara, and regions of the Caucasus Mountains. Thus, various subgroups developed new cultural ways which influenced their language and religious customs. Biological mixing with the "host" population in turn influenced physical appearance. Such factors are not unique to Oriental Jewry but can also be noted among the Sephardi and Ashkenazi groups.

Several important historical facts about Oriental Jewry are: (1) Oriental Jews represent the original "gene pool" of the Jewish people; (2) they never had to totally abandon their roots; Jews, although at times small in number, have always remained in the region; (3) for the past 1,300 years Oriental Jews have lived under the Islamic civilization; (4) many subgroups, with distinct environmental and genetic features, have evolved from Oriental Jewry; (5) the main languages of Oriental Jewry have been Arabic, Persian, and Judeo-Arabic.

With the rise of the Greco-Roman Empire, Oriental Jews began to migrate westward. With the advent of Islam and its westward thrust as far as Spain, a segment of Oriental Jewry evolved into what later came to be known as Sephardi Jewry. Centuries later, when the Moslems were defeated in the Iberian Peninsula and returned eastward, the Sephardi communities were expelled from Spain and moved mainly toward the eastern basin of the Mediterranean. Prior to this eastward refugee movement, portions of the Sephardi population had established themselves along the coast of North Africa.

Important historical facts about Sephardi Jewry include: (1) Sephardi Jewry is an outgrowth of Oriental Jewry; (2) it acquired the name Sephardi (in Hebrew *Sephardi* means "Spanish") after ceasing to exist in its main area of development (Spain); (3) most Sephardi Jews then came under Turkish Islamic rule; (4) many distinct subgroups evolved from Sephardi Jewry and established communities along the northern and southern shores of the Mediterranean and in parts of Western Europe and North and South America; (5) the main language of Sephardi Jewry was Ladino (Judeo-Spanish).

Ashkenazi Jewry also grew out of Oriental Jewry, mainly the Palestinian segment. While individual Jews made their way into Europe during the Romans' rule, most arrived in the Middle Ages and established themselves in France and Germany. Like the Sephardim, the Ashkenazim were eventually forced to abandon their roots and moved into Eastern Europe, where they became the largest of the Jewish communities. As they reached their peak in population, persecutions and economic difficulties in early modern times chipped away at their foundation, scattering parts of the community in all directions, but mainly westward. This westward migration culminated in the formation of American Jewry. The holocaust during World War II annihilated more than half of the Ashkenazi community.

Several important historical characteristics of Ashkenazi Jewry are: (1) It is an outgrowth of Oriental Jewry, mainly its Palestinian segment; (2) it acquired the name Ashkenazi Jewry from its early roots in Germany (*Ashkenazim* is Hebrew for "Germans"), but after a period of time moved into Central and Eastern Europe; (3) the majority of Ashkenazi Jews grew up within the framework of Christian society; (4) although it developed various regional and ethnic differences, it never established the degree of distinct subgroups that is found within Oriental and Sephardi Jewry; (5) the main language among Ashkenazi Jews was Yiddish.

ORIENTAL JEWRY

Since the time of Babylonian captivity Jews have been scattered in various parts of the Orient, but mainly in the Middle East and parts of the Mediterranean basin (North Africa). Today the term *Oriental Jews* refers mainly to those Jewish communities which have existed within the territorial and cultural bounds of Islamic civilization.

Jews in the Orient were predominantly agrarian until the advent of Islam. Then, during the 7th and 8th centuries C.E.,* important changes took place within the Jewish communities that came under Moslem influence. The Moslems were eager to have both Jews and Christians convert to their religion, and one way to accomplish this was to impose discriminatory taxes on the non-Moslem population. Jews and Christians were forced to pay a degrading poll-tax and a heavy land tax which amounted to a 20 percent tax on their yield. Conversion to Islam brought exemption from these taxes. The response to this discrimination was twofold. A great number of Christians and Jews decided to convert to Islam. It was not difficult from a religious viewpoint, due to the many similarities in customs, and it was most advantageous from a financial standpoint. This was not forced conversion. However, the majority of Jews decided not to convert. They migrated to new cities that offered many opportunities and a chance to continue their Jewish way of life.

Colonial cities were a necessity to the Arab conquerors, but later Islamic rulers built new garrison and administration cities to protect the integrity of their dynasties. For example, in early Islamic times (716) the Umayyad dynasty built Fustat or Old Cairo. The city of Baghdad was built in 762 under the auspices of the Abbasid dynasty, which deposed the Umayyads. In 969 the Fatimids (a Shiite ruling sect) built the city Al-Kahra or Cairo (City of Victory) on the other side of the Nile. The Fatimids also built in the early 10th century Mahdiya, in North Africa, close to the earlier Islamic garrison-city Kairuwan. Other cities built in the same way included Kufa, Basra, Rabbat, Fez, and Ramle in Palestine, to mention a few. From the 8th century onward, these cities were great Jewish centers, and some members of these communities were outstanding international merchants. In the late 8th century Baghdad became the main center of Islam and at the same time the

---

* *C.E.*, "Common Era," is the term used by Jews for the Christian era A.D.

focal point of Eastern Jewry. However, in the late 9th century, fragmentation began in Islam, followed by fragmentation within the Oriental Jewish communities. For example, in Fustat in the second half of the 9th century Ibn Tulun declared himself the independent ruler of Egypt, Palestine, and Syria. The Jewish communities there also separated themselves from the Jewish authorities in Baghdad, and an Egyptian-Palestinian-Syrian federation was formed for the Islamic people and the Jewish people. Under the Tulunids, and later under the Fatimids, Jewry flourished in Egypt, and in Palestine a Gaonate was established, thus providing a source of spiritual leadership. Excellent documentation for this period can be found in the Cairo Geniza (discarded Jewish manuscripts and books stored for burial). In 1071 the Seljuks invaded Palestine, bringing an end to the Palestinian Gaonate. The Palestine Gaonic Academy moved to Tyre and later to Damascus. In 1096 the Fatimids reconquered Palestine, but in 1099 the Crusaders captured Jerusalem. Not until the 13th century did the Palestinian Jews succeed in substantially rebuilding their settlements.

Egyptian Jewry continued to flourish, despite the fall of the Fatimids in 1171. The Ayyubid rulers, who followed the Fatimid dynasty, treated the Jews favorably, but by 1250 a new type of government had been established in Egypt under the Mamluks. The Mamluks ruled Egypt, Palestine, and Syria until the Ottoman conquest in 1516/1517. Having stopped the Mongol invaders in 1258 and having ultimately ousted the Crusaders, they provided a strong government from a military standpoint, but being a military feudal cast, they destroyed the country economically and brought the Jewish population to a very low point. With the Mongol conquest of Baghdad in 1258 and the corrupt economic system of the Mamluks there was a constant movement of Jews from east to west. The decline of Oriental Jewry must therefore be correlated with the deterioration and general decline of the Arab world from the 13th century onward. The story of the changing fortune of Oriental Jews following the advent of the Turks in the 16th century belongs to a later chapter.

ARABIAN JEWRY

Arabian Jewry, which is part of Oriental Jewry, can be divided into North and South Arabian Jewry. Jews from Palestine settled in North Arabia (in ancient times known as Hijaz; today known as Saudi Arabia) after the destruction of the Second Temple. Prior to this some Jews from Babylonia may have come to the area via the Taima Oasis. The Jews were the first settlers to introduce agricultural plantations to this region. These plantations were surrounded by various nomadic Arab tribes. Over the years the Jews became the leaders in trade and agriculture, but accepted the Arabic language and certain Arab customs, including a tribal mode of life. Until about a hundred years prior to Mohammed, Jews made up the majority of the population of the main city of Hijaz, Medina. When Mohammed left Mecca and came to Medina, he entered the city with the hope that the Jews of Medina would join him in the new-found religion of Islam. He encouraged them by offering to change the direction of prayer from Mecca to Jerusalem, to make the 10th day of the first month the great fast like Yom Kippur, and to incorporate other Jewish traditions into the new religion. Some Jews did convert; the majority, however, were unwilling to follow him. Mohammed then withdrew his pro-Jewish injunctions and began an armed struggle against the Jews of Medina and the northern regions. Many Jews were killed; others were taken into slavery or driven into exile. Some may have sought refuge in Palestine. In any event Jews disappeared from North Arabia.

The story of South Arabian Jewry is much different. South Arabia, which today makes up North and South Yemen, is a much lusher part of the Arabian peninsula. From the time of the 2nd century C.E., Jews resided in several cities of South Arabia (then known as Himyar). The area was well populated and the Jewish communities of that region were in close contact with those in Palestine. Trade with India and the Mediterranean countries constituted an important part of the economy of the region and Jews actively participated in it. In the 5th century two superpowers, Persia and the Byzantine Empire, vied for control of South Arabia. As a countermeasure, King Dhu Nuwas of Himyar decided to accept Judaism, and thus a Jewish kingdom was formed which lasted until forces from Ethiopia conquered the territory in 525 C.E. The Abyssinians ruled for 50 years, followed by the Persians and finally the Arabs. Unlike the Jews of Hijaz, however, the Jews of Himyar remained, notwithstanding the victory of Islam.

In the latter part of the 12th century, with the conquest of Yemen by the Ayyubid dynasty, the conditions of Jewry in Himyar deteriorated markedly. The dynasty's 80-year rule oppressed the Jews as never before, and it seemed that the community would be threatened with extinction. The leaders of the community contacted Maimonides, who responded with the "Epistle to Yemen." His words of inspiration gave strength to the community and he is regarded as the one who saved the Yemenite Jewish community from disaster.

The city of Sana then became the main center of South Arabian Jewry, and by the 19th century one-third of all the Jews living in Yemen resided there. But the position of Jews in Yemen was steadily downgraded under various fanatic Islamic sects and in 1882 a small number of Yemenite Jews left their country to settle in Palestine. In the 20th century, through the efforts of the Zionist pioneer movement, the Yemenite Jewish community was rediscovered, and in 1949–1950 almost the entire Jewish population of Yemen and Aden was flown (Operation Magic Carpet) to the newly formed state of Israel.

SEPHARDI JEWRY

During the Middle Ages the biblical term *Sefarad* was reinterpreted to mean "Spain," while the name Sephardi was given to the Jews of Spain (and thereafter to their descendants, wherever they resided). The term was used particularly for those Jews who were expelled from Spain in 1492 and settled along the North African coast and in Italy, Egypt, Palestine, and Syria. However, the majority of the Sephardim settled in the Balkans and the central provinces of the Ottoman Empire, where they established many communities, notably in Salonica and Constantinople.

During the Roman period some Hebrews may have settled in Spain along with the Phoenicians. They definitely came to the country after the destruction of the Second Temple of Jerusalem in 70 C.E. According to some accounts, they settled there after the destruction of the First Temple in 586 B.C.E. Other historians speculate that the ancient Hebrews spread out along the shores of the Mediterranean, mingling and developing a sense of kinship with early Semitics (Phoenicians) along the coast. In either case, they were in Spain in considerable numbers by 300 C.E., for in 301 the Council of Bishops in the city of Elvira issued decrees prohibiting Christians from calling a rabbi to bless their fields, from attending Jewish festivals, from marrying a Jewess (though they were allowed to marry pagan women), and from mingling with Jews. These laws show that by the early 4th century Jews carried significant weight in Spain.

In spite of the Christianization of Spain in the early part of the 4th century it was difficult for the authorities to ignore the Jewish influence that existed there. During the 5th century the western part of the Roman Empire was overrun by Germanic tribes. The Visigoths, nonorthodox Christians of the Arian creed and themselves a minority, tolerated the Jewish religion. Mutual trust also existed between the Gothic masters and their Jewish subjects, for those Jews who lived at the foot of the Pyrenees effectively guarded the frontier against repeated invasions by their Frankish neighbor to the north. The situation changed in 588 when the Visigoth ruler of Spain, King Reccared IV, converted to Catholicism, the religion of the majority population, and established the Catholic faith as the religion of the state. This had the immediate effect of isolating Jews from the mainstream of Spanish society. Although a number of prohibitions were passed against the Jews, the nobles and other authorities remained well disposed toward them, and under Reccared's immediate successors the severe anti-Jewish measures fell largely into abeyance. In 613, however, Visigoth king Sisebut ordered the forced conversion of Jews to Christianity and for approximately 100 years thereafter the Jews of Spain faced constant and ruthless persecution.

In 711 the Moslem commander Al-Tarik crossed the Strait of Gibraltar and invaded Spain. Within four short years practically the entire country was under Islamic control. Thus, the Jews of Spain moved out of an era of persecution into a period of great enlightenment and prosperity. By the 10th century, Spain had separated herself from the Eastern Caliphate and had formed her own caliphate in Cordova. The nation became the most advanced, cultured, and prosperous country of Western Europe. The society of Spain was a pluralistic one, with Jews, Christians, and Moslems developing their own cultural identities under the supreme government of Islam. Judaism flourished in this environment and great scholars, physicians, poets, diplomats, courtiers, and financiers were to be found in the Jewish community during this period.

By the mid-11th century, however, the War of (Christian) Reconquest had begun, with the Christians in northern Spain consolidating and beginning their march southward. Spain became the home of two state religions, Christianity and Islam, each ruling over a fragmented camp. This fragmentation kept the Jews alive in Spain until 1480, when the nation united under Christianity.

In the latter part of the 11th century the Moslem Almoravides from North Africa invaded Spain and succeeded in unifying certain Moslem principalities but they did not capture Christian territory. The year 1148 saw the invasion of Spain by the Almohades, a fanatical Moslem sect from Morocco which forced both Jews and Christians to convert to Islam. It was during this period that the family of Maimonides (the Rambam) fled from Spain to Morocco and later to Egypt. These

Moslem invasions of Spain did not prevent the reconquest of the country by Christian forces, however, and by the mid-13th century all of Spain except the southern province of Granada was under the rule of Christendom. The function of Jews as intermediaries between Christians and Moslems came to an end. From 1391 until their expulsion from Spain in 1492, Jews were subjected to forced baptism and constant threats and acts of persecution.

As a result of the Spanish Inquisition approximately 150,000 Jews were expelled from Spain in 1492 and three Jewish groups emerged. In order to understand these groups it is important to note that Spanish Jewry at this time was a society torn by deep class divisions.

The first group consisted primarily of lower middle class Jews who were committed to their religious beliefs and who left Spain for Morocco, Italy, and the Ottoman Turkish Empire. From Turkey some moved on to settle in Palestine, which was conquered by the Turks in 1516. For those who chose to settle in various parts of the Ottoman Empire it was like closing the circle. Returning to Islamic rule, they flourished as in centuries past.

The second group, the elite and prominent upper-class segment of Jewish society, felt equal to their Christian counterparts and many decided to maintain their status by voluntarily converting to Christianity. Many intermarried and, because they were not strongly committed to a Jewish way of life, easily reconciled themselves to their fate. These Jews were called *Conversos*.

Between these two extremes was a third class of Jews who had a great deal to lose if they accepted expulsion. Because they were stronger believers in Judaism than the elite upper-class Jews, they decided to accept Christianity outwardly, but to live clandestinely as Jews. These Jews became known as *Marranos*. In Hebrew the term is *anusim*, meaning "coerced."

While "coercion" to accept Christianity was the policy of the Spanish Church, the Spanish people felt endangered by the influx of Jews into their ranks, for converted Jews competed with them even more intensely politically and economically. Thus, by the mid-15th century, pogroms were launched in Toledo, not against professing Jews, but against the *Conversos* and even against second- and third-generation Christians. Some *Conversos* and *Marranos* left Spain and settled as Christians in southern France, Holland, and England, where professing Jews were not allowed to reside.

When in 1497 Spain and Portugal were united through a marriage alliance, the Jews of Portugal were ordered to leave the country or convert to Christianity. As it turned out, they were never permitted to leave and were forced to convert. Some Jews fully converted while others elected to live like the *Marranos* of Spain. With the Portuguese Inquisition in 1536, many *Marranos* left Portugal for Holland, Italy, parts of the Ottoman Empire, and the New World.

By the 16th century officially there were no Jews living in Spain, Portugal, France, England, Southern Italy and Sicily, and some parts of Germany. However, behind this facade thousands of *Conversos* and *Marranos* were living under the guise of Christianity. With the defeat of the Spanish Armada in 1588 and the independence of the Netherlands from Spain, it became possible for the clandestine Jewish communities of Western Europe to cast off their Christian garb and return to their true identities. Sephardi communities sprang up in such cities as Amsterdam, London, Hamburg, Bordeaux, Bayonne, and elsewhere in Western Europe, as well as in the West Indies and on the mainland of North America. Although these communities were not exceptionally large, they were of great significance economically and politically.

The differentiation between Sephardi Jewry and Ashkenazi Jewry became marked from the 16th century onward. Basically, the difference was one of synagogal rite and tradition, that of the Sephardim going back ultimately to the Babylonian tradition, and that of the Ashkenazim to Palestinian roots. It was reflected also in the pronunciation of Hebrew and in social habits, literary fashions, costume, etc. The Sephardim spoke a Judeo-Spanish vernacular Ladino while the Ashkenazim spoke Yiddish. The great cultural center of Sephardi life until modern times was Salonica, which was destroyed by the Nazis in 1943.

JEWRY UNDER BYZANTINE AND OTTOMAN RULE

While the religious unity of Western Europe, heir to the Western Roman Empire, was preserved under the popes, the area fragmented politically into several states as a result of the Germanic invasions. On the other hand, the Eastern Byzantine Empire succeeded in withstanding the attacks of the barbarians but was torn from within by various heretical movements which in fact were expressions of rebellious tendencies in the eastern regions. When these eastern regions (Syria, Palestine, Egypt, and North Africa) were finally conquered by the Arabs in the first half of the 7th century, the Byzantine Empire became, for all intents and purposes, a Greek state, with the Greek language and the Greek Orthodox Church being the hallmarks of its identity. For some 300 years this Greek state was in constant confrontation with Islam, and strengthening its Christian identity from within seemed to several emperors the necessary means of safeguarding the survival of Byzantium. Hence, sporadic attacks were directed against minorities in the state, primarily against Jews. From the 7th to the 10th century, Byzantine Jews were subjected to four waves of forced conversion, at the end of which they reached a low point numerically, politically, and economically. The survivors were segregated and relegated economically to the profession of hide tanners. Some sought refuge in Khazaria and neighboring countries. However, by the second half of the 10th century, with the decline of the Eastern Caliphate, there was a new upsurge of Byzantine military might after 300 years of constant tug-of-war with Islam. Byzantium became a great commercial and military power and reconquered several northeastern regions. Thus many Jewish communities of the east were incorporated into the Byzantine Empire. Jews immigrated to the principal towns and cities of the empire, thereby reviving old centers and creating new ones. By the 12th century approximately 85,000 Jews were living under Western Byzantine rule. With the parallel influx of Italian merchants from the West and the establishment of trading colonies in Constantinople and other cities, Jews became but one of many minorities in a pluralistic society and partook of the prosperity that characterized the era. However, the Crusades and the hegemony of the Italian maritime republics brought a drastic change in the international position of Byzantium.

In 1204 Constantinople was conquered by the Christian forces of the 4th Crusade and the Byzantine Empire was partitioned among the conquering Western Allies. In 1261 it partly regained its sovereignty, but in truth the empire never recovered from the attack in 1204. With the rise of Turkish forces in Anatolia—first the Seljukid Turks in the 11th century, then the Ottoman Turks in the 14th century— the fate of the empire was sealed. In 1453 Constantinople fell to the Ottoman Turks.

By 1516 Palestine and Syria had come under Ottoman rule and in 1517 Egypt was conquered by the Turks. A renaissance of Sephardi Jewry developed in Palestine at this time and the city of Safed became a great center of Jewish learning and culture. Ottoman expansion in the 16th century brought Romania and Hungary under Turkish influence, thus interlocking the two main bodies of Jews—the Ashkenazim living in Central Europe and the Sephardim living under Ottoman rule. The close proximity of these two communities during the 16th and 17th centuries was beneficial to both. The Ottoman Empire became a place of refuge for the persecuted Ashkenazim of Central Europe. Culturally the two communities stimulated each other to better define their identities and traditions. Joseph Caro, a Sephardi Jew living in Safed, wrote the *Shulkan Arukh* [The Prepared Table], recodification of Jewish Law according to Sephardi tradition, while Moses Isserles in Cracow wrote *Ha-Mappah* [The Tablecloth], an incorporation of Ashkenazi traditions concerning Jewish Law. Thus the *Shulkan Arukh* and *Ha-Mappah* became the authoritative code for Orthodox Jewry throughout the world.

The 18th century brought the deterioration of the Ottoman Empire and subsequent decline in the status of Jews. This process culminated in the first Balkan War and World War I, when the Turkish Empire was destroyed.

ASHKENAZI JEWRY

Ashkenazi Jews make up approximately 82 percent of the world's Jewish population. During the Middle Ages the Hebrew term *Ashkenaz* became identified with Germany, and thus, in a narrow sense, Ashkenazim are German Jews. However, the designation also encompasses their descendants in other countries.

As mentioned earlier, some Jews followed the Roman legions beyond the Alps. The reestablishment of tranquility in northern Europe under the Carolingians (751– 987) afforded the founders of Ashkenazi Jewry new and broader opportunities. Successive emperors appreciated the value of Jews in the economic sphere and accorded them special privileges and protection under charters. Thus, some international Jewish merchants from Moslem Spain and other countries settled in France. In the 10th century Jewish families from Italy settled in the Rhineland, forming the nuclei of later prominent communities in the area. In the 11th century several Jewish communities scattered throughout France and western Germany participated in the general upsurge of urbanization. Charters of protection were issued to these communities, bringing many opportunities for growth and prosperity. Ashkenazi Jewry as it is known today stems from these early Franco-German communities.

By the end of the 11th century, however, a movement had begun which was to be a turning point in the destiny of the Jews of Christian Europe. The Crusades marked the beginning of a series of murderous outbreaks prompted as much by economic jealousy as by religious fanaticism. The 1st Crusade in 1096 signaled a series of sanguinary onslaughts on the Jews of the Rhineland in such places as Speyer, Mainz, Worms, and Cologne. Thereafter massacre accompanied each Crusade and was regularly associated with Jewish life in Europe. The 2nd Crusade in 1147 was signaled by the spread of that infection to northern France. The 3rd Crusade consisted of a series of outbreaks in England. The massacre at York, on the day preceding Palm Sunday in 1190, became notorious in English as well as Jewish annals. In addition a blood libel in England, France, and Germany, accused Jews of killing Christians and of using their blood for ritual purposes. Individual Jews and whole Jewish communities were thereby exposed to the dangers of mob assault.

Events of the 13th century finally brought West European Ashkenazi Jewry to the brink of disaster. Great heretical movements within the Roman Church caused the latter to establish the Holy Office of Inquisition, the purpose of which was to guard over the standards of Christianity in the Christian world. Although originally not directed against Jews, the Inquisition eventually proved to be the scourge of Jewry under Western Christendom. Simultaneously, the economic function of the Jew was degraded, as he was relegated to the role of a money lender, a role which excited anti-Semitic feelings. The further alienation of Jews was signaled by the canon passed by the 4th Lateran Council of the Church which ordered all Jews to wear the yellow badge.

These events and actions culminated in the expulsion of Jews from various West European countries. In 1290 Jews were expelled from England, and between 1306 and 1394 they were driven out of France three times.

While these developments brought much misery to Jews in the West, a new life awaited Jews in Poland. This new-found opportunity came about as a result of the devastating Tartar invasions. In 1241 the Tartar inroads were checked and in 1264, seeking much-needed skills and manpower, the Duke of Kalish called upon foreign settlers to come in and rebuild the Polish cities on the basis of charters of protection. With the deterioration of Jewish life in the West, many Jews joined non-Jewish settlers in Poland. In 1333 the Polish duchies were united into a kingdom and by 1334 the charter safeguarding Jewish liberties was extended to the whole country. This was confirmed and amplified by King Casmir the Great in 1364. The new Jewish settlers provided a much-needed middle class between the landed proprietors and the peasantry.

In the latter part of the 14th century, to secure succession by a male heir, the Polish crown entered into a personal union with the Grand Duchy of Lithuania (the Lublin Union), thereby opening Lithuania as well to the influx of Jews. Lithuania was at this time a huge territory consisting mainly of forest lands sprinkled with small villages; it had undergone almost no urban development. Early in the 15th century only a few Jews elected to move into this wilderness. Following the Lublin Union, Polish noblemen became the feudal lords of great tracts of land in Lithuania, and Jews were sent into this region to help develop the country economically. Jews went into this wilderness in *very small groups* and it was not uncommon for *one or two families* to settle in villages that were far apart from each other. The Jews did not work in agriculture but were involved in small businesses such as innkeeping, dealing in furs and lumber, and the manufacture of vodka. Because of their economic interests and their cultural and linguistic differences, the local population was often hostile toward them.

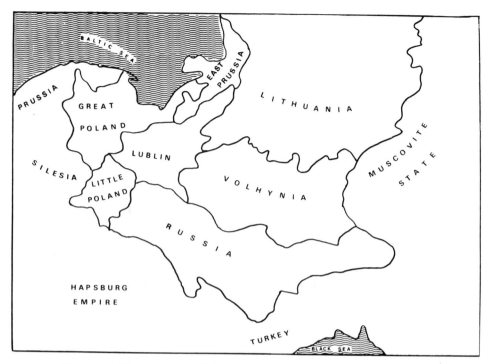

Figure 1.2. The area of Polish Jewry encompassing the "Four Lands,"
1667–1764. Note the vast size of Lithuania during this period.

By the end of the 16th century, Polish-Lithuanian Jewry and Ottoman Jewry
had become the most important Jewish communities both numerically and
intellectually.

The great autonomy and high cultural achievements of the Polish and Lithuanian
Jews at this time found expression in the famous Council of Four Lands (the
provinces of Great Poland, Little Poland, Podolia, and Volhynia), with its
elaborate organization and quasi-parliamentary powers (see Figure 1.2), and in the
parallel, independent council held in Lithuania.

The effects of the Lublin Union of 1569 and the resulting oppression by the
Poles of the local East European populations, from the Baltic Sea to the Ukraine,
had an indelible impact on the Jews who moved into these regions. When the local
populations rose in revolt under the Cossack leader Chmielnicki in 1648–1649,
Jews as well as Poles were massacred, but the Jews—the immediate go-betweens
and agents of the Polish landlords—sustained the greater tragedy. In the 1650s the
Swedes invaded Poland from the north while the Cossacks devastated the land
from the east. The ensuing wave of massacres ended the days of tranquility that had
hitherto been the rule.

Poland and Polish Jewry never recovered from the 17th-century "deluge."
Further tragic developments were in store for them throughout the 18th century.
The first partitioning of Poland—agreed upon by Austria, Prussia, and Russia—
occurred in 1772, with all of eastern Poland, Lithuania, Byelorussia, Podolia, and
the Ukraine being incorporated into Russia. The czar did not want the Jews to

infiltrate Russia proper, where they had hitherto been nonexistent, so in 1804 the Pale (Figure 1.3) was established. A huge ghetto-like territory, it confined the Jews to 13 regional governments: 5 in Lithuania and White Russia, 5 in the Ukraine, 1 in Little Russia, and 3 in New Russia (on the Black Sea). Within the confines of the Pale began the great biological multiplication of Ashkenazi Jewry. Aided by the relative absence of war and by improved health conditions, the Jewish population of Eastern Europe grew tremendously for three generations.

In 1881 a wave of pogroms began in Russia on a scale and of a character typical of the Middle Ages. These pogroms were accompanied by the May Laws, various economic and social restrictions of unprecedented scope. The first *aliyah* (modern-day immigration of Jews to Israel) in 1882 followed in the wake of the pogrom of Odessa, the second in 1903 after the pogroms of Kishinev and Homel, and the third after the Ukrainian pogrom in 1920. Waves of emigration to other parts of the world followed these pogroms on a vast scale. The face of European Jewry changed entirely within a few decades. The Jewish communities of Western Europe—particularly that of England—were greatly reinforced, but far more important than this was the transatlantic migration to America. The years between 1870 and 1880

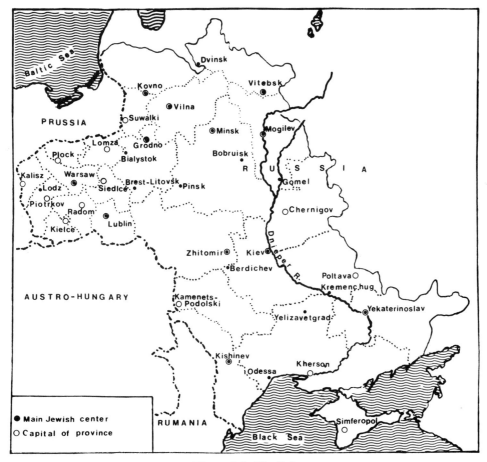

Figure 1.3. The Pale.

witnessed the great migration of Ashkenazi Jews from Europe to America. After the 1880s the United States was to become the second, and in due course the primary, center of Jewish life in the world. Thus, in terms of population, the relative role of European Jewry diminished.

World War I signaled the beginning of the end of European Jewish life. The revolution of 1917 brought emancipation to Russian Jews, but the Bolshevik regime in the long run severed the mass of Russian Jews from their brethren abroad and from Judaism in general. In the early days of the revolution Jews previously restricted to residence in the Pale were allowed to disperse to various parts of Russia, but some sought refuge in South America and in Palestine. The doors of North America were barely open to European Jews during the 1920s.

The defeat of the Germans in World War I and the physical and moral distress that ensued gave an enormous impetus to anti-Semitism in Germany. When the Nazi Party came to power in 1933, anti-Semitism was a cardinal principle. The persecution that followed drove large numbers of Jews from Germany and other parts of Europe to various places throughout the world—often to countries not of their choosing but the only ports of entry open to them.

During World War II the German army overran almost all of continental Europe and systematically carried out a campaign of exterminating Jews. By the end of the war in 1945, some 6 million of the 9 million Jews who had lived in Europe in 1933 had perished in the holocaust. Entire countries and great Jewish centers of learning were now devoid of Jews.

Over the post–World War II years a few Jews have returned to Europe, but that continent is no longer the center of Ashkenazi Jewry. Two and a half million Jews still live in the Soviet Union, but they are for the most part sealed off from the mainstream of Judaism, and in the 1970s several thousand Russian Jews have emigrated to Israel or North America. Romania is the only other country behind the Iron Curtain which has a substantial Jewish population, and Jews there know a relative degree of freedom. The only country on the European continent which has a larger Jewish population now than it had prior to World War II is France. The large influx of non-Ashkenazi Jews from North Africa explains this phenomenon.

Ashkenazi Jews now find their home mainly on the ancient soil of Israel or in the Western World, principally in the United States.

THE ROLE OF THE KHAZARS IN ASHKENAZI JEWRY

The author Arthur Koestler has recently revived the theory that the Khazars were the main populating force in the development of modern-day Ashkenazi Jewry. Koestler was not the first to propose such an idea, but most scholars have rejected it. The Khazars were a Turkish tribe which settled in the lower Volga region. Their capital was Itil. From the 8th to the 10th century they were a powerful kingdom, extending westward as far as Kiev. In 740 their king, along with a few thousand of his notables, accepted Judaism. The reason is thought to have been more political than religious, since the Kingdom of Khazaria formed a buffer state between countries adhering to Islam and Christianity. Very little is known about the extent to which these people practiced Judaism. In 1083 the kingdom fell to the Russians and in 1237 it disappeared with the Tartar invasion. It is possible, of course, that some of these people fled westward and established communities in Poland and Hungary, but their overall contribution to Ashkenazi Jewry is thought by most scholars to have been minimal. Furthermore, the development of Ashkenazi Jewry with the eastward migration of Franco-German Jewry is well documented and is thus considered to be the primary basis for today's Ashkenazi Jewish population.

OTHER COMMUNITIES

Falashas

The term *Falashas* is derived from the Ge'ez (Old Ethiopic) root *falasa*, which means "to emigrate" or "to wander." The Falashas live in Ethiopia in the provinces north of and surrounding Lake Tana. They claim to be of Jewish origin and according to their tradition were among the notables of Jerusalem who accompanied Menelik, the son of King Solomon and the Queen of Sheba, when he returned to his country.

According to various scientific theories, they are of Hamitic (Cushitic) origin and belong to the Agau family of tribes that formed a part of the Ethiopian population prior to the arrival of the Semitic tribes from southern Arabia. Judaism was spread among them by Jews living in southern Arabia, but may have reached them through Egypt or even from Jews who were permanent residents of Ethiopia. It appears that in time these Jews were assimilated into the local population. Ethiopian chronicles show that Judaism was widespread before the conversion of the Axum dynasty to Christianity during the 4th century C.E. It is thought that after this time the elements of the population that remained faithful to Judaism were persecuted and compelled to retreat from the coastal region to the mountains of Lake Tana. For centuries these people have been subjected to waves of persecutions, forced conversions, slavery, and massacres, and yet they continue to think of themselves as Jews. There are persistent legends among them of a former independent status, and at one time they were certainly more powerful and more widespread than at present. Since 1904 an intensive effort has been under way to bring the Falashas into the mainstream of Jewish life. Pro-Falasha committees in Europe and America have trained teachers in Jewish studies and have helped to establish and maintain their schools. After World War II, the establishment of the state of Israel caused a great awakening among the Falashas. Some Falasha youth were sent to Israel to learn Hebrew and to improve their Jewish education.

The size of the Falasha population is not known. As of 1970 it was estimated that they numbered between 25,000 and 30,000.

Karaites

The Karaites are a Jewish sect which originated in Iraq and Persia in the 8th century. Their doctrine is characterized primarily by the denial of the Talmudic-rabbinical tradition. The religious, political, and economic fermentation caused by the Arab conquests and the collision of Islam with other religions; the amalgamation of various ancient heterodox trends in Babylonian-Persian Jewry; and the social and economic grievances of the poorer classes of Jews, especially those living away from the main centers in Babylonia, all helped to turn this sect into a powerful force in medieval times.

In the latter part of the 9th century a vibrant center was created by Persian Karaite emigrants in Palestine. In the 10th century additional Karaite communities sprang up in the Byzantine Empire (Asia Minor and the Balkans), Syria (Damascus), Cyprus, and Moslem Spain. The Palestinian, Egyptian, and Byzantine centers eventually surpassed those of Persia and Babylonia, which dwindled and degenerated. Their success may have been due in part to the lenient marriage regulations generally adopted among Palestinian, Egyptian, and Byzantine Karaites in the 11th century, for they superceded the stringent rules laid down by the early Babylonian Karaite leaders. Some Karaites lived a particularly austere life, settling in Jerusalem and adopting the customs of *Avele Zion* ("Mourners for Zion").

At the end of the 11th century the Karaite center in Palestine came to an abrupt end as the result of the 1st Crusade (1099). During the 12th century the spread of Karaism in Spain was checked. However, in Egypt and Byzantium the sect flourished for many generations thereafter. This growth continued with the advent of the Ottoman Turks: Turkish Constantinople and Adrianople became the leading centers of Karaite life and scholarship. From Byzantium Karaism spread to the Crimea in the 12th century and to Lithuania and Volhynia in the 13th century. After the Russian annexation of Lithuania and the Crimea in the 18th century, the Crimeans, Karaites, and others received from the czars privileges and rights that were denied to those who adhered to the regular Jewish faith.

In 1932 the total Karaite population was estimated to be 12,000, with approximately 2,000 living outside Russia—in Poland, Constantinople, Jerusalem, Cairo, and Hit (on the Euphrates). In January 1939 the German Ministry of the Interior expressly stated that the Karaites did not belong to the Jewish religious community; their "racial psychology" was considered non-Jewish. Thus the Karaites enjoyed favorable treatment within the Polish and Russian territories conquered by the Germans in World War II.

After the establishment of the state of Israel Karaites as well as Jews suffered from Moslem persecution in the Arab states. Those in Egypt, Iraq (Hit), and elsewhere emigrated and settled in Israel, where they were given government assistance in accordance with the Law of Return on a par with traditional Jews. In 1970 approximately 7,000 Karaites were living in Israel.

Samaritans

It is generally postulated that the Samaritans are a mixture of the ancient Israelites who lived in Samaria and of other peoples brought into the country in the wake of the conquest of Samaria by Assyria (722–721 B.C.E.). The Samaritans themselves maintain that they are the direct descendants of the ancient tribes Ephraim and Manasseh; until the 17th century C.E. they possessed a high priesthood which claimed direct descent from Aaron. The Samaritans also claim to have continuously occupied their ancient territory in central Palestine. It was Eli, they say, who disrupted the northern cult by moving from Shechem to Shiloh and attracting some northern Israelites to his new cult there. For the Samaritans this was the "schism" *par excellence.*

In the Persian period (6th–4th century B.C.E.) Nehemiah foiled the Samaritan Sanballat's attempt to obtain political and religious influence over Judah. When his son-in-law was driven from Jerusalem (Nehemiah 13:28) Sanaballat built a rival temple on Mount Gerizim which was destroyed by John Hyrcanus in 128 B.C.E. However, the land between Judea and Galilee still remained under Samaritan control. The Samaritans did not participate in the Jewish revolt of 66–70 C.E. but rose independently from time to time against the Romans. In 486 Emperor Zeno destroyed the second Samaritan temple on Gerizim and built a church in its place. In 529 Emperor Justinian outlawed the Samaritans, and thereafter their autonomous existence under Byzantium practically ended. Under various Islamic rulers they suffered greatly and their numbers dwindled rapidly. In addition to the parent body in Palestine, a Samaritan diaspora existed in Egypt from the time of the Ptolemies until the 18th century.

In ancient times the Samaritan community numbered more than 100,000 people. At the time of the Arab conquest in the 7th century C.E. they numbered about 300,000, but by the end of the Ottoman rule only 146 Samaritans remained in Shechem. Their numbers gradually increased through marriage to Jewish women and in 1934 they numbered 206. Today they are the world's smallest ethnic community. Until their reunification in 1967 they were divided by political realities between two cities—Nablus (Shechem), on the West Bank of the Jordan River, with a population of 230 Samaritans, and Holon, Israel, with 240 members.

SIZE OF THE JEWISH POPULATION, PAST AND PRESENT

Throughout history the size of the Jewish population has been subjected to forces that at times have permitted growth, but that more frequently have brought a reduction in numbers. Periods of growth occurred when proselytism was in vogue or during those times when all populations generally expanded. The forces that brought a reduction in the number of Jews have been many and varied and include assimilation, forced and voluntary conversions, persecutions, plagues, wars, and massacres, of which the Nazi holocaust was the deadliest. Table 1.1, which presents estimates of the size of world Jewry from the time of King David to the present, shows an accordian-like pattern.

Tables and information presented later in this chapter show that Jewish population centers in Europe during the Middle Ages were quite small by comparison to the large centers found in the Middle East. They also indicate the present size of world Jewry, the effects of recent events on the Jewish communities, the proportional make-up of the various communities, and the present-day centers of the Jewish population. The last two sections deal with those places in which one is most likely to encounter genetic diseases in Jews.

Table 1.1. Estimates of the size of world Jewry during various historical periods

Years	Period	Influencing factors	Population in millions by end of period
1006–928 B.C.E.	Kingdom of David and Solomon	Growth of the Jewish people from desert wanderers to founders of a kingdom	1
100 B.C.E.– C.E. 70	Persian and Roman Empires	Widespread Jewish proselytizing	8[a]
325–1100	Medieval Christian and Islam	Widespread conversion to Christianity and Islam; persecutions	Gradual diminution of Jewry (see next period)
1100–1300	Crusades	Forced conversions and persecutions	2
1300–1650	European expulsions; Spanish Inquisition; Chmielnicki massacres	Forced conversions and persecutions	1
1650–1800	Europe prior to Napoleon	Resettlement in Western Europe	2
1800–1900	Industrial Revolution	Biological growth in spite of pogroms in the latter period; great migrations	10
1900–1939	Pre–World War II	Continuation of biological growth; expansion of American Jewry	16.5
1939–1945	World War II	Nazi holocaust	10.5
1945–1955	Post–World War II and establishment of modern Israel	Renewed growth; population explosion	14
1955–1977	Postwar population boom	Gradual decline in family size	14.4

[a] This figure is divided into 4 million Jews in the Roman Diaspora, 2.5 million in Palestine, and 1.5 million in the Persian Empire.

Benjamin of Tudela

Benjamin of Tudela, the great medieval Jewish traveler, left us *Itinerary*, the Hebrew *Sefer ha Massa'ot* [Book of Travels]. A resident of Tudela, Spain he set out on his travels around the year 1165 and in the next 8–9 years visited approximately 300 places in France, Italy, Greece, Palestine, Iraq, the Persian Gulf, Egypt, and Sicily. His book serves as a major source of Jewish history during that period and as an important work in geographical literature. He was interested in all phases of Jewish life, especially those pertaining to the political and economic conditions of that time. His estimates of the size of the various Jewish communities are controversial and require scholarly analysis, but it can be concluded with some degree of certainty that the Oriental communities had much larger Jewish populations than most of the places he visited in southern Europe.

France

From the 11th to the 15th century the Jewish communities of France, as in the rest of Christian Europe, remained very small. In such large centers as Aix, Avignon, Arles, and Narbonne the Jewish population numbered no more than 1,000 persons or 200 families. In other places, such as Capentras, Dijon, Tarascon, and Toulouse, there were 10–100 families. Paris in 1292 had only 124 Jews, comprising 86 households. Troyes at the time of Rashi (the great 11th-century Jewish commentator) had only 100 Jews. At the time of the expulsion of Jews from France in 1394 it is estimated that the average Jewish community was no larger than 200 persons.

Italy

Baron estimated that the total number of Jews in Italy was 50,000 in 1300 and 120,000 in 1490. Deducting the known figures for the large Jewish communities from this total, not more than 100–200 Jews, on the average, lived in each of the 100–200 smaller Jewish communities of Italy.

Germany

During the early Middle Ages only a few cities had relatively large concentrations of Jews. Most Jews lived in small groups in towns and hamlets. Moreover, the number of Jews in the large communities was subject to rapid fluctuations. Prior to the 1st Crusade it is estimated that the entire Jewish population of Germany was 20,000.

Poland and Lithuania

The Jewish population of Eastern Europe remained very small until the end of the Middle Ages. In 1300 there were only about 5,000 Jews in all of Poland and Lithuania. By 1490 their number had reached 30,000. In 1648, just before the Chmielnicki massacres, the population of 115 Jewish communities in the districts of Volhynia, Podolia, Kiev, and Bratslav totaled 51,000—an average of 444 Jews

Table 1.2. Jewish population and total population of Europe, 1300 and 1490

	1300		1490	
Country	No. of Jews	Total population	No. of Jews	Total population
France	100,000	14,000,000	20,000	20,000,000
Holy Roman Empire (including Switzerland and the Low Countries)	100,000	12,000,000	80,000	12,000,000
Italy	50,000	11,000,000	120,000	12,000,000
Spain	150,000	5,500,000	250,000	7,000,000
Portugal	40,000	600,000	80,000	1,000,000
Poland-Lithuania	5,000	500,000	30,000	1,000,000
Hungary	5,000	400,000	20,000	800,000
Total in Christian Europe	450,000	44,000,000	600,000	53,800,000

Source: S. W. Baron, 1952–1976, *A social and religious history of the Jews,* 2nd ed. (New York: Columbia University Press), 12:25.

Table 1.3. Development of three centers of world Jewry, 1840–1945

Year	Eastern Europe[a]		North America		Palestine	
	Absolute (no.)	% of world Jewry	Absolute (no.)	% of world Jewry	Absolute (no.)	% of world Jewry
1840	3,200,000	71.1	40,000	0.9	10,000	0.2
1900	7,400,000	67.3	1,100,000	10.0	50,000	0.5
1939	7,000,000	41.9	4,900,000	29.5	480,000	2.9
1945	1,000,000	9.1	5,400,000	49.0	580,000	5.3

Source: J. Lestschinsky, 1949, Jewish migrations, 1840–1946, in *The Jews: Their history, culture, and religion*, vol. 2, ed. L. Finkelstein (New York: Harper and Brothers).
[a] Figures exclude the Jews of Russia proper.

per community. The important point is that during this period the overwhelming majority of Jews lived in communities of fewer than 500 persons, or about 100 families. It is estimated that during the Middle Ages 300,000 Jews lived in the Kingdom of Poland (including the vast region of Lithuania) while not more than 100,000 Jews resided in all the rest of Europe. Table 1.2 presents a rough estimate of the Jewish population of Europe in 1300 and 1490.

The Pale

The Pale refers to the region in Eastern Europe where Jews were confined as of 1791 under the czars of Russia (see Figure 1.3). The borders were arbitrarily imposed by the oppressive 1835 "Statute concerning the Jews." In 1882 the "May Laws" excluded Jews from rural areas inside the Pale. As a result of these restrictions, Jewish economic development was severely hampered. The Pale was effectively abolished in August 1915 but remained in existence legally until March 1917.

The Pale covered an area of about 1,000,000 square kilometers from the Baltic Sea to the Black Sea. According to the census of 1897, 4,899,300 Jews lived there, forming 94 percent of the total population of that part of Russia and 11.6 percent of the general population of the area. The Jews were a minority in every province

Table 1.4. Jewish immigration by country, 1840–1942 (absolute numbers)

Years	U.S.	Canada	Argentina	Brazil	Uruguay
1840–1880	200,000	1,600	2,000	500	—
1881–1900	675,000	10,500	25,000	1,000	—
1901–1914	1,346,400	93,500	87,614	8,750	—
1915–1920	76,450	10,450	3,503	2,000	1,000
1921–1925	280,283	14,400	39,713	7,139	3,000
1926–1930	54,998	15,300	33,721	22,296	6,370
1931–1935	17,986	4,200	12,700	13,075	3,280
1936–1939	79,819	900	14,789	10,600	7,677
1940–1942	70,954	800	4,500	6,000	1,000
1840–1942	2,801,890	153,150	223,540	71,360	22,327

Source: U. Z. Engelman, 1949, Sources of Jewish statistics, in *The Jews: Their history, culture,*

(from 17.5 percent in the province of Grodno to 3.8 percent in the province of Crimea), but their concentration (82 percent) in the towns and townlets of the Pale was prominent. They formed 36.9 percent of the urban population and in nine provinces made up the majority of the urban population. The ten largest Jewish communities were in Warsaw (219,149), Odessa (138,915), Lodz (98,677), Vilna (64,000), Kishinev (50,237), Minsk (47,562), Bialystok (41,900), Berdichev (41,617), Yekaterinoslav (40,009), and Vitebsk (34,470).

According to the 1897 census, 99 percent of the Jews of the Pale spoke Yiddish. For all its obvious hardships, one positive aspect of the Pale should not be forgotten —namely, that it provided Ashkenazi Jewry with the cohesion and cultural creativity which subsequently led to the establishment of Ashkenazi Jewish centers in the Americas, Israel, South Africa, and many other countries.

DEVELOPMENT OF NEW CENTERS OF MODERN JEWRY

Persecutions and economic difficulties in Eastern Europe in the 19th century culminated in a massive shift of Ashkenazi Jewry mainly in a westward direction but also to other parts of the world. Table 1.3 shows the build-up of Ashkenazi Jewry and its shift to North America and Palestine, while Table 1.4 gives a more detailed account in terms of actual places and numbers.

Table 1.5 provides an estimate of the size of European Jewry prior to World War II and in three periods after the war—1946, 1969, and 1975.

The present-day Jewish population is estimated to be 14,400,000 and Table 1.6 shows the world-wide distribution of Jews according to their three major ethnic groups. As noted in this table, 82 percent of world Jewry is Ashkenazi, while the Sephardi and Oriental groups comprise 11 and 7 percent, respectively. In Israel, however, 47 percent of the Jewish population is Ashkenazi while 53 percent is Sephardi and Oriental (30 percent and 23 percent, respectively).

Table 1.7 lists the countries that are thought to have the largest Jewish populations, while Table 1.8 notes the cities outside Israel that have a Jewish population of over 100,000.

Other countries of the Americas	South Africa	Palestine	All other countries	Total	Years
1,000	4,000	10,000	2,000	221,000	1840–1880
1,000	23,000	25,000	4,000	764,500	1881–1900
3,000	21,377	30,000	10,000	1,602,441	1901–1914
5,000	907	15,000	5,000	89,310	1915–1920
7,000	4,630	60,765	10,000	426,930	1921–1925
10,000	10,044	10,179	10,000	172,908	1926–1930
15,000	4,507	147,502	20,000	238,250	1931–1935
15,000	5,300	75,510	60,000	269,595	1936–1939
2,000	2,000	35,000	10,000	131,954	1940–1942
59,000	75,765	378,956	131,000	3,916,988	1840–1942

and religion, vol. 2, ed. L. Finkelstein (New York: Harper and Brothers).

Table 1.5. Estimated Jewish populations of Europe by country
before and after World War II

Country	1939	1946	1969	1975
Albania	204	300	300	300
Austria	60,000	16,000	8,200	13,000
Belgium	100,000	30,000	40,500	40,500
Britain	340,000	350,000	410,000	410,000
Bulgaria	50,000	46,500	7,000	7,000
Czechoslovakia	360,000	55,000	14,000	12,000
Denmark	7,000	5,500	6,000	7,000
Estonia	5,000	500	?	?
Finland	1,755	1,800	1,450	1,320
France	320,000	180,000	535,000	550,000
Germany	240,000	85,000	30,000	33,000
Gibraltar	886	?	650	625
Greece	75,000	10,500	6,500	6,000
Hungary	403,000	200,000	80,000	80,000
Ireland	4,000	4,500	5,400	4,000
Italy	51,000	52,000	30,000	35,000
Latvia	95,000	12,000	?	?
Lithuania	260,000	20,000	?	?
Luxembourg	3,500	500	1,000	1,000
Malta	35	?	50	50
Netherlands	150,000	30,000	30,000	30,000
Norway	3,000	1,000	750	950
Poland	3,250,000	120,000	15,000	6,000
Portugal	3,500	4,000	650	600
Romania	900,000	300,000	100,000	60,000
Spain	4,500	3,500	7,000	9,000
Sweden	7,500	22,000	15,000	15,000
Switzerland	25,000	35,000	20,000	21,000
Turkey	80,000	80,000	39,000	30,000
U.S.S.R.	3,020,000	2,000,000	2,620,000	2,680,000
Yugoslavia	75,000	10,500	7,500	6,000
Total	9,894,880	3,676,100	4,030,950	4,059,345

Source: Based on figures from *American Jewish Yearbook*, 1940, 1947, 1970,
and 1977.

Table 1.6. Estimated number and world-wide distribution of
Jews according to their three major ethnic groups, 1978

Location	Ashkenazi	Sephardi	Oriental	Total
Asia and Oceania				
Israel	1,400,000	900,000	700,000	3,000,000
Other countries	70,000	50,000	100,000	220,000
Africa				
North	—	40,000	—	40,000
South	110,000	10,000	—	120,000
Europe				
U.S.S.R.	2,600,000	0	80,000	2,680,000
Other countries	1,100,000	250,000	20,000	1,370,000
America				
North	5,890,000	210,000	90,000	6,190,000
South	570,000	180,000	30,000	780,000
Total	11,740,000	1,640,000	1,020,000	14,400,000
Percentage	82	11	7	

Source: Modified from A. Adam, 1977, *Israel J. Med. Sci.* 9:1383.

Table 1.7. Countries with the largest
Jewish populations (1977 estimates)

Country	Population
United States	5,840,000
Israel	3,059,000
Soviet Union	2,680,000
France	550,000
Argentina	475,000
Great Britain	410,000
Canada	320,000

Source: Based on figures from *American Jewish year book*, 1977.

Table 1.8. Cities outside Israel with 100,000 or more Jews, 1976

Country	City (including suburbs)	No. of Jews (rough 1976 estimates)
Argentina	Buenos Aires	350,000
Canada	Montreal	105,000
	Toronto	110,000
England	London	280,000
France	Paris	300,000
U.S.	Baltimore	100,000
	Boston	180,000
	Chicago	270,000
	Essex County	100,000
	Los Angeles	500,000
	Miami	225,000
	New York	3,226,000
	Philadelphia	350,000
	Washington	115,000
U.S.S.R.	Kiev	170,000
	Leningrad	165,000
	Moscow	285,000
	Odessa	110,000

Source: Compiled from *American Jewish year book*, 1976.

REFERENCES

Jewish communities

Adler, M. N., ed. 1907. *The itinerary of Benjamin of Tudela.* Reprint ed., n.d. New York: Feldheim.

Ankori, Z. 1959. *Karaites in Byzantium.* New York: Columbia University Press.

Baer, Y. 1961. *A History of the Jews in Christian Spain*, vols. 1 and 2. Philadelphia: Jewish Publication Society of America.

Baron, S. W. 1952–1976. *Social and religious history of the Jews.* 2nd ed. 16 vols. New York: Columbia University Press.

———. 1956. The Modern Age. In *Great ages and ideas of the Jewish people*, ed. L. Schwartz, pp. 315–484. New York: Random House.

———. 1964. *The Russian Jews under Tsars and Soviets.* New York: Macmillan.

Bonné, B. 1966. The Samaritans: A demographic study. *Am. J. Hum. Genet.* 18:61.

———. 1966. Genes and phenotypes in the Samaritan isolate. *Am. J. Phys. Anthropol.* 24:1.

Brockelmann, C. 1960. *History of the Islamic peoples.* New York: Capricorn Books.

Dubnow, S. M. 1916. *History of the Jews in Russia and Poland,* vols. 1–3. Philadelphia: Jewish Publication Society of America.

Goitein, S. D. 1964. *Jews and Arabs: Their contacts through the ages.* New York: Schocken Books.

Heller, J. E., and Nemoy, L. 1972. Karaites. In *Encyclopaedia Judaica,* vol. 10, ed. C. Roth and G. Wigoder, pp. 762–82. Jerusalem: Keter Publishing House.

Hitti, P. K. 1961. *History of the Arabs.* New York: Macmillan.

Koestler, A. 1976. *The thirteenth tribe: The Khazer Empire and its heritage.* New York: Random House.

Kushner, G. 1973. *Immigrants from India in Israel.* Tucson: University of Arizona Press.

Leslau, W., trans. 1951. *Falasha anthology: Black Jews of Ethiopia.* New Haven: Yale University Press.

Lesourd, P., and Ismojik, M. 1966. *On the path of the Crusaders.* Israel: Massada Press.

Lewis, B. 1960. *The Arabs in history.* New York: Harper and Row.

Mahler, R. 1971. *A history of modern Jewry, 1780–1815.* New York: Schocken Books.

Margolis, M., and Marx, A. 1958. *History of the Jewish people.* Philadelphia: Jewish Publication Society of America.

Strizower, S. 1971. *The Bene Israel of Bombay.* New York: Schocken Books.

Tcherikover, V. 1959. *Hellenistic civilization and the Jews.* Philadelphia: Jewish Publication Society of America.

Tesdaka, B., and Lowenstamm, A. 1972. Samaritans. In *Encyclopaedia Judaica,* vol. 14, ed. C. Roth and G. Wigoder, pp. 726–58. Jerusalem: Keter Publishing House.

Weinryb, B. D. 1972. *The Jews of Poland.* Philadelphia: Jewish Publication Society of America.

Wurmbrand, M. 1972. Falashas. In *Encyclopaedia Judaica,* vol. 6, ed. C. Roth and G. Wigoder, pp. 1143–54. Jerusalem: Keter Publishing House.

Jewish populations

Adam, A. 1977. Genetic diseases among Jews. *Israel J. Med. Sci.* 9:1383.

Baron, S. W. 1952–1976. *Social and religious history of the Jews.* 2nd ed. 16 vols. New York: Columbia University Press.

Engelmann, U. Z. 1949. Sources of Jewish statistics. In *The Jews: Their history, culture, and religion,* vol. 2, ed. L. Finkelstein, pp. 1172–97. New York: Harper and Brothers.

Fine, M., and Himmelfarb, M. 1976. *American Jewish year book, 1976.* Philadelphia: Jewish Publication Society of America.

———. 1977. *American Jewish year book, 1977.* Philadelphia: Jewish Publication Society of America.

Goodman, R. M. 1975. Genetic disorders among the Jewish people. In *Modern trends in human genetics,* vol. 2, ed. A. E. H. Emery, pp. 270–307. London: Butterworths.

Israel government year book, 1975–76. 1975. Jerusalem: Government Printing Press.

Lestschinsky, J. 1949. Jewish migrations, 1840–1946. In *The Jews: Their history, culture, and religion,* vol. 2, ed. L. Finkelstein, pp. 1198–238. New York: Harper and Brothers.

Patai, R., and Wing, J. P. 1975. *The myth of the Jewish race.* New York: Charles Scribner's Sons.

Ruppin, A. 1946. The Jewish population of the world. In *The Jewish people: Past and present.* New York: Jewish Encyclopedic Handbooks.

Schmelz, O. S. 1972. Demography. In *Encyclopaedia Judaica,* vol. 5, ed. C. Roth and G. Wigoder, pp. 1493–522. Jerusalem: Keter Publishing House.

Statistical Abstract of Israel, 1972. 1972. Jerusalem: Central Bureau of Statistics.

2

Genetic heterogeneity and homogeneity among the Jewish people

MANY REFERENCES in the Bible indicate the mixed ancestral origins of the ancient Hebrews. The words of the prophet Ezekiel clearly serve as a reminder of this fact:

Thy birth and thy nativity is of the land of Canaan; thy father was an Amorite and thy mother a Hittite (Ezekiel 16:3).

The purpose of this chapter is to discuss a few selected studies that reflect the genetic heterogeneity and homogeneity of the Jewish people. Because this text is mainly concerned with genetic diseases among Jews rather than with the gene frequencies of the numerous genetic polymorphic systems, no effort will be made to present the extensive data that have been amassed regarding the latter. This information is readily available in the sources listed at the end of the chapter.

ANTHROPOMORPHIC FEATURES

Some people maintain that Jews share a variety of morphologic traits that make possible their identification by appearance alone. Numerous studies have been published on distinguishing "Jewish features"—height, hair form and color, eye color, shape of nose and lips, and cephalic index. However, even though some Jews have what may be called a "Semitic appearance," the variability in expression of the above-mentioned traits is as broad as the corresponding ranges among the non-Jewish majority populations with whom Jews have lived for thousands of years. Furthermore, many anthropomorphic traits tend to measure adaptation to climate and other environmental factors and thus tell more about a population's geographical surroundings than about its evolutionary origin. For example, alterations in height can reflect rapid, short-term changes in the environment rather than the genetic make-up of a population.

Those who have visited Israel know that Jews differ tremendously in physical

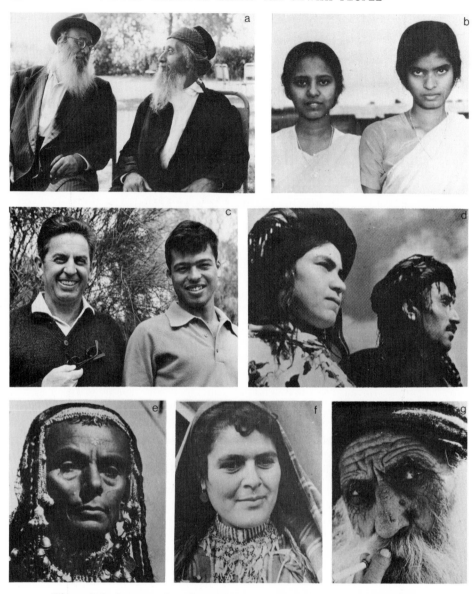

Figure 2.1. A composite of Jewish faces reflecting various countries of origin: (a) Yemen; (b) India; (c) Romania; (d) Kurdistan; (e) Hadramaut (South Arabia); (f) Libya; and (g) Iraq. Sections b, d, e, f, and g are from D. Hacohen and M. Hacohen, *One people: The story of the eastern Jews* (New York: Funk and Wagnalls, 1969).

appearance (see Figure 2.1). Today most physical anthropologists agree that it is impossible to construct a characteristic "Jewish phenotype." What, then, makes possible the recognition of Jews? Some contend that Jewish cultural patterns give rise to this form of recognition. I do not intend to define here the cultural characteristics of Jewish ethnicity, but I acknowledge that they exist and that in some instances they provide a means of identification. This synthesis in thought has been reached by various scholars and was stated well by Ashley Montagu in 1945:

> There undoubtedly exists a certain quality of looking Jewish, but this quality is not due so much to any inherited characters of the person in question, as to certain culturally acquired habits of expression, facial, vocal, muscular, and mental. Such habits do to a very impressive extent influence the appearance of the individual and determine the impression which he makes on others. . . . It is possible to distinguish many Jews from members of other cultural groups for the same reason that it is possible to distinguish Englishmen from such groups, or Americans, Frenchmen, Italians and Germans. . . . Members of one cultural group do not readily fit into the pattern of another.

However, the cultural habits of Jews have been changing and will continue to change, especially with regard to the once stigmatized "Jewish look."

GENETIC POLYMORPHIC SYSTEMS

The term *polymorphism* refers to the occurrence of two or more common genetic variants of the same trait within a given population. The vast majority of these variants are not directly disease producing—e.g., they are blood groups and electrophoretic variants of certain plasma proteins. Geneticists use these numerous polymorphic systems in man as genetic markers to trace the evolution, migration, and structure of populations.

As discussed in Chapter 1, the present-day Jewish communities represent mixtures of a common ancestral Jewish population with the various populations within which Jews have lived since their dispersion from ancient Israel. The key question that continues to be asked is, To what extent do the present-day Jewish communities reflect their admixture and at the same time their Middle Eastern origin? In the effort to answer this question an enormous amount of data has been collected on the comparative gene frequencies of a number of human polymorphic systems. However, important comparative information is still missing on certain non-Jewish populations of the areas where Jews formerly resided. Nevertheless, current interpretations stress two main trends: (1) an extrinsic admixture of different non-Jewish populations with Jews, resulting in great heterogeneity among the Jewish ethnic groups; and (2) a common Middle Eastern origin. For example, comparative gene frequencies for such polymorphic systems as the ABO blood groups, group-specific component (GC), phosphoglucomutase (PGM), and glutamicpyruvic transaminase (GPT) have been used to show great admixture of non-Jewish genes among the Jewish people. In contrast, the Rh system with allele CDe, adenylate kinase (AK), acid phosphatase (AP), the haptoglobins and HLA-Bw35, and haplotypes (A1, Bw17 and Aw 26, Bw16) have tended to show the Middle Eastern ancestral origin of most of the Jewish communities.

Differing gene frequencies of other polymorphic systems, such as pseudocholinesterase deficiency (see page 190), glucose-6-phosphate dehydrogenase deficiency (see page 163), and color vision (see page 376), demonstrate the marked genetic variability among the Jewish communities.

As more comparative information on genetic markers becomes available and is critically analyzed in light of the historical and cultural features of the Jewish community in question, it may be possible to better understand the degree of genetic heterogeneity versus homogeneity detected in a given community. An excellent example of this point is illustrated in a recent study by Bonné-Tamir and co-workers. These investigators examined a random sample of 148 Libyan Jews now living is Israel. Using blood groups, serum proteins, and red-cell enzyme frequencies, they compared their observations with data on non-Jewish Libyans. Their results showed significant differences between the two groups in most systems, thus indicating a high degree of genetic isolation of the Jewish community from the surrounding populations. The relative lack of the African component in the Libyan Jewish community further showed that this group interbred very little, if at all, with its non-Jewish neighbors. Although much genetic heterogeneity is known to exist among the various Jewish communities, studies like this one tend to support the genetic homogeneity of Jews within their individual communities.

DERMATOGLYPHICS

Fingerprint patterns are polygenically inherited and because they have little adaptive significance are particularly useful in anthropological studies.

In 1957 Sachs and Bat-Miriam studied the fingerprints of members of eight different Jewish ethnic groups and compared their findings with those from an unselected group of Israeli Arabs and with non-Jews. They found that the mean values for the frequencies of whorls and loops in the different Jewish ethnic groups were very similar and close to the average for Israeli Arabs, but were different from the figures reported for the non-Jewish populations.

Data on pattern indices (obtained by adding the percentage of loops to twice the percentage of whorls and dividing by 10) of Jews and non-Jews are given in Figure 2.2. Whereas the non-Jews from Europe and North America had indices ranging from 11.85 to 12.59, none of the Jewish groups, not even those who lived for long periods in the same countries, had such low indices. The indices for the various Jewish ethnic groups ranged from 13.30 for the Jews from Bulgaria to 13.98 for those from Poland. The mean index for all Jewish communities was 13.67. In a more recent study by Bonné-Tamir and co-workers the Habbanite Jews (a small Jewish isolate from South Arabia) were found to have an index of 13.13, which is close to that of the Bulgarian Jews.

High indices were also found among some non-Jews from the eastern Mediterranean area, e.g. in Egyptian Copts, non-Jewish Lebanese, and Syrian Arabs.

Sachs and Bat-Miriam concluded that the similarity of pattern indices among Jews to those of non-Jewish ethnic groups of the eastern Mediterranean area suggests a common origin from what may be called an "eastern Mediterranean gene pool."

CYTOGENETIC STUDIES

It has been suggested that differences in the frequencies of chromosomal variants may be due to racial, ethnic, or related parameters. For example, a long Y

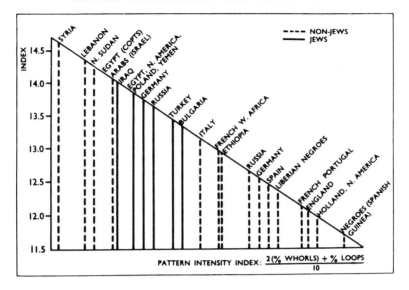

Figure 2.2. Fingerprint pattern indices of Jews and non-Jews. Courtesy of M. Bat-Miriam, Israel.

chromosome has been noted in Japanese males, a small additional metacentric fragment was found in 24 of 25 Hottentots investigated, and pericentric inversion of chromosome no. 9 has been demonstrated in various populations.

In 1975 Cohen and co-workers published cytogenetic studies (including an analysis of banding patterns) on the cord blood lymphocytes of 500 normal, healthy newborns representing the various Jewish ethnic groups. No numerical chromosomal aberrations were observed, but 10 percent of the individuals manifested cytogenetic variants. Six of the inherited abnormalities were structural (4 inversions and 2 deletions), while the remainder were classified as minor variants. The chromosomal variants were randomly distributed among the population and no particular variant was characteristic of a given ethnic group. Cohen then extended this study to include 500 more newborn Jewish infants, but still no characteristic chromosomal variants were observed in any of the Jewish communities studied. From this investigation it seems relatively safe to conclude that Jews do not manifest a characteristic chromosomal pattern.

SUMMARY

The main themes of a multitude of genetic polymorphic studies (most of which have not been discussed in this brief section) are (1) that the great admixture of different non-Jewish populations with Jews accounts for much heterogeneity among the various Jewish communities, and (2) that genetic evidence has been found to support the historic fact of the Jews' common Middle Eastern ancestry. In addition, recent studies using various genetic polymorphic systems show that some Jewish communities are quite homogeneous and differ greatly from their former surrounding non-Jewish populations.

REFERENCES

Anthropomorphic features

Coon, C. S. 1939. *The races of Europe.* New York: Macmillan.
———. 1962. *The origin of races.* New York: Alfred A. Knopf.
Fishberg, M. 1911. *The Jews: A study of race and environment.* New York: Charles Scribner's Sons.
Gates, R. R. 1923. *Heredity and eugenics.* New York: Macmillan.
———. 1948. *Human ancestry: From a genetical point of view.* Cambridge, Mass.: Harvard University Press.
Hacohen, D., and Hacohen, M. 1969. *One people: The story of the eastern Jews.* New York: 1969, Funk and Wagnalls.
Jacobs, J. 1885. On the racial characteristics of modern Jews. *J. Anthropol. Instit.* 15:31.
Judt, I. M. 1903. *Die Juden als Rasse.* Berlin: Judischer Verlag.
Montagu, M. F. A. 1945. *Man's most dangerous myth: The fallacy of race.* New York: Columbia University Press.
Patai, R., and Wing, J. P. 1975. *The myth of the Jewish race.* New York: Charles Scribner's Sons.
Salaman, R. N. 1910–1911. Heredity and the Jew. *J. Genet.* 1:273.
Shapiro, H. I. 1960. *The Jewish people.* Brussels: UNESCO.

Genetic polymorphic systems

Adam, A. 1977. Genetic diseases among Jews. *Israel J. Med. Sci.* 9:1383.
Bodmer, J., and Bodmer, W. F. 1973. Population genetics of the HL-A system: A summary of data from the Fifth International Histocompatibility Testing Workshop. *Israel J. Med. Sci.* 9:1257.
Bodmer, W. F., and Cavalli-Sforza, L. I. 1976. *Genetics, evolution, and man.* San Francisco: W. H. Freeman.
Bonné, B. 1966. Genes and phenotypes in the Samaritan isolate. *Am. J. Phys. Anthropol.* 24:1.
Bonné, B.; Ashbel, S.; Modai, M.; Godber, M. J.; Mourant, A. E.; Tills, D.; and Woodhead, B. G. 1970. The Habbanite isolate. 1: Genetic markers in blood. *Hum. Hered.* 20:609.
Bonné-Tamir, B.; Ashbel, S.; and Modai, J. 1977. Genetic markers in Libyan Jews. *Hum. Genet.* 37:319.
Bonné-Tamir, B.; Bodmer, J. G.; Bodmer, W. F.; Pickbourne, P.; Brautbar, C.; Gazit, E.; Nevo, S.; and Zamir, R. 1978. HLA polymorphism in Israel: An overall comparative analysis. *Tissue Antigens* 11:235.
Carmelli, D., and Cavalli-Sfonza, L. L. 1979. The genetic origin of the Jews: A multivariate approach. *Am. J. Hum. Genet.,* in press.
Cavalli-Sforza, L. L., and Bodmer, W. F. 1971. *The genetics of human populations.* San Francisco: W. H. Freeman.
Cleve, H.; Ramot, B.; and Bearn, A. G. 1962. Distribution of the serum group-specific components in Israel. *Nature* 195:86.
Cohen, T. 1971. Genetic markers in migrants to Israel. *Israel J. Med. Sci.* 7:1509.
Giblett, E. R. 1969. *Genetic markers in human blood.* Oxford: Blackwell.
Goldschmidt, E.; Bayani-Sisoson, P.; Sutton, H. E.; Fried, K.; Sandor, A.; and Bloch, N. 1962. Haptoglobin frequencies in Jewish communities. *Ann. Hum. Genet.* 26:39.
Harris, H. 1976. Enzyme variants in human populations. *Johns Hopkins Med. J.* 138:245.

Mourant, A. E. 1963. Blood groups of Jewish communities. In *The genetics of migrant and isolate populations*, ed. E. Goldschmidt, p. 256. Baltimore: Williams and Wilkins.

Mourant, A. E.; Kopeć, A. C.; and Domaniewska-Sobczak, K. 1978. *The genetics of the Jews*. London: Oxford University Press.

Nelken, D. 1963. Blood groups in Jewish communities. In *The genetics of migrant and isolate populations*, ed. E. Goldschmidt, p. 18. Baltimore: Williams and Wilkins.

Ramot, B.; Zikert-Duvdvani, P.; and Tauman, G. 1961. Distribution of haptoglobin types in Israel. *Nature* 192:765.

Sheba, C.; Szeinberg, A.; Ramot, B.; Adam, A.; and Ashkenazi, I. 1962. Epidemiologic survey of deleterious genes in different population groups in Israel. *Am. J. Public Health* 52:1101.

Steinberg, A. G. 1973. Contribution of the Gm and Inv allotypes to the characterization of human populations. *Israel J. Med. Sci.* 9:1383.

Szeinberg, A. 1963. G6PD deficiency among Jews: Genetical and anthropological considerations. In *The genetics of migrant and isolate populations,* ed. E. Goldschmidt, p. 69. Baltimore: Williams and Wilkins.

———. 1973. Investigation of genetic polymorphic traits in Jews. *Israel J. Med. Sci.* 9:1171.

Szeinberg, A.; Pipano, S.; Assa, M.; Medalie, J. H.; and Neufeld, H. N. 1972. High frequency of atypical pseudocholinesterase gene among Iraqi and Iranian Jews. *Clin. Genet.* 3:123.

Szeinberg, A.; Pipano, S.; Rozansky, Z.; and Ravia, N. 1971. Frequency of red cell adenosine deaminase phenotypes in several population groups in Israel. *Hum. Hered.* 21:357.

Szeinberg, A., and Tomashevsky-Tamir, S. 1971. Red cell adenylate kinase and phosphoglucomutase polymorphisms in several population groups in Israel. *Hum. Hered.* 21:289.

Tills, D.; Van Den Branden, J. L.; Clements, V. R.; and Mourant, A. E. 1971. The distribution in man of genetic variants of 6 phosphogluconate dehydrogenase. *Hum. Hered.* 21:305.

Dermatoglyphics

Bat-Miriam Katznelson, M., and Ashbel, S. 1973. Dermatoglyphics of Jews. I: Normal Ashkenazi population. *Z. Morphol. Anthropol.* 65:14.

Sachs, L., and Bat-Miriam, M. 1957. The genetics of Jewish populations. I: Fingerprint patterns in Jewish populations in Israel. *Am. J. Hum. Genet.* 9:117.

Slatis, H. M.; Bat-Miriam Katznelson, M.; and Bonné-Tamir, B. 1976. The inheritance of fingerprint patterns. *Am. J. Hum. Genet.* 28:280.

Cytogenetics

Cohen, M. M.; Dahahan, S.; and Shaham, M. 1975. Cytogenetic evaluation of 500 Jerusalem newborn infants. *Israel J. Med. Sci.* 11:969.

3

Family history
and modes of genetic
inheritance

THE CRUCIAL ROLE of the family history in evaluating patients with genetic diseases is discussed, and for those unfamiliar with the features of the different modes of genetic transmission, basic guidelines are presented.

IMPORTANCE OF THE FAMILY HISTORY

The family history plays an important role in the diagnosis of any genetic disorder, but when one speaks of genetic disorders among the various Jewish ethnic groups its role is further enhanced. It will become evident that Jews from different ethnic communities suffer from different genetic diseases. Knowing this, one would hesitate to diagnose in a Jewish patient of Sephardi or Oriental ancestry a genetic disease characteristically found in the Ashkenazi community.

Effective use of information obtained from the family history depends on one's knowledge of, and interest in, medical genetics and the hereditary diseases of various ethnic groups. As taught in many medical schools, the method of taking a family history lacks the proper orientation to be useful in approaching a genetic problem. Merely to ask "Does anybody else in your family have such a disease?" is far from adequate. Why, then, is a family history important?

Although the genetic mode of inheritance of many disorders is known, it is often impossible to diagnose a given disease accurately without a thorough knowledge of the patient's family history. Frequently it is necessary to examine members of the patient's family before diagnosis of a genetic disorder can be made with certainty. For example, a physician considering the diagnosis of Marfan syndrome in a patient with only arachnodactyly and ectopia lentis must obtain a history of similar findings in other members of the family to support this diagnosis. If such a history is doubtful due to lack of precise information, as is frequently the case, the physician must examine family members directly. Exception to this approach is taken when a

34

known autosomal dominant disease appears solely in one member as a result of a new mutation.

In addition to enhancing the accuracy of diagnosis, a complete family history is also helpful in genetic counseling. Genetic counseling should concern itself not only with the question of the probability of other family members' being affected but also with aspects of prognosis, treatment, and emotional adjustment. These can be achieved only with a full history of the proband and his kindred. For additional remarks on genetic counseling see Chapter 11.

The number of new genetic diseases that have been recognized within the past two decades is great, and new disorders will continue to be recognized, depending upon the astuteness of physicians and new methods of investigation. Paramount to the recognition of a new genetic entity is the role of genetic transmission. Thus, the family history helps the investigator initiate research to better understand the disease in question.

TAKING A FAMILY HISTORY

Before taking a family history, one should have some knowledge of the genetic problem that confronts the patient and his family. Does the genetic disorder involve cytogenetics or biochemical genetics, or is the precise defect unknown? What procedure, if any, will be needed to further evaluate the proband and his family? If the genetic disease is known, one should be familiar with the entity in question. Lack of knowledge of a given genetic disorder makes proper questioning of the family difficult. One needs to know that in autosomal dominant disorders the range of expression of symptoms and physical findings may vary markedly. Unless one is cognizant of this difference in expression (*expressivity*), it is possible to consider a minimally affected individual as not having the disorder.

As one begins to take a family history, it often becomes apparent that all the information needed cannot be obtained in a single interview. Perhaps the most common reason is that the patient or family members present are not sufficiently knowledgeable about the medical histories of other relatives. In obtaining information from family members it is customary, when possible, to start with the proband and proceed in an orderly fashion to the parents, sibs, etc. The information obtained should be recorded using the standard pedigree symbols shown in Figure 3.1. (These symbols are not universally used, however; the English prefer ♂ for the male and ♀ for the female.) In eliciting information from mothers it may be useful to say, "Let us start with your first pregnancy, and proceed to the last." This enables one to obtain birth order and also helps the informant to concentrate her thoughts on each individual. Specific information frequently needed on each member includes full name, age, sex, address, and present and past states of health. Further questioning depends on the disorder in question and its possible relationship to other disease entities. After gathering information on a given sibship, one must ask about abortions, stillbirths, miscarriages, children who died during infancy, and other members of the sibship who have died. In addition, a thorough prenatal history should always be obtained. Such a history includes questions pertaining to the use of drugs, consumption of alcohol, exposure to various infectious diseases, and

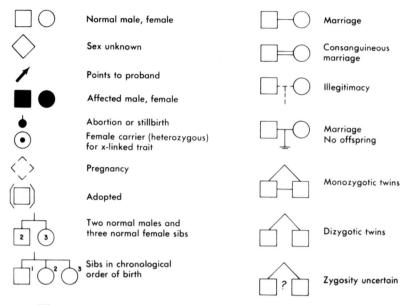

Figure 3.1. Symbols commonly used in drawing human pedigrees.

teratogenic and mutagenic agents in both parents. Some individuals tend to repress certain facts regarding these matters and unless questioned may unconsciously withhold information. One should always be concerned about the presence of congenital anomalies in the family as well as the clustering of any traits or diseases. As in any doctor-patient relationship, the physician or counselor must always be in control of the interview and must endeavor to communicate in language that the patient understands. Once again, one cannot be satisfied with a negative answer to a question such as, "Do any members of your family have congenital anomalies?" The need for being precise and using terms that the patient can understand cannot be overemphasized. Keeping one's ear attuned to family folk tales and observations pertaining to unusual members may be exceedingly informative from a diagnostic viewpoint.

In dealing with genetic disorders that are known to affect various ethnic groups, be they Jewish or otherwise, certain particulars should be recorded. These include the racial, religious, and ethnic background of the family, as well as the place of birth of the parents, grandparents, and frequently the great-grandparents. Place of birth should include not only the country but also the city or region and when appropriate the name of the hospital.

An important aspect of the family history that has not been mentioned is consanguinity. If consanguinity is present at the parental level or is even further removed in the case of the proband, it may serve as a clue to the mode of genetic transmission. Close parental consanguinity in a patient with a puzzling disease suggests autosomal recessive inheritance. Although consanguineous marriages are not as common today as they once were, it is still important to ask this question. Consanguinity among the Jewish people will be discussed in greater detail in Chapter 12.

DOMINANT AND RECESSIVE PHENOTYPES

Although most of the genetic disorders that afflict Jews are autosomal recessive traits and diseases, a few remarks will be made regarding the various modes of genetic transmission applicable to human diseases.

The distribution of certain hereditary traits and diseases in families produces characteristic genetic patterns. These pedigree patterns depend upon gene dosage and chromosomal location of the mutant gene. The mutant gene may be located on an autosome or on either of the sex chromosomes, X or Y. The term X-linked (sex-linked) is used to describe genes located on the X chromosome. For practical purposes the Y chromosome carries little information other than that which determines maleness. The presence of a single mutant gene is spoken of as the heterozygous state, while recessive traits are most often homozygous. Exceptions to the latter are X-linked recessive disorders in which a recessive gene on the single X-chromosome in the male produces a given trait or disease. Such males are referred to as *hemizygous*. Strictly speaking, the terms *dominant* and *recessive* refer to the phenotype of the individual, not to the genotype. This can be illustrated by analyzing the conditions produced by the gene for sickle hemoglobin. The sickling trait is dominant because the gene is expressed only in the heterozygous state, whereas the disease sickle cell anemia is recessive because the gene is expressed only in the homozygous state. The term *incompletely dominant* indicates an intermediate situation at the clinical level.

Codominant is used to describe traits that are jointly expressed in the heterozygote. For instance, those individuals who are of blood group AB have the genes for antigen A and antigen B; neither gene is dominant over the other. The same holds true for individuals having both hemoglobin S and hemoglobin C, which can be phenotypically identified by paper electrophoresis. Thus, *dominant* and *recessive* are somewhat arbitrary terms, since they depend on various methods of determining the products of gene action.

AUTOSOMAL DOMINANT INHERITANCE

A patient who has a disease caused by an autosomal dominant gene will usually be *heterozygous,* having received the mutant gene from one affected parent. Gametes from such a person will have an equal chance of carrying or not carrying the mutant gene. Some of the features of a rare autosomal dominant disease are: (1) one of the parents of an affected proband must also have the disorder (unless one is dealing with a new mutation or with an illegitimate child); (2) an affected parent will transmit the disease to approximately half of his or her offspring, regardless of sex; and (3) an unaffected child (not carrying the mutant gene) cannot transmit the disease. An autosomal dominant disorder produces a vertical pattern of transmission, as noted in Figure 3.2.

Diseases involving autosomal dominant inheritance are frequently associated with gross clinical alterations. For example, hereditary hemorrhagic telangiectasia is associated with visible telangiectasia, while neurofibromatosis is associated with visible café-au-lait spots and usually with neurofibromas.

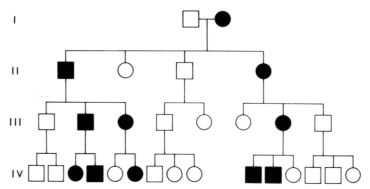

Figure 3.2. Pattern of transmission of an autosomal dominant disorder.

Another clinical feature of dominant traits, as stated previously, is the wide variability in expression of signs and symptoms. If the expressivity is reduced to such a degree that the gene cannot be detected by presently available means, the trait is said to be *nonpenetrant*. This nonpenetrance accounts for few of the expected 50 percent affected offspring.

In contrast to patients with recessive disorders, who frequently show symptoms early in life, patients with a dominant disease often develop clinical manifestations later in life. Examples of dominant diseases with delayed onset are Huntington disease and the adult type of polycystic renal disease. Dominant disorders may also be less severe in terms of ultimate prognosis compared to recessive disorders. A possible explanation for this, in terms of natural selection, is that a life-threatening mutation may make reproduction impossible. Under such conditions a dominant mutation would tend to be eliminated. On the other hand, genes for deleterious recessive conditions are protected in the carrier, or heterozygous, state and thus are maintained in the population.

If a known autosomal dominant genetic disease appears as an isolated case, one must consider the following possibilities: (1) it may be the result of a new mutation; (2) it may appear isolated because of nonpenetrance in one of the parents; and (3) it may be the result of illegitimacy.

Few autosomal dominant traits occur in the homozygous state. For this to happen, both parents must be affected with the disorder, and in theory 25 percent of their offspring will be homozygous. Such a case has been reported for achondroplasia, but the infant was so severely affected that it died. It is believed that the homozygous state in dominant disorders produces a more severe or even lethal form of the disease.

Two additional features commonly ascribed to autosomal dominant disorders should be mentioned—*skipped generations* and *anticipation*. As stated previously, dominant disorders may show wide variability in clinical manifestation. If expressivity is so markedly reduced that the gene cannot be detected, the trait is considered to be nonpenetrant. Skipped generations may seem to appear in a dominant pedigree, but when individuals in a given generation are closely studied, some will show definite but mild expression of the trait in question.

The idea of anticipation also is based largely on the wide variability in severity of dominant disorders. A genetic disease may manifest itself earlier, be more severe, and lead to earlier death in the present or in each successive generation than in the immediately preceding one. This theory has been advanced for Huntington disease, myotonic dystrophy, and other disorders. It is conceivable that the individual affected in generation I is less severely afflicted than individuals in generation II. Assuming that there are more affected offspring in generation II, they will most likely display a wider range of severity. However, bias may be introduced into a study by the fact that those offspring in generation II who are more severely affected are more prone to seek medical care. It is generally believed that there is no biological basis for the concept of anticipation.

AUTOSOMAL RECESSIVE INHERITANCE

Genetic diseases that are transmitted as autosomal recessives require the mutant gene in a double dose known as the *homozygous state*. The affected individual inherits one mutant gene from each parent. Although these heterozygous parents are usually clinically normal, in some cases they demonstrate a given biochemical alteration. For example, it has been shown that in classical phenylketonuria the heterozygous parents of affected individuals are not able to metabolize phenylalanine as rapidly as normal individuals when given a loading dose. A similar situation has also been found in the heterozygous parents of children with galactosemia and other rare recessive metabolic diseases. The precise recognition of a heterozygous individual further enhances the armamentarium of the genetic counselor.

Each parent who is heterozygous for a mutant gene has a 50 percent chance of transmitting that gene. In theory, when two heterozygous individuals mate, 25 percent ($\frac{1}{2} \times \frac{1}{2}$) of their offspring will be affected. The expected ratio of affected to normal children is $1:3$, and two-thirds of those children who appear normal will be heterozygous for the mutant gene, like their parents. In general, both sexes are affected equally in autosomal recessive disorders.

In contrast to the vertical transmission observed in autosomal dominant disorders, autosomal recessive diseases produce a horizontal pattern of transmission. One therefore sees affected members in sibships. In small families, however, autosomal recessive diseases frequently appear as single cases.

If an individual with an autosomal recessive disease marries a homozygous normal person, all their children will be carriers of the mutant gene. A dominant, or vertical, pattern of transmission will be produced if an individual affected with an autosomal recessive disorder marries a heterozygous carrier. In this same instance theoretically half of their children will be affected.

Emphasis is placed on consanguinity in recessive inheritance, particularly in individuals with rare recessive diseases. However, in the case of more common autosomal recessive diseases such as cystic fibrosis, no greater frequency of consanguineous matings has been found than in the general population. Additional comments on consanguinity are made in Chapters 12 and 13.

Clinically and biochemically, autosomal recessive disorders can be divided into two groups. One group makes up the so-called inborn errors of metabolism, in

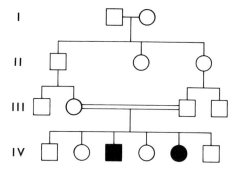

Figure 3.3. Pattern of transmission of an autosomal recessive disorder. Note the close consanguinity.

which the basic defect usually involves an alteration in a specific enzyme. In these disorders the physical findings are frequently secondary to the altered metabolism. The second group accounts for a large number of the malformation syndromes. In contrast to our understanding of many of the inborn errors of metabolism, essentially nothing is known about the basic defect in these autosomal recessive malformation disorders. In both of these groups, the disease manifestations tend to be more severe than in dominant disorders and often lead to early death. Figure 3.3 illustrates a typical pedigree pattern for a rare autosomal recessive disease.

X-LINKED INHERITANCE

In understanding X-linked (sex-linked) inheritance, it is necessary to recall that the mother receives an X chromosome from each of her parents and gives either one or the other to her sons and daughters. A daughter receives one X chromosome from her mother and a second X chromosome from her father. The pattern of transmission for X-linked recessive diseases is from female carriers to affected males, producing an oblique pattern in the pedigree (Figure 3.4). Women who are

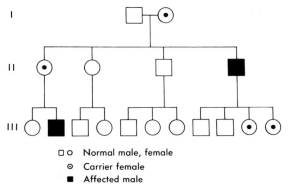

Figure 3.4. Pattern of transmission of an X-linked disorder.

carriers transmit the mutant gene to half their daughters, who also will be carriers, and to half their sons, who will be affected. Affected males transmit the mutant gene to all their daughters, who will be carriers, but father-to-son transmission (male-to-male) never occurs in X-linked inheritance, whether it is recessive or dominant. The only way male-to-male transmission may appear to take place in X-linked disorders is if the affected male marries a woman who is a carrier for the same mutant gene and they then have an affected son (Figure 3.5).

One difficult question concerning X-linked recessive disorders is whether or not an isolated affected male represents a new mutation. In a few X-linked recessive disorders it is possible to detect the female carrier state, but in the majority of cases this is not possible. In the Duchenne form of progressive muscular dystrophy the presence of normal muscle enzymes and a negative muscle biopsy does not totally exclude the possibility that the mother is a carrier. Without helpful linkage studies such a situation makes genetic counseling difficult.

Although there are relatively few X-linked dominant traits or diseases, their distinguishing features should be mentioned. The pedigree pattern of an X-linked dominant disorder such as vitamin D–resistant rickets superficially resembles that of an autosomal dominant disease. The distinguishing features of X-linked dominant disorders are as follows: (1) in X-linked disorders male-to-male transmission does not occur; (2) all the daughters of an affected father will have the disorder, since the father transmits his mutant X chromosome solely to his daughters; and (3) as a result of (2) there is usually an excess of affected females (Figure 3.6).

Other features of X-linked dominant inheritance (excluding new mutation and decreased penetrance) show that affected males always have an affected mother, while affected females have an affected father half of the time and an affected mother half of the time.

Evidence is accumulating in a few X-linked dominant disorders (incontinentia

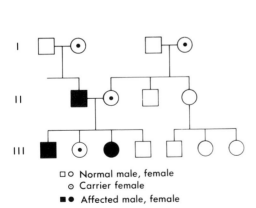

□○ Normal male, female
○ Carrier female
■● Affected male, female

Figure 3.5. Pattern of transmission of an X-linked recessive disorder whereby affected male and carrier female have an affected son. The son is affected because his mother is a carrier. Note that this mating can also produce an affected female.

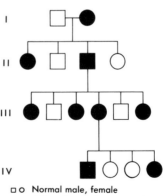

□○ Normal male, female
■● Affected male (hemizygous), female (heterozygous)

Figure 3.6. Pattern of transmission of an X-linked dominant disorder. Male-to-male transmission does not occur. Since all daughters of an affected male have the condition, more females than males are affected.

pigmenti, focal dermal hypoplasia, and oral-facial-digital syndrome I) that the condition is lethal in the male (hemizygotes). This lethality then accounts for the 2:1 ratio of females to males among the progeny of affected women and transmission solely in the female line.

At times it is impossible to determine from pedigree analysis whether the disorder affecting several sibs resulted from X-linked or autosomal recessive inheritance. When all efforts to detect carriers for a given trait have failed, provisional counseling may be offered the sisters in question; the likelihood of obtaining the observed distribution of healthy offspring is compared assuming autosomal recessive and X-linked inheritance.

In terms of genetic diseases in humans and the precise chromosomal location of the mutant gene causing the disease, more is known about X-linked disorders than about any other form of genetic transmission. In 1966 McKusick cataloged over 119 X-linked diseases or traits in which X-linkage was considered proved or extremely likely. The most recent revision of this catalog lists 205 X-linked disorders.

SEX-INFLUENCED AND SEX-LIMITED INHERITANCE

In any discussion of X-linked inheritance it is important to understand the terms *sex-influenced* and *sex-limited* autosomal inheritance. Baldness is considered a sex-influenced trait. Its expression in the male is autosomal dominant, whereas in the female it occurs only when the gene is in the homozygous state as a recessive.

Sex-limited refers to an autosomal trait that is expressed in only one sex. When the expressing sex is male, it is often difficult to distinguish sex-limited autosomal dominant from X-linked recessive inheritance.

Y-LINKED INHERITANCE

In most cases the Y chromosome confers maleness on an individual, for generally the presence of a Y chromosome indicates the presence of testes. Presently only one trait is known in which a given gene is located on the Y chromosome, and that trait is "hairy ears," or hypertrichosis of the pinna. This condition was originally described in men from India but has subsequently been found in other parts of the world (see page 385). As expected, the father transmits this gene to all his sons but to none of his daughters (Figure 3.7). This is sometimes referred to as holandric

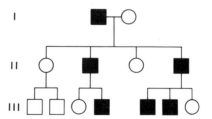

Figure 3.7. Pattern of transmission of a Y-linked trait.

inheritance. It is necessary to distinguish this mode of inheritance from autosomal dominant traits that are expressed only in males (sex-limited). In the latter, half of the daughters of an affected male, although not affected themselves, could transmit the trait to their sons.

There is some indication that genes on the Y chromosome may also be responsible for delayed skeletal maturation and other signs of physical maturity in the male.

MULTIFACTORIAL INHERITANCE

Numerous diseases and traits such as weight, height, and intelligence appear to be controlled by multiple genes. This type of transmission is variously termed multifactorial, polygenic, or quantitative inheritance. When a polygenic trait such as intelligence is studied in a population, a continuous curve shaped like any other probability curve is obtained. This is in contrast to the bimodal distribution curve noted in conditions transmitted by a single gene. In addition to multiple genes, other factors such as environment may play a vital role in the ultimate clinical picture. Some prefer the term *multifactorial* for conditions in which the environment seems to play the most obvious role. Common diseases such as atherosclerosis and essential hypertension are most probably caused by multiple genetic factors. Certainly environment can play a significant role in influencing such disease states.

Multifactorial inheritance is believed to play a causative role in some of the conditions discussed in Chapter 8. Such disorders tend to have the following characteristics: (1) the rarer the trait in the population, the greater the difference in risk between first- and second-degree relatives and between second- and third-degree relatives; (2) the more severe the malformation in the proband, the greater the risk to relatives; (3) if there is a sex difference in frequency of the trait, the risk will be higher in relatives of affected members of the less frequently affected sex; and (4) the risk to relatives of an index patient will be higher if there is another affected near relative.

In cases of multifactorial inheritance the family history is an important tool in studying and understanding the trait in question and in estimating the risk for other family members. Unfortunately, at the present time it is possible to give only empirical risks of recurrence for most multifactorial disorders. Research efforts in this area are directed not only at identifying the specific environmental factors involved but also at attempting to prevent recurrence by eliminating those factors from the environments of genetically susceptible individuals.

REFERENCES

Bodmer, W. F., and Cavalli-Sforza, L. L. 1976. *Genetics, evolution, and man.* San Francisco: W. H. Freeman.

Fraser, F. C. 1963. Taking the family history. *Am. J. Med.* 34:585.

Goodman, R. M. 1970. The family pedigree and genetic counseling. In *Genetic disorders in man*, ed. R. M. Goodman, pp. 87–104. Boston: Little, Brown.

Levitan, M., and Montagu, A. 1977. *Textbook of human genetics.* 2nd ed. New York: Oxford University Press.

McKusick, V. A. 1978. *Mendelian inheritance in man.* 5th ed. Baltimore: The Johns Hopkins University Press.

Murphy, E. A. 1975. Clinical genetics: Some neglected facets. *N. Engl. J. Med.* 292:458.

Slatis, H. H. 1966. Mendelian genetics and genetic problems. In *Lectures in medical genetics,* ed. David Yi Yung Hsia, pp. 143–66. Chicago: Year Book Medical Publishers.

Stern, C. 1973. *Principles of human genetics.* 3rd ed. San Francisco: W. H. Freeman.

4

Genetic disorders in
the Bible and Talmud

THIS CHAPTER is not meant to be an exhaustive study of all the
human genetic disorders recorded in the Bible and Talmud, but
rather is intended to introduce the reader to the fact that these
two sources contain a wealth of medical genetic material that
warrants further study.

BACKGROUND

Physicians and medical historians have long been interested in the medical
diseases mentioned or alluded to in the Bible and Talmud; however, little attention
has been given to the genetic factors that may have been responsible for some of
these disorders. Although there is evidence to suggest that the ancient Hebrews
were aware of the familial nature of certain diseases, they probably had little or no
knowledge of the genetic principles governing the transmission of these disorders.
Moreover, in the past many of the medical scholars who wrote about diseases in
the Bible and Talmud were likewise not oriented to consider the genetic etiology of
disease. This is understandable when we realize that genetic thinking as applied
to diseases is still in its infancy and has come to the forefront of medicine only
during the past 25 years.

A great pitfall in dealing with any form of medical material from the Bible and
Talmud is that the interpretation or diagnosis made may involve an extrapolation
beyond normal limits. This holds true not only for genetic disorders but for disorders of any nature; thus the term *postulated diagnosis* has been used in those
instances where any doubt prevails. Errors in interpretation and diagnosis are
likely to be made, for the Bible and Talmud were never intended to be used as
manuals for making medical diagnoses.

The actual descriptions of diseases in the Bible and Talmud can be divided into
two categories. The first may be called the *case history description*, in which an
actual case history is presented. The second is referred to as the *formal description*,
in which a general account of a pathological process is presented. Each of these
forms has inherent advantages and disadvantages. For example, the case history of
a disease may appear easier to diagnose than a diffuse formal account. The danger

lies in regarding legendary material as diagnostic. The historical validity of case history descriptions must be assessed before a diagnosis can be made, and this assessment should include an examination of the motive for writing the passage.

Formal descriptions, on the other hand, present problems in differentiation, for different disorders have similar presenting signs and symptoms and are often considered to be the same disease. In addition, the lack of technical terminology makes the interpretation of some formal descriptions difficult in modern terms; where the ancients used technical terminology, only philological methods can be used to decipher it, unless parallel usage is found elsewhere.

Talmudic sources are somewhat easier to assess than biblical ones, mainly because their purpose is to explain the Old Testament. Thus, Talmudic descriptions tend to be more extensive and frequently provide sufficient information for diagnosis. However, in using Talmudic texts to clarify an Old Testament source, one must keep in mind that the Talmudic suggestion may be a supposition and not a conclusion.

THE TALMUD

Before discussing some of the genetic disorders mentioned in the Bible and Talmud it may be useful to explain briefly the meaning and organization of the Talmud. The Talmud is the oral law of the Jews that was passed down through the centuries by sages living in Palestine and Babylonia until the beginning of the Middle Ages. It has two main components: the *Mishnah*; and the commentary on the Mishnah, the *Gemarah*. The Mishnah (from the Hebrew *shonah*, "to repeat," and therefore "to study by repetition") is the recorded oral law of the Jews that was in use about the year 200 C.E., the time when the Mishnah was finally compiled and edited by Judah Ha Nasi (Judah the Prince). There are two Talmuds, the Palestinian and the Babylonian, each being a record of the comments on and discussions of the Mishnah by different schools of rabbis, sages, and scholars. The Mishnah of Judah Ha Nasi and the Gemarah of the Palestinian scholars make up the *Talmud Yerushalmi*, or the Jerusalem (Palestinian) Talmud. The Mishnah of Judah Ha Nasi and Gemarah of the Babylonian academies make up the *Talmud Babli*, or the Babylonian Talmud. The Jerusalem Talmud was completed by 400 C.E., the Babylonian Talmud around 500 C.E. During the compilation period and for 500 years afterward, Babylonia was the main center of world Jewry. Thus the more extensive, Babylonian Talmud became the dominant work. Reference to the Talmud herein is to the Babylonian Talmud; reference to the Jerusalem Talmud includes the place-name adjective.

The Jerusalem and Babylonian versions of the Talmud are quite different in size, content, and, according to some scholars, in purpose. The Jerusalem Talmud is about one-sixth the size of the Babylonian text. It is more direct and simpler in language, while its Babylonian counterpart has greater depth. The two versions also use different dialects, the Jerusalem being written in a mixture of Hebrew and west-Aramaic, the Babylonian in a mixture of Hebrew and east-Aramaic.

In terms of content the Talmud is a conglomerate of law, legend, and philosophy, a blend of unique logic and shrewd pragmatism, of history, medicine, science, anecdotes, and humor. It is a collection of paradoxes. Its framework is orderly and logical, with every word and term having been subjected to a meticulous editing completed centuries after the actual work of composition ended. The objectives of the authors and compilers of the Talmud can best be understood in the interpretation of the Hebrew word *Talmud*, which means "teaching."

DISEASES AND MALFORMATIONS

Table 4.1 lists the various genetic traits and diseases discussed in this chapter. As mentioned previously, the list is far from complete.

In order to explain some of the gaps and the unusual concern for certain conditions mentioned in the Bible and the Talmud, it is necessary to say a few words about the practice of medicine in each of these periods.

Table 4.1. Genetic traits and diseases mentioned or alluded to in the Bible and Talmud

Diagnosis or postulated diagnosis of trait or disease	Mode of transmission[a]	Source[b]
Alopecia	AD in males	Bible
Anosmia	V	Talmud
Asthma (P)[c]	M	Bible
Congenital cataract (P)	V	Talmud
Cranial malformations	V	Talmud
Deaf-mutism	V	Bible & Talmud
Dwarfism	V	Talmud
Esophageal fistula and atresia	V	Talmud
External eye malformations	V	Talmud
Facial and body malformations	V	Talmud
Familial cardiac conduction defect (P)	AD	Talmud
Familial epilepsy	AD & M	Talmud
Gout (P)	M	Bible
Gynecomastia	V	Talmud
Hemophilia A	XR	Talmud
Hermaphroditism	V	Talmud
Hirsutism	V	Bible
Hypertrophy and atrophy of the upper extremities (P)	V	Talmud
Hypothyroidism (P)	V	Talmud
Imperforate anus	V	Talmud
Left-handedness	M	Bible
Male genital defects, including cryptorchidism	V	Talmud
Nightblindness (P)	AD & XR	Talmud
Pigmented hairy nevus	AD	Talmud
Red hair	AR?	Bible
Syndactyly and polydactyly	AD & V	Talmud
Tall stature and polydactyly	V	Bible
Testicular feminization (P)	XR	Talmud
Thrombocytopenia purpura (P)	V	Talmud
Urolithiasis	M	Talmud

Note: This list should in no way be considered complete. It includes only the disorders discussed in this text.

[a] AD = autosomal dominant; AR = autosomal recessive; M = multifactorial; V = variable; XR = X-linked recessive.

[b] The exact reference is given in the text.

[c] (P) = postulated diagnosis.

In ancient times medicine and religion were closely interwoven. The priests were the custodians of public health. The problem of the propriety of human interference in sickness, regarded as divine retribution, lessened as the Jews came to regard the physician as the instrument through whom G-d could effect the cure. Physicians were considered to be spiritually endowed. Healing was in the hands of G-d and physicians were helpers or instruments of G-d. The numerous references to physicians throughout the Bible imply that man may administer treatment, but G-d heals: "I am the Lord that healeth thee" (Exodus 15:26).

Biblical medicine was concerned chiefly with hygiene and prophylaxis, and thus the stress was on prevention of epidemics, suppression of prostitution and venereal diseases, frequent washing, care of the skin, strict dietetic and sanitary regulations, rules for sexual life, isolation and quarantine, and many other regulations. Of the 613 commandments in the Bible, 213 are medical in nature.

During the period in which the Talmud was compiled, a number of external factors greatly influenced Jewish medical thinking; however, the central theme in Talmudic medicine was the same as that during the Biblical period—the prevention of disease and the safeguarding of community health. The study of medicine was included in the curriculum of Talmudic schools and many Talmudic scholars were also physicians. Furthermore, the Talmud mentions research-oriented individuals who concerned themselves more with the study of animal and human anatomy and physiology than with the actual practice of medicine. Through their special interest in the ritual fitness of animals and in the extremely high physical qualifications for priesthood, they acquired an extraordinary knowledge of anatomy and physiology. In the Talmud one finds detailed descriptions of malformations that disqualify a man from serving in the temple as a priest, or an animal from use in a sacrificial rite. Discussions in the Talmud pertaining to marriage, sexual relations, and problems of fertility and sterility account for the recognition of various disease states of possible genetic etiology.

Despite the fact that animal dissection was performed during the Talmudic period, little was known about the nervous system in either animals or man. Neither the Bible nor the Talmud mentions a single disease of man involving the brain, spinal cord, or nerves. Lack of knowledge regarding other systems was also apparent during these times, but the area of greatest ignorance was the nervous system. It is somewhat paradoxical that today many of the characteristic genetic disorders affecting Ashkenazi Jews involve the nervous system.

In conclusion, it can be stated that no direct link has been found between the genetic traits and diseases mentioned or alluded to in the Bible or Talmud and those known to be common among Jews today; however, so much has not been touched upon (e.g. the *Midrashim*) that a search for such links seems indicated, despite the difficult and speculative nature of such an endeavor.

DIAGNOSIS: Alopecia

SOURCE: Bible, 2 Kings 2:23

TRANSLATION: And he [Elisha] went up from thence unto Beth-el: and as he was going up by the way, there came forth little children out of the city, and mocked him, and said unto him, go up, thou bald head; go up, thou bald head.

COMMENT: The ordinary form of baldness is thought to be autosomal dominant in males; it is autosomal recessive in females, who transmit the trait if heterozygous but are bald only if homozygous. The transmission of baldness through many successive generations implicates a single major gene.

REFERENCES

Osborne, D. 1916. Inheritance of baldness. *J. Hered.* 7:347.

Snyder, L. H., and Yingling, H. C. 1935. The application of the gene-frequency method of analysis to sex-influenced factors, with special reference to baldness. *Hum. Biol.* 7:608.

DIAGNOSIS: Anosmia

SOURCE: Talmud, order Nezikin, tractate Baba Batra, 146a

TRANSLATION: Rabbi Yehuda said in the name of Rav: It once happened that a certain person was told that his wife could not smell. The man took his wife into a building to test her with radishes he had in his lap. He said to her, "I smell radishes from the Galilee," and she said, "I wish I had some dates from Jericho."

COMMENT: From the inappropriate response of the wife in the above passage, it would seem logical to assume that indeed she could not smell. The partial or complete absence of the sense of smell (anosmia) is a genetic defect that can be transmitted as an autosomal or X-linked dominant trait. In some individuals it is present from birth, while in others it occurs later in life. Certain affected persons lack the sense of smell for only one given substance. Anosmia in males may be associated with hypogonadism (see Kallmann syndrome, page 413).

REFERENCES

Brown, K. S.; MacLean, C. M.; and Robinette, R. R. 1968. The distribution of the sensitivity to chemical odors in man. *Hum. Biol.* 40:456.

Glaser, O. 1918. Hereditary deficiencies in the sense of smell. *Science* 48:647.

Mainland, R. C. 1945. Absence of olfactory sensation. *J. Hered.* 36:143.

Males, J. L.; Townsend, J. L.; and Schneider, R. A. 1973. Hypogonadotropic hypogonadism with anosmia—Kallmann's syndrome. *Arch. Intern. Med.* 131:501.

Singh, N.; Grewal, M. S.; and Austin, J. H. 1970. Familial anosmia. *Arch. Neurol.* 22:40.

POSTULATED DIAGNOSIS: Asthma

SOURCE: Bible, Deuteronomy 2:20

TRANSLATION: The land was also called the land of Rephaim: Rephaim dwelt therein previously, and the Ammonites called them Zamzummin.

COMMENT: In modern Hebrew the word *zomzom* means "wheezing," and it is thought that the people referred to as Zamzummin or Zomzoomin were called this because of their wheezing. It could thus be inferred that they suffered from asthma. The fact that an entire group of people had asthma suggests a familial feature of the disease which is known to exist today. The genetics of asthma is not a simple matter and is not well understood (see asthma, page 304). If one considers asthma to be a part of atopic hypersensitivity, which also includes hay fever and eczema, there is some evidence that the heritability of atopy is dominant. Many investigators consider asthma to be multifactorial in cause.

REFERENCES

Brim, C. J. 1936. *Medicine in the Bible*, pp. 109, 168. New York: Froben Press.

Lubs, M. L. E. 1972. Empiric risks for genetic counseling in families with allergy. *J. Pediatr.* 80:26.

Schwartz, M. 1952. *Heredity in bronchial asthma*. Copenhagen: Munksgaard.

Tips, R. L. 1954. A study of the inheritance of atopic hypersensitivity in man. *Am. J. Hum. Genet.* 6:328.

POSTULATED DIAGNOSIS: Congenital cataract

SOURCE: Talmud, order Moed, tractate Megillah, IV, 6

TRANSLATION: An individual born blind can not represent the congregation in the recital of the *Shema* portion of the service, for that includes a blessing for the creation of light.

COMMENT: Various forms of congenital cataract are genetically determined and may be inherited as either autosomal dominant or autosomal recessive traits. In addition, congenital cataract may be associated with a number of malformation syndromes and metabolic disorders, some of which also are known to be of genetic etiology. In all infants with congenital cataract, proper diagnostic studies must be done in order to provide adequate care.

REFERENCES

Fraser, G. R., and Friedmann, A. I. 1968. *The causes of blindness in childhood: A study of 767 children with severe visual handicaps.* Baltimore: The Johns Hopkins Press.

Goldberg, M. F., ed. 1974. *Genetic and metabolic eye diseases.* Boston: Little, Brown.

Goodman, R. M., and Gorlin, R. J. 1977. *An atlas of the face in genetic disorders.* 2nd ed. St. Louis: C. V. Mosby.

DIAGNOSIS: Cranial malformations

SOURCE: Talmud, order Kodashim, tractate Bekhorot, 44a

TRANSLATION: These are the physical defects that disqualify a priest from serving in the temple. In addition to these are various defects of the head such as *kilon*, when the head resembles the cover on a barrel, pointed on the top and wide at the bottom; *liftan*, where the head resembles the head of a turnip, wide on the top and narrow at the bottom; *makkaban*, one whose head resembles a hatchet, is angular in front; and *sekifas*, as if a piece is missing in back.

COMMENT: Many of the genetically caused congenital malformations seen today were obviously recognized in ancient times. The priest and his advisers were called upon to evaluate individuals with various physical and mental defects, so it was natural for them to note abnormal findings and to include them among the various conditions that would disqualify a man from serving as a priest in the temple.

In certain cases the description leaves little doubt as to the exact malformation. For example, a head shaped like a hatchet, being angular in front, almost certainly denotes the form of craniostenosis referred to as trigonocephaly, while a head that is pointed on top and wide at the bottom could refer to acrocephaly. A skull that is wide at the top and narrow at the bottom could be the expression of brachycephaly.

The skull configuration "as if a piece is missing in back" could indicate a flat occiput or a defect in the occipital bone or in the posterior fontanel. Most of these cranial defects are of genetic etiology and are frequently seen in combination with other malformations, thereby producing a distinct syndrome.

REFERENCES

Goodman, R. M., and Gorlin, R. J. 1977. *An atlas of the face in genetic disorders.* 2nd ed. St. Louis: C. V. Mosby.

Gorlin, R. J.; Pindborg, J. J.; and Cohen, M. M., Jr. 1977. *Syndromes of the head and neck.* 2nd ed. New York: McGraw-Hill.

McKusick, V. A. 1972. *Heritable disorders of connective tissue.* 4th ed. St. Louis: C. V. Mosby.

DIAGNOSIS: Deaf-mutism
SOURCES: (a) Bible, Psalms 38:14
          (b) Talmud (Jerusalem), order Moed, tractate Hagigah, 2a
          (c) Talmud, order Moed, tractate Hagigah, 3a

TRANSLATION: (a) But I, as a deaf man, heard not; and I was as a dumb man that openeth not his mouth.

(b) All males should come to rejoice with G-d. The word *all* includes minors, but the Talmud then asks does the word *all* also include one who is *cheresh* (one who is a deaf-mute). The Talmud responds that *all* who come, come to hear and to learn; this would then exclude the *cheresh* (deaf-mute). Let us say that would also exclude the minor who is not capable of learning.

Rabbi Yoseh responded, "Since the word *all* is inclusive and the words 'in order they learn' exclude, I therefore chose to include the average minor, who can eventually achieve adult learning, and I chose to exclude the deaf-mute, because generally he is not capable of attaining adult learning."

(c) What is the law regarding a person who can speak but not hear, or hear but not speak? According to the Talmud, "in order that thou shalt hear" excludes a person who speaks but cannot hear, and the words "in order that thou shalt learn" exclude the person who can hear but not speak. Shall it be said that a person who cannot speak cannot attain scholarship? Obviously this is incorrect, for two brothers who could not speak (*ilimim*) once lived in the neighborhood of the rabbi. They were sons of the daughter of Rabbi Johanan ben Gudgada (according to others, sons of the sister of Rabbi Johanan). Whenever the rabbi entered the place of learning and sat down, they nodded their heads and moved their lips and the Rabbi prayed for them and they were cured, and it was found that they were versed in Halachah, Sifra and Sifre, and the whole Talmud.

COMMENT: Congenital deafness is frequently of a genetic etiology. If not given proper treatment from a very early age, children with this disorder are destined to have great difficulties with speech. In the not-too-distant past, speech therapy and hearing instruments were unknown. Deaf individuals never acquired speech and were considered among the unlearned. The above quotations distinguish between those who can hear but not speak, and those who can speak but not hear.

If deafness occurs at a later age, after speech has been acquired, it still may be due to a genetic cause. Deafness should be considered a symptom and not a diagnosis. In addition to the various environmental causes, there are a multitude of genetic syndromes that also can account for hearing loss. The importance of early diagnosis and treatment of hearing loss in children cannot be overemphasized. For a discussion of deafness in Jews see page 149.

REFERENCES

Brown, K. S. 1967. The genetics of childhood deafness. In *Deafness in childhood*, ed. F. McConnell and P. H. Ward, pp. 177–202. Nashville: Vanderbilt University Press.

Konigsmark, B. W., and Gorlin, R. J. 1976. *Genetic and metabolic deafness*. Philadelphia: W. B. Saunders.

Lindenov, H. 1945. *The etiology of deaf-mutism, with special reference to heredity*. Copenhagen: Munksgaard.

DIAGNOSIS: Dwarfism
SOURCE: Talmud, order Kodashim, tractate Bekhorot, 45b
TRANSLATION: A male dwarf should not marry a female dwarf, for they may have a dwarfed child.
COMMENT: Because dwarfism is one of the main features of numerous genetic disorders, the above advice was certainly sound, considering the period in which it was expounded. The amount of information given in the translation precludes additional remarks.

REFERENCES

Bailey, J. A. 1973. *Disproportionate short stature*. Philadelphia: W. B. Saunders.

Bergsma, D., ed. 1974. *Skeletal dysplasias*. White Plains, N.Y.: The National Foundation–March of Dimes.

McKusick, V. A. 1972. *Heritable disorders of connective tissue*. 4th ed. St. Louis: C. V. Mosby.

DIAGNOSIS: Esophageal fistula and atresia
SOURCE: Talmud, order Toharot, tractate Nidah, 23b
TRANSLATION: Rava states that where the esophagus has a hole [fistula] the laws of childbirth apply [inferring that this is a viable birth]; where the esophagus is blocked [atresia] the laws of childbirth do not apply [inferring this is a nonviable state].
COMMENT: Although most infants born with an esophageal fistula or atresia are isolated cases, familial aggregation involving these defects has been reported. The precise mode of inheritance when there is familial aggregation is not known. During the Talmudic period, infants born with a fistula had a chance of surviving if the fistula closed, whereas with atresia life was not possible. Today most of these defects can be repaired surgically.

REFERENCES

Dennis, N. R.; Nicholas, J. L.; and Kovar, I. 1973. Oesphageal atresia: 3 cases in 2 generations. *Arch. Dis. Child.* 48:980.

Grieve, J. C., and McDermott, J. G. 1939. Congenital atresia of the oesophagus in two brothers. *Can. Med. Assoc. J.* 41:185.

Schimke, R. N.; Leape, L. L.; and Holder, T. M. 1972. Familial occurrence of esophageal atresia: A preliminary report. *Birth Defects* 13:22.

DIAGNOSIS: External eye malformations such as hypertelorism, orbital asymmetry, strabismus, photophobia, eyebrow and eyelash abnormalities, and excess tearing
SOURCE: Talmud, order Kodashim, tractate Bekhorot, 43b
TRANSLATION: What is *charom* [defect]? Where one can paint the eyes blue in a straight line; where the eyes are elevated and also where the eyes are lower than they should be; where one is high and one is low; where one eye sees the attic and the other eye sees the room; where one cannot see well in strong sunlight; where the eyebrows are long and thick; where the eyes are round almost like a circle; where the eyes tear excessively; where the eyelashes are too heavy and where there are no eyelashes.
COMMENT: These eye malformations exempted a man from serving as a priest in the temple. The above descriptions and details are fascinating. For example, hypertelorism (increased interpupillary distance) is commonly associated with a broad, flat nasal bridge. The description "where one can paint the eyes blue in a straight line" certainly fits a broad, flat nasal bridge and perhaps extends to include hypertelorism. There can be no mistake about strabismus, "where one eye sees the attic and the other eye sees the room." These external eye malformations may be isolated defects or they may be associated with a number of syndromes. In both cases the cause is frequently genetic.

REFERENCES
François, J. 1961. *Heredity in ophthalmology*. St. Louis: C. V. Mosby.
Goodman, R. M., and Gorlin, R. J. 1977. *An atlas of the face in genetic disorders.* 2nd ed. St. Louis: C. V. Mosby.
Waardenburg, P. J.; Franceschetti, A.; and Klein, D. 1961 and 1963. *Genetics and ophthalmology*, vols. 1 and 2. Springfield, Ill.: Charles C Thomas.

DIAGNOSIS: Facial and body malformations
SOURCE: Talmud, order Kodashim, tractate Bekhorot, 44a
TRANSLATION: If a man has eyes as big as a calf's or as small as a goose's; if his body is out of proportion to his organs [limbs] or smaller in proportion to his organs [limbs]; if his nose is out of proportion, whether too large or too small; if his ears are out of proportion, either too big or too small; if his upper lip overlaps his lower lip, or if the lower lip overlaps the upper lip—these are all defects which make it impossible for a man to serve as a priest in the temple.
COMMENT: Rather specific malformations are listed in this section. Eyes as big as a calf's is a most fitting description of bupthalmos, which can be noted in congenital glaucoma or keratoglobus, each of which may be of genetic etiology. Eyes as small as a goose's, or microphthalmia, may be an isolated genetic defect or one associated with a number of genetic syndromes. Altered body proportions involving discrepancies between trunk and limbs is characteristic of a number of genetic skeletal dysplasias. Micrognathia, prognathism (Hapsburg jaw), and alterations in the size and shape of the ears and nose also are observed as isolated malformations or are seen in association with other defects in a variety of genetic syndromes.

REFERENCES
Bergsma, D., ed. 1974. *Skeletal dysplasias*. White Plains, N.Y.: The National Foundation–March of Dimes.

Goodman, R. M., and Gorlin, R. J. 1977. *An atlas of the face in genetic disorders.* 2nd ed. St. Louis: C. V. Mosby.

McKusick, V. A. 1978. *Mendelian inheritance in man.* 5th ed. Baltimore: The Johns Hopkins University Press.

POSTULATED DIAGNOSIS: Familial cardiac conduction defect

SOURCE: Talmud, order Nashim, tractate Yevamot, 105a

TRANSLATION: There was a certain family in Jerusalem whose members used to die when they were about the age of 18 years.

COMMENT: The Talmud goes on to state that the premature deaths in this family were due to a curse inflicted on their great-grandfather, the son of Eli the High Priest.

Rather than list all those genetic diseases which could account for death before the age of twenty, I have chosen to discuss only one. Sex is not mentioned in the above passage, so it is assumed that both males and females were affected by the condition, and it is also most likely that more than one generation was involved. For these reasons I selected an autosomal dominant disorder, disturbance in cardiac conduction.

In 1965 Green and co-workers described a family in which 21 members over eight generations since the early 1800s had died suddenly and unexpectedly. The age of sudden death ranged from 3 to 58 years, with a mean age of 33 years. In a subgroup of this family 10 such deaths had occurred, with the average age at death being 17 years. Post-mortem examinations of two of the affected individuals showed the only abnormal finding to be a striking malformation of the cardiac conducting system with hypoplasia of the right bundle branch and spurious branches of the His bundle. In one individual the artery of the atrioventricular node was absent. Green and co-workers postulated that this alteration predisposed affected members to ventricular fibrillation and death. In the mother of 3 children who died unexpectedly, mild exercise provoked frequent ventricular premature contractions. Since deafness is not mentioned in the above passage, I have ruled out the genetic syndrome of Jervell and Lange-Nielsen characterized by congenital deaf-mutism, syncope, prolonged QT interval, and sudden death. The above is, of course, speculative, and other genetic diseases must be considered in the differential diagnosis.

REFERENCES

Green, J. R., Jr.; Krovetz, L. J.; Shanklin, D. R.; de Vito, J. J.; and Taylor, W. J. 1965. A pathological basis for sudden death in eight generations. *Ann. Intern. Med.* 63:906.

Harris, W. S. 1970. The cardiovascular system. In *Genetic disorders of man,* ed. R. M. Goodman. Boston: Little, Brown.

POSTULATED DIAGNOSIS: Familial epilepsy

SOURCE: Talmud, order Nashim, tractate Yevamot, 64b

TRANSLATION: A man should not marry a woman who comes from a family of epileptics or from a family of lepers; this is applicable only when the illness repeats itself three times in the same family.

COMMENT: Seizures were known during the Talmudic period, and in another portion of the Talmud (order Kodashim, tractate Bekhorot, 44b) it is stated that a man cannot serve as a priest in the temple if he is subject to seizures, even if they are infrequent. It is impossible to draw any conclusions regarding the form of seizures mentioned in the above quotation except that a familial type was undoubtedly recognized. It is noteworthy that three family members must be affected before a restraint is issued. The same thinking is displayed in the Talmudic referral to hemophilia and is based on Halachic probability (*hazaka*), which warns an individual to avoid engaging in an event that has occurred three times.

Hereditary factors do play a role in some of the more common forms of epilepsy, and multifactorial inheritance is probably involved. However, autosomal dominant transmission has been noted in certain instances of centrencephalic epilepsy, focal temporal lobe seizures, and various reflex seizures induced by auditory, visual, tactile, or even visceral stimuli.

REFERENCES

Harvald, B. 1958. Hereditary factors in epilepsy. *Med. Clin. North Am.* 42:345.

Paulson, G., and Allen, N. 1970. The nervous system. In *Genetic disorders of man*, ed. R. M. Goodman, pp. 581–83. Boston: Little, Brown.

Pratt, R. T. C. 1967. *The genetics of neurological disorders*, pp. 98–118. London: Oxford University Press.

Slater, E., and Cowie, V. 1971. *The genetics of mental disorders*, pp. 160–84. London: Oxford University Press.

POSTULATED DIAGNOSIS: Gout
SOURCES: (a) Bible, 1 Kings 15:23
                (b) Bible, 2 Chronicles 16:12

TRANSLATION: (a) Now the rest of all the acts of Asa and all that he did and the cities which he built, are they not written in the book of chronicles of the Kings of Judah? But in the time of his old age, he was diseased in his feet.

(b) And Asa in the thirty and ninth year of his reign was diseased in his feet, and his disease was exceedingly great; yet in his disease he sought not to the Lord, but to the physicians.

COMMENT: Although the first modern description of gout was made by Thomas Sydenham in the 17th century, its occurrence has been recognized since ancient times. Various medical authorities seized on the above account of King Asa's illness and were quite satisfied to make the diagnosis of gout. In the Talmud one can find two separate discussions (order Nashim, tractate Sotah, 10a, and order Nezikin, tractate Sanhedrin, 48b) that elaborate on King Asa's gout, and in the 11th century the famous Talmudic commentator Rashi speaks of the king's illness, stating that the name of this illness, podagra, "is the same even in our language" (i.e. French, Rashi's native tongue).

In 1975 de Vries and Weinberger challenged this long-held diagnosis: "We conclude that the biblical case report does not provide sufficient data to diagnose King Asa's illness accurately but that, considering the course of his disease, gout seems improbable. Taking into account the patient's sex, the advanced age at which he became ill, and the severity of his disease leading to his death within two years from the onset, the diagnosis of peripheral obstructive vascular disease with ensuing gangrene seems a more probable assumption." Although the latter interpretation seems more acceptable, the beauty of such a debate is that it can continue, for no one will ever know what illness afflicted the feet of King Asa.

Perhaps a more intriguing Biblical allusion to gout is that found in the ritual of consecration of the priesthood. In Exodus 29:20 the command is given to Moses that from the sacrificial ram he "take of the blood and put it upon the *t'nooch ozen* [concha of the ear] of Aaron's right ear and that of his sons, and upon the *bohen* [thumb] of their right hand and upon the *bohen* [great toe] of their right foot."

Those who favor this as a description of gout contend that the blood signifies the etiology and that its application to the various parts of the body represents the sites involved in the disease. In the majority of cases, the initial attack involves the basal joint of the big toe. This occurs more commonly on the right than the left. The feet are usually affected first, followed by the hands. Concomitant with these lesions, tophi, or nodules, appear in the ears. This ritual may have had a prophylactic meaning, for the sons of Aaron were exposed to the same rites. Some have argued that this point reflected ancient knowledge of a genetic factor in gout. Most authorities today consider the inheritance of the most common form of gout to be multifactorial.

REFERENCES

Brim, C. J. 1936. *Medicine in the Bible*, pp. 90–91. New York: Froben Press.

De Vries, A., and Weinberger, A. 1975. King Asa's presumed gout. *N.Y. State J. Med.* 75:452.

Rosner, F. 1969. Gout in the Bible and Talmud. *JAMA* 207:151.

Wyngaarden, J. B., and Kelly, W. N. 1972. In *The metabolic basis of inherited disease*, ed. J. B. Stanbury, J. B. Wyngaarden, and D. S. Fredrickson, 3rd ed., pp. 889–968. New York: McGraw-Hill.

DIAGNOSIS: Gynecomastia

SOURCE: Talmud, order Kodashim, tractate Bekhorot, 44b

TRANSLATION: A man is disqualified from serving as a priest in the Temple if he has breasts like a woman.

COMMENT: Among the various causes of gynecomastia one must consider a genetic etiology. When this finding is associated with hypogonadism other genetic disorders should be thought of, such as the Klinefelter and Reifenstein syndromes. In normally virile men there is evidence to suggest that in some cases isolated gynecomastia may be transmitted as a male-limited autosomal dominant, autosomal recessive, and X-linked trait.

REFERENCES

Bowen, P.; Lee, C. N. S.; Migeon, C. J.; Kaplan, N. M.; Whalley, P. J.; McKusick, V. A.; and Reifenstein, E. C. 1965. Hereditary male pseudohermaphroditism with hypogonadism, hypospadias, and gynecomastia (Reifenstein's syndrome). *Ann. Intern. Med.* 62:252.

Ljungberg, T. 1960. Hereditary gynecomastia. *Acta Med. Scand.* 168:371.

Rosewater, S.; Gwinup, G.; and Hamwi, G. J. 1965. Familial gynecomastia. *Ann. Intern. Med.* 63:377.

Wallach, E. E., and Garcia, C. R. 1962. Familial gynecomastia without hypogonadism: A report of three cases in one family. *J. Clin. Endocrinol. Metab.* 22:1201.

DIAGNOSIS: Hemophilia A

SOURCE: Talmud, order Nashim, tractate Yevamot, 64b

TRANSLATION: For it was taught that if she circumcised her first son and he died, and she had the second one circumcised and he died, she must not circumcise her third son. So stated Rabbi Judah Ha Nasi. Rabbi Shimon ben Gamliel, however, said: "She may circumcise the third child, but must not circumcise the fourth if the third child dies." It once happened with four sisters from Tzippori that the first had her son circumcised and he died, the second sister had her son circumcised and he died, the third sister had her son circumcised and he also died, and the fourth sister came before Rabbi Shimon ben Gamliel and he told her, "You must not circumcise your son." (See frontispiece for the original in Hebrew.)

COMMENT: Classical hemophilia, or hemophilia A as it is known today, was accurately described by an American physician, Otto, in 1803. He wrote that it is a familial disorder affecting only males, although females transmit the disorder. In 1820 Nasse better formulated the manner of transmission and in 1839 the name hemophilia was coined by Schönlein.

The above quotation from the Talmud is the earliest record of the disorder. The fact that the disease presented itself during the ritual of circumcision to the three sons of one woman and later to the sons of her three sisters strongly supports the genetic features of X-linked recessive hemophilia A.

In the above discussion the two Rabbis did not differ as to the matter of maternal transmission of the disease, but disputed the number of repetitions necessary to establish a pattern and to remove a subsequent similar event from the category of chance. This, then, is a technical point in Talmudic Law. In general, three repetitive events are required to establish a pattern, but in matters of life and death the view of Rabbi Judah is upheld that two such events suffice.

Maimonides, the great physician and Talmudist of the 12th century, carried on the discussion of hemophilia in his *Mishneh Torah*:

> If a woman had her first son circumcised and he died as a result of the circumcision, which enfeebled his strength, and she similarly had her second circumcised and he died as a result of the circumcision—whether [the latter child was] from her first husband or from her second husband—the third son may not be circumcised at the proper time [on the eighth day of life]. Rather one postpones the operation for him until he grows up and his strength is established. One may circumcise only a child that is totally free of disease, because danger to life overrides every other consideration. It is possible to circumcise later than the proper time, but it is impossible to restore a single [departed] soul of Israel forever.

Maimonides may have been referring to the mode of death when he wrote "enfeebled his strength"—i.e. exsanguination. This conclusion was perhaps unwarranted, however, for he may have grouped circumcision mortality with numerous causes such as prematurity and anemia in addition to bleeding disorders. As a physician, his aim was to delay circumcision until health was established.

Maimonides went on to set a specific time limit—i.e. circumcision may be performed when the child is declared medically fit. He thus seemed to believe that spontaneous remission or perhaps medical therapy could produce control of the disease or even its cure. He rightly recognized that a woman could transmit the disease to her male offspring by different fathers.

These ancient Jewish writings do not consider the question of circumcision of a child whose maternal uncles died of bleeding after circumcision. Only the direct maternal transmission of the disease was recognized, whether demonstrated in sibs or in maternal cousins.

Even with modern-day treatment it is not recommended that a newborn hemophiliac male be circumcised, for the risk of his bleeding after the operation is substantially greater than that faced by a normal infant. A woman who has a family history of hemophilia cannot have her son circumcised until coagulation studies show her son to be perfectly normal. Thus, by Jewish Law, one must today withhold circumcision and abide by the wisdom enunciated by Maimonides: "One may circumcise only a child that is totally free of disease, because danger to life overrides every other consideration."

REFERENCES

Castiglioni, A. 1941. *A history of medicine*, p. 107. New York: Alfred A. Knopf.

Maimonides, M. 1957. Laws of circumcision: Book of Adoration [Sefer Ahavah]. In *Code of Maimonides* [Mishneh Torah], chap. 1, par. 18. Jerusalem: Pardes Publisher.

Major, R. H. 1954. *A history of medicine*, vol. 1, p. 252. Springfield, Ill.: Charles C Thomas.

Nasse, C. F. 1820. Von einer erblichen Neigung zu todtlichen Blutungen. *Arch. Med. Erfahr.* 1:385.

Otto, J. C. 1803. An account of an hemorrhagic disposition existing in certain families. *Med. Respository* 6:1.

Rosner, F. 1969. Hemophilia in the Talmud and rabbinic writings. *Ann. Intern. Med.* 70:833.

DIAGNOSIS: Hermaphroditism
SOURCES: (a) Talmud, order Zeraim, tractate Bikurin, chapter 4, 5th Mishnah
         (b) Talmud, order Nashim, tractate Yevamot, 80b
TRANSLATION: (a) Rabbi Yossi says *androgenous* is a unique person and the sages could not decide if he is a male or female. But this is not so with one whose sex is partially concealed, for such a one is at times a man and at other times a woman.

(b) What woman is deemed to be incapable of procreation? Any woman who has reached 20 years of age and has not produced two pubic hairs. And even if she produces them afterwards she is still thought to be incapable of procreation. And these are her features. She has no breasts and suffers pain during intercourse. Rabbi Shimon ben Gamliel states she has no mons veneris like other women. Rabbi Shimon also states that the voice is deep, so that one cannot distinguish whether it is that of a man or a woman.

COMMENT: It is apparent from the above descriptions that the Talmudic sages were well aware of the problems that can arise in human sexual differentiation. Various

---

types of hermaphroditism, be they the true form (involving testicular and ovarian tissue) or the pseudo forms, may be of genetic etiology. Included among the genetic types are those caused by alterations in the sex chromosomes, but even with present-day methods of chromosomal examination, it is not always possible to make an accurate diagnosis of the type of hermaphroditism without the benefit of a laporatomy.

REFERENCES
Gardner, L. I., ed. 1969. *Endocrine and genetic diseases of childhood*. Philadelphia: W. B. Saunders.
Rimoin, D. L., and Schimke, R. N. 1971. *Genetic disorders of the endocrine glands*. St. Louis: C. V. Mosby.
Rosenberg, H. S.; Clayton, G. W.; and Hsu, T. C. 1963. Familial true hermaphrodism. *J. Clin. Endocrinol.* 23:203.

DIAGNOSIS: Hirsutism
SOURCES: (a) Bible, Genesis 25:25
(b) Bible, Genesis 27:11
(c) Bible, 2 Kings 1:8
TRANSLATION: (a) And when the first came forth, he was red, full of hair like a woolen cloth; and they called his name Esau.

(b) And Jacob said to Rebekah his mother, "Behold, Esau my brother is a hairy man, and I am a smooth man."

(c) And they answered him, "He was a hairy man, and girt with a girdle of leather about his loins." And he said, "It is Elijah the Tishbite."

COMMENT: Esau and Jacob were dizygotic twins and among their many differences was the fact that Esau was hairy and Jacob was not. Hirsutism is also mentioned with regard to Elijah the Tishbite. Although there is no account of the degree of hairiness of the fathers of these two men, body hairiness is usually genetically determined. Some populations are known to have sparse body hair, while others are exceptionally hairy. There are certain genetic syndromes in which an increase in body hair is a key feature of the disorder. Along this line of thinking some have postulated that Esau had a form of congenital adrenal hyperplasia. The great Talmudic scholar Rashi commented that Esau appeared like a child of years with well-developed parts. The findings of generalized hirsutism, enlarged genitalia, unusually rapid growth, abnormal strength, and precociousness provide for some interpreters a rather complete physical description of Esau. Certainly Esau was a virile man, but whether or not his virility was due to a genetic form of adrenal hyperplasia is a moot point. Certain forms of congenital adrenal hyperplasia are known to be common in some Jewish ethnic groups, as discussed on page 131 of this text.

REFERENCES
Brim, C. J. 1936. *Medicine in the Bible*, pp. 102–3. New York: Froben Press.
Ebling, F. J. G., and Rook, A. 1968. Hair. In *Textbook of dematology*, ed. A. Rook, D. S. Wilkinson, and F. J. G. Ebling. Philadelphia: F. A. Davis.
Felgenhauer, W. R. 1969. Hypertrichosis lanuginosa universalis. *J. Genet. Hum.* 17:1.

Greenblatt, R. B. 1963. *Search the Scriptures*, pp. 11–15. Philadelphia: J. B. Lippincott.

POSTULATED DIAGNOSIS: Hypertrophy and atrophy of the upper extremities
SOURCE: Talmud, order Kodashim, tractate Bekhorot, 3b
TRANSLATION: If there are two very big arms or two very small arms, this is considered a defect. If they are too large it is a sign of strength, and if they are too small it is a sign of weakness.
COMMENT: Hypertrophy and atrophy of the upper extremities are not diagnoses but physical findings. Various muscular and neurological diseases of genetic etiology could account for such findings. For example, the autosomal dominant disorder facioscapulohumeral muscular dystrophy could produce atrophic changes in the arms, causing weakness, while neurofibromatosis, also an autosomal dominant disease, might cause the overgrowth of an extremity, producing a hypertrophic appearance. Increased strength, however, is not always associated with hypertrophic changes.

REFERENCES
Crowe, F. W.; Schull, W. J.; and Neel, J. V. 1956. *A clinical, pathological, and genetic study of multiple neurofibromatosis.* Springfield, Ill.: Charles C Thomas.
Pratt, R. T. C. 1967. *The genetics of neurological disorders.* London: Oxford University Press.
Tyler, F. H., and Stevens, F. S. 1950. Studies in disorders of muscle. Part II: Clinical manifestations and inheritance of facioscapulohumeral dystrophy in a large family. *Ann. Intern. Med.* 32:640.
Walton, J. 1969. *Diseases of the muscles.* 2nd ed. Boston: Little, Brown.

POSTULATED DIAGNOSIS: Hypothyroidism
SOURCE: Talmud, order Nashim, tractate Nedarim, 66b
TRANSLATION: A man said to his wife, "I vow that you will not have benefit of me until you show some pleasing attribute of yourself to Rabbi Ishmael, the son of Rabbi Yossi." So Rabbi Ishmael asked of those who viewed her, "Perhaps her head is beautiful?" His students answered that her head is round. "Perhaps her hair is attractive?" They replied, "It resembles strands of flax." "Perhaps her eyes are beautiful?" "They are round." "Perhaps her ears are attractive?" "They are large." "Perhaps her nose is attractive?" "It is swollen and closed." "Perhaps her lips are beautiful?" "They are thick and puffy." "Perhaps her neck is attractive?" "It is short." "Perhaps her abdomen is nice?" "It is swollen and protrudes." "Perhaps her feet are nice?" "They are wide like a duck."
COMMENT: Hypothyroid individuals may be classified as having cretinism, juvenile myxedema, adult myxedema, and hypothyroidism without myxedema. Clinical findings are determined by the degree and duration of thyroid failure and the time of life at which it occurs. Translating the above quotation into medical findings, it is possible to conjure up a picture of a short, lethargic woman with a puffy face, straight dry hair, protruding abdomen, and edema of the feet, all of which suggest that she may have had hypothyroidism, possibly to the extent of being myxedematous. Certainly other conditions could also explain her appearance, but if

indeed she was hypothyroid, a number of genetic syndromes could account for an alteration in thyroid metabolism.

REFERENCES

Beierwaltes, W. H. 1964. Genetics of thyroid disease. In *The thyroid*, ed. J. B. Hazard and D. E. Smith. Baltimore: Williams and Wilkins.

Hall, P. F. 1965. Familial occurrence of myxedema. *J. Med. Genet.* 2:173.

Rimoin, D. L., and Schmike, R. N. 1971. *Genetic disorders of the endocrine glands.* St. Louis: C. V. Mosby.

Stanbury, J. B.; Wyngaarden, J. B.; and Fredrickson, D. S., eds. 1972. *The metabolic basis of inherited disease.* 3rd ed. New York: Blakiston Division, McGraw-Hill.

DIAGNOSIS: Imperforate anus

SOURCE: Talmud, order Moed, tractate Shabbat, 134a

TRANSLATION: And Abaya said, "My mother told me, if this infant was born without a noticeable anal opening, rub the area with oil and hold the child up in the brightness of the day, and that part which appears transparent should be pierced with the shaft from a barley plant, but not with a metal object because that causes inflammation."

COMMENT: The sagaciousness noted in the above quotation cannot help but make one appreciate the medical knowledge contained in the Talmud. Imperforate anus has been reported in multiple family members, but no consistent pattern of transmission has been observed. Autosomal dominant, recessive, and X-linked recessive inheritance have all been suggested. In one family involving a mother and two daughters, a rectovaginal fistula also was present.

REFERENCES

Kaijser, K., and Malmstrom-Groth, A. 1957. Anorectal abnormalities as a congenital familial incidence. *Acta Paediatr.* 46:199.

Weinstein, E. D. 1965. Sex-linked imperforate anus. *Pediatrics* 35:715.

Winkler, J. M., and Weinstein, E. D. 1970. Imperforate anus and heredity. *J. Pediatr. Surg.* 5:555.

DIAGNOSIS: Left-handedness

SOURCES: (a) Bible, Judges 3:15

(b) Bible, Judges 20:15–16

TRANSLATION: (a) But when the children of Israel cried unto the Lord, the Lord raised them up a deliverer, Ehud the son of Gera, a Benjamite, a man left-handed.

(b) And the children of Benjamin were numbered at that time out of the cities twenty and six thousand men that drew sword, beside the inhabitants of Gibeah, which were numbered seven hundred chosen men.

Among all these people there were seven hundred chosen men left-handed; every one could sling stones at a hair's breadth and not miss.

COMMENT: The frequent occurrence of left-handedness among members of the tribe of Benjamin seems to be well documented in the above quotation. Although the genetics of handedness is far from clear, we know that men are more left-handedness than women by a factor of two. In Israel the frequency of left-handedness was recorded among school children from various Jewish ethnic groups and a relatively high rate was found compared to some non-Jewish populations (see page 393). Handedness is probably a multifactorial trait.

REFERENCES

Annett, M. 1973. Handedness in families. *Ann. Hum. Genet.* 37:93.

Coren, S., and Porae, C. 1977. Fifty centuries of right-handedness: The historic record. *Science* 198:631.

Huheey, J. E. 1977. Concerning the origin of handedness in humans. *Behav. Genet.* 7:29.

Levy, J. 1976. A review of evidence for a genetic component in the determination of handedness. *Behav. Genet.* 6:429.

Rife, D. C. 1940. Handedness with special reference to twins. *Genetics* 25:178.

DIAGNOSIS: Male genital defects, including cryptorchidism
SOURCE: Talmud, order Kodashim, tractate Bekhorot, VII, 5
TRANSLATION: A man is disqualified for serving as a priest in the temple if his scrotum goes down to his knees, or if his penis reaches his knees, or if he has no testicles, or if he has only one testicle.
COMMENT: Enlargement of the external male genitalia may be due to infection (filariasis manifested as elephantiasis), herniation (in some cases caused by a genetic disorder in connective tissue), trauma, or congenital lymphedema, which may be of genetic cause. An enlarged penis can also be present due to certain endocrine disorders of genetic etiology. A hydrocele is a common cause for scrotal enlargement, and such an entity was known in ancient times by the name *meroach oschech* (Leviticus 21:20). *Oschech* means "large testes" and *meroach* means "air-filled"; thus the scrotum appears blown up and enlarged. When not associated with other malformations, cryptorchidism (unilateral and bilateral) is seldom due to a genetic cause; nevertheless, familial cases of such a defect have been reported.

REFERENCES

Corbus, B. C., and O'Connor, V. J. 1922. The familial occurrence of undescended testes: Report of six brothers with testicular anomalies. *Surg. Gynecol. Obstet.* 34:237.

McKusick, V. A. 1972. *Heritable disorders of connective tissue.* 4th ed. St. Louis: C. V. Mosby.

Perrett, L. J., and O'Rourke, D. A. 1969. Hereditary cryptorchidism. *Med. J. Aust.* 1:1289.

Rimoin, D. L., and Schimke, R. N. 1971. *Genetic disorders of the endocrine glands.* St. Louis: C. V. Mosby.

DIAGNOSIS: Night blindness (nyctalopia)
SOURCE: Talmud, order Nashim, tractate Gittin, 69a
TRANSLATION: If a man has night blindness he should take a strong rope made from hair [the tail of a horse] and tie one end to his foot and the other to the foot of a dog.
COMMENT: The above passage from the Talmud is found in a section dealing with mystical cures, but the idea is not so far removed from our present-day use of the

seeing-eye dog. Because Rashi states that this form of blindness comes upon an individual at night, it is safe to assume that the problem is night blindness.

Night blindness by itself is a symptom of multiple episodes of chorioretinal degenerations, which usually begin in childhood and continue into advanced life before the patient becomes disabled. Autosomal dominant inheritance has been well documented in many families.

Night blindness associated with myopia is transmitted as an X-linked recessive condition and occurs only in males.

REFERENCES

François, J. 1961. *Heredity in opthalmology*. St. Louis: C. V. Mosby.

Fraser, G. R., and Friedmann, A. I. 1967. *The causes of blindness in childhood: A study of 776 children with severe visual handicaps*, p. 72. Baltimore: The Johns Hopkins Press.

Morton, A. S. 1893. Two cases of hereditary congenital night-blindness without visible fundus change. *Trans. Ophthalmol. Soc. U.K.* 13:147.

DIAGNOSIS: Pigmented hairy nevus

SOURCE: Talmud, order Nashim, tractate Ketubot, 75a

TRANSLATION: A mole that has hair in it is considered a bodily defect; if it does not have hair in it, only a large mole is deemed to be a bodily defect. What is considered to be a large mole? Rav Shimon ben Gamliel said, "If it is as large as the Issar Italki" [a certain coin of that time].

COMMENT: Here, as in other passages from the Talmud in this chapter, one detects the concern of the sages for detail. Obviously, in matters of health nothing should be vague and every effort should be made to define the problem clearly.

Small pigmented nevi, with or without hair, have not been considered to be of genetic origin; however, there is evidence that a certain type of giant pigmented hairy nevus (GPHN) may be of genetic etiology. GPHN is almost always associated with multiple small pigmented hairy nevi and is often observed in other family members. Autosomal dominant transmission has been postulated for some forms of GPHN.

REFERENCES

Goodman, R. M.; Caren, J.; Ziprkowski, M.; Padeh, B.; Ziprkowski, L.; and Cohen B. E. 1971. Genetic considerations in giant pigmented hairy naevus. *Br. J. Dermatol.* 85:150.

Russell, J. L., and Reyes, R. G. 1959. Giant pigmented nevi. *JAMA* 171:2083.

DIAGNOSIS: Red hair

SOURCES: (a) Bible, 1 Samuel 16:12
(b) Bible, 1 Samuel 17:42

TRANSLATION: (a) And he sent and brought him [David] in. Now he was ruddy, and withal of a beautiful countenance, and goodly to look to.

(b) And when the Philistine looked about and saw David, he disdained him, for he was but a youth, and ruddy, and of a fair countenance.

COMMENT: It is generally agreed that King David had red hair and a ruddy complexion. Geneticists, however, are not certain of the exact mode of transmission of red hair. Some contend that red hair is an expression of autosomal recessive inheritance, while others argue that the frequency of red-haired offspring in families in which one or both parents are red-haired is too high to support a simple recessive hypothesis. Some state that red pigment in the hair is hypostatic only to brown or black pigment.

REFERENCES

Neel, J. V. 1943. Concerning inheritance of red hair. *J. Hered.* 34:93.
Reed, T. E. 1952. Red hair colour as a genetical character. *Ann. Eugen.* 17:115.
Rife, D. C. 1967. The inheritance of red hair. *Acta Genet. Med. Gemellol.* 16:342.

DIAGNOSIS: Syndactyly and polydactyly

SOURCE: Talmud, order Kodashim, tractate Bekhorot, 45a

TRANSLATION: If his fingers lie next to each other as if they have grown together at the root, he is unfit; if he tries to separate them by cutting them, he is also unfit. If he has an additional finger and he cuts it off and if there was bone in it, he is unfit; but if there was no bone in it, he is fit. If he has additional fingers and additional toes on each hand and foot, six fingers and six toes, twenty four, Rabbi Yehudah declared such a priest fit, whereas the sages declared him unfit.

COMMENT: There are various forms of syndactyly and polydactyly, depending on location and degree of involvement, and most cases involve a genetic etiology. When the defect appears as an isolated malformation, it is usually transmitted as an autosomal dominant trait. Webbing, or syndactyly, between the second and third toes is one of the most common of all genetic malformations and is inherited in an autosomal dominant manner. Polydactyly is also discussed on page 65.

REFERENCES

McKusick, V. A. 1978. *Mendelian inheritance in man.* 5th ed. Baltimore: The Johns Hopkins University Press.
Temtamy, S. A., and McKusick, V. A. 1975. *The genetics of hand malformations.* White Plains, N.Y.: The National Foundation–March of Dimes.

DIAGNOSIS: Tall stature and polydactyly

SOURCES: (a) Bible, Numbers 13:32–33
            (b) Bible, Deuteronomy 2:10–11
            (c) Bible, Deuteronomy 3:11
            (d) Bible, 2 Samuel 21:20–22

TRANSLATION: (a) . . . and all the people that we saw in the land were men of great stature. And we saw the giants, the sons of Anak, which come of the giants; and we were in our own sight as grasshoppers, and so we were in their sight.

(b) The Emims dwelt therein in times past, a people great and many, and tall as the Anakims; which also were accounted giants, as the Anakims; but the Moabites called them Emims.

(c) For only Og king of Bashan remained of the remanent of giants; behold, his bed is a bed of iron; is it not in Rabbath of the children of Ammon? Nine cubits is the length thereof and four cubits the breadth of it, after the cubit of a man.

(d) And there was yet a battle in Gath, where there was a man of great stature, that had on every hand six fingers, and on every foot six toes, four and twenty in number; and he also was born to the giant. And when he defied Israel, Jonathan the son of Shimeah the brother of David slew him. These four were born to the giant in Gath and fell by the hand of David and the hand of his servants.

COMMENT: Although there are various genetic and nongenetic disease states in which tall stature is a main finding, quotations a and b probably refer to tall tribal groups (such as the Watusi of Africa) in which a nonpathological genetic component accounts for height. However, quotation (c) refers to an exceptionally tall man. A cubit is the length from the elbow to the tip of the middle finger—approximately 1½ feet. The bed of Og, king of Bashan, measured 13½ feet in length and was made of iron (a material not commonly used in the construction of beds in ancient times). It has been postulated that Og's great height was due to over-production of growth hormone by the pituitary gland rather than to a nonpathological genetic cause.

The "Giant of Gath" also had polydactyly involving all four extremities. Although I am not aware of a genetic syndrome involving polydactyly and gigantism, such a possibility must be considered. In this regard it is interesting to note that one form of postaxial polydactyly is about 10 times more frequent in blacks than in whites. Since some black African tribes are known for their height, such an association may be common in the absence of a genetic disease. For other remarks on polydactyly see page 64.

REFERENCES

Brim, C. J. 1936. *Medicine in the Bible*, pp. 109–10. New York: Froben Press.

Frazier, T. M. 1960. A note on race-specific congenital malformation rates. *Am. J. Obstet. Gynecol.* 80:184.

Hook, E. B., and Reynolds, J. W. 1967. Cerebral gigantism: Endocrinological and clinical observations of six patients including a congenital giant, concordant monozygotic twins, and a child who achieved adult gigantic size. J. Pediatr. 70:900.

Seip, M. 1959. Lipodystrophy and gigantism with associated endocrine manifestation: A new diencephalic syndrome? *Acta Paediatr.* 48:555.

POSTULATED DIAGNOSIS: Testicular feminization syndrome
SOURCE: Talmud, order Nashim, tractate Ketubot, 10b
TRANSLATION: A man came before Rabbi Gamliel the Elder and said to him, "Rabbi, I have had intercourse with my wife and no virginal blood resulted." So the wife said to the Rabbi, "I am from the family *Dorkati*, where the women have neither menstral flow nor virginal bleeding." Rabbi Gamliel examined her family and verified what she had stated.

COMMENT: There are a number of chromosomal and endocrine disorders that can produce primary amenorrhea, but the testicular feminization syndrome has been selected to be the most likely diagnosis in this instance. The reasons are as follows: (a) although genotypically these individuals are males, phenotypically they are noted for their very attractive female appearance, with luxuriant head hair, smooth skin, and a well-proportioned body; (b) because of their beauty it seems logical to assume that they would have no problem finding a marriage partner; (c) all have primary amenorrhea; and (d) since this condition is genetically transmitted as an X-linked recessive disorder, it is not uncommon to find other affected "female" members in the same family.

Even more interesting is the reference to the Hebrew family name Dorkati. *Dor* in Hebrew means "generation," while *kati* comes from the Hebrew verb *lachtoch,* which means "to cut." Thus, because it was well known that some "women" in this family could not have children, the family was called Dorkati, referring to the fact that some "female" members were "cut off from producing a new generation."

REFERENCES

Morris, J. M. 1953. The syndrome of testicular feminization in male pseudoher-maphrodites. *Am. J. Obstet. Gynecol.* 65:1192.

Southern, A. L. 1965. The syndrome of testicular feminization. In *Advances in metabolic diseases*, ed. R. Levine and R. Luft, pp. 227–56. New York: Academic Press.

POSTULATED DIAGNOSIS: Thrombocytopenia purpura
SOURCE: Talmud, order Moed, tractate Shabbat, 134a
TRANSLATION: Rabbi Nathan said, "Once I traveled abroad and a woman came before me who had circumcised her first son and he died, and the same happened to her second son. The third son she brought before me and I saw that he was red [according to Rashi, his blood was between his skin and flesh (purpura)]. I told her to wait until his blood was absorbed. She waited, then circumcised him, and he lived and he was called Nathan the Babylonian, after my name."
COMMENT: In 1969 Ehrlich discussed this Talmudic passage and concluded that the affected sons most probably had neonatal thrombocytopenia due to maternal-fetal incompatibility of platelet antigens. Such a clinical entity has been well documented and its multiple occurrence in sibships may simulate autosomal recessive inheritance. However, genetics is one of the many causes of thrombocytopenia purpura. Numerous forms of thrombocytopenia with diverse genetic, clinical, and laboratory features have been reported, but some are not associated with well-defined ancillary clinical or laboratory findings. In the latter group the mode of transmission is quite variable, and X-linked and autosomal recessive types do exist. Such a form of hereditary thrombocytopenia should also be considered in the cases mentioned above.

REFERENCES

Ehrlich, D. 1969. Neonatal purpura in the Talmud. *Harefuah* 76:1.

Pagonelli, V. H. 1969. Thrombocytopenia in newborn siblings. *JAMA* 208:1703.

Roberts, M. H., and Smith, M. H. 1950. Thrombopenic purpura: Report of four cases in one family. *Am. J. Dis. Child.* 79:820.

Wintrobe, M. M. 1974. *Clinical hematology*, 7th ed., pp. 1100–1101. Philadelphia: Lea and Febiger.

DIAGNOSIS: Urolithiasis
SOURCE: Talmud, order Nashim, tractate Gittin, 69b
TRANSLATION: If someone has a stone in the bladder let him take three drops of sap (from a certain tree) and three drops of juice (from a certain vegetable) and three

drops of clear wine and apply it to the penis or the corresponding place in a woman. COMMENT: The excruciatingly painful condition of renal stones was a well-known disorder in Talmudic times. In fact, Rabbi Judah the Prince, an editor of the Mishnah, is known to have been a sufferer of urolithiasis (Talmud, order Nashim, tractate Baba Metzia, 85a). Later in the above Talmudic section one finds the ingenious suggestion that patients with urinary stones urinate on the doorsteps to watch for the passage of the stone.

The causes of urolithiasis are many and include a number of inborn errors of metabolism. It is thought that the etiology of calcium oxalate renal stones (one of the most common forms) is multifactorial and that the risk of their occurrence is greater for males than for females.

REFERENCES

Resnick, M.; Pridgen, D. B.; and Goodman, H. O. 1968. Genetic predisposition to calcium oxalate renal calculi. *N. Engl. J. Med.* 278:1313.

Stanbury, J. B.; Wyngaarden, J. B.; and Fredrickson, D. S., eds. 1972. *The metabolic basis of inherited disease.* 3rd ed. New York: McGraw-Hill.

5

Genetic disorders among Ashkenazi Jews

THE GENETIC disorders discussed in this chapter occur most commonly among Ashkenazi Jews, but their frequency varies tremendously. Although a few of these diseases were described in the 1880s, the majority have been recognized only during the past three decades, with the most recent one being reported in 1974.

Two interesting observations can be made concerning these disorders. First, most of them involve the central nervous system, either primarily or secondarily. Second, in three of them (Tay-Sachs, Gaucher, and Niemann-Pick disease) the enzymatic alterations involved share a common metabolic pathway. It is not known whether these findings are merely random or are indicative of a particular genetic relationship. For further comments on this subject the reader is referred to Chapter 12.

ABETALIPOPROTEINEMIA
(BASSEN-KORNZWEIG SYNDROME)

Historical note

In 1950 Bassen and Kornzweig described an 18-year-old Ashkenazi Jewish female with a syndrome characterized by retinitis pigmentosa, ataxic neuropathy, and circulating red blood cells that appeared to be crenated. A few years later her brother was found to be similarly affected and his case was reported by the same authors. The parents of these sibs were cousins. In 1959 Druez suggested the term *acanthocytosis* for the deformed erythrocytes involved and in the early literature this disorder was referred to as *acanthocytes, acanthocytosis*, or Bassen-Kornzweig syndrome. In 1960 various investigators independently demonstrated the absence of low-density lipoproteins (LDL) from the serum of these patients. Also at this time unique changes in the small intestine and the absence of plasma chylomicrons were reported. On the basis of these new observations the terminology was further modified on the supposition that this lipoprotein abnormality might be the basic defect; the term congenital beta-lipoprotein deficiency was employed. However, upon further study the deficiency of beta-lipoproteins appeared to be complete, and in an effort to distinguish those patients with complete absence of beta-lipoprotein from a group with hypobetalipoproteinemia, the term *abetalipoproteinemia* (ABL) was coined. Early reports suggested that ABL was more common in Ashkenazi Jews, but other ethnic groups are known to be affected.

Clinical features

The earliest manifestation of ABL is failure to grow and gain weight during the first year of life. Subsequent symptoms are diarrhea and steatorrhea. The steatorrhea may be either moderate or severe. Associated with the frequent loose, pale, and bulky stools are vomiting and abdominal distention. Usually by the fourth or fifth year of life the steatorrhea becomes less marked. Between the ages of 5 and 10 years atypical retinitis pigmentosa and neurological findings resembling Friedreich ataxia develop.

By adolescence most patients experience some decrease in visual acuity, visual field defects, night blindness, and pigmentary degeneration of the retina (including the macular region). Lenticular opacities, choriditis, opthalmoplegia, and ptosis also have been described.

The earliest neurological manifestation of this disorder is unsteadiness in walking, which may appear by the age of 2 years. Other clinical findings in order of frequence are areflexia, proprioceptive deficit, cerebellar signs of ataxia, titubation and dysarthria, muscle weakness, opthalmoparesis, Babinski sign, and cutaneous sensory loss. Athetoid movements occur in rare instances. Muscle weakness may involve the lower extremities as the disease progresses. Associated with the progressive neuromuscular dysfunction are kyphoscoliosis, lordosis, abdominal protrusion, and pes cavus deformity. Intellectually these patients are usually without impairment, although mental retardation has been reported in a few cases where the parents were consanguineous.

Other clinical findings include dyspnea, cardiomegaly, and cardiac arrhythmias (multifocal premature beats), and signs of congestive heart failure may develop during the course of the disease.

Diagnosis

This disorder should be considered in any child who presents with the following symptoms: severe malabsorption of fat, retinitis pigmentosa or macular degeneration, and unexplained neurological alterations simulating Fredreich ataxia. The most important laboratory screening test is the plasma cholesterol determination. If this value is subnormal (below 100 mg per 100 ml), the test should be followed by a triglyceride determination and lipoprotein electrophoresis. A definitive diagnosis is based on the immunochemical demonstration of the absence of low-density lipoproteins.

Other diagnostic aids include the detection of "burr-cell" malformation of the red cells (acanthocytes), which has been observed as early as 17 months of age and presumably continues throughout life. These acanthocytes do not form rouleaux and their sedimentation rate is low. Osmotic fragility is normal or slightly decreased, while mechanical fragility is increased.

A jejunal biopsy shows a pathognomonic mucosal abnormality (Figure 5.1). In contrast to the atrophic villi of celiac disease, the villi in this disorder are normal

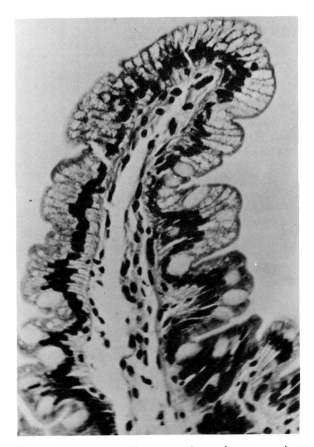

Figure 5.1. Jejunal biopsy specimen from a patient
showing foamy accumulation of clear material in the
epithelial cells near the villus tip. From M. A.
Weinstein, 1973, *Radiology* 108:269.

in shape, length, and thickness of the mucosa. The cytoplasm of the intestinal
epithelial cells appear foamy and vacuolated. There are no lipid droplets outside
the mucosal cells—i.e. there are none in the intracellular spaces, in the villous
cores, or in the lacteals.

Electron microscopic studies of the small bowel mucosa reveal normal microvilli,
mitochondria, endoplasmic reticulum, and lipid droplets throughout the epithelial
cells.

In one child with ABL and hepatomegaly, light microscopic studies of the liver
hepatocytes showed large fat droplets rupturing to form centrilobular fatty lakes.
Ultrastructurally, the Golgi were completely deficient in trans-Golgi vacuole formation. Endogenous triglyceride particles were not observed, and the circum-Golgi
smooth endoplasmic reticulum was absent.

More recently roentgenographic studies of the small bowel have shown thickening of the intestinal folds, most markedly in the duodenum and jejunum, but
throughout the entire ileum. The large bowel also showed thickening of the haustra
and abnormally prominent mucosal folds.

Basic defect

The basic defect in this disorder is not known; however, the alteration appears to be an inability to transport preformed triglyceride from the epithelial cells of the small intestinal mucosa and apparently also from the liver.

In 1971 Gotto and co-workers showed that both low-density lipoprotein and its principal protein component, apoLP-ser (referring to its carboxyl-terminal serine residue), were absent from a patient with ABL. However, the major protein constituents of the very low density lipoproteins other than apoLP-ser, as well as the two predominant proteins of high-density lipoproteins, are normally present in the plasma of abetalipoproteinemic patients. These investigators acknowledge that their results do not conclusively establish the exact nature of the defect, because the possibility remains that undetected apoLP-ser (either in modified or in incomplete form) is present in the plasma of these patients. Their finding suggests that apoLP-ser is necessary for the release of triglyceride from the small intestine and lymph into the plasma, which will result in the accumulation of triglyceride in the small intestinal mucosa and the delayed appearance of chylomicrons in the bloodstream, followed eventually by hypolipidemia. Since these patients are unable to form chylomicrons, it seems paradoxical that they excrete only a moderate amount of fat, rather than demonstrate a complete inability to absorb fat. It has been proposed that an alternate pathway is used to a greater extent than normal to transport long-chain fatty acids—unesterified and complexed with albumin—by way of the portal vein.

The cause of the acanthocytosis is unknown. It may occur in the absence of beta-lipoprotein deficiency. Likewise, our understanding of the neurological and retinal changes that occur is shrouded in ignorance, despite the various explanations that have been proposed.

Genetics

Originally this rare metabolic disorder was thought to affect mainly Ashkenazi Jews, but by 1972 a review of all 28 cases showed that only 29 percent of the patients were Jewish and of Ashkenazi origin. Presently, the number of reported cases is less than 45, with approximately 25 percent occurring in Ashkenazi Jews. In Israel, at least 3 cases have been reported from 3 different Jewish families. Of these, 1 family is Ashkenazi; the other 2 are of Oriental origin. No survey of ABL has been done in Israel.

The decrease in the proportion of Jews affected and in the occurrence of the disorder in non-Ashkenazi Jews raises many questions about the frequency of ABL among Jews which can be answered only by a well-designed genetic and epidemiological study.

ABL has been reported among many other populations, including several families of black African extraction and children whose parents were of French, Scottish, English, Dutch, and Italian backgrounds.

Analysis of the genetic data strongly supports autosomal recessive transmission of this disorder. Consanguinity is common in many of the affected families. Even among Ashkenazi Jews at least one-third of the patients have come from consanguineous matings, which suggests the extreme rarity of this mutant gene.

No abnormalities or partial defects have been observed in the heterozygous parents, although one report noted a reduction in the concentration of beta-lipoproteins in both parents and one grandparent of an affected child.

Prognosis and treatment

This is a progressively debilitating disease; death may occur in early childhood or as late as the age of 37 years. The ability to walk gradually declines and most patients are unable to stand by the age of 30 years. Cerebral findings are not considered to be relevant to this disorder, and sluggish responses are thought to be secondary to dysarthria rather than to intellectual impairment.

During the first few years of life the crucial problem is one of maintaining an adequate state of nutrition. As patients age, their tolerance to fat improves slightly. Efforts to improve fat absorption by the intravenous administration of human plasma or LDL have not been successful. This suggests that these individuals are not able to utilize exogenously administered apolipoprotein B to form chylomicrons.

Based on the observations that neurological lesions may be produced in animals with vitamin E deficiency, and that patients with ABL are markedly deficient in this vitamin, large amounts of vitamin E have been given as treatment for this disorder. No dramatic response has been noted, but it is thought that vitamin E may prevent some degree of deterioration.

ABL patients are also deficient in vitamin A, and administration of large doses of this vitamin may improve their night blindness, although it does not seem to affect the progression of their retinitis pigmentosa.

Musculoskeletal deformities present the most challenging problem to ABL patients as they grow older, and various means must be used to aid them in adapting to this severely deforming disease.

References

Bassen, F. A., and Kornzweig, A. L. 1950. Malformation of the erythrocytes in a case of atypical retinitis pigmentosa. *Blood* 5:381.
Berrebi, A., and Levene, C. 1976. Acanthocytes bearing the i antigen. *Vox Sang.* 30:396.
Brown, M. S.; Dana, S. E.; and Goldstein, J. L. 1975. Receptor-dependent hydrolysis of cholesteryl esters contained in plasma low density lipoprotein. *Proc. Natl. Acad. Sci. USA* 72:2925.
Dische, M. R., and Porro, R. S. 1970. The cardiac lesions in Bassen-Kornzweig syndrome: Report of a case, with autopsy findings. *Am. J. Med.* 49:568.
Farquar, J. W., and Ways, P. 1972. Abetalipoproteinemia. In *The metabolic basis of inherited disease,* ed. J. B. Stanbury, J. B. Wyngaarden, and D. S. Fredrickson, 3rd ed. New York: McGraw-Hill.
Greenwood, N. 1976. The jejunal mucosa in two cases of abetalipoproteinemia. *Am. J. Gastroenterol.* 65:160.
Isselbacher, K. J.; Scheig, R.; Plotkin, G. R.; and Caulfield, J. B. 1964. Congenital beta-lipoprotein deficiency: An hereditary disorder involving a defect in the absorption and transport of lipids. *Medicine* 43:347.
Jampel, R. S., and Falls, H. F. 1958. Atypical retinitis pigmentosa, acanthrocytosis, and heredodegenerative neuromuscular disease. *Arch. Ophthalmol.* 59:818.
Kahlke, W. 1967. A-β-lipoproteinemia. In *Lipids and lipidoses,* ed. G. Schettler, p. 382. New York: Springer-Verlag.
Kayden, H. J. 1972. Abetalipoproteinemia. *Ann. Rev. Med.* 23:285.

Kornzweig, A. L. 1970. Bassen-Kornzweig syndrome: Present status. *J. Med. Genet.* 7:271.

Lees, R. S. 1967. Immunological evidence for the presence of β protein (apoprotein of β-lipoprotein) in normal and a-beta-lipoproteinemic plasma. *J. Lipid Res.* 8:396.

Lees, R. S., et al. 1973. The familial dyslipoproteinemias. *Prog. Med. Genet.* 9:237.

McBride, J. A., and Jacobs, H. S. 1970. Abnormal kinetics of red cell membrane cholesterol in acanthocytes: Studies in genetic and experimental abetalipoproteinemia and in spur cell anemia. *Br. J. Haematol.* 18:383.

Mars, H.; Lewis, L. A.; Robertson, A. L.; Butkus, A.; and Williams, G. H., Jr. 1969. Familial hypo-β-lipoproteinemia: A genetic disorder of lipid metabolism with nervous system involvement. *Am. J. Med.* 46:886.

Ockner, R. K. 1971. Abetalipoproteinemia: Rarity and relevance. *N. Engl. J. Med.* 284:848.

Partin, J. S.; Partin, J. C.; Schubert, W. K.; and McAdams, J. 1974. Liver ultrastructure in abetalipoproteinemia: Evolution of micronodular cirrhosis. *Gastroenterology* 67:107.

Salt, H. B.; Wolff, O. H.; Lloyd, J. K.; Fosbrooke, A. S.; Cameron, A. H.; and Hubble, D. V. 1960. On having no beta-lipoprotein: A syndrome comprising a-beta-lipoproteinemia, acanthocytosis, and steatorrhoea. *Lancet* 2:325.

Schwartz, J. F.; Rowland, L. P.; Eden, H.; Marks, P. A.; Osserman, E. F.; Hirschberg, E.; and Anderson, H. 1963. Bassen-Kornzweig syndrome: Deficiency of serum β-lipoprotein. *Arch. Neurol.* 8:438.

Sobrevilla, L. A.; Goodman, M. L.; and Kane, C. A. 1964. Demyelinating central nervous system disease, macular atrophy, and acanthocytosis (Bassen-Kornzweig syndrome). *Am. J. Med.* 37:821.

Sperling, M. A.; Hengstenberg, F.; Yunis, E.; et al. 1971. Abetalipoproteinemia: Metabolic, endocrine, and electron-microscopic investigations. *Pediatrics* 48:91.

Weinstein, M. A.; Pearson, K. D.; and Agus, S. G. 1973. Abetalipoproteinemia. *Radiology* 108:269.

Yee, R. D., et al. 1976. Ophthalmoplegia and dissociated nystagmus in abetalipoproteinemia. *Arch. Ophthalmol.* 94:571.

BLOOM SYNDROME

Historical note

Bloom first reported on this syndrome in 1954, although he saw his first case in 1941. He termed the disorder "congenital telangiectatic erythema resembling lupus erythematosus in dwarfs." In 1963 Szalay presented evidence for a genetic etiology in this disorder. In 1966 German and co-workers described chromosomal breakage in patients with Bloom syndrome and noted that they have a predisposition for neoplasia. The first review article on the disease was published in 1969 by German, who by that time had determined from data on 27 cases that the disorder occurs most frequently among Ashkenazi Jews. German has since become the leading authority on this syndrome, and in 1977 he and his colleagues published their findings from a survey conducted in Israel.

Clinical features

The characteristic clinical features in this syndrome are growth retardation, sun-sensitive telangiectatic eruptions on the face, disturbance of the immune function, and a predisposition to cancer. Full-term infants tend to have a low birth weight (males average 2,094 g and females 1,841 g). During childhood these patients

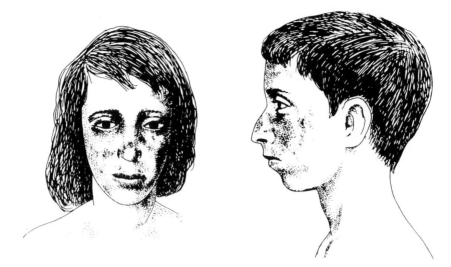

Figure 5.2. Composite drawings from several photographs of children with Bloom syndrome. Note the small, narrow face, dolicocephalic head, and skin lesions about the nose, lips, and malar area of the face. Courtesy of J. German, New York.

may present with dwarfism, although by the late teens sufficient growth has usually taken place and they are not true dwarfs. Adult height rarely exceeds 145 cm. The body proportions are normal and the patients appear delicate and slender. They show a striking resemblance to one another due to their small, narrow faces, dolichocephalic heads, facial skin lesions, and dwarfism. Figure 5.2 shows composite drawings from several photographs of children with Bloom syndrome depicting the typical head configuration and facies. A high-pitched voice has been noted in several male and female patients.

Although the skin is normal at birth, late in infancy or early in childhood telangiectatic erythema lesions begin to develop about the nose, lips, and malar area of the face. In approximately half the patients these lesions also involve the forearms, dorsa of the hands, back of the neck, and ears. Exposure to sunlight exacerbates the skin lesions. The erythema tends to fade after puberty, followed by scarring, atrophy, and depigmentation. More than half of the patients also have café-au-lait spots.

A recent observation indicates that some older patients may have reduced muscle strength accompanied by ultrastructural changes in skeletal muscle.

Sexual development is normal in both sexes with the exception that the testes of some affected men are disproportionately small. Azoospermia has been demonstrated in a few cases. In affected females menstrual periods are often irregular and infrequent.

Diagnosis

By childhood the clinical features of this disorder are usually characteristic and this, combined with chromosomal studies and the demonstration of diminished immunoglobulins, allows for a relatively easy diagnosis.

Regarding the specific chromosomal changes in this disorder, German states that the most characteristic aberration is a quadriradial configuration (Qr) present in 0.5–14.0 percent of all dividing PHA-stimulated lymphocytes (Figure 5.3). In addition to an increase in the number of chromatid gaps, breaks, and interchanges, German has noted the tendency for exchanges to occur between chromatids of homologous chromosomes at homologous sites. In 1974 his group reported an abnormal increase in the number of sister-chromatid exchanges (SCEs) in PHA-stimulated blood lymphocytes from patients with Bloom syndrome (Figure 5.4). In 1977 this same group observed that some patients with Bloom syndrome do not exhibit the increase in the number of SCEs that was previously thought to be characteristic of all patients with this disorder. The reason for and significance of these two different cytological responses in this disease are not understood at this time.

In 1977 Ahmad and co-workers studied two brothers with this disorder and noted that in one the growth hormone response to hypoglycemia was absent while in the other the levels of serum thyroid-stimulating hormone and serum follicle-stimulating and -luteinizing hormones were high. The significance of these observations must await further documentation in other patients.

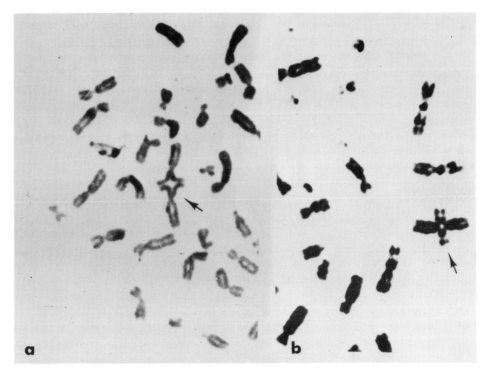

Figure 5.3. Chromosomes from two dividing lymphocytes showing quadriradial configurations (Qr's) of the type characteristic of Bloom syndrome. (a) The homologues of pair no. 1 (arrow) have undergone chromatid exchange at the same, or approximately the same, points near the middle of the long arm. Orcein stain. (b) The nos. 6 (arrow) have undergone exchange near or at the centromeric regions. Giemsa stain for G-bands. Courtesy of J. German, New York.

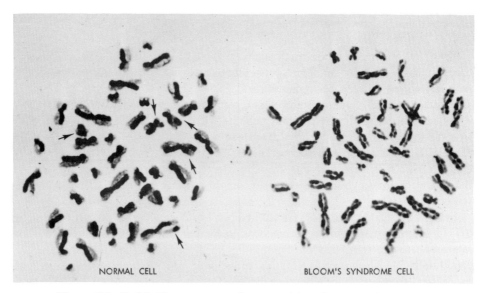

NORMAL CELL   BLOOM'S SYNDROME CELL

Figure 5.4. (Left) Chromosomes of a normal lymphocyte at the second metaphase after growth in bromodeoxyuridine, fluorodeoxyuridine, and uridine, stained first with 33258 Hoechst and a day later with Giemsa. Arrows indicate points of exchange between sister chromatids (SCE). (Right) Chromosomes of a cultured Bloom syndrome lymphocyte showing many more SCEs than normal. Courtesy of J. German, New York.

Since affected infants are small for birth, prenatal detection through the use of ultrasound may be of value in determining fetal size. Amniocentesis has been done in a few pregnancies known to be at risk for this disorder (using the previously mentioned chromosomal changes as a diagnostic aid), but no case has as yet been diagnosed *in utero*.

Basic defect

The biochemical alteration in this syndrome is unknown. Attempts to find an enzymatic defect involving the repair mechanism of DNA using ultraviolet light have been unproductive. In 1975 Hand and German observed a retarded rate of DNA chain growth in this syndrome. To explain this finding they suggested two possibilities: (a) a defective enzyme is concerned directly with semiconservative DNA replication; or (b) a defective enzyme is not directly concerned with replication but results in disturbed cellular metabolism, which in turn affects replication.

German's recent finding that some patients with Bloom syndrome have the normal number of SCEs in some of their cells indicates that the basic defect may be regulatory in nature and by some unknown mechanism results in the observed dimorphism.

Genetics

The formal genetic analysis of Bloom syndrome shows that this disorder is transmitted as an autosomal recessive condition. At the end of 1976, 71 patients with this syndrome had been recognized. Of these, 32 were Jewish.

During 1971 and 1972 German conducted a survey of all cases of this syndrome in Israel and found 8 affected individuals. One of the 8 had had an affected sib who died before the family's immigration to Israel. All the Israeli patients were of Ashkenazi Jewish descent. Most affected Jewish families in both Israel and the United States can trace their origins to the area of Eastern Europe lying between Warsaw and Crakow on the east and Kiev and Chernovtsy on the west—i.e. southeastern Poland (Galacia) and the southwestern Ukraine.

The gene frequency of this disorder among Ashkenazi Jews is estimated to be 0.0042 (minimum), implying a heterozygote frequency of greater than 1 in 120. There is no doubt that this gene is much more common in the Ashkenazi Jewish community than in any other ethnic group. The actual observed incidence of this syndrome among Ashkenazi Jews in Israel during 1971–1972 was 1 in 161,000.

Parental consanguinity was not present in any of the affected families from Israel and, in general, it has been low in all the Jewish families examined by German (Table 5.1). In the non-Jewish affected families the rate of parental consanguinity was high (Table 5.1), indicating that the expression of this gene in this population must be rare in contrast to its relatively common occurrence among the Ashkenazi Jewish population.

In German's study the sex ratio among all persons with Bloom syndrome appears to be distorted—41 males to 30 females (Table 5.2). The deficit in females is particularly striking among the cases seen in Israel, where 8 of the 9 patients were male. A possible explanation for the relatively low incidence in females is the disproportionately high death rate among females during fetal and early postnatal life. Affected Jewish females might be less viable because they have a lower mean birth weight: 1,740 g compared to 1,916 g for males. Underdiagnosis is another possible explanation for the low incidence of this syndrome among females. Because skin lesions are usually less severe in females than in the males, females may not consult a dermatologist as readily as males.

Table 5.1. Parental consanguinity in known cases of Bloom syndrome

Group	No. of sibships	Parental consanguinity	
		Yes	No
Jews in Israel, 1971–1972	8	0	8
Jews outside Israel	19	1	18
All Jews	27	1	26
Non-Jews	32	14	18
Jews and Non-Jews	59	15	44

Source: J. German et al., 1977, *Am. J. Hum. Genet.* 29:553. © 1977 by the American Society of Human Genetics. Reprinted by permission of The University of Chicago Press.

Note: The figures in this table are based on published and unpublished data.

Table 5.2. Sex ratio in Bloom syndrome

Group	No.	Male	Female	Ratio M/F
Jews in Israel, 1971–1972	9[a]	8	1	8.0
Jews outside Israel	23	11	12	0.9
All Jews	32	19	13	1.5
Non-Jews	39	22	17	1.3
Jews and non-Jews	71	41	30	1.4

Source: J. German et al., 1977, *Am. J. Hum. Genet.* 29:553. © 1977 by the American Society of Human Genetics. Reprinted by permission of The University of Chicago Press.

[a] Includes a male child who died in Europe before the family moved to Israel with his affected sister.

It is not possible to detect the heterozygous state, and parents of these affected individuals appear normal in size, intelligence, and health. Whether or not the heterozygous individual is more susceptible to neoplasia is not known at this time.

There is no evidence at present to suggest that the course of this disorder in non-Jews is any different from that in Jews.

Prognosis and treatment

Intelligence appears to be normal in most Bloom syndrome patients. The fact that married male patients have not had children raises the question of possible sterility in the males. More studies are needed to assess the fertility of female patients.

The crucial problem in this syndrome is the propensity these patients have to develop cancer. Thirteen cancers have already been diagnosed in 12 of the 71 affected individuals, and 10 of the 12 have died from the cancers. The types of neoplasia include acute leukemia (type not specified), reticulum cell sarcoma, sqamous cell carcinoma of the tongue, and various neoplastic lesions involving the gastrointestinal tract. Some patients have died from infection during infancy.

Individuals with this disorder have a shortened life span; the mean age of the present group of living patients is 16.4 years. Each of the 4 individuals who have reached the age of 30 developed at least one cancer between the ages of 30 and 40. Early cancer detection is of prime importance in this disease, as is proper treatment of all infections during infancy and childhood. Patients should avoid exposure to sunlight, and wearing a hat and using various protective creams tends to reduce the severity of the facial lesions. Bloom syndrome patients often have psychological problems stemming from their physical appearance, and psychiatric help may be indicated.

References

Ahmad, U.; Fisher, E. R.; Danowski, T. S.; Nolan, S.; and Stephan, T. 1977. Endocrine abnormalities and myopathy in Bloom's syndrome. *J. Med. Genet.* 14:418.

Bloom, D. 1954. Congenital telangiectatic erythema resembling lupus erythematosus in dwarfs. *Am. J. Dis. Child.* 88:754.

———. 1966. The syndromes of congenital telangiectatic erythema and stunted growth: Observations and studies. *J. Pediatr.* 68:103.

Chaganti, R. S. K.; Schonberg, S.; and German, J. 1974. A manyfold increase in sister chromatid exchanges in Bloom's syndrome lymphocytes. *Proc. Natl. Acad. Sci. USA* 71:4508.

German, J. 1969. Bloom's syndrome. I: Genetical and clinical observations in the first twenty-seven patients. *Am. J. Hum. Genet.* 21:196.

———. 1974. Bloom's syndrome. II: The prototype of human genetic disorders predisposing to chromosome instability and cancer. In *Chromosomes and cancer,* ed. J. German, pp. 601–17. New York: John Wiley.

German, J.; Bloom, D.; Passarge, E.; Fried, K.; Goodman, R. M.; Katznellenbogen, I.; Laron, Z.; Legum, C.; Levin, S.; and Wahrman, J. 1977. Bloom's syndrome. VI: The disorder in Israel, and an estimation of the gene frequency in the Ashkenazim. *Am. J. Hum. Genet.* 29:553.

German, J.; Crippa, P.; and Bloom, D. 1974. Bloom's syndrome. III: Analysis of the chromosome aberration characteristic of this disorder. *Chromosoma* 48:361.

German, J.; Schonberg, S.; Louie, E.; and Chaganti, R. S. K. 1977. Bloom's syndrome. IV: Sister-chromatid exchanges in lymphocytes. *Am. J. Hum. Genet.* 29:248.

Hand, R., and German, J. 1975. A retarded rate of DNA chain growth in Bloom's syndrome. *Proc. Natl. Acad. Sci. USA* 72:758.

Sawitsky, A.; Bloom, D.; and German, J. 1966. Chromosomal breakage and acute leukemia in congenital telangiectatic erythema and stunted growth. *Ann. Intern. Med.* 65:487.

Szalay. G. C. 1963. Dwarfism with skin manifestations. *J. Pediatr.* 62:683.

FAMILIAL DYSAUTONOMIA
(RILEY-DAY SYNDROME)

Historical note

Although Riley, Day, Greeley, and Langford are credited with first describing this disorder in 1949, the first actual case report was that of Aring and Engel in 1945. In 1964 and 1965 Smith and Dancis described additional clinical features, noting unusual responses of the autonomic nervous system and observing abnormalities in the urinary excretion of catecholamine metabolites in these patients. It was early recognized that this disorder affects primarily Ashkenazi Jews, and in 1967 McKusick and co-workers conducted a survey in the U.S. which documented 200 cases in 164 families. All families were of Ashkenazi Jewish ancestry except two, in which the mothers were not Jewish. In 1967 Moses and co-workers presented a detailed report on 23 Israeli patients with this disorder. All were of Ashkenazi Jewish descent. In 1970 Brunt and McKusick published a detailed account of 210 patients in 172 families, the largest series reported to date. In 1971 Goodall and co-workers demonstrated a decrease in synthesis of noradrenaline in these patients. In conjunction with this observation Weinshilboum and Axelrod independently detected decreased activity of beta-hydroxylase (BDH), the enzyme that converts dopamine to norepinephrine. A more recent finding is a two- to threefold elevation of the beta fraction of nerve growth factor (NGE) in familial dysautonomia patients.

Clinical features

Familial dysautonomia usually manifests itself during infancy and is marked by feeding problems due to dysphagia, recurrent bouts of pneumonia, indifference to pain, absence of or masked diminution in tearing, and hypotonia. Growth retardation is usually evident by early childhood. As affected children begin to develop, a number of abnormal symptoms and findings reflecting abnormalities in the autonomic, sensory, and central nervous systems become apparent. Such symptoms include the following: absence of reduction in tearing, hypoactive corneal reflex, dysarthria, hypersalivation, excessive perspiration, erratic temperature control, cyclic vomiting, difficulty in swallowing, vasomotor instability as manifested by labile blood pressure, postural hypotension, hypertension with excitement, skin blotching with excitement or eating, emotional lability, cold hands and feet, diarrhea and constipation, absence or hypoactivity of deep-tendon reflexes, ataxia, poor motor coordination, convulsions, and a relative indifference to pain.

A pathognomonic feature of familial dysautonomia is the complete absence of the fungiform papillae and taste buds on the tongue (Figure 5.5). The circumvallate papillae also have been noted to be hypoplastic or absent in some patients. Most patients show a marked resemblance in facial expression, which has been described as sad, empty, and frightened. They also tend to have a thin face and transverse mouth and to grimace. Often facial asymmetry and hypertelorism are manifested. Patients may appear pale or have a grayish complexion. Kyphoscoliosis is a common finding as these children begin to develop.

Table 5.3 shows the frequency of clinical features noted in 210 patients with this disorder by Brunt and McKusick.

Several other clinical findings should be mentioned. For example, the speech of these patients is often monotonous, slurred, and dysarthric, with a peculiar nasal quality. Multiple ocular findings are frequently observed in addition to alacrima or hypolacrima. Corneal hypesthesia, exodeviation, and methacholine-induced miosis may be noted. Seventy-seven percent of McKusick's patients were myopic, but this may be an unrelated finding (see section on myopia). Several patients had anisometropia, a few had anisocoria, while pronounced retinal vascular tortuosity was a common finding. A number of gastrointestinal phenomena have been reported in this disease, including disturbed esophageal motility, megaesophagus,

Table 5.3. Familial dysautonomia: Frequency of
clinical features in 210 patients

Feature	%
Absence of fungiform papillae	100[a]
Absence of overflow tears	100
Vasomotor disturbance (blotching)	98
Abnormal sweating	97
Episodic fever	92
Incoordination and unsteadiness	90
Swallowing difficulty in infancy	85
Physical retardation	78
Episodic vomiting	67
Breath-holding attacks	66
Marked emotional instability	65
Scoliosis	55[a]
Bowel disturbance	49

Source: P. W. Brunt and V. A. McKusick, 1970,
Medicine 49:343. © 1970 The Williams & Wilkins Co.,
Baltimore.
[a] Percentage of those examined for this defect.

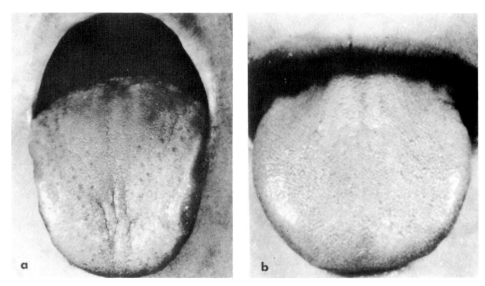

Figure 5.5. (a) Normal tongue with fungiform papillae. (a) Tongue without these papillae in a patient with familial dysautonomia.

pylorospasm, gastric ulcer, jejunal distention, and megacolon. In terms of oral pathology, malocclusion and crowding of teeth associated with comparatively small maxillary and mandibular areas have been noted frequently. Because of reduced taste sensibility and the lack of craving for sweets, these patients have few caries. Nevertheless, periodontal disease and oral ulcerations are common findings which can probably be attributed to poor oral hygiene and diminished sensation. Salivation is thought to be excessive in these patients.

It is a myth that familial dysautonomia patients are impaired intellectually. They may appear to have lower IQs, but this is usually a reflection of their behavior and an anticipation by others of below-normal achievement. It has been observed that these individuals have difficulty in maturing; many do not fully enter the adolescent world, let alone that of the adult. It has been suggested that if these children were less sheltered and given more exposure to the outside world, they would mature more easily.

Diagnosis

Early diagnosis of familial dysautonomia is becoming more common now that the neonatal manifestations of the disease are known, and cases have been detected as early as six weeks and even 24 hours after birth. This disease should be considered in any Ashkenazi Jewish infant who has feeding problems due to dysphagia and shows an indifference to pain and the absence of or diminution in tearing. The most striking feature of this disorder is the absence of fungiform papillae. In 1,275 control tongues seen in dental reviews, complete absence of fungiform papillae was never noted, but only one report of visible fungiform papillae in a probable case of familial dysautonomia exists.

In 1975 Grünebaum described the roentgenographic finding of what he termed the "chest-abdomen sign" in 6 patients with familial dysautonomia who had aspiration pneumonitis. In addition to the roentgenographic pattern of aspiration pneumonia, he observed distended intestinal loops. This distention was not accompanied by acute clinical symptoms and was not related to the respiratory distress or to periodic episodes of vomiting. In all 6 cases the lung and intestinal findings were evident on chest films that included the upper abdomen. Such a combination of findings in an undiagnosed patient may be an important clue in making the correct diagnosis and have been noted as early as the first few days of life.

A number of functional abnormalities have been described in these patients and may be useful in making a diagnosis. They include: (a) diffuse pain and absence of a red flare after an intradermal injection of histamine; (b) hyperreactivity to administered methacholine; (c) inappropriate or prolonged hypoglycemic response to insulin; (d) pressor hyperreactivity to administered norepinephrine; (e) absence of cardiovascular autonomic reflexes; (f) reduced respiratory sensitivity to experimentally induced hypercapnia and hypoxia; (g) decreased vanillylmandelic acid excretion in the urine; (h) decreased dopamine-beta- hydroxylase activity; (i) abnormal release of renin with high plasma renin activity. The histamine and methacholine tests are relatively simple to administer and are exceedingly dependable diagnostically.

HISTAMINE TEST

In the normal individual the intradermal injection of histamine phosphate 1:1,000 produces intense pain and erythema followed within minutes by the development of a central wheal surrounded by the axon flare, a zone of erythema 1–3 cm in radius, which is maintained for over 10 minutes. In the patient with familial dysautonomia the pain is markedly reduced and there is no axon flare. Since the infant's skin reacts more intensely to intradermal histamine, a dilution of 1:10,000 may provide a more clearly defined difference between the normal and the dysautonomic reaction. No false negative results have been observed, and the only false positive response requiring serious consideration occurs in congenital sensory neuropathy.

METHACHOLINE (MECHOLYL) TEST

The instillation of 2.5 percent methacholine into the conjunctival sac produces miosis in almost all patients with familial dysautonomia but has no observable effect on the normal pupil. This is a sign of parasympathetic denervation and will occur in any condition involving such denervation. Both pupils are carefully examined for symmetry under proper lighting after which a drop of methacholine is applied locally to one eye while the other eye serves as a control. The pupils are compared at 5-minute intervals for 20 minutes.

In 1976 Ziegler and co-workers demonstrated that patients with familial dysautonomia have no norepinephrine response to standing or exercise, while normal individuals show a consistent increase in plasma levels of norepinephrein after such activities. This observation supports the view that hypertension and hypotension in familial dysautonomia are related to the rate of norepinephrine release.

Another observation that may have diagnostic significance stems from recent studies on nerve growth factor in this disease. Siggers and co-workers have reported a two- to threefold increase ($p < 0.001$) in serum antigen levels of the biologically active subunit beta-NGF in patients with familial dysautonomia compared with normal subjects. By all other assays the groups were alike. This marked discrepancy in beta-NGF levels between antigenic and functional (biological and binding) measurements suggests a qualitative abnormality of beta-NGF in this disease.

Basic defect

The basic defect in familial dysautonomia is not known. Post-mortem studies have shown no consistent pathological changes in the central nervous system. While some investigators have commented on degenerative changes in reticular formation and others have noted demyelination in the dorsal columns and dorsal nerve roots, a third group has wholly exonerated the central nervous system. Recent neuropathological studies by the group at the New York University Medical Center have shown rather specific findings, such as a decrease in unmyelinated fibers from the sural nerve and a reduction of cells in autonomic and sensory ganglia. These observations are consistent with a previously held hypothesis that the primary defect may involve developmental arrest due to an insufficiency or alteration in some factor that controls differentiation, e.g. NGF.

However, the role of NGF in familial dysautonomis is far from clear. Levi-Montalcini, the leading authority on NGF, has pointed out that it is not known whether the discrepancies in NGF radioimmunoassays and other assays noted in familial dysautonomia are distinct features of the disease or may be due to the fluctuations in cross-reacting material to beta-NGF which normally occur in healthy people as well as in patients with dysautonomia and other disorders. Furthermore, she suggests that since familial dysautonomia involves a marked deficiency in sympathetic function, one would expect a decrease rather than a normal level or an increase in the binding of beta-NGF.

Genetics

Although a few cases of this disease have been well documented in non-Jews, the vast majority of cases (99 percent) occur in children of Ashkenazi Jewish descent. Family studies strongly support autosomal recessive inheritance of this disorder.

The largest reported series of patients—that of Brunt and McKusick—consists of 210 affected children from 172 families. The sex difference (97 males and 113 females) is not significant, but the ethnic distribution of these cases is striking. Of the 344 parents only 1 (a mother) was not Jewish or did not have Jewish ancesters; all the others were of Ashkenazi background. Brunt and McKusick compared the geographical origins of these families with the data compiled by Aronson and Myrianthopoulos on families with Tay-Sachs disease and with a limited "control" group representing a number of urban and suburban synagogues in the U.S. As seen in Table 5.4, the differences in area of origin were significant. In particular, familial dysautonomia was most prevalent among families from Galica, Bukovina, the Ukraine (around Kiev), Romania, and areas of Austro-Hungary. When the three groups were analyzed from the viewpoint of Yiddish linguistic variations, the differences were even more striking, with the families of familial dysautonomia patients coming predominatly from southeastern Central Europe (Romania, the Ukraine, etc.).

Table 5.4. Comparison of cases of Tay-Sachs disease (TSD) and familial dysautonomia (FD) with a "control group by country or area of origin"

Country or area of origin	Control No.	%	TSD No.	%	FD No.	%
Latvia, Lithuania	113	4.3	83	9.9	41	6.6
Grodna, Vilna, Suwalki, Lumza	182	7.0	90	10.8	42	6.8
Byelorussia	190	7.3	68	8.1	41	6.6
Central Poland	143⎫		69⎫		53⎫	
Western Poland	49⎭	7.4	13⎭	9.8	7⎭	9.7
Poland (area not stated)	74	2.8	71	8.5	22	3.6
Gracow, Galicia, Bucowina	151	5.8	66	7.9	82	13.3
The Ukraine	258	9.9	79	9.5	99	16.0
Russia (other areas)	22	0.8	9	1.1	4	0.6
Russia (area not stated)	317	12.2	101	12.1	61	9.9
Romania, Moldavia	127	4.9	37	4.4	47	7.6
Austria	91⎫		22⎫		19⎫	
Hungary	110⎭	7.7	27⎭	5.9	48⎭	10.9
Germany	155	5.9	23	2.8	18	2.9
Other European areas	102	3.9	41	4.9	17	2.8
North America	523	20.1	36	4.3	16	2.6
Total	2,607		835		617	

Source: P. W. Brunt and V. A. McKusick, 1970, *Medicine* 49:343. © 1970 The Williams & Wilkins Co., Baltimore.

Note: In Cracow, Galicia, Bucowina, the Ukraine, Romania, Moldavia, Austria, and Hungary the FD figures differ from those of both the control group and the TSD group. The composite $\chi^2 = 387.8$ ($p < 0.001$). Excluding ancestors from the U.S., the $\chi^2 = 165.2$ ($p < 0.001$).

Nine families in the Brunt-McKusick series showed close consanguinity. Thus, the rate of marriage of close relatives for the series was 5.3 percent (2.9 percent for first-cousin marriages).

Based on the calculations of Brunt and McKusick, the frequency of familial dysautonomia in North American Jews is between 1:10,000 and 1:20,000 live births, which yields a gene frequency of 0.01 at the highest.

In 1967 Moses and co-workers published extensive studies on 23 Israeli patients with this disease, although their genetic calculations are based on 30 cases diagnosed as of 1965. They estimated the incidence of the disease in Israel to be 8.3 per 100,000 Ashkenazi Jews, which gives a gene frequency of 0.0091 and a carrier frequency of 18 per 1,000 or 1:55. All cases were Ashkenazi Jews, despite the fact that in Israel the Sephardi and Oriental communities comprise over 50 percent of the Jewish population.

At present it is not possible to detect the heterozygote accurately either clinically or biochemically, even though some investigators have reported lower than normal levels of VMA in the urine of known carriers while others have found a decrease in DBH activity in the mothers of affected patients. Likewise, prenatal diagnosis is not possible at this time.

Prognosis and treatment

Death during infancy and childhood is usually due to aspiration or bronchopneumonia. With improved care, patients are now living longer. The main area of improvement has been in respiratory care. Postural drainage and suctioning of excessive mucous have given patients a better appetite by relieving the nausea associated with the presence of mucous. Such respiratory care has also decreased the episodes of acute and chronic respiratory infections experienced by these patients.

Thought must also be given to the other problems of familial dysautonomia patients: corneal ulceration, vasomotor instability, vomiting, and excessive perspiration. Early institution of a Milwaukee brace and orthopedic surgery (spinal fusion) should be considered for treatment of their kyphoscoliosis. Attention must be given to older patients, who may develop Charcot neuropathic joints with severe involvement of the knees and milder alterations in the shoulders and elbows.

Some individuals have married and have had normal children. It is crucial that these patients be helped with their emotional problems and given job training.

References

Aguayo, A. J.; Martin, J. B.; and Bray, G. M. 1972. Effects of nerve growth factor antiserum on peripheral unmyelinated nerve fibers. *Acta Neuropathol.* 20:288.
Aguayo, A. J.; Nair, C. P. V.; and Bray, G. M. 1971. Peripheral nerve abnormalities in the Riley-Day syndrome: Findings in a sural nerve biopsy. *Arch. Neurol.* 24:106.
Aring, C. D., and Engel, G. L. 1945. Hypothalamic attacks with thalamic lesions. 2: Anatomic considerations. *Arch. Neurol. Psychiatr.* 54:37.
Axelrod, F. B., and Moloshok, R. E. 1975. Familial dysautonomia. In *Current pediatric therapy,* ed. S. C. Gellis and B. M. Kagan, pp. 96–97. Philadelphia: W. B. Saunders.
Axelrod, F. B.; Nachtigal, R.; and Dancis, J. 1974. Familial dysautonomia: Diagnosis, pathogenesis, and management. *Adv. Pediatr.* 21:75.
Brunt, P. W., and McKusick, V. A. 1970. Familial dysautonomia: A report of genetic and clinical studies, with a review of the literature. *Medicine* 49:343.
Grünebaum, M. 1975. The "chest-abdomen" sign in familial dysautonomia. *Br. J. Radiol.* 48:23.
Hochberg, Z.; Kahana, L.; Spindel, A.; and Diengott, D. 1976. Plasma renin activity in familial dysautonomia: Unresponsiveness to a beta-adrenergic blocker. *Pediatrics* 58:618.
Levi-Montalcini, R. 1976. Nerve-growth factor in familial dysautonomia. *N. Engl. J. Med.* 295:671.
Levine, S. L., et al. 1977. Familial dysautonomia: Unusual presentation in an infant of non-Jewish ancestry. *J. Pediatr.* 90:79.
Moses, S. W.; Rotem, Y.; Jogoda, N.; Talmor, N.; Eichhorn, F.; and Levin, S. 1967. A clinical, genetic, and biochemical study of familial dysautonomia in Israel. *Israel J. Med. Sci.* 3:358.
Pearson, J.; Axelrod, F. B.; and Dancis, J. 1974. Current concepts of dysautonomia: Neuropathological defects. *Ann. N.Y. Acad. Sci.* 228:288.
Rabinowitz, D.; Landau, H.; Rösler, A.; et al. 1974. Plasma renin activity and aldosteron in familial dysautonomia. *Metabolism* 23:1.
Riley, C. M.; Day, R. L.; Greeley, D. McL.; and Langford, W. S. 1949. Central autonomic dysfunction with defective lacrimation: Report of five cases. *Pediatrics* 3:468.
Rogers, J. G.; Siggers, D. C.; Boyer, S. H.; et al. 1975. Serum nerve growth factor levels in familial dysautonomia. *Pediatr. Res.* 9:384.
Rubenstein, A. E., et al. 1977. Adult onset autonomic dysfunction co-existent with familial dysautonomia in a consanguineous family. *Neurology* 27:168.
Siggers, D. C.; Rogers, J. G.; Boyer, S. H.; Margolet, L.; Dorkin, H.; Banerjee, S. P.;

and Shooter, E. M. Increased nerve-growth-factor beta-chain cross-reacting material in familial dysautonomia. *N. Engl. J. Med.* 295:629.

Smith, A. A., and Dancis, J. 1964. Exaggerated response to infused nor-epinephrine in familial dysautonomia. *N. Engl. J. Med.* 270:704.

————. 1964. Peripheral sensory deficits in familial dysautonomia. *J. Pediatr.* 65:1035.

————. 1964. Taste discrimination in familial dysautonomia. *Pediatrics* 33:441.

————. 1967. Cathecholamine release in familial dysautonomia. *N. Engl. J. Med.* 277:61.

Smith, A. A.; Farbman, A.; and Dancis, J. 1965. Tongue in familial dysautonomia: A diagnostic sign. *Am. J. Dis. Child.* 110:152.

Smith, A. A.; Hirsch, J. I.; and Dancis, J. 1965. Responses to infused methacholine in familial dysautonomia. *Science* 147:1040.

Weinshilboum, R. M.; Raymond, F. A.; and Elveback, L. R. 1973. Serum dopamine-β-hydroxylase activity: Sibling-sibling correlation. *Science* 181:943.

Ziegler, M.; Lake, R.; and Kopin, I. J. 1976. Deficient sympathetic nervous response in familial dysautonomia. *N. Engl. J. Med.* 294:630.

GAUCHER DISEASE TYPE I
(CHRONIC ADULT NONCEREBRAL FORM)

Historical note

In 1882 Gaucher first reported a patient with the clinical features of hepatosplenomegaly and bone involvement that are characteristic of the type I form of this disorder. Multiple theories were put forth regarding the nature of these peculiar large cells involving the reticuloendothelial system. In 1924 Lieb isolated from the spleens of Gaucher patients large amounts of cerebrosides (enzymes found in the brain 50 years before and thus so named). In 1934 Aghion determined that glucocerebroside, not galactocerebroside, is the compound that accumulates in this disorder. In 1965 Brady and co-workers demonstrated the deficiency of beta-glucosidase (glucocerebrosidase) activity in fibroblasts from homozygotes with the adult form of the disease and found an intermediate level of enzyme activity in a heterozygote. In 1974 Brady's group reported encouraging findings on the treatment of this disease using intravenous infusion of purified placental glucocerebrosidase.

Clinical features

The chronic adult noncerebral form of the disease may manifest itself at any age, but symptoms usually appear during the late teens or early in adulthood. Cases have been reported in infants, however, and at least one patient was an octogenarian before the diagnosis was made. The earlier the onset, usually the more severe the clinical course. The spleen, liver, and bone are the main areas of involvement in this form, and the symptoms usually correspond to the degree of pathology present. Splenomegaly is usually the earliest finding and with very few exceptions is always present. Although pain is not a common complaint, the splenomegaly does give the patient a feeling of discomfort. Thrombocytopenia, leukopenia, and mild microcytic anemia are common findings. Splenic enlargement, coupled with hypersplenism and epistaxis, purpura, and various bleeding episodes, eventually leads to a splenectomy in more than half the patients with this disorder.

Hepatomegaly and symptoms of portal hypertension, including the presence of ascites, occur in many patients. Jaundice is not a feature of Gaucher disease.

Although the kidney is occasionally involved, renal function usually is not disturbed.

Bone symptoms, mainly bone pain and fractures, may occur later in the course of the disease. The most common site of pathological fractures is the hip, particularly the region of the acetabulum and the head and neck of the femur. Other portions of the pelvis, as well as the long bones, phalanges, and ribs, also are frequently involved. Skull and mandibular lesions tend to be less common. Vertebral destruction sometimes produces complete spinal fusion and gibbus formation.

Children and adolescents often suffer from episodes of severe bone pain that last for days or weeks. This pain usually involves the end of a long bone, with local swelling, redness, tenderness, and muscle spasms.

Cardiac and pulmonary involvement are not common, but when children are affected they frequently suffer from a productive cough, chest pain, and recurrent pulmonary infections.

Pingueculae are usually seen in the eyes, and Gaucher-like cells have been reported in these lesions.

A peculiar yellow pallor to the skin which is not correlated with anemia has been reported in some children and adults. In addition, a diffuse yellow-brown pigmentation develops on exposed skin surfaces in older patients. It may be localized or unilateral, symmetrically distributed over the lower portion of the legs or apparent only on the face. The etiology of this pigmentation is not well understood, but after splenectomy the yellowing of the skin has been known to lessen.

Neurological findings have been noted only in the infantile neuropathic varieties of the disease.

Diagnosis

Clinically Gaucher disease should be considered in any patient with splenomegaly. Roentgenographic abnormalities of bone are present in up to 75 percent of all patients, and the most common radiographic sign is an expansion of the cortex at the lower end of the femur, producing the shape of an Erlenmeyer flask (Figure 5.6). Alteration of bony trabecular pattern with infiltration and collapse of the femoral (Figure 5.7) or humeral heads also may be apparent. Evidence of pulmonary involvement may be found later.

A number of biochemical abnormalities have been reported, but in almost every case the levels of serum acid phosphatase and serum angiotensin—converting enzyme are elevated.

The presence of Gaucher cells from a bone marrow aspirate is characteristic enough to permit a satisfactory diagnosis. The best method of viewing these cells is with supravital preparations using phase microscopy. The cells are from 20 to 100 microns in size, with a nucleus that is often eccentric. The cytoplasm appears to contain many fibrils of different lengths, giving the appearance of wrinkled tissue paper. Figure 5.8 is a micrograph of a lymph node sinus filled with typical Gaucher cells. Occasionally Gaucher cells are not found or are present in such small numbers that their significance or authenticity is questionable. Moreover, "secondary" Gaucher cells have been observed in some leukemia patients.

The most definitive diagnostic test is the demonstration of a deficiency of beta-glucosidase activity in peripheral leukocytes or cultivated skin fibroblasts from affected patients.

Cultured amniotic fluid cells, whose enzyme activity is similar to that of cultured skin fibroblasts, have been used in the prenatal diagnosis of the infantile form of the disorder.

Basic defect

The basic defect in all three types of Gaucher disease is the deficient activity of beta-glucosidase (glucocerebrosidase). Inadequate activity of this enzyme accounts for the accumulation of glucocerebrosides in various organ systems of the body. It has been shown that the level of beta-glucosidase activity in patients with Gaucher disease is about 15 percent of that in normal individuals. The level of residual enzyme activity is inversely related to the rate of progression of the disease. Thus, patients with higher levels of enzymatic activity show a slower rate of organ involvement.

Studies on the enzyme glucocerebrosidase are difficult because it is firmly bound to the lysosomal membrane. Furthermore, it tends to aggregate even when it has been solubilized. The reaction of the enzyme to its natural substrate, glucocerebroside, and artificial substrates differs with changes in assay conditions. A heat-stable protein effector that seems to activate the enzyme has been discovered, and it has been suggested that deficiency in this factor rather than glucocerebrosidase could account for some cases of Gaucher disease. However, the physiological function of this factor remains uncertain.

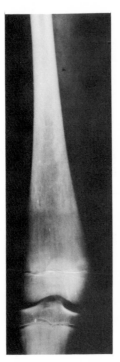

Figure 5.6. Erlenmeyer deformity of the femur. Courtesy of M. Hertz, Israel.

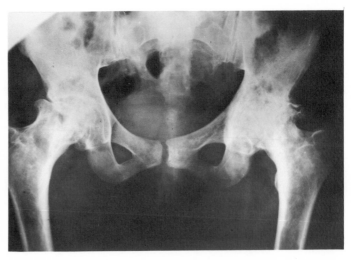

Figure 5.7. Severe osteolytic changes and deformity of head and neck of femurs. Courtesy of M. Hertz, Israel.

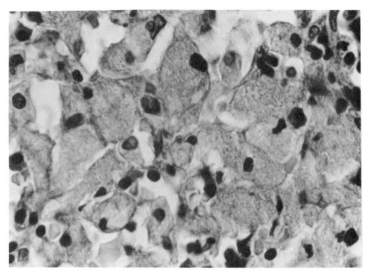

Figure 5.8. Micrograph of a lymph node sinus filled with typical Gaucher cells. The abundant cytoplasm appears granular or striated. Courtesy of G. Seltzer, Israel.

Genetics

There are three distinct genetic forms of this disease: type I (chronic adult noncerebral), type II (acute neuronopathic), and type III (subacute neuronopathic, juvenile). Family studies support autosomal recessive transmission in all three types. Type I is the most common of the three forms and although it has been described in many ethnic groups, it tends to occur most commonly in Ashkenazi Jews.

One study in Israel estimated the frequency at birth for the homozygous state in the Ashkenazi community to be 1:2,500, with a gene frequency of 0.02. The carrier frequency for this disorder among Ashkenazi Jews has been estimated to be from 1:50 to 1:70. It has been calculated that approximately 50 infants with type I Gaucher disease are born yearly in the U.S. and that at any one time there are between 1,000 and 1,200 patients with this disorder in the U.S. Although it has been reported that 80 percent of the patients with this form are of Ashkenazi Jewish descent, proper genetic and epidemiological surveys of this disease among the Jewish communities have not been made. For example, we now know that in Israel Gaucher disease also occurs among the Oriental and Sephardi communities. Of 17 patients reported from South Africa 14 were Jewish; of these, 13 were of Ashkenazi origin, 1 of Sephardi background. In 1970 Drukker and co-workers reported a case of the infantile form in an infant of Sephardi Jewish background. Fried has estimated that the gene frequency of the adult form of Gaucher disease in the non-Ashkenazi Jewish communities is probably less than 0.005.

In 1973 Fried reported 105 patients with Gaucher disease, 100 of whom were Ashkenazi Jews. The age distribution at the time of diagnosis in 98 of the Ashkenazi patients is given in Figure 5.9. In only 38 percent was the diagnosis made before the age of 15, while in 12 percent it was made between the ages of 45 and 60. In only 20 percent was the diagnosis made before the age of 5, and almost all cases

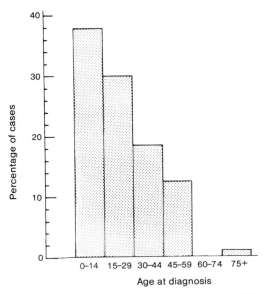

Figure 5.9. Age distribution of patients with Gaucher disease at time of diagnosis. From K. Fried, 1973, *Israel J. Med. Sci.* 9:1396.

were diagnosed before the age of 50. Such an age distribution suggests incomplete penetrance of the gene. Thus, it should be expected that some individuals identified as homozygotes on a biochemical basis will be essentially healthy.

Detection of the heterozygous states has been difficult, for considerable overlap has been noted in the range of enzyme activity between normal individuals and those who are presumed to be heterozygous. More recently, Beutler and co-workers have found that if the lymphocyte-rich fraction of the cells to be assayed is further fractioned into a component consisting almost entirely of monocytes and one consisting of lymphocytes, better differentiation between normal subjects and heterozygotes for Gaucher disease can be obtained. These investigators point out that this fractionation and assay technique is too complex for large population surveys, however. Its primary usefulness lies in the study of families specifically at risk for Gaucher disease.

Prognosis and treatment

The prognosis for Gaucher disease type I can be quite variable, depending on the age of onset. The later the onset, the more favorable the prognosis. The disease is usually slowly progressive and is marked by exacerbations and remissions. Splenectomy is a useful operation to combat the findings of hypersplenism and the discomfort produced by marked splenomegaly. Nonspecific arthritis, bone pain, pathological fracture, and bony deformity are usually treated in accordance with accepted orthopedic principles. Prosthetic replacement of a diseased hip joint has proved to be a satisfactory procedure, and the long-term results of this operation have been excellent.

In the Israeli cases studied by Fried, those patients who survived to the age of 45 seemed to be as fertile as healthy members of the Ashkenazi population. Both sexes tend to marry and show no evidence of marked sterility, either voluntary or involuntary.

Enzyme replacement may prove to be a useful tool in the treatment of this disorder. Recently this approach has shown that exogenous glucocerebrosidase causes definite decreases in the quantity of accumulated lipids in patients with Gaucher disease. It should be emphasized, however, that the effectiveness of this form of therapy remains unproven.

References

Aghion, A. 1934. La Maladie de Gaucher dans l'enfance. Thesis, Paris.

Beighton, P., and Sacks, S. 1974. Gaucher's disease in southern Africa. *S. Afr. Med. J.* 48:1295.

Beutler, E.; Dale, G. L.; Guinto, E.; and Kuhl, W. 1977. Enzyme replacement therapy in Gaucher's disease: A rapid high-yield method for purification of glucocerebrosidase. *Proc. Natl. Acad. Sci. USA* 74:4620.

Beutler, E., and Kuhl, W. 1970. The diagnosis of the adult type of Gaucher's disease and its carrier state by demonstration of deficiency of beta-glucosidase activity in peripheral blood leukocytes. *J. Lab. Clin. Med.* 76:747.

Beutler, E.; Kuhl, W.; Matsumoto, F.; and Pangalis, G. 1976. Acid hydrolases in leukocytes and platelets of normal subjects and in patients with Gaucher's and Fabry's disease. *J. Exp. Med.* 143:975.

Beutler, E.; Kuhl, W.; Trinidad, F.; Teplitz, R.; and Nadler, H. 1971. Beta-glucosidase activity in fibroblasts from homozygotes and heterozygotes for Gaucher's disease. *Am. J. Hum. Genet.* 23:62.

Brady, R. O., and King, F. M. 1973. Gaucher's disease. In *Lysosomes and storage diseases,* p. 382. New York: Academic Press.

Brady, R. O.; Pentchev, P. G.; and Gal, A. E. 1975. Investigations in enzyme replacement therapy in lipid storage diseases. *Fed. Proc.* 34:1310.

Brady, R. O.; Pentchev, P. G.; Gal, A. E.; Hibbert, S. R.; and Dekaban, A. S. 1974. Replacement therapy with purified glucocerebrosidase in Gaucher's disease. *N. Engl. J. Med.* 291:989.

Desnick, R. J.; Dawson, G.; Desnick, S. J.; Sweeley, C. C.; and Krivit, W. 1971. Diagnosis of glycosphingolipidoses by urinary-sediment analysis. *N. Engl. J. Med.* 284:739.

Drukker, A.; Sacks, M. I.; and Gatt, S. 1970. The infantile form of Gaucher's disease in an infant of Jewish Sephardi origin. *Pediatrics* 45:1017.

Frederickson, D. S., and Sloan, H. R. 1972. Glucosyl ceramide lipidoses: Gaucher's disease. In *The metabolic basis of inherited disease,* ed. J. B. Stanbury, J. B. Wyngaarden, and D. Fredrickson, 3rd ed. p. 730. New York: McGraw-Hill.

Fried, K. 1973. Population study of chronic Gaucher's disease. *Israel J. Med. Sci.* 9:1396.

Fried, K.; Matoth, Y.; and Goldschmidt, E. 1963. Gaucher's disease: Chronic adult type. In *Genetics of migrant and isolate populations,* ed. E. Goldschmidt, p. 292. Baltimore: Williams and Wilkins.

Gaucher, P. 1882. De l'épithélioma primitif de la rate. Thesis, Paris.

Groen, J. J. 1964. Gaucher's disease: Hereditary transmission and racial distribution. *Arch. Intern. Med.* 113:543.

Ho, M. W., and O'Brien, J. S. 1971. Gaucher's disease: Deficiency of acid-glucosidase and reconstitution of enzyme activity in vitro. *Proc. Natl. Acad. Sci. USA* 68:2810.

Lieb, H. 1924. Cerebrosidspeicherung bei Morbus Gaucher. *Z. Physiol. Chem.* 140:305.

Lieberman, J., and Beutler, E. 1976. Evaluation of serum angiotensin-converting enzyme in Gaucher's disease. *N. Engl. J. Med.* 294:1442.

Matoth, W., and Fried, K. 1965. Chronic Gaucher's disease: Clinical observations on 34 patients. *Israel J. Med. Sci.* 1:521.

Matoth, Y.; Zaizov, R.; Hoffman, J.; and Klibansky, Ch. 1974. Clinical and biochemical aspects of chronic Gaucher's disease. *Israel J. Med. Sci.* 10:1523.

Schneider, E. L.; Epstein, C. J.; Kaback, M. J.; and Brandes, D. 1977. Severe pulmonary involvement in adult Gaucher's disease: Report of three cases and review of the literature. *Am. J. Med.* 63:475.

MUCOLIPIDOSIS TYPE IV

Historical note

In 1974 Berman and co-workers first described this disorder in a 7-month-old Israeli boy of Ashkenazi Jewish descent who presented with congenital corneal clouding. Enzymatic analysis of cultured fibroblasts excluded any of the already described mucolipidoses and thus the name "mucolipidosis type IV" was assigned to this form. Since then, this group of investigators has noted a marked increase and altered distribution of GM_3 and GD_3 gangliosides in patients with this disorder. Furthermore, they have devised a method for making a prenatal diagnosis of the disease on the basis of the ultrastructural appearance of cultured amniotic cells. More recently other cases of this disorder have been diagnosed in Ashkenazi Jewish children outside the state of Israel. In 1976 Tellez-Nagel and co-workers reported extensive ultrastructural, histochemical, and chemical results from their study of a 7-year-old Ashkenazi Jewish boy with this condition.

Clinical features

The main clinical features of this disorder are corneal opacities in infancy and severe psychomotor retardation. In addition, affected children frequently have strabismus (esotropria) and later show signs of retinal degeneration. As a result, their visual acuity is extremely poor. Hypotonia and hyperactive deep-tendon reflexes also are common findings. Psychomotor retardation is severe; affected children usually do not speak or say only a few words, show no response to verbal commands, are unable to feed themselves, and pay little attention to their surroundings. If they are able to walk, they do so only with support. These children show no skin, joint, or bone abnormalities and have no organomegaly. A mild kyphosis has been noted in one patient, but no scoliosis or gibbus has been observed. The facial features of some patients have been described as full but not coarse.

The following case report on a 3-year-old female illustrates the characteristic clinical features of the disorder.

Born to unrelated Ashkenazi Jewish parents after a full-term, uneventful pregnancy, the infant weighed 3,040 g. At the age of 4 months she developed a squint, and ophthalmological examination revealed photophobia, increased lacrimation, and bilateral corneal opacities. A right corneal transplant was performed when the child was 18 months old. Her psychomotor development was markedly retarded. At 3 years of age she sat without support but could not assume a sitting position alone and walked only with support. Her vocabulary consisted of 3 words. There were no signs of regression. Physical examination showed a well-developed, passive child whose head circumference was 47 cm (44 cm at 11 months, 47 cm at 23 and 32 months), height was 96 cm, and weight was 15 kg. Her facial features were full but not coarse. Both corneas, including the transplanted one, were opaque. The fundi were normal. There was no evidence of organomegaly, obvious skeletal anomalies, or restrictions of joint movements. Neurological examination showed hypotonia with increased reflexes. The Babinski reflex was positive bilaterally. A radiological skeletal survey was within normal limits.

Diagnosis

The clinical diagnosis of this disorder should be suspected in any Ashkenazi Jewish infant who presents with clouding of the corneas and psychomotor retardation.

The diagnosis can easily be confirmed by ultrastructural examination of a biopsy from the conjunctiva. Affected conjunctival epithelial cells show large cytoplasmic vacuoles containing both fibrillogranular and membranous lamellar inclusions in myelin-like figures.

In the electron microscope these storage bodies appear as orderly arranged lamellae with a granular component usually present within large membrane-bound cytoplasmic vacuoles. Frequently the vacuoles are empty, but they may contain small amounts of moderately electron-dense material. Tellez-Nagel's group has shown that these granular-lamellar bodies resemble the compound bodies found in the brain of a child with this disorder. Their presence within the vacuoles in apparently different stages of morphological development suggests that they form within the vacuoles and eventually occupy and replace them.

In patients with this disorder different tissues, both *in vivo* and *in vitro*, seem to possess varying propensities for the storage of the abnormal material. While corneal and conjunctival biopsies show primarily single-membrane-limited vesicles filled with fibrillogranular material, cultured fibroblasts from amniotic fluid contain inclusion bodies that are almost exclusively of the lamellar type (Figure 5.10). The hepatocytes of one patient showed inclusions composed primarily of concentric lamellae, while the single-membrane vacuoles in the Kupfer cells were mainly clear.

Electron microscopic studies have been done on one affected aborted fetus. Cells from the brain and spinal cord contained numerous inclusions similar to those observed in the amniotic fluid cultures. Such inclusions were also found in epithelial (skin, cornea, conjunctiva) and endothelial cells. However, mesodermally derived cells such as cardiac muscle, kidney, and placenta (excluding the endothelium of blood vessels) did not contain these inclusions. The adrenals, liver, and pancreas were not available for study.

Mucolipidosis IV patients show no abnormalities in urinary amino acid or mucopolysaccharide excretion.

Basic defect

The basic defect in this lysosomal storage disease is not known. Bach and co-workers have postulated that since GD_3 and GM_3 gangliosides accumulate in affected fibroblasts in this disorder (GD_3 to 3 times the normal level, GM_3 to a lesser extent), and since both serve as substrates for the enzyme ganglioside

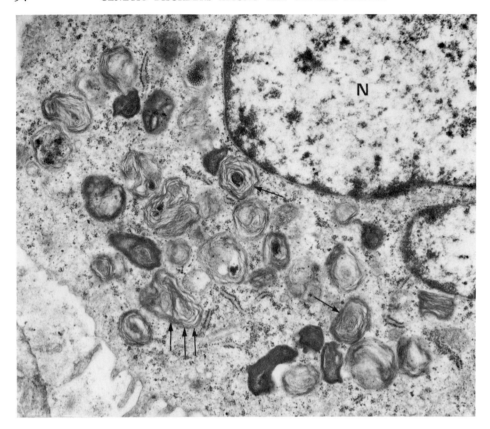

Figure 5.10. Electron micrograph of part of a cultured amniotic fluid cell. Note unicentric myelinated bodies (single arrow) with granular or amorphous contents and multicentric myelinated bodies (arrows). Cells were glutaraldehyde and OsO_4 fixed. N = nucleus. Courtesy of G. Kohn, Israel.

sialidase, the possibility exists that the basic defect is due to a sialidase deficiency. This group has also noted increased mucopolysaccharide accumulation in cultured fibroblasts from these patients.

Biochemical studies from a brain biopsy in the case reported by Tellez-Nagel and co-workers showed that the major abnormality in both gray and white matter was the ganglioside content, which was elevated approximately 50 percent in gray matter and at least threefold in white matter. In neither sample was there a specific notable elevation in any individual ganglioside.

Additional biochemical studies are needed to determine the precise defect responsible for the storage of several complex saccharide- and lipid-containing compounds.

Genetics

Since the original report of this disorder in 1974, 11 unrelated Ashkenazi Jewish families are known to have had affected children. Six of these families reside in Israel; the others are mainly from the United States.

Family studies support autosomal recessive inheritance of this disease. Although most of the affected families can trace their origins to eastern Poland, no information is available regarding a possible clustering effect. Consanguinity has not been observed in any of these families. At present the heterozygous state cannot be detected.

In one Israeli family two pregnancies have been interrupted following *in utero* diagnosis of the disorder. In two other cases where the amniotic fluid cells did not show any abnormalities, the pregnancies were carried to term and healthy children were born.

Prognosis and treatment

Since mucolipidosis IV patients suffer from a severe degree of mental retardation and a marked loss in visual acuity, their capabilities are extremely limited. The youngest patient known today is 2 years old; the oldest is 23. All the patients diagnosed during the past 4 years are alive.

Treatment is symptomatic. Corneal transplant does not help, for the transplant also becomes cloudy.

It is worthwhile to point out again that prenatal diagnosis is possible, despite the lack of knowledge concerning the basic defect.

References

Bach, G.; Cohen, M. M.; and Kohn, G. 1975. Abnormal ganglioside accumulation in cultured fibroblasts from patients with mucolipidosis IV. *Biochem. Biophys. Res. Commun.* 66:1483.

Bach, G.; Zeigler, M.; Kohn, A.; and Cohen, M. M. 1977. Mucopolysaccharide accumulation in cultured skin fibroblasts derived from patients with mucolipidosis IV. *Am. J. Hum. Genet.* 29:610.

Berman, E. R.; Livni, N.; Shapira, E.; Merin, S.; and Levij, I. S. 1974. Congenital corneal clouding with abnormal systemic storage bodies: A new variant of mucolipidosis. *J. Pediatr.* 84:519.

Kohn, G.; Livni, N.; and Beyth, Y. 1975. Prenatal diagnosis of mucolipidosis IV by electron microscopy. *Pediatr. Res.* 9:314.

Kohn, G.; Livni, N.; Ornoy, A.; Sekeles, E.; Beyth, Y.; Legum, C.; Bach, G.; and Cohen, M. M. 1977. Prenatal diagnosis of mucolipidosis IV by electron microscopy. *J. Pediatr.* 90:62.

Merin, S.; Livni, N.; Berman, E. R.; and Yatziv, S. 1975. Mucolipidosis IV: Ocular, systemic, and ultrastructural findings. *Invest. Ophthalmol.* 14:437.

Newell, F. W.; Matalon, R.; and Meyer, S. 1975. A new mucolipidosis with psychomotor retardation, corneal clouding, and retinal degeneration. *Am. J. Ophthalmol.* 80:440.

O'Brien, J. S.; Wiessmann, U.; Herschkowitz, N.; and Sipe, J. 1977. Mucolipidosis 4: Phospholipid storage. *Clin. Res.* 25:114A.

Sekeles, E.; Ornoy, A.; and Kohn, G. 1977. Mucolipidosis IV. Fetal and placental pathology: A report on two subsequent interruptions of pregnancy. *Hum. Hered.* 27:212.

Tellez-Nagel, I.; Rapin, I.; Iwamoto, T.; Johnson, A. B.; Norton, W. T.; and Nitowsky, H. 1976. Mucolipidosis IV: Clinical, ultrastructural, histochemical, and chemical studies of a case, including a brain biopsy. *Arch. Neurol.* 33:828.

NIEMANN-PICK DISEASE
(TYPE A: ACUTE NEUROPATHIC FORM)

Historical note

In 1914 Niemann reported the case of an 18-month-old Jewish infant who died after progressive deterioration associated with hepatosplenomegaly, lymphadenopathy, edema, and pigmentation of the skin. Although he thought the histopathological features were consistent with Gaucher disease, he doubted this diagnosis because of the very rapid demise of the patient. From 1922 to 1927 Pick collected and studied similar case reports of Gaucher disease and noted the distinguishing features of the new syndrome, which he called lipoid cell splenomegaly. In 1934 Klenk demonstrated that the predominant phospholipid accumulated is sphingomyelin. In 1961 Crocker and Mays showed that the sphingomyelin formed in the tissues of these patients is normal and postulated that the defect is due to a lack of the enzyme that aids in the metabolism of sphingomyelin. In 1966 Brady and co-workers discovered a deficiency in the activity of the enzyme that catalyzes cleavage of sphingomyelin to phosphorylcholine and ceramide in the classic infantile form of the disease. In 1967 Uhlendorf and co-workers found that the metabolic defect persists in cell culture, making possible the prenatal diagnosis of this disorder. Six distinct forms of Niemann-Pick disease are known, but only the classic infantile form (type A of Crocker) is found in Ashkenazi Jews.

Clinical features

Most infants with the type A form of Niemann-Pick disease appear normal at birth but within the first few months of life develop feeding problems. Before the age of 6 months they have hepatosplenomegaly and lymphadenopathy and show a definite failure to thrive. Vomiting and severe feeding problems become more pronounced. Various skin lesions have been described, including Mongolian spots, generalized thickening of the skin, suppurative lesions about the face, and a peculiar brownish-yellow hue to the skin. Edema about the face and legs also may be present. By the age of one year a generalized loss of motor and intellectual functions is apparent. A cherry-red spot in the macula is present in approximately half the patients, but it may not be evident until late in the illness. Neurological deterioration is progressive in Niemann-Pick disease and death usually occurs by the fourth year.

Some affected infants are abnormal at birth, and stillbirths demonstrate that severe manifestations may develop *in utero*. A few children appear healthy for a year or more but then develop symptoms and deteriorate rapidly.

In addition to type A, there are five other forms of Niemann-Pick disease. Type B is characterized by marked visceral involvement, and the manifestations of the disease become apparent during infancy or childhood. The nervous system is spared and many patients reach adulthood in relatively good health. Type C is characterized by both visceral and nervous system involvement, and the condition is usually fatal before the age of 20. Patients with type D have a common Nova Scotian ancestry and their clinical presentation is similar to that of type C. The level of cholesterol in the tissues of these patients is high, but the quantity of sphingomyelin that accumulates is not impressive. Adults who are found incidentally to have a moderate accumulation of sphingomyelin in their tissues have been classified as having type E. Recently type F has been described in a case involving childhood onset of splenomegaly, lack of neurological manifestations, and diminished sphingomyelinase activity.

Diagnosis

Niemann-Pick disease can be diagnosed on the basis of the clinical finding of hepatosplenomegaly, central nervous system damage (in types A, C, and D), and the characteristic histology of the foam cell, particularly as revealed by electron microscopy (Figures 5.11–5.13). Foam cells are observed in many tissues and their vacuolation is easily recognizable in peripheral leukocytes and in aspirated bone marrow examined with a supravital stain under a phase microscope.

A definitive diagnosis of Niemann-Pick disease can be made by showing deficient activity of the enzyme sphingomyelinase in extracts of sonicated fresh leukocyte preparations. This technique can also be applied to cultivated skin fibroblasts. Ease in obtaining skin fibroblasts makes biopsy of the liver, brain, or lymph nodes unnecessary.

It has also been found that sphingomyelinase activity is readily detectable in cultivated amniotic fluid cells; thus, prenatal diagnosis of this disorder is possible. Such a diagnosis has been confirmed on fetal tissues after therapeutic abortion.

Determinations of sphingomyelinase activity once required the use of sphingomyelin labeled with radiocarbon or radiohydrogen. These materials are expensive, and their use is restricted to laboratories with radioactive counting facilities. Recently, however, an analogue of sphingomyelin, 2-hexadecanoylamino-4-nitrophenylphosphorylcholine, was synthesized by Gal and co-workers. This substance is hydrolyzed by highly purified sphingomyelinase and by sphingomyelinase in extracts of human liver tissue, cultured skin fibroblasts, cultured amniotic cells, and washed leukocyte preparations. Extracts of tissues and cells from patients with Niemann-Pick disease type A do not hydrolyze this compound, and heterozygotes and patients with Niemann-Pick disease type C show only an intermediate level of hydrolytic activity.

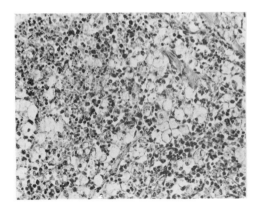

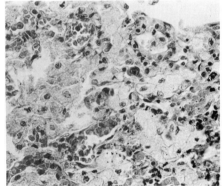

Figure 5.11. Spleen containing large numbers of foam cells with small, dark nuclei at the periphery of the cells. Courtesy of U. Sandbank, Israel.

Figure 5.12. Lung showing alveoli filled with foam cells. Courtesy of U. Sandbank, Israel.

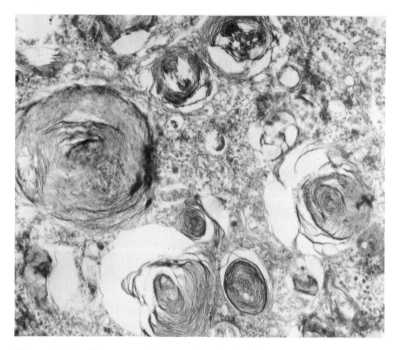

Figure 5.13. Electron micrograph of the liver showing numerous cytoplasmic vacuoles with concentric membranous formation. Courtesy of U. Sandbank, Israel.

Thus, the analogue is a reliable chromogenic reagent for the diagnosis of patients with Niemann-Pick disease and the detection of heterozygous carriers of the Niemann-Pick trait.

Basic defect

The basic defect in Niemann-Pick disease (types A–C and F) is a deficiency in the activity of the lysosomal enzyme sphingomyelinase, which catalyzes cleavage of sphingomyelin into phosphorylcholine and ceramide. Types D and E may not be sphingomyelin lipidoses, since the storage of sphingomyelin often is not impressive and frequently is overshadowed by the degree of cholesterol storage.

It is thought that sphingomyelin, which is a constituent of all cells and extracellular lipoproteins, accumulates in many cells that have phagocytic potential, since the demand for its catabolism exceeds the capacity of the degradative system. Organs containing a preponderance of these cells enlarge and the excess sphingomyelin causes both physical destruction and inactivation of cellular organelles.

When these events occur in the brain and other parts of the nervous system the neurons involved are not able to regenerate damaged components and the phagocytosis of lipids by the glial cells and other macrophages becomes secondary to the defective metabolism of sphingomyelin within the neurons. Although much is known about Niemann-Pick disease, much remains to be learned about the events that initiate and sustain brain damage in patients with this disorder.

Genetics

Family studies strongly support the autosomal recessive nature of type A Niemann-Pick disease. It has been estimated that approximately two-thirds of all infants with this form of the disease are of Ashkenazi Jewish descent. The incidence among Ashkenazi Jews is between 1:20,000 and 1:30,000 births per year, or approximately 60 new patients per year, about 25 of whom are born in the United States. The gene frequency of this disorder among Ashkenazi Jews is thought to be greater than 1:100,000, with the frequency for the heterozygote state ranging between 1:100 and 1:140.

Partial deficiency in sphingomyelinase activity in cultured fibroblasts indicates the heterozygote state.

Prognosis and treatment

Type A Niemann-Pick disease is lethal and most patients die by the age of four years. Various symptomatic approaches have been tried—splenectomy, chemotherapy, radiation therapy, and steroids—but all to no avail.

Sufficient quantities of purified sphingomyelinase have not been available to properly assess its role in the treatment of this disease. A procedure was recently developed for purifying sphingomyelinase from human placental tissue, but the yield of pure enzyme obtained was exceedingly small.

Recently an animal model of Niemann-Pick disease was developed by injecting neonatal rats with AY-9944 (an inhibitor of F-dehydrocholesterol reductase). This model will make it possible for investigators to conduct a number of critical experiments concerning enzyme replacement in this disease.

References

Brady, R. O. 1977. Heritable catabolic and anabolic disorders of lipid metabolism. *Metabolism* 26:329.

Brady, R. O.; Johnson, W. G.; and Uhlendorf, B. W. 1971. Identification of heterozygous carriers by lipid storage diseases. *Am. J. Med.* 51:423.

Brady, R. O.; Kanfer, J. N.; Mock, M. B.; and Fredrickson, D. S. 1966. The metabolism of sphingomyelin. II: Evidence of an enzyme deficiency in Niemann-Pick disease. *Proc. Natl. Acad. Sci. USA* 55:366.

Brady, R. O.; Pentcher, P. G.; and Gal, A. E. 1975. Investigations in enzyme replacement therapy in lipid storage diseases. *Fed. Proc.* 34:1310.

Crocker, A. C. 1961. The cerebral defect in Tay-Sachs disease and Niemann-Pick disease. *J. Neurochem.* 7:69.

Crocker, A. C., and Farber, S. 1958. Niemann-Pick disease: A review of eighteen patients. *Medicine* 37:1.

Epstein, C. J.; Brady, R. O.; Schneider, R. M.; Bradley, D.; and Shapiro, D. 1971. *In utero* diagnosis of Niemann-Pick disease. *Am. J. Hum. Genet.* 23:533.

Fredrickson, D. S., and Sloan, H. R. 1972. Sphingomyelin lipidoses: Niemann-Pick disease. In *The metabolic basis of inherited disease,* ed. J. B. Stanbury, J. B. Wyngaarden, and D. Fredrickson, 3rd ed., p. 783. New York: McGraw-Hill.

Gal, A. E.; Brady, R. O.; Hibbert, S. R.; and Pentchev, P. G.: A practical chromogenic procedure for the detection of homozygotes and heterozygous carriers of Niemann-Pick disease. *N. Engl. J. Med.* 293:632.

Holtz, A. I.; Uhlendorf, B. W.; and Fredrickson, D. S. 1964. Persistence of a lipid defect in tissue cultures derived from patients with Niemann-Pick disease. *Fed. Proc.* 23:129.

Klenk, G. 1934. Uber die Natur der Phosphatide der Milz bei der Niemann-Pickschen Krankheit. *Z. Physiol. Chem.* 229:151.

Knudson, A. G., Jr., and Kaplan, W. D. 1962. Genetics of the sphingolipidoses. In *Cerebral sphingolipidoses: A symposium on Tay-Sachs disease,* ed. S. M. Aaronson and B. W. Volk, p. 395. New York: Academic Press.

Niemann, A. 1914. Ein unbekanntes Krankheitsbild. *Jahrb. Kinderheilk.* 79:1.

Pentchev, P. G.; Brady, R. O.; Gal, A. E.; and Hibbert, S. R. 1977. The isolation and characterization of sphingomyelinase from human placental tissue. *Biochim. Biophys. Acta* 488:312.

Pick, L. 1927. Uber die lipoidyellige splenohepatomegalie typus Niemann-Pick als Stoffwechselerkrankung. *Med. Klin.* 23:1483.

———. 1933. Niemann-Pick's disease and other forms of so-called xanthomatoses. *Am. J. Med. Sci.* 185:601.

Sakuragawa, N.; Sakuragawa, M.; Kuwabara, T.; Pentchev, P. G.; Barranger, J. A.; and Brady, R. O. 1977. Niemann-Pick disease experimental model: Sphingomyelinase reduction induced by AY-9944. *Science* 196:317.

Schneider, E. L.; Pentchev, P. G.; Hibbert, S. R.; Sawitsky, A.; and Brady, R. O. 1978. A new form of Niemann-Pick disease characterized by temperature-labile sphingo-myelinase. *J. Med. Genet.* 15:370.

PRIMARY TORSION DYSTONIA
(DYSTONIA MUSCULORUM DEFORMANS)

Historical note

In 1908 Schwalbe reported dystonia in three Jewish sibs and suggested a genetic etiology for this disorder. In 1911 Flatau and Sterling noted the susceptibility of Jews to torsion dystonia (TD) and suggested that it may be genetically transmitted. They also made several astute clinical observations about dystonia and coined the term "progressive torsion spasm of childhood," which according to Eldridge may be the most accurate description of this form of the disease. In the same year, Von Oppenheim referred to the condition as "dystonia musculorum deformans," a widely used but inaccurate term. In 1929 Mankowsky and Czerny postulated the existence of two distinct genetic forms of dystonia.

For several years the ethnic and genetic features of this disease were ignored, and in a large review published by Hertz in 1944 importance was given instead to the disease's psychogenic aspects.

With the pioneering work of Cooper and co-workers during the late 1950's, neurosurgery became the popular therapeutic approach to the relief of torsion dystonia. In 1970 Eldridge reviewed the entire subject of the torsion dystonias and further clarified the clinical and genetic features of the recessive form, which is particularly common among Ashkenazi Jews.

Clinical features

The autosomal recessive form of TD is characterized by irregular involuntary movements usually in association with an increase in muscle tone. The average age of onset of this form is 10:6 years. The limbs—usually the hand and/or foot on the dominant side—are generally involved earlier and more severely than the axial musculature, and the course of the disease in the early stages is often rapid. Following adolescence, symptoms may remit or actually improve, but the earlier the age of onset, the more severe the symptoms.

The degree of muscle involvement varies greatly. Some patients may suffer from only the dragging of one foot, while others may make bizarre involuntary movements of the arms, legs, head, and torso. Involvement of facial muscles and speech is seldom noted in this disorder. The disease generally progresses in stages. In the first stage the movements are sporadic, usually initiated by a stressful event. Later the dystonic postures and movements persist and permanent deformities result from a shortening of the tendons.

In addition to sustained contortional spasms, these patients may make a variety of abnormal movements simulating tremor, chorea, athetosis, tic, etc. The torsion spasms may be painful, especially when the axial musculature is involved.

During sleep the involuntary movements and postural deformities disappear unless they are fixed due to contractures. The duration of sleep may be affected, with some patients requiring less sleep than their unaffected sibs.

Diagnosis

The diagnosis of this form of TD is solely clinical. It should be considered in any Ashkenazi Jewish child who experiences spontaneous onset of involuntary torsion spasms involving the muscles of one or more limbs. No characteristic biochemical or pathological changes have been noted. In 1973 Wooten and co-workers observed that plasma activity of dopamine-beta-hydroxylase (DBH), the enzyme that converts dopamine to norepinephrine, is elevated in patients with the dominant form of TD but normal in those with the recessive type. More recently, however, other investigators have maintained that the dominant and recessive forms cannot be differentiated by DBH levels.

Basic defect

The basic defect in this disorder is not known. However, certain observations suggest that the biochemical alteration in the hereditary forms of torsion dystonia may involve the basal ganglia. For example, dystonic movements are a prominent feature of several disorders that involve these structures, and especially of those conditions associated with the abnormal accumulation of heavy metals (copper, iron, and manganese). Furthermore, dystonia may be produced by drugs that influence the supposed neurotransmitters concentrated in this region of the brain. Lastly, focal injuries to those thalamic nuclei with major connections to one or more of these structures may dramatically relieve existing symptoms.

In 1976 Grossman and Kelly reviewed the physiology of the basal ganglia in relation to dystonia and suggested two main areas for future study. The first involves the basal ganglia–thalamocortical circuit, the second the descending brainstem motor projections, mainly those in the tegmentum. Whether or not these are indeed the primary sites of alteration remains to be determined.

Genetics

Family studies provide evidence for an autosomal dominant, recessive, and even an X-linked form of TD. The autosomal recessive form is particularly frequent among Ashkenazi Jews, while the autosomal dominant and X-linked recessive types affect the non-Jewish population.

In the 63 families that Eldridge and co-workers studied in 1970 there were no apparent environmental causes for dystonia and no instances in which parent and child were affected. Thirty-seven of these families were Jewish. A high rate of occurrence among Ashkenazi Jews was later noted in a survey of cases throughout the U.S. Of 578 families surveyed, at least 148 were of Jewish descent. Segregation analysis of the Jewish sibships involved confirmed autosomal recessive inheritance. Consanguinity was not present in any of these Jewish families originally surveyed, but it was in 3 of the 77 additional affected Jewish families Eldridge reported in 1976. Consanguinity tends to be a factor more frequently in non-Jewish cases of this form of the disease.

Eldridge obtained information on the European origins of the affected Jewish families from 116 grandparents of 38 patients. Thirty-five were from Lithuania, Latvia, Grodno, Suwalki, Vilna, Kovno, and Courland; 24 were from Volhynia, Kiev, Podolia, Bessarabia, Moldavia, and Bukovina; and the remainder were from other regions of Russia, Poland, and Central Europe. In only 1 family was there a suggestion of Sephardi lineage. According to the report of Eldridge and Gottlieb in 1976, the incidence of this disorder among Ashkenazi Jews in the U.S. is estimated to be 1:17,000. Thus, among U.S. Ashkenazi Jews the gene frequency would be 1:130 and the frequency for carriers would be 1:65.

In 1976 Alter and co-workers reported data collected on 23 Israeli TD patients from 1969 to 1972. Of these patients, 18 were of Ashkenazi descent and 5 were of Sephardi-Oriental origin. Table 5.5 shows that in both groups the age of onset was between 10 and 19 years. The age-adjusted annual incidence of TD was over four times as great in the Ashkenazi group as in the Sephardi-Oriental group (4.82 and 1.05 per 10^5 population, respectively). The rate of TD was higher among the Ashkenazim than among the Sephardim and Orientals in all but the oldest age

Table 5.5. Torsion dystonia: Number of Israeli Jewish cases, 1969–1972, by age at onset and ethnic group

Age at onset (years)	Ethnic group		
	Ashkenazi	Sephardi-Oriental	Total
0–9	2	—	2
10–19	8	3	11
20–29	4	—	4
30–39	2	1	3
40–49	1	—	1
50–59	1	1	2
Total	18	5	23

Source: M. Alter et al., 1976, Differences in torsion dystonia among Israeli ethnic groups, in *Advances in neurology*, vol. 14: *Dystonia* (New York: Raven Press).

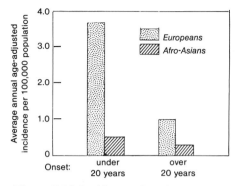

Figure 5.14. Incidence of torsion dystonia Israel, 1969–1972, by ethnic group and age (under or over 20 years) at onset. From M. Alter et al., 1976, Differences in torsion dystonia among Israeli ethnic groups, in *Advances in neurology*, vol. 14: *Dystonia* (New York: Raven Press).

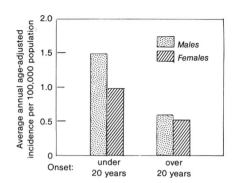

Figure 5.15. Incidence of torsion dystonia in Israel, 1969–1972 by sex and age (under or over 20 years) at onset. From M. Alter et al., 1976, Differences in torsion dystonia among Israeli ethnic groups, in *Advances in neurology*, vol. 14: *Dystonia* (New York: Raven Press).

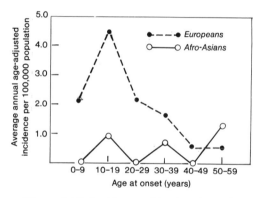

Figure 5.16. Incidence of torsion dystonia in Israel, 1969–1972, by ethnic group and age at onset. From M. Alter et al., 1976, Differences in torsion dystonia among Israeli ethnic groups, in *Advances in neurology*, vol. 14: *Dystonia* (New York: Raven Press).

group (Figure 5.14). The greatest difference was observed in the age group 10–19 years. The excess of Ashkenazi Jews among patients in whom the onset of TD was earlier is shown in Figure 5.15. As seen in Figure 5.16, there were more males than females among the early-onset patients, while among the late-onset patients this ratio was almost equal.

Family studies were not done in this Israeli study, but the authors postulate that the same gene is responsible for the TD observed in the Israeli Ashkenazi community and in Ashkenazi Jews in the United States. They also suggest that the TD noted in the Sephardi-Oriental Jewish community of Israel may be similar to the later-onset dystonia observed among non-Jews in the United States. There is little evidence to support the latter suggestion, however, for late onset occurred in only 2 of their 5 Sephardi-Oriental patients. The number of cases is too small to warrant proposing at this time TD heterogeneity among the Jewish communities.

Although the studies from the United States and the recent survey conducted in Israel certainly support the concept that the autosomal recessive form of TD occurs primarily among Ashkenazi Jews, additional genetic studies are needed to achieve a better understanding of the possible differences in TD within the various Jewish ethnic groups.

At present it is not possible to identify the carrier state in this form of dystonia. Some patients with recessive dystonia have noted increased dystonic movements while under the influence of phenothiazine, and their unaffected relatives have observed mild temporary dystonic movements while on such drugs. This observation suggests that a drug challenge may be useful in detecting the heterozygous state, but it should be stressed that such an approach to detecting the gene may be fraught with many dangers.

An interesting observation made by Eldridge and co-workers suggests that Jewish patients with the autosomal recessive form of the disease may have a high intelligence quotient. Their data (using control studies) were statistically significant at the level of $p < 0.03$. The validity of the finding that the TD gene, whether in single or double dose, confers high intellect, and the theory that such a factor would have survival advantage for the heterozygote, remain to be tested.

Prognosis and treatment

The prognosis in this disorder depends on the severity of its expression, and this can be quite variable. In general the disorder is not fatal, but few affected individuals lead normal, productive lives.

Numerous therapeutic approaches have been tried, but few are totally effective.

Neurosurgery has provided significant relief to a number of patients. According to the most recent survey by Eldridge, 180 of 257 patients who had had neurosurgery reported beneficial long-term results, 63 were no better or were worse, and 14 were reported improving during the short period they were observed. The most effective operative site appears to be the region of the ventrolateral nucleus of the thalamus (cryothalamectomy). Multiple operations may be necessary in this disorder, but good results have been achieved after three or more procedures. Neurosurgery seems to be most beneficial to those patients who have minimal torticollis or truncal involvement. In contrast, it poses the greatest risks and yields the poorest results in those in whom axial involvement predominates.

Various pharmacological agents have been used in the treatment of torsion dystonia. During recent years varying results have been achieved with orphenadrine, ACTH, large doses of chloropromazine, and diazapam. Of these diazapam has proved the most useful, but patient response has varied. Haloperidol, in combination with other drugs or alone, also has been reported to be useful in improving dystonic symptoms. When first tested, L-dopa appeared to be a useful drug, but recent studies suggest that because of its uncertain long-term effects it should be reserved for older patients. At present there is no specific drug therapy for torsion dystonia.

Hypnosis, electroconvulsive shock, psychotherapy, transcendental meditation, and acupuncture have been tried in these patients, but there is little evidence that these approaches have any long-lasting benefit. Bio-feedback is currently being evaluated. The nerve impulses detected above the affected muscles are amplified and fed back to the patients on visual or auditory screens. This method of feedback has helped some patients control muscles that had previously been uncontrollable due to some neurological defect. Again, it should be stressed that this approach is in its infancy and much remains to be learned before this method of therapy can be advocated.

It is crucial that torsion dystonia patients be diagnosed as early as possible and be given the help of various professional people to aid them in their emotional adjustment to the illness.

References

Alter, M.; Kahana, E.; and Feldman, S. 1976. Differences in torsion dystonia among Israeli ethnic groups. In *Advances in neurology*, vol. 14: *Dystonia*, pp. 115–20. New York: Raven Press.

Barbeau, A. 1970. Rationale for the use of L-dopa in the torsion dystonias. *Neurology* 20:96.

Barrett, R. E.; Yahr, M. D.; and Duvoisin, R. C. 1970. Torsion dystonia and spasmodic torticollis: Results of treatment with L-dopa. *Neurology* 20:107.

Cooper, I. S. Twenty-year follow-up study of the neurological treatment of dystonia musculorum deformans. In *Advances in neurology,* vol. 14: *Dystonia,* pp. 423–52. New York: Raven Press.

Ebstein, R. P.; Freedman, L. S.; Lieberman, A.; et al. 1974. A familial study in serum dopamine-beta-hydroxylase levels in torsion dystonia. *Neurology* 24:684.

Eldridge, R. 1970. The torsion dystonias: Literature review and genetic and clinical studies. *Neurology* 20:1.

Eldridge, R. 1976. Flautau-Sterling torsion spasm in Jewish children, and the early history of human genetics. In *Advances in neurology,* vol. 14: *Dystonia,* pp. 105–14. New York: Raven Press.

Eldridge, R., and Gottlieb, R. 1976. The primary hereditary dystonias: Genetic classification of 768 families and revised estimate of gene frequency, autosomal recessive form, with selected bibliography. In *Advances in neurology,* vol. 14: *Dystonia,* pp. 457–74. New York: Raven Press.

Eldridge, R.; Harlan, A.; Cooper, I. S.; and Riklan, M. 1970. Superior intelligence in recessively inherited torsion dystonia. *Lancet* 1:65.

Flatau, E., and Sterling, W. 1911. Progressiver Torsions-spasmus bei Kindern. *Z. Ges. Neurol. Psychiatr.* 7:586.

Grossman, R. G., and Kelly, P. J. 1976. Physiology of the basal ganglia in relation to dystonia. In *Advances in neurology,* vol. 14: *Dystonia,* pp. 49–57. New York: Raven Press.

Hertz, E. 1944. Dystonia. I. Historical review: Analysis of dystonic symptoms and physiologic mechanisms involved. *Arch. Neurol. Psychiatr.* 51:305.

Kartzinel, R., and Chase, T. N. 1977. Pharmacology of dystonia. In *Clinical neuropharmacology,* ed. H. L. Klawans, 2: 43–53. New York: Raven Press.

Mandell, S. 1970. The treatment of dystonia with L-dopa and haloperidol. *Neurology* 20:103.

Mankowsky, B. N., and Czerny, L. I. 1929. Zur Frage über die Heredität der Torsionsdystonie. *Mschr. Psychiatr. Neurol.* 72:165.

Schwalbe, W. 1908. Eine eigentümliche tonische Krampfform mit hysterischen Symptomen. In *Medicin und Chirurgi*. Berlin: Universitäts-Buchdruckerei von Gustav Schade.

Von Oppenheim, H. 1911. Über eine eigenartige Kranpfkrankheit des kindlichen und jugendlichen Alters (dysbasia lordotica progressiva, dystonia musculorum deformans). *Neurol. Abl.* 30:1090.

Wooten, G. F.; Eldridge, R.; Axelrod, J.; and Stern, R. S. 1973. Elevated plasma dopamine-beta-hydroxylase activity in autosomal dominant torsion dystonia. *N. Engl. J. Med.* 288:284.

Zeman, W. 1970. Pathology of the torsion dystonias (dystonia musculorum deformans). *Neurology* 20:79.

Zeman, W. 1976. Dystonia: An overview. In *Advances in neurology*, vol. 14: *Dystonia*, pp. 91–103. New York: Raven Press.

PTA DEFICIENCY
(PLASMA THROMBOPLASTIN ANTECEDENT, OR FACTOR XI, DEFICIENCY)

Historical note

In 1953 Rosenthal and co-workers first described PTA deficiency, which is characterized by a mild-to-moderate bleeding tendency. It was early recognized that almost all patients who have this bleeding diathesis are of Ashkenazi Jewish origin. In 1974 Muir and Ratnoff surveyed the Jewish community in the Cleveland area and estimated the minimal prevalence for the homozygous affected individual and the heterozygous carrier state. In 1978 Seligsohn and co-workers reported data from their 11-year study of this disorder in Israel.

Clinical features

Clinically, PTA deficiency is usually associated with a rather mild hemorrhagic episode with minimal bleeding following dental extractions, minor surgical procedures, or trauma. Occasionally a prolonged partial thromboplastin time leads to detection of the disorder during routine hematological studies. Some patients are known to experience spontaneous and severe bleeding as manifested by hematuria, epistaxis, and menorrhagia, while others are completely asymptomatic.

Diagnosis

The diagnosis of this coagulation disorder is totally dependent upon laboratory confirmation. The entire blood coagulation process—prothrombin consumption test, partial thromboplastin time, thromboplastin generation test, recalcification times, and factor XI assay—is abnormal. When PTA levels are less than 20 percent of normal, patients are considered to be severely deficient and to represent the homozygous state. Levels of PTA ranging from 20 to 70 percent indicate a mild deficiency and these individuals are thought to be heterozygous. Clinically there may be no relationship between the PTA factor level and the bleeding manifestation.

Basic defect

Using antibodies to factor XI, Rimon and co-workers recently demonstrated that this disorder is a true glycoprotein deficiency.

Factor XI participates in the initial phases of the contact activation of the intrinsic clotting system. It is composed of a 2-chain zymogen which is cleaved by activated factor XII in the presence of high molecular weight rininogen. The cleaved molecule (activated factor XI) then activates factor IX by a proteolytic reaction.

Genetics

Ashkenazi Jews have a striking predisposition for PTA deficiency, while only a few cases have been described in the non-Ashkenazi Jewish communities. In their survey of the Jewish community in Cleveland, Muir and Ratnoff estimated the minimal prevalence of the homozygous individual to be 1:12,000 and that of the heterozygous carrier state to be 1:56. Since PTA deficiency in most instances produces few symptoms, it is likely that these investigators overlooked some cases and that the prevalence of both the affected patient and the carrier state is higher than they estimated.

The dividing line between the homozygous and heterozygous states in this condition cannot always be clearly defined and this discrepancy must be considered when gene frequencies for the homozygous and heterozygous states are estimated. Furthermore, PTA deficiency should not be thought of as a totally recessive disorder, for heterozygotes may have a mild but definite bleeding tendency.

In the 1978 study by Seligsohn's group in Israel, the diagnosis of factor XI deficiency was made in 36 unrelated probands (12 females and 24 males), all of whom were from Ashkenazi Jewish families. Twenty-two individuals had severe factor XI deficiency (less than 0.15 μ/ml) and 14 had partial deficiency (0.15–0.49 μ/ml). Knowledge regarding parental consanguinity was available in only 22 of the probands; in 1 case the parents were first cousins.

In an effort to determine the frequency of this disorder in the Israeli Ashkenazi community, Seligsohn and co-workers measured the level of factor XI in 428 healthy adult Ashkenazi Jews randomly selected from participants in a Tay-Sachs disease carrier-detection program. Severe deficiency was noted in 1 individual (3 percent of the normal level), partial deficiency was detected in 35 subjects (24–29 percent), and a normal level was recorded in the remaining 392 subjects. The frequency of the mutant gene in this surveyed population was calculated to be 0.043. On the basis of these findings, the 95 percent confidence limit of the frequency of severely factor XI–deficient subjects (homozygotes) among the Ashkenazi Jewish population would be 0.1–0.3 percent, while that for partially deficient individuals (heterozygotes) would be 5.5–11.0 percent. It should be stressed, however, that even this data may be an underestimation, since only subjects with factor XI levels below the lower limit of the normal range were considered heterozygous carriers.

The Seligsohn group then tried to determine whether or not geographical clustering is a factor in this disease. The countries of origin of the grandparents of 66 PTA-deficient patients, as well as those of 289 normal subjects, are shown in Table 5.6. No significant differences were observed in the geographical origins of the two groups of grandparents except that fewer grandparents of PTA-deficient patients were from Romania. A further breakdown by province of birth did not disclose a particular area with a high concentration of possible carriers.

Table 5.6. PTA deficiency: Origin of grandparents of individuals with deficient and normal factor XI levels

Country of origin[a]	Grandparents of 289 individuals with normal factor XI level		Grandparents of 66 individuals with deficient factor XI level[b]	
	No.	% of total	No.	% of total
Poland	597	51.6	149	56.4
U.S.S.R.	215	18.6	54	20.5
Czechoslovakia	47	4.1	13	4.9
Hungary	44	3.8	11	4.2
Romania	180	15.6	18	6.8
All others	73	6.3	19	7.2
Total	1,156	100.0	264	100.0

Source: U. Seligsohn, Israel.
[a] Present-day boundaries.
[b] Thirty-four patients were known previously and 32 were detected in the survey.

Prognosis and treatment

The high gene frequency of this disorder warrants performing the appropriate tests in all Ashkenazi Jewish patients who are to undergo surgery. In most cases the prognosis is excellent. Hemorrhagic episodes respond well to the administration of fresh plasma or whole blood.

References

Biggs, R., and MacFarlane, F. G. 1962. *Human blood coagulation and its disorders.* 3rd ed. Oxford: Blackwell.

Dodds, W. J., and Kull, J. E. 1971. Canine factor XI (plasma thromboplastin antecedent) deficiency. *J. Lab. Clin. Med.* 78:746.

Leiba, H.; Ramot, B.; and Many, A. 1965. Heredity and coagulation studies in ten families with factor XI (plasma thromboplastin antecedent) deficiency. *Br. J. Haematol.* 2:654.

Muir, W. A., and Ratnoff, O. D. 1974. The prevalence of plasma thromboplastin antecedent (PTA, factor XI) deficiency. *Blood* 44:569.

Ramot, B., and Fisher, S. 1960. Plasma thromboplastin antecedent deficiency and its association with pseudohemophilia. *Israel Med. J.* 19:85.

Rapaport, S. I.; Proctor, R. R.; Patch, M. J.; and Yettra, M. 1961. The mode of inheritance of PTA deficiency: Evidence for the existence of major PTA deficiency and minor PTA deficiency. *Blood* 18:149.

Ratnoff, O. D. 1967. Genetic disorders of blood coagulation. *Seminars Hematol.* 4:93.

Rimon, A.; Schiffman, S.; Feinstein, D.; and Rapaport, S. I. 1976. Factor XI activity and factor XI antigen in homozygous and heterozygous factor XI deficiency. *Blood* 48:165.

Rosenthal, R. L. 1964. Haemorrhage in PTA (factor XI) deficiency. *Proc. 10th Int. Cong. Soc. Hematol.* Stockholm.

Rosenthal, R. L.; Dreskin, H. O.; and Rosenthal, M. 1953. New hemophilia-like disease caused by deficiency of third plasma thromboplastin factor. *Proc. Soc. Exp. Biol. Med.* 82:171.

———. 1955. Plasma thromboplastin antecedent (PTA) deficiency: Clinical, coagulation, therapeutic, and hereditary aspects of a new hemophilia-like disease. *Blood* 10:120.

Seligsohn, U., et al. 1978. High gene frequency of factor XI (PTA) deficiency in Ashkenazi Jews. *Blood* 87:165.

Zacharski, L. R., and French, E. E. 1978. Factor XI (PTA) deficiency in an English-American kindred, in press.

SPONGY DEGENERATION OF THE CENTRAL NERVOUS SYSTEM

Historical note

The first reported case of this disease was probably that of Globus and Strauss in 1928. In 1931 Canavan reported a similar case and stressed that macroephalus could be caused by a diffuse degenerative disease of the brain as well as by hydrocephalus or tumor. In 1937 Eiselsberg called attention to the familial occurrence of this disorder. In 1942 and 1954 Jervis reported six cases of spongy degeneration but referred to the disorder as Krabbe disease. It was Van Bogaert and Bertrand in 1949 who established spongy degeneration of the central nervous system as a nosological entity, describing its occurrence in 3 Jewish infants. In 1964 Banker and co-workers reviewed the literature and reported on the clinical and pathological features of 7 new cases. This excellent review not only further delineated the clinical and pathological features of this disease but stressed its genetic etiology and Jewish ethnic distribution.

Clinical features

Spongy degeneration of the central nervous system (CNS) usually begins during the second or third month of life. The most common presenting symptoms are inability to support the head, seizures, and spasticity. By the age of 5 months there is definite impairment of motor function, with a change in muscle tone from flaccidity to spasticity. Abnormal postures of the hands and feet are early manifestations of the spasticity. Increased tendon reflexes, clonus, and a positive Babinski are common findings. Eventually these children develop pseudobulbar palsy and decerebrate or decorticate postures.

Enlargement of the head is a common feature in this disease and is usually evident by the fifth month. This slowly progressive symmetrical enlargement of the calvarium is associated with delay in closure of the anterior fontanelle.

By the age of 8–10 months these patients usually develop an internal strabismus of one eye and then the other. Progressive eye involvement results in optic atrophy and blindness, with roving movements of the eyes and nystagmus. The pupillary light reflex may be preserved but it usually is not of normal briskness.

Some physicians have called attention to the contrast between the fair complexion, blue eyes, and blond or red hair that characterize some of these affected children and the darker hair and complexion of their normal sibs. However, this interesting and perhaps significant clinical observation needs further documentation.

Diagnosis

Clinically the presence of megalencephaly, blindness, spasticity and progressive psychomotor deterioration in an infant, especially one of Ashkenazi Jewish descent, strongly suggests the diagnosis of spongy degeneration of the CNS.

Various laboratory studies, including serum and urine amino acid analyses, have failed to disclose any distinctive abnormalities. Examination of the spinal fluid may reveal a slight elevation in protein content. Electroencephalographic studies usually show a diffuse, abnormal pattern.

Distinct histopathological changes can be observed either by examining tissue from a brain biopsy while the child is living or by noting these changes in post-mortem studies. More specifically, it is the particular topography of the spongy changes and the presence of Alzheimer type 2 astrocytes, the paucity of myelin degradation products, and the disorder's unique ultrastructural features which, taken together, constitute the neuropathological entity of spongy degeneration of the CNS in infancy. The most characteristic feature of these changes is the widespread vacuolation involving the lower layers of the cerebral cortex and the subcortical white matter; the more central zones are relatively or entirely spared. There is widespread disintegration of myelin not only in the areas of spongy degeneration but far beyond them. Despite the severe myelin loss, fatty by-products of myelin degradation have not been noted. There is a conspicuous increase in the number and size of protoplasmic astrocytes scattered throughout the cerebral cortex and basal ganglia. The astrocytic nuclei are frequently enlarged and lobulated. Many of the astrocytes contain dark-staining, eccentrically placed nucleoli. In the white matter there is an increase in small fibrillary astrocytes. Figures 5.17–5.20 show various pathological findings in this disease.

Electron microscopic studies reveal that the astrocytes contain peculiar elongate mitochondria. These abnormal mitochondria contain a central core of filaments surrounded by cristae. Homogeneous osmiophilic densities are occasionally seen

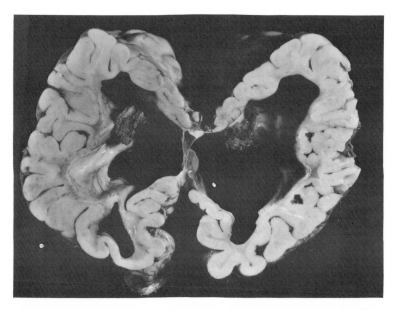

Figure 5.17. Coronal section through parietal lobes of formalin-fixed brain. Ventricles are markedly dilated; white matter is greatly reduced in amount and darker than normal. From B. Banker et al., 1964, *Neurology* 14:981.

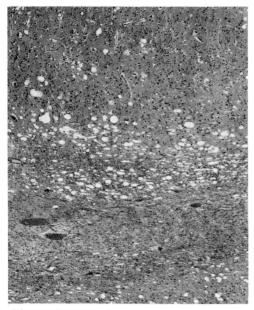

Figure 5.18. Band of vacuolation occupies
deep layers of frontal cortex and subjacent
white matter. From B. Banker et al., 1964,
Neurology 14:981.

within the filamentous matrix. Such abnormal mitochondria are observed only in
astrocytes. A striking finding is the normal appearance of the majority of the
oligodendroglia in regions of expanded extracellular space and disintegrating myelin
sheaths. Vacuolated cells resembling macrophages and containing ingested myelin
sheaths are evident in areas of most extensive demyelination.

Although vacuolation of cerebral tissue occurs in several neurological disorders,
only in spongy degeneration of the CNS in infancy is the topography of the vacuolation so characteristic or the spongy change so diffuse or severe. In a recent report
of the ultrastructural findings in 5 cases of this disorder, a team of Israeli investigators noted these changes and stressed that the ultrastructural abnormalities in the
astrocytic mitochondria are pathognomonic for the disease (Figure 5.21). They also
demonstrated that, using the electron microscope, one can detect these changes in
the early stages of the disease, a time when findings from the light microscope may
be equivocal. Electron microscopic study of brain tissue is suggested for all suspected
patients.

Biochemical studies have been done on brain tissue in connection with the
diagnosis of this disease, but no characteristic abnormality has been recognized.

Basic defect

The basic defect in spongy degeneration of the CNS is unknown. Various theories
have been postulated, but the most consistent hypothesis is that demyelination and
vacuolation are secondary to edema formation. The presence of swollen astrocytes

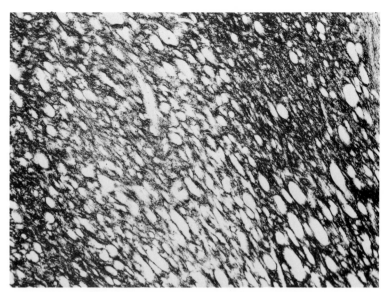

Figure 5.19. Inferior cerebellar peduncle showing advanced spongy state. From B. Banker et al., 1964, *Neurology* 14:981.

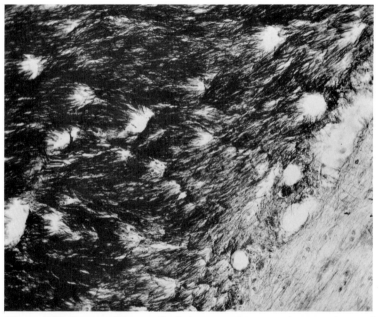

Figure 5.20. Intense fibrous gliosis in zone of spongy degeneration and demyelination. From B. Banker et al., 1964, *Neurology* 14:981.

in otherwise morphologically normal neurophils and the recognized role of astrocytes in osmotic regulation suggest that a defect in this cell may be responsible for the edema. The mitochondrial changes noted in the astrocytes lends support to the theory that the basic defect may involve abnormal mitochondrial metabolism.

Mitochondrial studies from biopsied tissue and tissue culture explants from affected patients should provide greater insight into the pathogenesis of this disorder.

Genetics

The most extensive genetic studies on this disease have been done by Banker and co-workers. In 1978 Banker and Victor reviewed the literature and according to their strict criteria found 83 cases in 48 families. Of these 48 affected families, 28 were Jewish and 20 were known to be of Ashkenazi origin. In her original study Banker noted that the Ashkenazi Jewish families came from two specific regions of Eastern Europe: the Vilna-Kovno section of Lithuania and the adjacent Bialystok area of Poland, and the Volyhnia area of the Ukraine (Figure 5.22).

Family studies support an autosomal recessive mode of inheritance in this disease. Consanguinity was present in 11 of the 48 affected families mentioned above— i.e. in 21 percent of the Jewish families and in 36 percent of the non-Jewish families.

The ratio of affected males to affected females in this study was 39:41 (sex was not stated in 3 cases). In the Jewish families the male to female ratio was 29:17, while in the non-Jewish group the ratio was 7:19. Ethnicity was not stated for 8 patients. Although the difference in sex distribution between the two groups was significant ($p < 0.005$), it cannot be adequately explained. Clinically the disease was the same in both groups.

In Israel at least 9 families are known to have had affected children and all have

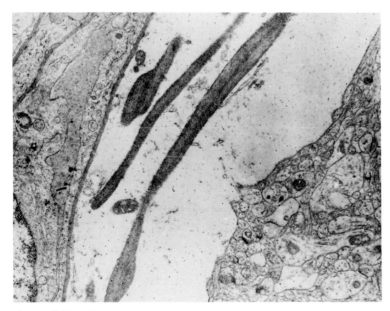

Figure 5.21. Electron micrograph from brain tissue of an affected Israeli child showing swollen and water-clear cytoplasmic projection of an astrocyte. Within the astrocytic process note the long mitochondria characteristically found in spongy degeneration of the brain. Courtesy of C. Bubis, Israel.

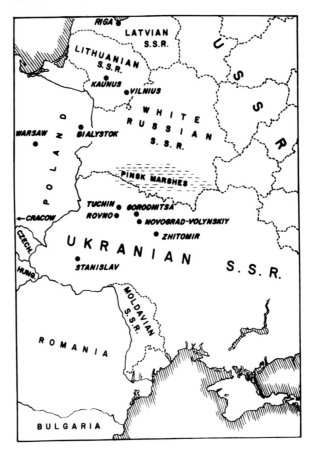

Figure 5.22. Geographical origins of the cases studied by Banker and co-workers in 1964. From B. Banker et al., 1964, *Neurology* 14:981.

been of Ashkenazi descent. Data on 6 of these families has been published; in 2 the parents are consanguineous.

There is no evidence that the heterozygous carriers have any abnormalities. Prenatal disgnosis is not possible at this time.

Prognosis and treatment

Most affected infants with this disorder die at the age of 4 years, although one patient is known to have reached the age of 10 years. Unfortunately, only supportive care can be given to those who suffer from this disease.

References

Adachi, M.; Torii, J.; Schneck, L., and Volk, B. W. 1972. Electron microscopic and enzyme histochemical studies of the cerebellum in spongy degeneration. *Acta Neuropathol.* 20:22.

Adachi, M.; Wallace, B.; Schneck, L.; et al. 1966. Fine structure of spongy degeneration of the central nervous system (Van Bogaert and Bertrand type). *J. Neuropathol. Exp. Neurol.* 25:589.

Adornato, B. T.; O'Brien, J. S.; Lampert, P. W.; Roe, T. F.; and Neustein, H. B. 1972. Cerebral spongy degeneration of infancy: A biochemical and ultrastructural study of affected twins. *Neurology* 22:202.

Banker, B. Q.; Robertson, J. T.; and Victor, M. 1964. Spongy degeneration of the central nervous system in infancy. *Neurology* 14:981.

Banker, B. Q., and Victor, M. 1979. Spongy degeneration of infancy. In *Genetic diseases in Ashkenazi Jews*, ed. R. M. Goodman and A. G. Motulsky. New York: Raven Press, forthcoming.

Buchanan, D. S., and Davis, R. L. 1965. Spongy degeneration of the nervous system: A report of 4 cases with a review of the literature. *Neurology* 15:207.

Canavan, M. M. 1931. Schilder's encephalitis periaxialis diffuse: Report of a case in a child aged sixteen and one-half months. *Arch. Neurol. Psychiatr.* 25:299.

Eiselsberg, F. 1937. Über frühkindliche familiäre diffuse Hirnsklerose. *Z. Kinderheilk.* 58:702.

Globus, J. H., and Strauss, I. 1928. Progressive degenerative subcortical encephalopathy (Schilder's disease). *Arch. Neurol. Psychiatr.* 20:1190.

Hogan, G. R., and Richardson, G. P., Jr. 1965. Spongy degeneration of the nervous system (Canavan's disease): Report of a case in an Irish-American family. *Pediatrics* 35:284.

Jervis, G. A. 1942. Early infantile acute diffuse sclerosis of the brain (Krabbe's type). *Am. J. Dis. Child.* 64:1055.

———. 1954. Early infantile acute diffuse sclerosis of brain (Krabbe's disease). *Mod. Probl. Paediatr.* 1:781.

Kamoshita, S.; Rupin, I.; Suzuki, K.; et al. 1968. Spongy degeneration of the brain: A chemical study of two cases including isolation and characterization of myelin. *Neurology* 18:975.

Mahloudji, M.; Daneshbod, K.; and Karjoo, M. 1970. Familial spongy degeneration of the brain. *Arch. Neurol.* 22:294.

Van Bogaert, L., and Bertrand, I. 1949. Sur une idiote familiale avec dégénérescence spongieuse de nevraxe. *Acta Neurol. Belg.* 49:572.

———. 1967. *Spongy degeneration of the brain in infancy.* Amsterdam: North Holland.

Varsano, I.; Lerman, P.; and Sandbank, U. 1977. Ultrastructural examination in the early diagnosis of spongy degeneration of the brain. *Harefuah* 192:533.

Wolman, M. 1958. The spongy type of diffuse sclerosis. *Brain* 81:243.

Zu Rhein, G. M.; Eichman, P. L.; and Puletti, F. 1960. Familial idiocy with spongy degeneration of the central nervous system of Van Bogaert-Bertrand type. *Neurology* 10:998.

TAY-SACHS DISEASE
(GM$_2$ GANGLIOSIDOSIS TYPE I)

Historical note

In 1881 Tay, an ophthalmologist, first described the cherry-red macular degeneration in the fundus of an affected infant. He later reported 2 affected patients from the same family. In 1887 Sachs, a neurologist, published clinical and pathological findings in an infant with blindness and severe psychomotor retardation. A few years later he reported 8 patients with retinal change and progressive neuro-logical deterioration and referred to the syndrome as "amaurotic family idiocy." It soon became apparent that this disorder affects primarily Ashkenazi Jewish in-fants, although later a few non-Jewish cases were reported. In the early 1940s Klenk and co-workers discovered that the disease manifests itself in the brain in greatly increased amounts of gangliosides. Over the years various investigators have at-tempted to identify the GM_2 ganglioside, but it was Makita and Yamakawa who in 1963 first reported its correct structure. In 1969 Okada and O'Brien demonstrated that the isoenzyme hexosaminidase A was deficient in this disease. In 1970 Schneck and co-workers diagnosed the first case *in utero* and the diagnosis was confirmed on fetal tissues after a therapeutic abortion. During the early 1970s a number of carrier-detection screening programs for Tay-Sachs disease (TSD) were estab-lished in several metropolitan centers of the United States, and soon thereafter similar programs were developed in other countries with a large Ashkenazi Jewish population.

Clinical features

Infants with TSD usually appear normal at birth but by the age of 6 months parents may note that their affected child is unusually quiet, listless, and apathetic. Early in the disease parents may also note difficulty in feeding and hypotonia (particularly of the pectoral muscles). Soon these infants develop spasticity, fail to hold up their heads, and show abnormal limb movements. Accompanying these early signs is an exaggerated startle response. On hearing a sharp sound, infants respond with a rapid extension of both arms and a startled expression. The motor response of affected infants resembles decerebrate posturing and myoclonus. Eye involvement is detected early in the disease; findings include inattentiveness, fixed gaze, and abnormal eye movements. By the age of 3 or 4 months fundiscopic findings indicate the development of the classic cherry-red spot. The spot itself is not the abnormal finding, but merely represents the color of the choroidal vessels, which at the depth of the relatively acellular fovea are covered only by the pigment epithelium. The characteristic feature of the cherry-red macula is the whitish halo surrounding the fovea. This halo consists of lipid-laden biopolar ganglion cells, which are most dense in this region of the retina. Blindness occurs between the ages of 12 and 18 months. Optic atrophy may either precede or follow the blind-ness, but is usually present by the age of 2 years. As the neurological symptoms progress, the cranium becomes enlarged. Epileptiform seizures are common and are frequently associated with episodes of abnormal laughter and autonomic dys-function. Hypothalamic involvement may lead to precocious puberty after the age of 2 years. In the terminal stage of the disease affected children are quiet and hypotonic and the startle reaction is much less exaggerated. If these children sur-vive to the age of 3 years, their hands become pudgy, with tapering of the fingers, and their skin takes on a faint yellowish hue. Eventually the seizures decrease in frequency and severity, but progressive cachexia and aspiration pneumonia usually lead to death before the age of 4 years. There is little or no organomegaly except for an increase of about 40 percent in head size compared with children of the same age.

Diagnosis

Clinically this diagnosis should be suspected in any Ashkenazi Jewish infant with progressive psychomotor retardation, exaggerated startle response, and visual difficulties. The findings of a cherry-red spot, hypotonia, and apathy in the absence of hepatosplenomegaly makes the diagnosis of TSD highly probable.

Confirmation of the diagnosis is easily made in the laboratory through detection of a deficiency in the activity of the isoenzyme hexosaminidase A in serum, leukocytes, skin fibroblasts, urine, saliva, tears, and a number of other tissues (Figures 5.23 and 5.24).

Prenatal diagnosis of TSD can be made using a variety of techniques. One of the most recent methods is acrylamide gel electrophoresis of the cell-free amniotic fluid. At the present time it is still essential to confirm the prenatal diagnosis by analysis of cultured amniotic fluid cells. Currently efforts are being devoted to

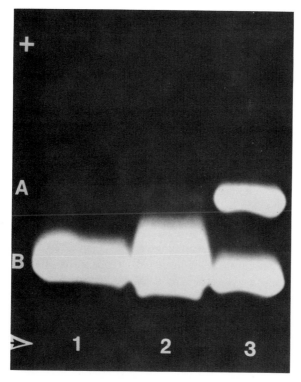

Figure 5.23. Fluorescent bands of beta hexosaminidase activity after electrophoresis of cultured fibroblasts on cellulose acetate gel at pH 6.0 and development with fluorogenic substrate. (Lane 1) Patient with Tay-Sachs disease (note absence of hexosaminidase A). (Lane 3) A normal individual with hexosaminidase A and B. (Lane 2) A variant individual showing a minor band of enzyme activity migrating between hexosaminidase B and the point of application. Exposure time necessary for the photographic documentation of the hexosaminidase A band in lane 2 caused this minor slow-moving band, quite distinct visually, to appear as part of the hexosaminidase B band. Courtesy of M. C. Rattazzi, Buffulo, N.Y. For a discussion of this variant see R. Navon et al., 1976, *Am. J. Hum. Genet.* 28:339.

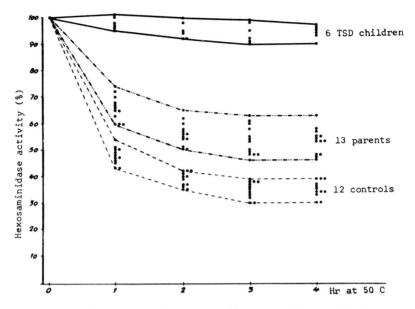

Figure 5.24. Heat inactivation curves of hexosaminidase activity from peripheral leukocytes. Note that in affected cases there was practically no inactivation of the enzyme, while the heterozygous parents showed an intermediate level compared to those affected and to the normal controls. Enzyme activity is expressed as the percentage of initial activity in nonheated samples. The range of initial activities was 1.5–2.0 nmol of substrate cleaved by 1 ml of leukocyte solution diluted 1:100. From B. Padeh and Navon, 1971, *Israel J. Med. Sci.* 7:259.

improving the rapid-tissue-culture and microbiochemical methods for the purpose of reducing the time required to diagnose this disease using cultured amniotic cells.

It has been demonstrated that in a few families at risk for TSD, healthy members may appear to be lacking hexosaminidase A (Figure 5.23). Thus, the absence of this isoenzyme from cultured amniotic cells and amniotic fluid may produce an uninterpretable situation. In such a case hexosaminidase A levels should be determined in both parents before the prenatal diagnosis is made.

The histopathological changes that occur in the brain of a patient with TSD are striking. The gross brain weight in a child over the age of 1:6 years may be 20–50 percent greater than normal, with diffusely broadened cortical gyri and an edematous, necrotic white matter. A diffuse neuronal storage process causes the neurons to lose their angular, pyramidal shape. The nerve cell body increases two- to three-fold in diameter and develops a blunt ballooned-out or pear shape, with its nucleus displaced to one side and its Nissl substance reduced (Figures 5.25 and 5.26). In cases of longer survival there is a marked reduction in neurons, and those that remain contain pyknotic nuclei in various stages of disintegration. Within the white matter there is an intense astrofibrosis with marked proliferation of proto-plasmic astrocytes and microglia. Myelin deficiency occurs, marked by a 50–85 percent decrease in cerebrosides caused by arrested myelinogenesis and secondary demyelination. Cerebellar atrophy occurs, accompanied by severe loss of Purkinje and granule cells.

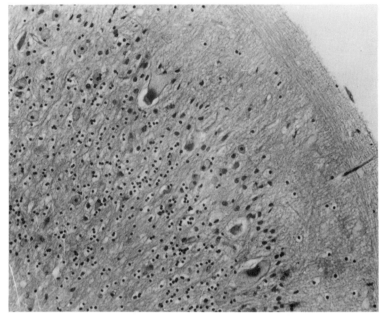

Figure 5.25. Low-resolution micrograph of the cerebellar cortex of a patient with TSD showing a ballooning of the cytoplasm of many nerve cells, especially the Purkinje cells. Courtesy of C. Bubis and G. Seltzer, Israel.

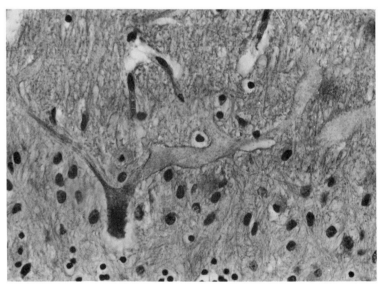

Figure 5.26. High-resolution micrograph of a ballooned nerve cell. Courtesy of C. Bubis and G. Seltzer, Israel.

Nerve cells outside the central nervous system show similar changes.

Ultrastructural studies have shown that the pale-staining, finely granular cytoplasm contains numerous bodies, approximately 1 micron in diameter, composed of concentrically arranged electron-dense arrays of membranes. In 1963 Samuels and co-workers reported the following breakdown for the dry weight of these bodies: 55 percent gangliosides, 20–25 percent cholesterol, approximately 10 percent phospholipid, 4–5 percent cerebrosides, and the remaining 5 percent amino acids and protein.

Basic defect

In 1968 Robinson and Stirling observed two hexosaminidase components in the lysosomal fraction of human spleen which, because they differed in charge, could easily be separated from each other by ion exchange chromatography and starch gel electrophoresis. The following year Okada and O'Brien noted that the more negatively charged enzyme component hexosaminidase A was absent from the tissues of patients with TSD.

Immunochemical studies suggested that hexosaminidases A and B (hex A and hex B) share at least one common antigenic determinant. Later it was demonstrated that hex A has a specific antigen not found in hex B. These findings led Srivastava and Beutler to propose that hex A might be a heteropolymer composed of two different types of subunits, alpha and beta, whereas hex B is probably a homopolymer made up of identical subunits of only the beta variety.

In 1976 Geiger and Aron dissociated the placental enzymes (hex A and hex B) into 25,000-dalton polypetide chains and determined their amino acid composition. Their proposed model for each enzyme consisted of 4 polypeptide chains linked together by disulfide bridges. In the same year Beutler and co-workers reported similar findings. They dissociated hex A into subunits and showed their recombination into enzymatically active hex A, hex B, and hex S. Hex S is a minor hexosaminidase whose activity is increased by Sandhoff disease (gangliosidosis type II). By hybridizing hex S from Sandhoff liver with placental hex B, Geiger and Aron formed a hex A which upon electrophoresis was indistinguishable from placental hex A. Their observations supported the 2-gene theory they had proposed in 1973, namely that hex B was a homopolymer of beta subunits, while hex A was a heteropolymeric structure with alpha and beta subunits. According to this theory, TSD represents a defect in the alpha subunit which results in a deficiencey of hex A and leads to an excess of hex B. Sandhoff disease involves a mutation of the beta chain such that neither hex A nor hex B is formed. Instead, the alpha chain homopolymer hex S is formed and is present in increased amounts in Sandhoff disease.

Both hex A and hex B show GM_2-ganglioside cleaving activity, but that of hex A has been shown to be 8 times greater than that of hex B. It has therefore been concluded that the $beta_2$ subunit is responsible for most of the catalytic activity while the $alpha_2$ subunit is involved in overcoming the hinderance imposed on the breakdown of GM_2 by its sialic acid moiety.

Linkage studies have shown that the gene for hex A is located on chromosome no. 15 while that for hex B is on chromosome no. 5.

Despite our sophisticated knowledge of TSD, several questions remain unanswered from both a biochemical and a clinical viewpoint.

Genetics

Although this disease has been reported from every continent and in many ethnic groups, 90 percent of all affected children are of Ashkenazi Jewish descent (primarily from the Lithuanian and Polish provinces of Korno and Grodno). A few Israeli TSD families are of Sephardi origin.

Family studies show that the disorder is transmitted as an autosomal recessive trait with nearly complete penetrance. The sexes are equally affected.

It is now possible to identify the heterozygous carrier of TSD. The genetic surveys that have been conducted in the past few years among the Ashkenazi Jewish communities of the U.S., Canada, South Africa, and Israel suggest a carrier rate of about 1:27, although in some communities it is as high as 1:15 and in others as low as 1:30. The estimated carrier rate in non-Jewish Americans is 1:300. The consanguinity rate among Ashkenazi Jewish parents is not significantly elevated compared to that observed in non-Jewish parents with affected children. Although the reported incidence among Ashkenazi Jewish newborns is 1:6,000, the actual number may be much higher, for some cases are not reported. It is thought that the true incidence among Ashkenazi Jews may be close to 1:3,600 births. For a discussion of the reasons why the TSD gene is so common among Ashkenazi Jews, the reader is referred to Chapter 12.

In 1977 Kaback reported some of the results of the TSD carrier-screening programs. As of late 1976 more than 160,000 young adults had volunteered for the serum hexosaminidase A screening test and nearly 7,000 heterozygotes had been identified. Of the 101,000 American Ashkenazi Jews screened (without known carriers or affected offspring in their families) 1 in 27.3 were carriers of the TSD gene (heterozygote frequency = 0.037). Critically, 125 couples who had not had offspring with TSD were identified as being "at risk" for the occurrence of the disease in their children (both parents being carriers). Prenatal monitoring for TSD has occurred in at least 12 countries. Four hundred sixty "at risk" pregnancies have been studied—371 in couples with 1 or more previously affected children and 89 in "at risk" couples identified through carrier screening. One hundred twenty affected fetuses have been identified (99 and 21, respectively, in the two "at risk" groups) and 115 have been electively aborted. One TSD infant was missed *in utero* and 339 unaffected children were born as predicted.

A crucial problem in all the screening programs for the detection of TSD carriers is the discrimination between those who are true carriers and those who are normal homozygotes. Even a small percentage of "false positives" among the normal homozygotes will considerably increase the proportion of couples defined as carriers and at risk for TSD, exposing them to unnecessary emotional stress and the pregnant women to amniocentesis. In a recent report on the screening of 3,629 Israelis for TSD carriers, Padeh and co-workers estimated the rate of "false positive" individuals at risk for TSD to be 1:13.5 couples while the rate of "true positives" who are missed or are "false negatives" is 1:20. As laboratory methods continue to improve, there will be better separation of the genotypes, thus eliminating this overlap. Not all screening programs have the same degree of difficulty in differentiating genotypes, but the problem does exist.

A number of genetic, social, and psychological questions have arisen as a result of TSD screening programs and these will be discussed in Chapter 11.

Prognosis and treatment

TSD is a lethal disease and most affected children die between the ages of 2 and 2:6 years, although 1 patient is known to have reached the age of 6 years. Frequently the length of survival depends upon the quality of nursing care and the treatment of multiple respiratory infections.

Enzyme replacement has been tried in a few TSD patients using both intravenous and intrathecal routes, but neither has improved the clinical course of the disease. There are a number of problems involved with enzyme replacement therapy and these are discussed in Chapter 11.

References

Aaronson, S. M.; Valsamis, M. P.; and Volk, B. W. 1960. Infantile amaurotic family idiocy: Occurrence, genetic considerations, and patho-physiology in the non-Jewish infant. *Pediatrics* 26:229.

Beutler, E.; Yoshida, A.; Kuhl, W.; and Lee, J. E. S. 1976. The subunits of human hexosaminidase A. *Biochem. J.* 159:541.

Brady, R. O.; Pentchev, P. G.; and Gal, A. E. 1975. Investigations in enzyme replacement therapy in lipid storage diseases. *Fed. Proc.* 34:1310.

Geiger, B., and Arnon, R. 1976. Chemical characterization and subunit structure of human N-acetylhexosaminidases A and B. *Biochemistry* 15:3484.

Geiger, B.; Navon, R.; Ben-Yoseph, Y.; and Arnon, R. 1975. Specific determination of N-acetyl-β-D-hexosaminidase isozymes A and B by radioimmunoassay and radial immunodiffusion. *Eur. J. Biochem.* 56:311.

Gilbert, F.; Kucherlapati, R.; Creagan, R. P.; Murnane, N. J.; Darlington, G. J.; and Ruddle, R. H. 1975. Tay-Sachs' and Sandhoff's diseases: The assignment of genes for hexosaminidase A and B to individual chromosomes. *Proc. Natl. Acad. Sci.* 72:263.

Kaback, M. M. 1977. Heterozygote screening and prenatal diagnosis in the control of Tay-Sachs disease. *Hum. Hered.* 27:186.

Kaback, M. M.; Nathan, T. J.; and Greenwald, S. 1977. Tay-Sachs disease: Heterozygote screening and prenatal diagnosis—U.S. experience and world perspective. In *Tay-Sachs disease: Screening and Prevention,* ed. M. M. Kaback, pp. 13–36. New York: Alan R. Liss.

Kaback, M. M.; Zeiger, R. S.; Reynolds, L. W.; and Sonneborn, M. 1974. Approaches to the control and prevention of Tay-Sachs disease. *Prog. Med. Genet.* 10:103.

Klenk, E. 1942. Über die Ganglioside des Gehirins bei der infantilen amaurotischen Idiotie vom Typus Tay-Sachs. *Ber. Deutsch Chem. Ges.* 75:1632.

Kolodny, E. H. 1979. Tay-Sachs disease. In *Genetic diseases in Ashkenazi Jews,* ed. R. M. Goodman and A. G. Motulsky. New York: Raven Press, forthcoming.

Makita, A., and Yamakawa, T. 1963. The glycolipids of the brain of Tay-Sachs disease: The chemical structures of a globoside and main ganglioside. *Jpn. J. Exp. Med.* 33:361.

Navon, R.; Geiger, B.; Ben-Yoseph, Y.; and Rattazzi, M. C. 1976. Low levels of beta-hexosaminidase A in healthy individuals with apparent deficiency of this enzyme. *Am. J. Hum. Genet.* 28:339.

Navon, R., and Padeh, B. 1971. Prenatal diagnosis of Tay-Sachs genotypes. *Br. Med. J.* 4:17.

Navon, R.; Padeh, B.; and Adam, A. 1973. Apparent deficiency of hexosaminidase A in healthy members of a family with Tay-Sachs disease. *Am. J. Hum. Genet.* 25:287.

O'Brien, J. S.; Okada, S.; Fillerup, D. L.; Veath, M. L.; Adornato, B.; Brenner, P. H.; and Leroy, N. G. 1971. Tay-Sachs disease: Prenatal diagnosis. *Science* 172:61.

Okada, S., and O'Brien, J. S. 1969. Tay-Sachs disease: Generalized absence of β-D-N-acetyl-hexosaminidase component. *Science* 160:698.

Padeh, B. 1973. A screening program for Tay-Sachs disease in Israel. *Israel J. Med. Sci.* 9:1330.

Robinson, D., and Stirling, J. L. 1968. N-Acetyl-β-glucosaminidases in human spleen. *Biochem. J.* 107:321.

Sachs, B. 1887. On arrested cerebral development, with special reference to its cortical pathology. *J. Nerv. Ment. Dis.* 14:541.

Sandhoff, K.; Conzelmann, E.; and Nehrkorn, H. 1977. Specificity of human liver hexosaminidases A and B against glycosphingolipids GM_2 and GA_2: Hoppe-Seyler's 2. *Physiol. Chem.* 358:779.

Schneck, L.; Valenti, C.; Amsterdam, D.; Friedland, J.; Adachi, M.; and Volk, B. W. 1970. Prenatal diagnosis of Tay-Sachs disease. *Lancet* 1:582.

Srivastava, S. K., and Beutler, E. 1973. Hexosaminidase A and hexosaminidase B: Studies in Tay-Sachs' and Sandhoff's disease. *Nature* 241:463.

Tallman, J. F.; Brady, R. O.; Navon, R.; and Padeh, B. 1974. Ganglioside catabolism in hexosaminidase A–deficient adults. *Nature* 252:254.

Tallman, J. F.; Brady, R. O.; Quirk, J. M.; Villalba, M.; and Gal, A. E. 1974. Isolation and relationship of human hexosaminidases. *J. Biol. Chem.* 249:3489.

Tay, W. 1881. Symmetrical changes in the region of the yellow spot in each eye of an infant. *Trans. Ophthalmol. Soc. U.K.* 1:155.

Volk, B. W., and Schneck, L., eds. 1976. *Current trends in sphingolipidoses and allied disorders.* New York: Plenum Press.

6

Genetic disorders among Sephardi and Oriental Jews

MOST OF THE GENETIC diseases and the few polymorphisms mentioned in this chapter occur in the Sephardi and Oriental Jewish communities but are also found in non-Jewish populations of the world. Furthermore, these disorders tend to be found within individual Jewish ethnic subgroups rather than dispersed among the many communities that make up the two major non-Ashkenazi groups. There are some exceptions to this pattern of occurrence and they will be discussed accordingly.

ATAXIA-TELANGIECTASIA

Historical note

Although the initial description of this disorder was given by Syllaba and Henner in 1926, it was Madame Louis-Bar in 1941 who described its major clinical components. In 1958 Boder and Sedgwick reported 7 children with sino-pulmonary infection, progressive ataxia, and telangiectasis. They coined the term *ataxia-telangiectasia* (A-T) to describe this syndrome. Subsequent studies have shown that A-T patients have thymic abnormalities, an immunologic defect, an increase in malignancy, various endocrine abnormalities, and chromosomal instability.

In 1971 Levin and Perlov called attention to the remarkably large number of cases found among Jewish children of Moroccan ancestry. Most recently Levin and co-workers reviewed their experience with 47 Israeli cases.

Clinical features

Since the clinical features noted in the above-mentioned Israeli patients are similar to those seen in other patients with this disease, most comments will pertain to the recent observations made by Levin and co-workers.

The earliest sign of the disease, progressive cerebellar ataxia, can often be observed as the child begins to walk. This alteration frequently leads to marked invalidism before the age of 6 years and involves gait, motor coordination, and the ability to stand, walk, and speak. Chronically "red" eyes due to telangiectasis of

124

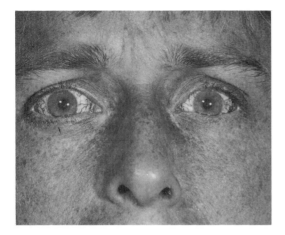

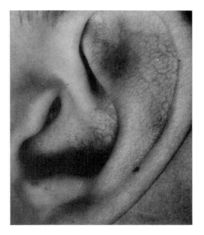

Figure 6.1. Telangiectasia involving the eyes.

Figure 6.2. Telangiectasia of the external ear.

the bulbar conjunctivae are often seen in the first few years of life and are eventually observed in all cases of A-T (Figure 6.1). Telangiectasia of the skin, cheeks, ears (Figure 6.2), or shoulders is less common, particularly in Israeli patients.

Most affected children suffer recurrent respiratory infections from early infancy and many develop purulent bronchiectasis and sinusitis.

Primary or secondary involvement of other systems may be noted. For example, nystagmus occurs early and is a prominent feature of oculomotor dyspraxia; malabsorption of unknown cause was observed in two Israeli infants but cleared spontaneously after a year or two; skin findings other than telangiectasia include pigmented nevi, café-au-lait spots, vitelligo, seborrhea, and sclerodermal-like changes. Other ectodermal findings include premature graying of the hair, loss of subcutaneous fat, and the appearance of atrophic scars. Lymphatic tissue is abnormally deficient, and tonsillar and glandular response to infections is minimal. Sexual development is fairly normal, although it may be delayed. Stunted growth is common but may be secondary to chronic infection. A third of the patients in the Israeli study were found to be mentally retarded; poor educational opportunities due to physical disabilities caused by the progressive and chronic nature of the disease may have been a major contributory factor in this finding.

Older patients show joint contractures, kyphoscolosis, absence of tendon reflexes, and myoclonic jerks.

Diagnosis

The clinical features of A-T are quite distinct. Cytogenetic studies have shown: (1) increased chromosomal instability with breakage and rearrangement in the majority of patients; (2) breakage and rearrangement in skin fibroblasts as well as lymphatic cells; and (3) specificity of damage, with chromosome no. 14 preferentially involved. The rearrangement of chromosome no. 14 in A-T patients usually involves a translocation between no. 14 and other chromosomes of the complement, but in some cases additional material has been detected on no. 14. G-banding has shown that the band 14q12 may be a highly specific exchange point. The exact interpretation of these chromosomal changes is not known, but changes involving no. 14 occur in other conditions leading to malignancies of lymphoid origin. Figures 6.3–6.5 show some of the chromosomal changes observed in A-T patients.

Serum IgA is low or absent in 70 percent of A-T patients, while secretory IgA is deficient in the saliva or duodenum in most cases. IgE also may be deficient, and most cases of A-T are marked by combined IgA and IgE deficiency.

Antibody response to bacterial and viral antigens is diminished, and autoantibodies are found in about half of the patients with A-T.

Peripheral blood lymphocyte counts are usually lower than normal; in the Israeli study about two-thirds of the patients had less than 2,000 lymphocytes/cm and one-third less than 1,000/cm.

The proportion of T-cells as studied by E Rosettes and T-cell cytotoxicity with anti-T-cell serum was normal or low normal in all the Israeli patients. Levin and co-workers feel that although some degree of diminished cellular immunity may be found in most patients with A-T, there is great variability in the type and degree of deficiency present. Table 6.1 shows the immunologic findings they have noted.

Of the Israeli patients studied, 10 out of 17 showed marked hypoglycemia, resistance to ketosis, absence of glycosuria, and elevated plasma insulin levels in response to the administration of glucose or tolbutamide. The amount of 17-ketosteroids and 17-hydroxysteroids present may be normal or diminished. Gonadotropin secretion in response to FSH and LSH was found to be diminished in 5 cases (2 boys and 3 girls), indicating a possible gonadal dysfunction. However, gonadotropin excretion in postpubertal females was noted to be within normal range. Thyroid function was normal.

Alpha-fetoprotein in the blood is usually elevated in A-T patients. This may be an important observation because it has recently been shown that alpha-fetoprotein in mice suppresses certain T-dependent functions.

Table 6.1. Ataxia-telangiectasia: Immunologic studies in Israeli cases

Immunologic factor	Normal	Slightly abnormal	Deficient
E Rosettes	6/11	4/11	1/11
T-Cytotoxicity	7/13	6/13	—
LIF			
PHA	3/13	2/13	8/13
PPD	3/13	3/13	7/13
Interferon			
"Nonimmune"	3/4	—	1/4
"Immune"	3/4	—	1/4
Cyc.-AMP (Lymphs)	1/2	1/2	—
EAC. Rosettes	12/12	—	—
SMI g			
IgG	6/7	1/7	—
IgA	3/6	3/6	—
IgM	4/6	2/6	—
IgE	3/3	—	—
IgD	2/2	—	—
Immunoglobulins			
IgG	15/15	—	—
IgA	9/15	2/15	4/15
IgM	14/15	1/15	—

Source: S. Levin, Israel.

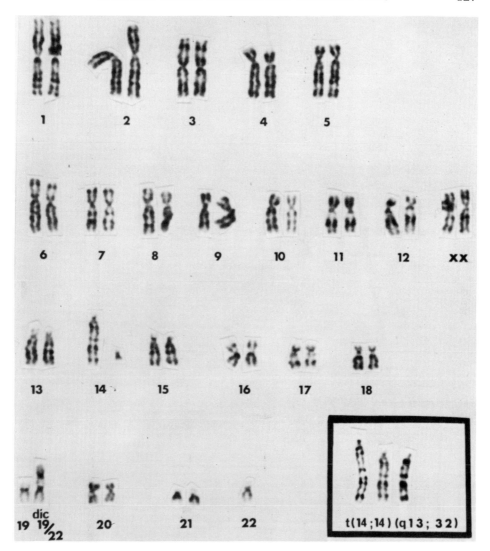

Figure 6.3. G-banded karyotype of clone cell from an A-T patient with clonal translocation (14;14) (q12;q32). In addition, a dicentric chromosome has formed from one chromosome no. 19 and one chromosome no. 22. The latter is a random change. Inset shows three clonal markers from other cells of the clone. From J. M. Oxford et al., 1975, *J. Med. Genet.* 12:251.

Electromyography may show a reduced nerve conduction velocity consistent with denervation. Electroencephalographic studies have not shown any consistent changes.

Basic defect

The basic defect in A-T is not known. In 1977, Joncas and co-workers found early antigen antibodies to the Epstein-Barr virus (E.B.V.) in 8 of 16 patients with

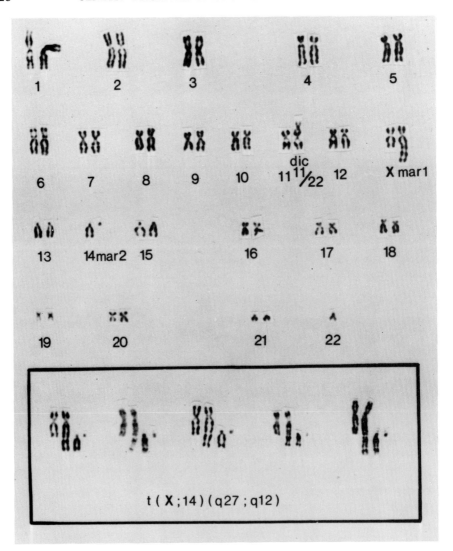

Figure 6.4. G-banded karyotype from an A-T patient with clonal translocation (X;14) (q27;q12). In addition a dicentric chromosome has
formed from one chromosome no. 11 and one chromosome no. 22.
The latter is a random change. The large marker is referred to as mar
1, the smaller one as mar 2. From J. M. Oxford et al., 1975, *J. Med.
Genet.* 12:251.

A-T. They postulated that the early antibody response, along with changes in
chromosome no. 14, could lead to transformation of lymphoid cells into the
malignant state following the cells' exposure to E.B.V. or other putative carcinogens.
Alternatively, with cell-mediated immunity being generally impaired in A-T patients,
a deficiency in the regulatory function of a T-cell subpopulation on B-cells could
contribute to the dysfunction of the target B-cell of the E.B.V. infection. The
target cell transformed in A-T may be a genetically defective, dysfunctional,
IgA-producing lymphoid cell.

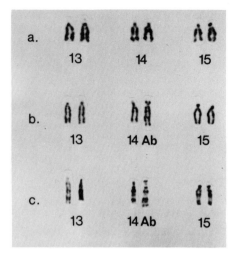

Figure 6.5. D-group chromosomes from
G-banded cells of an A-T patient showing (a) normal D-group chromosomes
and (b,c) the abnormal chromosome
probably derived from a chromosome no.
14. From J. M. Oxford et al., 1975, *J.
Med. Genet.* 12:251.

Genetics

A-T is considered to be an autosomal recessive disorder and family studies in
Israel confirm this mode of genetic transmission. In 23 Israeli families known to
have this disease, 47 affected individuals were observed, representing 31 percent of
the individuals at risk in these sibships. The sex ratio among the affected was 24
females and 23 males. The rate of consanguinity in these families was 52 percent,
which is significantly higher than that for the general population.

The ethnic distribution of this disorder in Israel is given in Table 6.2. Of the 23
families affected, 18 were Jewish. Of these 18, 17 originated in Morocco (36
affected members), 1 in Algeria (1 affected member). Of the 5 non-Jewish families
3 were Moslem Arabs (5 affected members), 1 was Christian Arab (2 affected
members), and 1 was Druze (3 affected members). No cases were observed among
Jewish families of Ashkenazi descent. The concentration of this disease in the

Table 6.2. Ethnic distribution of ataxia-telangiectasia in Israel

Ethnic origin of affected families	No. of affected families	No. of affected children	Consanguinity
Jewish Sephardi	18	37	7
Moroccan	17	36	
Algerian	1	1	
Arab (Israeli)	4	7	4
Druze (Israeli)	1	3	1
Total	23	47	12

Source: S. Levin, Israel.

Moroccan Jewish community is striking. The frequency of A-T homozygotes has been estimated to be about 1:40,000 in the general population. In 1971 Levin and Perlov estimated the frequency of this disease in the Moroccan Jewish community to be 1:8,000, but the true frequency in this community may be higher.

Prognosis and treatment

A-T is a fatal disease from which the majority of patients die before or during their teens. In rare cases individuals have survived to the age of 40 years. Progressive respiratory distress is a common cause of death during the first and second decades of life. As these patients grow older and the neurological defect progresses, they develop a mask-like face with diminished grimacing, drooling at the mouth, difficulty with speech, and choreoathetoid-like movements of the limbs. Older patients become bedridden and must depend on others for the performance of normal functions.

Malignancies occur in about 10 percent of A-T cases, the majority being lymphoreticular or leukemic, with the remainder involving epithelial, nervous, and mesenchymal tissues. The average age of onset of lymphatic tumors is 10 years, whereas nonlymphatic tumors occur at about 20 years. Malignant neoplasms are common in relatives of A-T patients, and in A-T heterozygotes under the age of 45 years the risk of dying from cancer is 5 times greater than that for the general population. In the Israeli series of 47 cases, 6 developed cancer (2 lymphosarcoma, 2 lymphoma, 1 acute lymphatic leukemia, and 1 basal-cell carcinoma of the scalp).

Treatment, unfortunately, is mainly palliative, with efforts being made to prevent the development of bronchiectasis or severe pulmonary disease. Control of ataxia and of involuntary movements has not been properly achieved, although recently *Dantrium*, a hydantoin compound, has been reported to be beneficial.

The use of transfer factor to stimulate the defective immune system has not proved to be useful in the majority of cases. Plasma infusions in IgA-deficient patients with acute infections have been tried with some success, although the level of secretory IgA is not affected. Bone marrow and thymus transplantation have not proved successful.

References

Boder, E. 1975. Ataxia-telangiectasia: Some historic, clinical, and pathological observations. In *Immuno-deficiency in man and animals*, ed. D. Bergsma, p. 255 (Stamford, Conn.): Sinauer Assoc.

Boder, E., and Sedgwick, R. 1958. Ataxia-telangiectasia: A familial syndrome of progressive cerebral ataxia, oculocutaneous telangiectasia, and frequent pulmonary infection. *Pediatrics* 21:526.

Cohen, M. M.; Shaham, M.; Dagan, J.; Shneli, E.; and Kohn, G. 1975. Cytogenetic investigation in families with ataxia-telangiectasia. *Cytogenet. Cell Genet.* 15:338.

Joncas, J., et al. 1977. Unusual prevalence of antibodies to Epstein-Barr virus early antigens in ataxia telangiectasia. *Lancet* 2:1160.

Levin, S., and Perlov, S. 1971. Ataxia-telangiectasia in Israel. *Israel J. Med. Sci.* 7:1535.

Levin, S.; Gottfried, E.; and Cohen, M. 1977. Ataxia-telangiectasia: A review, with observations on 47 Israeli cases, *Paediatr.* 6:135.

Louis-Bar, D. 1941. Sur un syndrome progressif comprenant des telangiectasies capillaires cutanées et conjonctivales symétriques à disposition naevoide et des troubles cérébelleaux. *Confin. Neurol.* 4:32, 1941.

McFarlin, D. E.; Strober, Q.; and Waldman, T. A. 1972. Ataxia-telangiectasia. *Medicine* 51:281.

Oxford, J. M.; Harnden, D. G.; Parrington, J. M.; and Delharity, J. D. A. 1975. Specific chromosome aberrations in ataxia-telangiectasia. *J. Med. Genet.* 12:251.

Reed, W. B.; Epstein, W. L.; Boder, E.; and Sedgwick, R. 1966. Cutaneous manifestation of ataxia-telangiectasia. *JAMA* 195:746.

Swift, M.; Shoman, L.; Perry, M.; and Chase, C. 1976. Malignant neoplasms in the families of patients with ataxia-telangiectasia. *Cancer Res.* 36:209.

Syllaba, L., and Henner, K. 1926. Contributions à l'indépendance de l'athethose double idiopathique et congénitale: Atteite familiale, syndrome dystrophique, signe du réseau vasculaire conjonctival integrite psychique. *Rev. Neurol.* 1:541.

CONGENITAL ADRENAL HYPERPLASIA

The genetic syndrome congenital adrenal hyperplasia (CAH) occupies a key position in the list of those disorders responsible for the clinical picture of intersex. The disease is caused by an enzymatic defect at one of the various stages of steroid hormone synthesis in the adrenal gland. As a result of this defect, cortisol production is impaired—i.e. it becomes uninhibited. ACTH release occurs and increased amounts of intermediary steroids are produced, many of which have an anabolic effect resulting in the clinical syndrome.

The characteristic clinical finding is increased androgen production. In the male this results in the picture of the "infant Hercules" and in the female in virilization of the external genitalia with a masculine habitus. The heterosexual picture in the female is usually more dramatic than the isosexual precocity of the male, and therefore diagnosis is usually made at an earlier stage in the female. This fact is of major importance in detecting the 21-hydroxylase deficiency variant, which appears in about one-third of the patients in the form of a life-threatening salt-losing crisis in the first weeks of life. The absence of abnormal external genitalia in the male makes clinical recognition of the problem less likely, unless there is a prior history of affected sibs to alert the physician. Lack of diagnosis in early infancy may also lead to problems in gender role definition. Prior to the understanding of the biochemical defect in this syndrome, genetic females were commonly reared as phenotypic males.

All forms of CAH are transmitted as an autosomal recessive disorder. The most common biochemical variant is 21-hydroxylase deficiency, with 11-hydroxylase deficiency and other forms being relatively rare. The 11-hydroxylase form is characterized by hypertension in addition to those features produced by excess androgen production.

The frequency of this syndrome is known to vary in different populations. In view of the large number of cases seen in one hospital in Israel, Porter and coworkers decided to review the number of cases diagnosed in Israel between the years 1957 and 1973. All cases were diagnosed on the basis of clinical findings and confirmation by laboratory studies. The survey covered 68 cases from 11 hospitals and was limited to two forms of CAH, 21- or 11-hydroxylase deficiency. Of the 68 cases, 54 had 21-hydroxylase deficiency while 14 had the 11-hydroxylase form. A

Table 6.3. Congenital adrenal hyperplasia: Distribution of Israeli cases

| | Type of CAH | |
	21-OH	11-OH
Number of cases	54	14
Male/female ratio	1.8	2.5
Consanguinity	7.4%	14.2%
Multiple sibs affected	22.2%	28.5%
Jewish North African origin	22.2%	64.2%

Source: S. Moses, Israel.

slight predominance of males was noted in both variants. In 6 cases some degree of parental consanguinity was present, and in 14 families more than 1 case was diagnosed. Twelve of the cases with 21-hydroxylase deficiency and 9 of the cases with 11-hydroxylase deficiency were Jews of North African ancestry. Table 6.3 shows the distribution of the Israeli patients according to enzymatic type, while Table 6.4 shows the incidence of the adrenogenital syndrome in Israel and in other population groups.

Among Jews, the North African Jewish community seems to have the highest occurrence of this disorder. In terms of population size it makes up approximately 12 percent of the total Israeli Jewish population, but it accounts for 22 percent of the cases of 21-hydroxylase deficiency and in 64 percent of the cases with 11-hydroxylase deficiency (Table 6.3). Further clarification and documentation of this syndrome among North African Jews is needed.

References

Childs, B.; Grumbach, M. M.; and Van Wyk, J. J. 1956. Virilising adrenal hyperplasia: A genetic and hormonal study. *J. Clin. Invest.* 35:213.

Gazi, Q. H., and Thompson, M. W. 1972. Incidence of salt-losing form of congenital virilising adrenal hyperplasia. *Arch. Dis. Child.* 47:302.

Hirschfeld, A. J., and Fleishman, J. K. 1969. An unusually high incidence of salt-losing congenital adrenal hyperplasia in the Alaskan Eskimo. *J. Pediatr.* 75:492.

Hubble, D. 1966. Congenital adrenal hyperplasia. In *Basic concepts of inborn errors and defects of steroid biosynthesis: Proceedings of the third symposium of the Society for the Study of Inborn Errors of Metabolism,* ed. K. S. Holt and D. N. Raine, p. 68. Edinburgh: Livingstone.

Table 6.4. Incidence of adrenogenital syndrome in different population groups

Author	Population	Type of AGS	Incidence	Heterozygote frequency
Childs, 1956	Maryland, U.S.	21-OH	1:67,000	1:128
Prader, 1972	Zurich, Switzerland	21-OH	1:18,500	1: 68
Hubble, 1966	Birmingham, England	21-OH	1: 7,255	1: 44
Rosenblum, 1966	Wisconsin, U.S.	21-OH	1:15,000	—
Hirshfeld, 1969	Alaska (Yupik Eskimos)	21-OH	1: 1,481 1: 490	1: 20 1: 11
Gazi, 1972	Toronto, Canada	21-OH	1:26,292	1: 82
Moses, 1973	Israel (North African Jewish community)	21-OH 11-OH	1:20,000 1:60,000	1: 90 1:150

Source: S. Moses, Israel.

Porter, B.; Finzi, M.; and Moses, S. 1978. The syndrome of congenital adrenal hyperplasia in Israel, in press.

Prader, A.; Anders, G. J. P. A.; and Habich, H. 1962. Zur Genetik des kongenitalen
adrenogenitalen syndrome. *Helv. Paediatr. Acta* 17:271.

Rosenbloom, A. L., and Smith, D. W. 1966. Congenital adrenal hyperplasia. *Lancet*
1:660.

CYSTINOSIS

Historical note

In 1903 Aberhalden described a marked increase in cystine content and cystine
crystals in the liver and spleen of a 21-month-old infant who died from "inanition."
Two of the child's sibs died of a similar disease which Abderhalden termed "familial
cystine diathesis." In 1924 Lignac reported widespread deposits of cystine in the
tissues of 3 children who had progressive renal insufficiency, wasting, dwarfism,
and severe rickets. During the 1930s several investigators elaborated on such features of the disease as rickets, dwarfism, glycosuria, albuminuria, and acidosis. In
1936 Fanconi demonstrated the increased excretion of organic acids and established the syndrome "nephrotic-glycosuric dwarfism with hypophosphatemic rickets." Although Fanconi thought that the disorder he described was distinct from
cystinosis, in actuality it was part of the same entity. However, not all cases of the
Fanconi syndrome show evidence of crystalline cystine deposits and, conversely,
not all patients with cystine deposits have the Fanconi syndrome. In 1973 Gadoth
and co-workers reported on the high frequency of the infantile form of cystinosis
among North African Jews.

Clinical features

Since the infantile form, not the adult or juvenile type, is common to Jewish
infants of North African origin, comments will be directed mainly to this group.

Children with the infantile form usually appear normal at birth but by the age
of 6 months most begin to show overt signs of the disease due to the renal tubular
defect in water reabsorption. The resulting polyuria and polydipsia make these
infants vulnerable to dehydration, which leads to recurrent fever. By the age of 1
year children usually show signs of growth retardation, rickets, acidosis, and other
chemical symptoms of renal tubular abnormalities. Other early manifestations of
the disease include recurrent episodes of acute prostration, weakness, and cardiovascular collapse, which can lead to sudden death.

Affected infants fail to thrive and are usually below the third percentile in both
height and weight throughout life. Rickets develops at an early age in most patients
and such skeletal changes as frontal bossing, genu valgum, thickening of the
wrists and ankles, and rachitic rosary are frequently observed.

Other clinical features not associated with renal problems include fair complexion and light-colored hair.

Eye involvement is common and severe photophobia is usually present within the
first few years of life. Slit-lamp examination shows homogeneously dispersed re-

fractile opacities in the cornea and conjunctiva. In the infantile and juvenile forms of cystinosis a peripheral retinopathy has been described. The pathological findings consist of a generalized pigment disturbance that assumes a depigmented patchy pattern with superimposed regularly distributed pigment clumps giving a fine pepper-like stippling. These changes occur more on the temporal side than the nasal side and are marked in the peripheral regions of the retina, whereas the central regions usually show no abnormal pigmentation. These retinal changes are perhaps the earliest findings of the disease and have been recognized during the first month of life.

There appears to be a direct relationship between the amount of crystine deposited in tissues and the clinical severity of the disease. In the late stage, patients suffer from the symptoms associated with severe renal failure and uremia.

Diagnosis

Clinically this disorder must be considered in any child with vitamin-D-resistant rickets, the Fanconi syndrome, or glomerular insufficiency. The retinal changes previously mentioned are most helpful in making an early diagnosis, as is looking for cystine crystals in the cornea (slit-lamp examinations), in unstained preparations of peripheral blood or bone marrow cells, or in biopsies of rectal mucosa. The diagnosis can be confirmed by chemical determination of the cystine content of peripheral leukocytes or cultured skin fibroblasts. Prenatal diagnosis is possible by demonstrating an increased amount of nonprotein cystine in cultured amniotic fluid cells.

Basic defect

The basic defect in this disorder is not known. Many hypotheses have been proposed but later discarded because of lack of support by subsequent investigations. Although the underlying cause of the accumulation of excessive quantities of cystine has not been identified, the site of crystal formation has been established as intracellular. The site has been further localized to a subcellular organelle—the lysosome.

Genetics

Family studies support autosomal recessive transmission of this disease. Homozygous patients have cystine deposits in one or many tissues, while heterozygous carriers apparently have moderately elevated cystine concentrations in cells but do not develop the cystine storage diathesis. The existence of three clinical forms of the disorder suggests genetic heterogeneity, but the nature of these different mutations is not well understood biochemically.

Of 20 Israeli cases of the infantile form, 15 were Sephardi Jewish children whose parents or grandparents were born in North Africa. Extensive family studies were not done in this study, but the investigators estimated the incidence in the North African Jewish community to be 1:20,000 in contrast to 1:40,000 or 1:60,000 in non-Jewish populations.

Prognosis and treatment

The prognosis in this disorder is directly related to the amount and distribution of cystine deposited in tissues.

Treatment of nephropathic cystinosis is mainly symptomatic and consists of providing adequate fluid intake, correcting the metabolic acidosis and potassium deficit, and healing the rickets. Such measures are effective in maintaining growth, development, and a feeling of "well-being" in affected children. More specific forms of therapy for the nephropathic problem involve the use of thiol reagents, cystine-poor diets, and renal transplantation. Of these three, renal transplantation seems to be the most promising, but a longer follow-up of the children who undergo this operation is needed to better evaluate the effectiveness of this therapeutic approach.

References

Abderhalden, F. 1903. Familiäre cystindiathese. *Z. Physiol. Chem.* 38:557.

Fanconi, G. 1936. Der nephrotisch-glykosurische Zwergwuchs mit hypophosphatämischer Rachitis. *Dtsch. Med. Wochenschr.* 62:1169.

Gadoth, N.; Moses, S. W.; and Boichis, H. 1975. Cystinosis in Israel. *Harefuah* 88:113.

Lignac, G. O. E. 1924. Über Störung des Cystinstoffwechsels bei Kindern. *Dtsch. Arch. Klin. Med.* 145:139.

Schulman, J. D., ed. 1973. *Cystinosis,* pp. 1–245. Washington, D.C.: Government Printing Office.

Scriver, C. R., and Rosenberg, L. E. 1973. *Amino acid metabolism and its disorder,* pp. 222–26. Philadelphia: W. B. Saunders.

CYSTINURIA

Historical note

Cystinuria is frequently confused with cystinosis, but the two disorders are very different. In cystinuria the problem is formation of cystine renal calculi, whereas in cystinosis it is the accumulation of intracellular cystine in various tissues.

Cystinuria is a well-recognized and rather common inborn error of metabolism. Highlights of the history of the disease begin in 1810 with Wollaston's first description of cystine bladder calculi. In 1908 Garrod postulated that this disease is an inborn error of metabolism. In 1955 Harris and co-workers documented recessive inheritance. In 1964 one group of investigators reported a defect in the uptake of dibasic amino acids by kidney slices, while another noted a defect in uptake of cystine and dibasic amino acids by gut mucosa. In 1967 Rosenberg confirmed genetic heterogeneity. In 1974 Weinberger and co-workers reported the high frequency of this disorder among Jews of Libyan origin.

Clinical features

Crystalluria and calculus formation are the major clinical symptoms in this disorder. Cystine calculi have been detected during the first year of life and as late as the ninetieth, but the initial symptoms of lithiasis appear most commonly during the third and fourth decades of life. Males and females are affected with about equal frequency, but as is true of all types of renal lithiasis, morbidity is more frequent in males.

Pure cystine stones are easy to recognize, for they are sand-colored, granular, and may be recovered from any part of the renal system. These stones are radiopaque but their roentgenologic density is less than that of calcium or magnesium stones. Stones in cystinuric patients have a tendency to grow to a large size and may form a cast of the entire pelvic system or grow to the size of an egg in the bladder.

Colic, the most common presenting symptom, may be associated with obstruction of the urinary tract, subsequent infection, and eventual loss of renal function. Infection, hypertension, and renal failure occur occasionally and may cause the patient to seek medical care.

Diagnosis

Not all cystinuric patients pass pure cystine stones. Almost 10 percent of the stones passed contain no detectable cystine. Thus, stone analysis per se is an unsatisfactory means of excluding the diagnosis of cystinuria in patients with renal lithiasis.

The diagnosis of cystinuria is not a difficult one. The appearance of hexagonal, flat crystals in the urine of a patient who has not been taking sulfa drugs is pathognomonic, but examination for these crystals should be carried out only on concentrated urine specimens.

The cyanide-nitroprusside test is a simple and useful diagnostic aid in this disorder. The addition of sodium cyanide to a urine sample made alkaline with ammonium hydroxide leads to the reduction of cystine to cysteine. The cysteine forms a magenta-red complex when sodium nitroprusside is added. The test will be markedly positive in homozygotes and weakly positive in those heterozygotes who excrete modest or moderate excesses of cystine. Acetone, various drugs, and homocystinuria also give a positive response, but all can easily be differentiated.

Diagnostic confirmation depends on demonstration of the characteristic amino acid pattern in the urine. Selective excessive excretion of cystine, lysine, arginine, and ornithine is not observed in other pathological aminoacidurias and can easily be detected by paper chromatographic or electrophoretic techniques. Homozygotes and heterozygotes can be distinguished using quantitative amino acid determinations obtained by column chromatography.

Stones generally form at cystine excretion rates of greater than 300 mg of cystine per g of creatinine in acid urine.

Basic defect

The basic defect in this disorder is not known. Recent studies have shown an intestinal defect similar but not identical to the renal lesion in this disorder. The lack of amino acid transport defects in the circulating leukocytes of cystinuric individuals precludes the use of leukocytes in discerning the genetic features of this disease. Furthermore, these findings attest to the variation in transport systems observed in a group of substances that exist in tissues with different morphological and functional characteristics.

Genetics

Differences in the pattern of the defect in the kidney and the intestine and in its manifestations among heterozygotes have led to the conclusion that there are at least three allelic mutations. Kindreds in which both types I and II are segregating demonstrate that the genes for these types are allelic. Cystinuria type I seems to be completely autosomal recessive, since heterozygotes for this type have a normal urinary amino acid profile. Heterozygotes for types II and III excrete excessive or moderately increased amounts of the characteristic amino acids—especially cystine and lysine—and intestinal absorption of these amino acids differs in types II and III. Homozygotes for all three types, as well as compound heterozygotes and probably some heterozygotes for type II, form urinary cystine stones and are clinically indistinguishable.

The incidence of homozygous cystinuria in the population of England has been estimated to be 1:20,000. In a comprehensive population survey in the United States in 1972, Levy and co-workers did chromatographic analyses of urine specimens from 141,903 newborns. They found the frequency of homozygous cystinurics to be 1:17,738. No estimates are presently available for the gene frequencies of the various alleles. The majority of cystinuria patients are considered to be homozygotes for type I.

In 1974 Weinberg and co-workers reported their evaluation of 24 Israeli patients with cystine lithiasis representing 24 cystinuric families and their screening survey for cystinuria in 385 school children (ages 6–14 years) of Jewish Libyan origin. Their studies revealed that 7 of 24 unrelated Israeli Jewish families affected with cystinuria were of Libyan descent. Five of these 7 families were intensively investigated. Heterozygotes were identified in 4 of them, indicating that, contrary to other populations, the cystinuria in this community is mainly type II or type III (Table 6.5). Among the randomly screened healthy school children of Libyan descent, 3–4 percent were found to be heterozygotes for cystinuria. It is estimated that in the Libyan Israeli community the overall frequency of mutant cystinuria alleles among Libyan Jews may be as high as 0.02. This would result in an incidence of about 1:2,500, which is among the highest reported. Further large-scale screening is underway in an attempt to clarify whether or not particularly high frequencies of cystinuria characterize specific subpopulations of Libyan Jews; several such isolates still maintain their identity within the Israeli society.

Table 6.5. Cystinuria: Ethnic distribution and type in
24 Israeli Jewish patients

Community	No. of probands	No. of families evaluated	Type of cystinuria	
			I	II or III
Ashkenazim	12	7	4	3
Libyan	7	5	1	4[a]
Others	5	3	2	1
Total	24	15	7	8

Source: A. Weinberger et al., 1974, *Hum. Hered.* 24:568.

[a] The parents in one of these families are compound heterozygotes.

Prognosis and treatment

The prognosis in this disorder is excellent when patients are identified early and placed on proper therapy. Treatment is directed at reducing the concentration of cystine in the urine by increasing urine volume, increasing cystine solubility by alkalinizing the urine, and reducing cystine excretion by the use of D-penicillamine. This last drug, although effective, is not without its complications and should be used only in those patients who fail to respond to more conservative therapy.

References

Garrod, A. E. 1908. The Croonian lecturer. *Lancet* 2:1, 73, 142, 214.

Gold, R. J. M.; Dobrinski, M. J.; and Gold, D. P. 1977. Cystinuria and mental deficiency. *Clin. Genet.* 12:329.

Harris, H.; Mittwoch, U.; Robson, E. B.; and Warren, F. L. 1955. Phenotypes and genotypes in cystinuria. *Ann. Hum. Genet.* 20:57.

Hershko, L.; Ben-Ami, E.; Paciorkovski, J.; and Levin, N. 1965. Allelomorphism in cystinuria. *Proc. Tel-Hashomer Hosp.* 4:21.

Levy, H. J.; Shih, V. E.; and MacCready, R. A. 1972. Massachusetts metabolic disorders screening program. In *Early diagnosis of human genetic defects,* ed. M. Harris, pp. 47–66. Washington, D.C.: Government Printing Office.

Rosenberg, L. E.: Genetic heterogeneity in cystinuria. 1967. In *Amino acid metabolism and genetic variation,* ed. W. L. Nyhan, pp. 341, 349. New York: McGraw-Hill.

Scriver, C. R., and Rosenberg, L. E. 1973. *Amino acid metabolism and its disorders,* pp. 156–77. Philadelphia: W. B. Saunders.

Weinberger, A.; Sperling, O.; Rabinovitz, M.; Brosh, S.; Adam, A.; and de Vries, A. 1974. High frequency of cystinuria among Jews of Libyan origin. *Hum. Hered.* 24:568.

Wollaston, W. H. 1810. On cystic oxide, a new species of urinary calculus. *Phil. Trans. R. Soc. Lond.* [*Biol.*]

DOWN SYNDROME
(MONGOLISM)

Down syndrome, or mongolism, is generally thought to have an incidence of 1:600 live births. In 1970 Wahrman and Fried published findings from their epidemiological study of this disorder in Jerusalem from July 1, 1965, to June 30, 1969. This study of Down syndrome in newborns included all hospital births in a well-defined geographical area. Possible stratification was counterbalanced by pooling the results obtained from the only 4 hospitals in the area. Accurate diagnosis was guaranteed by chromosome analysis, which was performed in all Down patients and in suspected cases of the disease. With the exception of 2 cases, all patients were Jewish. Altogether 53 cytologically proven cases were found among 24,248 live births, giving an incidence of 2.19/1,000 live births (1:457), which is among the highest rates yet reported. The frequency of translocation mongolism was 3/53 (5.7 percent). In 2 of these cases translocation chromosomes D/G and G/G were inherited from the mothers, whereas in the third, G/G appeared sporadically. The 10 best clinical signs were selected and their frequencies and usefulness in arriving at a clinical diagnosis were established.

Table 6.6. Mongolism: Annual incidence in Jerusalem, 1965–1969

| Period | No. of falsely suspected mongoloids[a] | No. of cytologically proven mongoloids | | | Total no. of live births | Incidence per 1,000 live births | Incidence |
		Regular trisomy-21 mongolism	Translocation mongolism	Total			
First year	1	16	1	17	5,969	2.68	1:351
Second year	7	13	—	13	5,940	2.19	1:457
Third year	4	12	1	13	5,972	2.18	1:459
Fourth year	—	9	1	10	6,364	1.57	1:636
Total and average	12	50	3	53	24,245	2.19	1:457

Source: J. Wahrman and K. Fried, 1970, *Ann. N.Y. Acad. Sci.* 171:341. Reprinted by permission of the New York Academy of Sciences.
Note: $\chi^2 = 2.30$; D.F. = 3; $p = 0.70$–0.50.
[a] All falsely suspected mongoloids had a normal karyotype except for 1, who was a normal/45 Turner mosaic.

In attempting to explain this high incidence, Wahrman and Fried made the following observations. The overall increase in incidence of Down syndrome in Jerusalem was rather evenly distributed among the various age groups and thus could be attributed to some factor operating in the same direction for all age groups. These investigators emphasized that this increase could well be due to the utilization of a prospective approach involving personal examination of all cases as well as chromosomal studies.

Table 6.7. Distribution of ages of all mothers and mothers of mongoloids and corresponding frequencies of mongoloids and normal births in Jerusalem, 1965–1969

Mother's age group	Estimated no. of live births[a]	No. of mongoloids observed	Incidence/1,000 births	Incidence	% of mongoloid births in mother's age group relative to total mongoloid births	% of births in mother's age group relative to total births
−19	1,101	2	1.82	1:550	3.77	4.54
20–24	6,522	6	0.92	1:1,087	11.32	26.90
25–29	7,465	8	1.07	1:933	15.09	30.79
30–34	5,543	12	2.17	1:462	22.64	22.86
35–39	2,708	11	4.06	1:246	20.75	11.17
40–44	773	12	15.52	1:64	22.64	3.19
45+	136	2	14.72	1:68	3.77	0.56
Total and average	24,248	53	2.19	1:457	99.98	100.01

Source: J. Wahrman and K. Fried, 1970, *Ann. N.Y. Acad. Sci.* 171:341. Reprinted by permission of the New York Academy of Sciences.
[a] Extrapolated from figures for the period 1964–1966 kindly supplied by Dr. A. M. Davies.

Table 6.8. Community and country of origin of mothers of mongoloids
and of 27 control newborns

Community and country of origin	Mothers of mongoloids	Mothers of controls
Jewish		
Morocco	11	9
Algeria	2	0
Tunisia	4	0
North Africa (unspecified)	1	0
Turkey	1	0
Iraq	7	4
Persia (Iran)	7	1
Kurdistan	1	2
Yemen	2	0
Sephardi (unspecified)	2	1
Ashkenazi	11	7
Unknown	2	2
Non-Jewish		
Finland	1	0
Unknown	1	1
Total	53	27

Source: J. Wahrman and K. Fried, 1970, *Ann. N.Y. Acad. Sci.* 171:341.
Reprinted by permission of the New York Academy of Sciences.

In attempting to compare their results with other findings reported in the literature Wahrman and Fried noted that the standards for recognition of Down syndrome vary tremendously from place to place. They concluded that the problem of the incidence of mongolism at birth in different populations can be properly evaluated only by careful, unbiased clinical screening of birth populations combined with chromosomal studies, preferably by one team of investigators. It may therefore be premature to state that Down syndrome is more common in Jews than in other populations.

Tables 6.6–6.9 and Figures 6.6–6.8 show some of the main findings of the Wahrman-Fried study.

Table 6.9. The ten best clinical signs of Down syndrome

Clinical sign	No. showing sign/ no. checked	Percentage showing sign
1. Abundant neck skin	48/51	94.1
2. Corner of mouth turned downward	42/50	84.0
3. General hypotonia	28/34	82.4
4. Flat face	39/49	79.6
5. At least one dysplastic ear	39/50	78.0
6. Epicanthus in at least one eye	38/50	76.0
7. Gap between toes one and two	35/52	67.3
8. Protruding tongue	32/51	62.7
9. Circumference of head at birth not more than 32 cm	20/47	42.6
10. Simian crease in at least one hand	22/52	42.3

Source: J. Wahrman and K. Fried, 1970, *Ann. N.Y. Acad. Sci.* 171:341. Reprinted by permission of the New York Academy of Sciences.

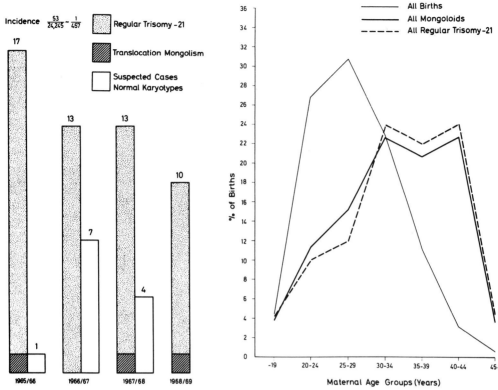

Figure 6.6. Annual distribution of regular trisomy-21 mongoloids, translocation mongoloids, and falsely suspected mongoloids who were found to have normal karyotypes. From J. Wahrman and K. Fried, 1970, *Ann. N.Y. Acad. Sci.* 171:341. Reprinted by permission of the New York Academy of Sciences.

Figure 6.7. Maternal age distribution for all births, all mongoloid births (including cases of translocation mongolism), and regular trisomy-21 births alone. From J. Wahrman and K. Fried, 1970, *Ann. N.Y. Acad. Sci.* 171:341. Reprinted by permission of the New York Academy of Sciences.

Reference

Wahrman, J., and Fried, K. 1970. The Jerusalem prospective newborn survey of mongolism. *Ann. N.Y. Acad. Sci.* 171:341.

DUBIN-JOHNSON SYNDROME

Historical note

This disorder consists of chronic idiopathic jaundice and was first described in 1954 by Dubin and Johnson. Since its original description numerous cases have been described throughout the world and it is now known that this condition has a wide ethnic and geographical distribution. In 1955 Klajman and Efrati first reported cases from Israel and soon thereafter it was noted that this disorder is especially prevalent among Iranian Jews. In 1970 Shani and co-workers reported the results of an extensive clinical and genetic study of this disease in 101 Israeli

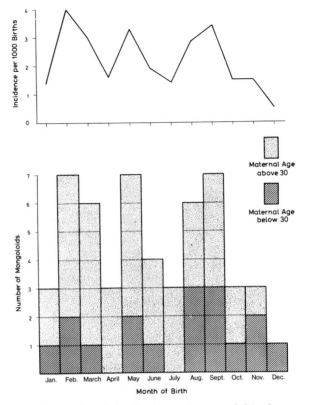

Figure 6.8. Distribution of mongoloids by month of birth and corresponding monthly incidence per 1,000 live births. In the histogram mongoloid births are divided by age of mother (above or below 30). From J. Wahrman and K. Fried, 1970, *Ann. N.Y. Acad. Sci.* 171:341. Reprinted by permission of the New York Academy of Sciences.

patients, which is the largest series ever reported from a single country. Their findings form the basis of the present-day understanding of this syndrome among Oriental and Sephardi Jews.

Clinical features

Chronic or intermittent jaundice is a finding common to all patients with Dubin-Johnson syndrome (DJS). The onset of jaundice generally occurs between the ages of 15 and 35 years, although it has been observed in an infant at 10 weeks and in an adult for the first time at the age of 56 years. The jaundice may be precipitated or aggravated by many factors, including pregnancy, surgery, severe physical strain, alcoholism, and infectious diseases. Shani and co-workers noted that 73 of their 101 patients complained of vague abdominal pains, while 28 patients were asymptomatic except for the jaundice. Among those complaining of abdominal pain, 59 patients also complained of weakness after slight effort, 32 had occasional nausea and vomiting, and 14 complained of recurrent diarrhea. Of these 101 patients, 54 had hepatomegaly and in 39 there was tenderness upon palpation of the liver.

In the Israeli series, 15 patients had mild bleeding manifestations such as epistaxis, ecchymoses, and excessive bleeding after tooth extractions. The significance of these findings will be discussed under the heading "Association with factor VII deficiency."

Diagnosis

Chronic or intermittent idiopathic hyperbilirubinemia and a liver biopsy showing pigmentary changes typical of this condition are adequate criteria for the diagnosis of DJS.

Biopsied liver tissues frequently appear dark-gray when discharged into fixative prior to microscopy. Microscopically the most striking finding in these tissues is the presence of a coarsely granular brownish-yellow pigmentation in the parenchymal cells (Figure 6.9). The pigment is located mainly in the centrilobular zones but may involve the entire lobule; at times the Kupffer cells also contain a small amount of brown pigment. The amount of abnormal pigment varies considerably, as does the size of the granules. The bile canaliculi are normal and the liver is free of fibrosis or inflammatory infiltrate.

In various nonspecific liver function studies the levels of serum proteins, transaminases, bile acids, and alkaline phosphatase are usually within normal limits or may be slightly elevated. Flocculation tests also are normal. In contrast, all DJS patients show a marked retention of such dyes as Bromsulphalein (BSP), rose bengal, methylene blue, and indocyanine green. This retention appears to be due to some defect in excretion by the hepatic cells. During the first 30 minutes after injection, BSP is cleared from the plasma at a rate similar to that noted in normal subjects; the level of the dye in the plasma then rises again and remains elevated for as long as 48–72 hours, although exceptions to this may occur. With BSP the proportion of dye conjugated with glutathione in the plasma gradually increases and an appreciable amount of the injected dye can be recovered from the urine. Oral cholecystography frequently fails to visualize the gall bladder or shows it only faintly. Intravenous administration of contrast medium may enhance visualization.

Measurements of serum bilirubin show elevated conjugated (direct) and total levels. These levels tend to fluctuate, depending on a variety of factors, some of which have been mentioned previously. For example, the levels of total serum bilirubin may range from normal to 19 mg per 100 ml of plasma. Values for conjugated bilirubin range from 26 to 86 percent of the total bilirubin, with a mean value of 60 percent.

The main laboratory findings in DJS patients are shown in Table 6.10.

Basic defect

The basic defect in this disorder is not known, but it is thought that it concerns the biliary secretory mechanism of the liver. It has been shown that the organic anions are secreted abnormally, while the organic cations are secreted normally. This altered secretory mechanism is most probably related to the abnormal accumulation of hepatic pigment.

Corriedale sheep have been found to have morphological and functional defects similar to those noted in DJS patients. They exhibit impaired excretion of organic anions but normal excretion of cations, which suggests that different mechanisms are involved in the excretion of these two groups of compounds.

Association with factor VII deficiency

In their study of DJS patients, Shani and co-workers noted that some patients (mainly those of Iranian origin) showed decreased levels of factor VII and some even had mild bleeding manifestations (see "Clinical features"). To properly evaluate this observation they screened 78 of 101 DJS patients for vitamin K–dependent clotting factors. In addition they examined 138 normal, non-DJS relatives from 24 unrelated families.

Since a great number of the DJS patients belonged to the Iranian Jewish community, two control groups were examined for factor VII levels: 52 non-Iranian Jews and 57 Iranian Jews. No difference was detected between the control groups.

Further studies showed no difference between the DJS and control groups' levels of factors II, IX and X, but a highly significant difference was observed in their factor VII levels (Table 6.11).

In 33 DJS patients the level of factor VII was below normal, and in 4 of them levels 2–10 percent of normal were noted. This deficiency was not confined to DJS patients, however, for 51 of 138 normal relatives also had decreased levels of factor VII.

Analysis of the pedigrees of the families studied showed various combinations of the two disorders among individual members (Figure 6.10). There were DJS patients with severe factor VII deficiency or no deficiency. Normal family members had normal, partially decreased, or severely decreased levels.

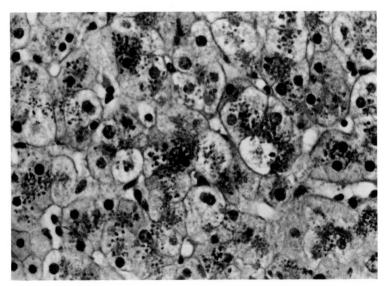

Figure 6.9. Micrograph of biopsied liver tissue from a DJS patient. Note the pigment (black granules) in the majority of the liver cells. Courtesy of G. Seltzer and C. Bubis, Israel.

Table 6.10. Dubin-Johnson syndrome: Main laboratory findings in Israeli patients, 1970

Laboratory test	Values	No. of patients	Total no. examined
Serum bilirubin, total maximal	1.8–3.9	52	
levels (% mg)	4.0–5.9	30	
	6.0–9.9	10	
	10.0+	9	101
Bilirubin in conjugated form (%	≤ 50	15	
of total bilirubin)	≥ 51	86	101
BSP retention at 45 min (%)	≤ 6	11	
	9–19	35	
	≥ 20	20	66
BSP level at 90–120 min (compared	Decreased	—	
to level at 45 min)	Unchanged	2	
	Increased	33	35
BSP maximal transport rate	> 1	—	
(Tm) mg/min	< 1	15	15
SGOT units	≤ 40	96	
	≥ 41	5	101
Alkaline phosphatase	Normal	79	
	Increased	4	83
Flocculation and turbidity tests	Normal	82	
	Abnormal	9	91
Visualization of gall bladder	Oral { clear	4	
upon cholecystography	faint	11	
	absent	46	61
	I.V. { clear	14	
	faint	7	
	absent	19	40
Prothrombin time (%)	≥ 71	32	
	41–70	55	
	≤ 40	9	96
Clotting factor VII (%)	≥ 42	45	
	13–41	29	
	3–12	4	78
Urinary coproporphyrin I (%	≤ 40	3	
of total)	≥ 60	59	62

Source: M. Shani et al., 1970, *Quart. J. Med.* 39:549.

Table 6.11. Dubin-Johnson syndrome: Factor II, VII, IX, and X levels in
Israeli patients and control subjects, 1970

	DJS patients			Control subjects			
	No.	Mean %	S.D.	No.	Mean %	S.D.	Significance of difference[a]
Factor II	66	88.9	18.1	40	96.6	16.9	$0.05 > p > 0.02$
Factor VII	78	51.9	25.5	109	85.2	31.3	$p < 0.00003$
Factor IX	59	80.4	32.3	21	85.0	27.1	$p > 0.5$
Factor X	63	98.9	26.1	40	100.6	25.2	$p > 0.05$

Source: U. Seligsohn et al., 1972, *Birth Defects* 8:133. Reprinted by permission of The National Foundation–March of Dimes, White Plains, New York.

[a] Statistical analyses for factor II, IX, and X levels were done by the t-test, whereas factor VII levels were analyzed by the Mann-Whitney U-test.

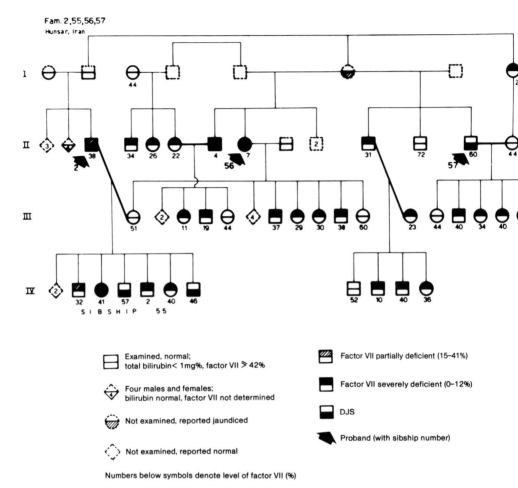

Figure 6.10. Pedigree of a family with 9 DJS patients demonstrating many combinations of DJS and factor VII deficiency. From U. Seligsohn et al., 1972, *Birth Defects* 8:133. Reprinted by permission of The National Foundation–March of Dimes, White Plains, New York.

    Factor VII deficiency in DJS patients was not limited to Iranian Jewish families but was also observed in 2 Iraqi and 4 out of 5 Moroccan Jewish families.

    What is the explanation for this association between DJS and factor VII deficiency? A number of ideas have been put forth, but the association still is not understood. McKusick has suggested that perhaps the DJS and factor VII loci are closely linked and that the 2 mutant genes are in coupling in a majority of the Iranian Jewish cases, not yet having attained equilibrium of linkage phase. Adam questions this linkage interpretation because the association has been seen in other Jewish ethnic groups as well as in Iranian Jews. Furthermore, he points to 1 family in which several recombinants of DJS and factor VII deficiency occurred among the children of a woman who must have been doubly heterozygous in coupling because her mother was doubly homozygous.

In terms of therapy, 4 factor VII–deficient patients received repeated intramuscular injections of vitamin K_1, but these had no effect on their factor VII levels.
Thus, many questions remain to be answered regarding the association of DJS with
factor VII deficiency.

Genetics

The recent survey of Israeli Jewish patients with DJS has shown, contrary to
previously held opinion, that the fully expressed condition is transmitted as an
autosomal recessive trait. Heterozygotes may have various subclinical symptoms of
the disorder. In tests with urinary coproporphyrin I, normals excreted 24.8 percent
of the coproporphyrin as coproporphyrin I, while homozygotes and heterozygotes
excreted 88.9 percent and 31.6 percent, respectively.

Sixty-four of the 101 cases studied by Shani's group were of Iranian origin
(Table 6.12). It has been calculated that 1 out of 1,300 Iranian Jews is affected,
compared with about 1 in 40,000 Sephardim and less than 1 in 100,000
Ashkenazim. The minimum prevalence of DJS in the Iranian Jewish community
(1:1,300) appears to be one of the highest rates in the world. To date, not a single
case of DJS has been found among the Yemenite Jews. The ancestors of the 64
Iranian patients came from at least 12 different cities in various parts of Iran
(Figure 6.11). Of these 12 cities, Isfahan seems to be the major source of the
syndrome. Before their mass migration to Israel the number of Jews in and around
Isfahan was estimated to be 10,000. The overall rate of consanguinity among
Iranian Jews was reported to be 26 percent, while among parents of the 39 Iranian
DJS sibships 46 percent were consanguineous.

From studies in Israel and other countries the sex ratio in DJS patients can now
be estimated (Table 6.13). In the Israeli study investigators found a ratio of 1.5
(61 males to 40 females), which is somewhat lower than that observed in other
published series. The slightly higher ratio 2.0 was noted in a Japanese study. A
possible explanation for the preponderance of diagnosed males may be the fact that
DJS occurs in males earlier than in females and also tends to be more symptomatic in males.

Table 6.12. Geographical origin of Israeli DJS patients, 1970

Country or community of origin	No. of unrelated kindreds	No. of probands	No. of patients
Iran	34	53	64
Iraq	6	9	9
Afghanistan	1	1	1
Morocco	6	9	9
Europe			
Ashkenazim	6	7	7
Sephardim	2	2	2
Israel			
Sephardim	2	2	6
Israel			
Arabs	2	3	3
Total	59	86	101

Source: M. Shani et al., 1970, *Quart. J. Med.* 39:549.

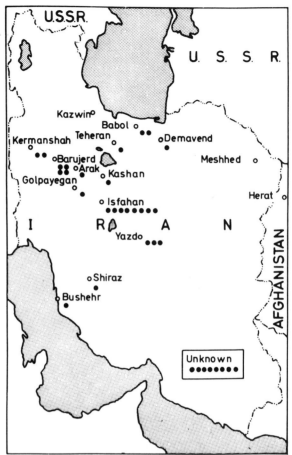

Figure 6.11. Origins of 34 Jewish Iranian kindreds
with DJS. Each solid dot indicates one kindred. From
M. Shani et al., 1970, *Quart. J. Med.* 39:549.

Prognosis and treatment

   Patients with DJS can live a normal life span and in general require no treatment. However, it is important to explain to these patients the benign nature of
their disease. In those who may have an associated factor VII deficiency mild
bleeding may occur, but these episodes respond well to symptomatic treatment.

References

Klajman, A., and Efrati, P. 1955. Prolonged jaundice with unidentified pigment in liver
    cells. *Lancet* 1:538.
McKusick, V. A. 1975. *Mendelian inheritance in man.* 4th ed., p. 454. Baltimore: The
    Johns Hopkins University Press.
Seligsohn, U.; Shani, M.; Ramot, B.; Adam, A.; and Sheba, C. 1970. Dubin-Johnson
    syndrome in Israel. II: Association with factor VII deficiency. *Quart. J. Med.* 39:569.

Table 6.13. Sex distribution and age of Israeli DJS patients at time of diagnosis

Age at time of diagnosis (yr)	Males		Females		Total
	Probands	Nonprobands	Probands	Nonprobands	
Birth–9	5	1	1	2	9
10–19	13	5	5	1	24
20–29	18		13	1	32
30–39	10		6	1	17
40–49	4	1	3	1	9
50+	4		4	2	10
Total	54	7	32	8	101

Source: M. Shani et al., 1970, *Quart. J. Med.* 39:549.

———. 1972. Association of hereditary factor VII deficiency and Dubin-Johnson syndrome. *Birth Defects* 8:133.

Shani, M.; Seligsohn, U.; and Adam, A. 1973. The inheritance of Dubin-Johnson syndrome. *Israel J. Med. Sci.* 9:1427.

Shani, M.; Seligsohn, U.; Gilon, E.; Sheba, C.; and Adam, A. 1970. Dubin-Johnson syndrome in Israel. I: Clinical laboratory and genetic aspects of 101 cases. *Quart. J. Med.* 39:549.

Wolkoff, A. W.; Cohen, L. E.; and Arias, I. M. 1973. Inheritance of the Dubin-Johnson syndrome. *N. Engl. J. Med.* 288:113.

FAMILIAL DEAFNESS

In 1969 Dar and Winter published a retrospective study of familial deafness in 430 deaf children from 319 northern Israeli families. In these 319 families familial deafness occurred in 209 children (48.6 percent) and was most prevalent among the North African Sephardi Jewish communities (Table 6.14), especially among Jews of Moroccan origin. Seventy-three percent of the familial cases had an autosomal recessive form of deafness (Table 6.15). The percentage of consanguineous matings among the deaf in the North African Jewish communities was 46 percent, compared to the normal overall rate of consanguinity in these communities of approximately 12 percent. Dar and Winter thought that consanguinity alone could not explain the high frequency of genetic deafness in the North African Jewish communities, since other Jewish ethnic groups have a much higher rate of consanguinity but a lower occurrence of deafness. Moreover, it has been noted that in the central part of Israel an autosomal recessive form of deafness is common in the Moroccan Jewish community.

A more complete genetic and audiological survey of familial deafness is needed to better assess this problem among the various Israeli Jewish communities in terms of detection, treatment, and genetic counseling.

References

Dar, H. and Winter, S. T. 1969. A genetic study of familial deafness. *Israel J. Med. Sci.* 5:1219.

Goldschmidt, E. A.; Ronen, A.; and Ronen, I. 1960. Changing marriage systems in the Jewish communities of Israel. *Ann. Hum. Genet.* 24:191.

Table 6.14. Ethnic origin, types of deafness, and percentage of consanguineous matings in families of 430 deaf children from northern Israel

Ethnic group	Type of deafness			Total no. and average rate	Overall rate of consanguineous matings by community[a]
	Familial	Acquired	Unknown		
North African Jews					
No. of affected children	118	36	25	179	12.0
No. of matings	46	36	25	107	
Consanguineous matings as percentage of total matings	46	19	12	26	
Ashkenazi Jews					
No. of affected children	26	29	18	73	2.5
No. of matings	18	29	18	65	
Consanguineous matings as percentage of total matings	0	4	6	3	
Arab and Druze					
No. of affected children	30	13	22	65	—
No. of matings	15	13	22	50	
Consanguineous matings as percentage of total matings	93	38	28	53	
Oriental Jews					
No. of affected children	32	15	9	56	25.0
No. of matings	16	15	9	40	
Consanguineous matings as percentage of total matings	56	27	22	35	
Unknown origin and Intercommunity matings					
No. of affected children	3	24	30	57	—
No. of matings	3	24	30	57	
Consanguineous matings as percentage of total matings	33	4	0	12	
Total and average					
No. of affected children	209	117	104	430	7.9
No. of matings	98	117	104	319	
Consanguineous matings as percentage of total matings	46	15	11	24	

Source: H. Dar and S. T. Winter, 1969, *Israel J. Med. Sci.* 5:1219.

[a] Data from E. A. Goldschmidt et al., 1960, *Ann. Hum. Genet.* 24:191.

FAMILIAL MEDITERRANEAN FEVER

Historical note

In 1945 Siegal was the first to recognize this disorder as a distinct entity and because of the nature of the abdominal attacks involved he termed the condition benign paroxysmal peritonitis. Siegal recognized the prevalence of the disorder among Jews and also called attention to its occurrence in Armenians. In 1948–1949 Reimann noted the periodic rhythmicity of the attacks and referred to the disorder as periodic disease. In the 1950s several French physicians published reports noting the familial occurrence of this disorder among the Jews of North

Table 6.15. Familial deafness: Mode of inheritance in relation to ethnic group

Mode of inheritance	Ethnic group					Total no. and average rate
	North African	Ashkenazim	Arab and Druze	Middle Eastern	Inter-community matings	
Autosomal recessive						
No. of deaf children	93	8	30	22	—	153
No. of matings	35	4	15	11	—	65
Percentage of children with familial deafness	79	31	100	69	—	55
Autosomal dominant						
No. of deaf children	25	11	—	10	2	48
No. of matings	11	9	—	5	2	27
Percentage of children with familial deafness	21	42	—	31	—	19
Both parents affected						
No. of deaf children	—	7	—	—	1	8
No. of matings	—	5	—	—	1	6
Percentage of children with familial deafness	—	27	—	—	—	5
Total						
No. of deaf children	118	26	30	32	3	209
No. of matings	46	18	15	16	3	98

Source: H. Dar and S. T. Winter, 1969, *Israel J. Med. Sci.* 5:1219.

Africa. In addition, they expanded the list of the disease's clinical manifestations and suggested that amyloidosis may be the cause of the renal manifestations. Beginning in 1952, Heller and co-workers further delineated the symptoms of this disease and confirmed its preferential occurrence in certain Jewish ethnic groups and its autosomal recessive mode of inheritance. Their studies further establish amyloidosis as the cause of the renal phase of the disease. From these investigations came the present-day term *familial Mediterranean fever* (FMF). In 1972 Goldfinger first reported the therapeutic use of colchicine in reducing the painful attacks in this disorder.

Clinical features

On the basis of their observations of 1,500 patients, Sohar et al. have divided the clinical features of this disease into two phenotypes. Phenotype I, the much more common form, consists of painful febrile attacks followed later in the course of the disease by amyloidosis. In a small percentage of cases amyloidosis presents as first or sole manifestation of the disease, and this form constitutes phenotype II.

More specifically, the diagnostic features of phenotype I are: (1) attacks of fever, usually of short duration, recurring at various intervals, sometimes over the course of many years; (2) pain in the abdomen, chest, joints, or skin, or in all, accompanying the fever; and (3) these findings in the absence of any known cause. The attacks usually continue with the appearance of amyloid nephropathy, but in some patients the attacks become less severe and less frequent.

In phenotype II the diagnosis can be established (1) if the amyloidosis occurs first, followed later by the attacks of fever, or (2) if amyloidosis is detected in a patient who gives a history of attacks in other family members. Table 6.16 lists the presenting signs in 470 patients with FMF.

Table 6.16. Familial Mediterranean fever: Presenting signs in
470 patients in the Tel Hashomer series

Presenting sign	Patients	
	Number	Percent[a]
Abdominal attacks	251	55.2
Joint attacks	120	26.1
Chest attacks	23	5.1
Simultaneous attacks	40	8.7
Fever attacks	14	3.0
Nephropathy	8	1.9
Unknown	14	—
Total	470	100.0

Source: E. Sohar et al., 1967, *Am. J. Med.* 43:227.
[a] Percentages calculated excluding unknowns.

The attacks of fever usually occur at an early age and have even been noted during the first few months of life. Two-thirds of the patients manifest symptoms by the age of 10 years and 90 percent by the age of 20. Usually pain in one of the previously mentioned sites precedes the fever by several hours. A temperature of 38–40 °C is reached in approximately 3–6 hours and may be accompanied by chills. The fever then rapidly subsides. Most attacks of pain regress completely in 12–24 hours, although they may last as long as 2 days and, when affecting the joints, even longer.

ABDOMEN

Abdominal attacks are the most dramatic and most common manifestation of FMF. The pain is localized at first but rapidly gains in intensity and spreads over the entire abdomen. Vomiting is frequent. Physical examination shows an exquisitely tender doughy abdomen which may progress to board-like rigidity with rebound tenderness, guarding, and absent bowel sounds. Roentgenographic studies may reveal fluid in the small bowel (Figure 6.12). Given these findings, it is understandable that many patients undergo abdominal surgery. Usually within a day the above symptoms abate and diarrhea follows.

CHEST

The chest pain associated with FMF tends to be unilateral and pleural in nature and radiates to the shoulder. Breathing is splinted, breath sounds are diminished, and in rare instances a friction rub is heard. A chest radiograph may show a small effusion, but this is absorbed within a day after the attack subsides.

JOINTS

Joint pains are episodic, recur at irregular intervals, and usually involve a single large joint. Sites of involvement in decreasing order of frequency are the knee (Figure 6.13), ankle, hip (Figure 6.14), shoulder, elbow, and sacroiliac joint. Most attacks terminate within a week, but some persist for a month and in rare cases much longer. The clinical picture is one of a rapidly evolving acute arthritis with exquisite tenderness and immobilization. The synovial fluid contains many leukocytes and is sterile. Roentgenographic findings show osteoporosis and, later,

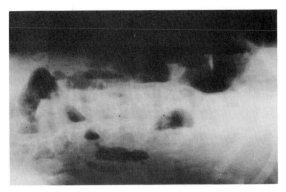

Figure 6.12. Horizontal flat plate of the abdomen in a patient with FMF. Note the typical paralytic ileus with distention of the intestine and fluid in the small bowel. Courtesy of M. Pras and J. Gafni, Israel.

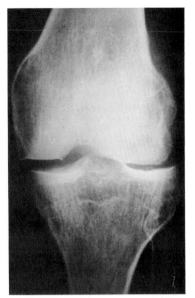

Figure 6.13. Chronic inflammation of the knee joint in a patient with FMF. Note the marked osteoporosis and narrowing of joint space. Courtesy of M. Pras and J. Gafni, Israel.

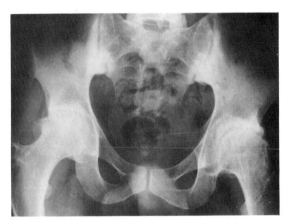

Figure 6.14. Hip involvement in a patient with FMF. Note the limitation of joint space, sclerosis, and destruction of the head of the left femur. Courtesy of M. Pras and J. Gafni, Israel.

mild osteoarthritic changes. However, in most cases these joint changes are reversible, the exception being the hip joint, which may develop aseptic necrosis and require replacement. Rheumatoid factor is consistently absent.

SKIN

An erysipelas-like erythema is a characteristic finding in FMF cases and may be the only manifestation of a febrile attack or may accompany one involving a joint. In general it appears around the ankle.

KIDNEY

Renal involvement with amyloidosis is independent of the appearance or severity of the clinical attacks of FMF. The nephropathy progresses through 4 stages. The presence of amyloidosis in the preclinical stage can be detected by either renal or rectal biopsy (Figures 6.15 and 6.16). The stage of proteinuria shows intermittent and, later, constant and massive proteinuria. The nephrotic

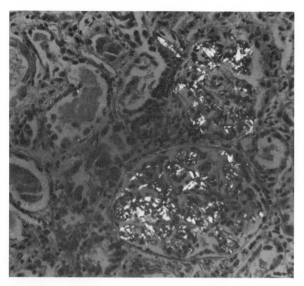

Figure 6.15. Amyloid deposits in an FMF patient as seen in the renal glomeruli after staining with congo red and examination with polarized light microscope. Courtesy of M. Pras and J. Gafni, Israel.

stage begins with a fall in serum albumin level and the appearance of edema. The final stage, uremia, follows after a variable, relatively short interval. Hypertension affects from one-third to one-half of these patients. Death due to renal failure occurs within 2–10 years after the onset of proteinuria, sometimes in the first decade of life, often in the second, and usually before the age of 40.

Diagnosis

No diagnostic test is presently available for FMF. A number of tests show consistently abnormal results at all stages of the disease and are the only significant findings until nephropathy appears. Cryofibrinogenemia has been observed in some patients during an acute attack. Increases in erythrocyte sedimentation rate, C-reactive protein, fibrinogen, hexosamine, IgM, haptoglobins, seromucoids, orosomucoids, and lipoproteins are the most common laboratory alterations observed. No specific deviations in the frequency of HLA antigens have been noted.

In the experience of the Tel Hashomer group, amyloidosis has been the most significant pathological finding during autopsy. The range of histopathological findings includes: vascular lesions of perireticulin amyloidosis throughout the body, except in the central nervous system, and amyloid involving the glomeruli, red pulp of the spleen, hepatic portal vessels, and alveolar capillaries of the lungs.

Amyloidosis in FMF

In 1968 Gafni and co-workers published a report on the role of amyloidosis in FMF. Of 316 actively followed-up living patients, 27 percent had developed amy-

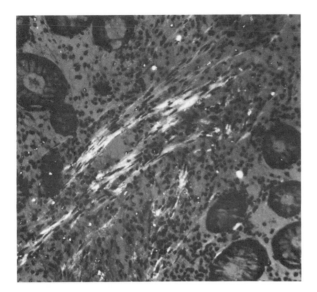

Figure 6.16. Amyloid deposits in an FMF patient seen upon rectal biopsy after staining with congo red and examination with polarized light microscope. Courtesy of M. Pras and J. Gafni, Israel.

loidosis. Of 85 FMF patients who had died, 83 had succumbed to amyloidosis. In a total of 401 actively followed-up cases, the frequency of amyloidosis increased progressively from 18 percent in patients born between 1955 and 1959 to 75 percent in those born before 1930. These investigators pointed out that the latter figure would presumably have been considerably higher had full ascertainment of the earlier cohorts been possible. They concluded that virtually all patients with FMF develop and die of amyloidosis. However, although amyloidosis is systemic, renal involvement accounts for the death of patients.

Basic defect

The basic defect in this disorder is unknown. Nevertheless, it has been shown that amyloid belongs to the fibrous class of proteins, consists of filaments that have periodicity, and is composed of helical strands. No significant findings were noted when the amino acid sequence of amyloid in FMF was compared to that in other disorders. Additional studies suggest that amyloid is produced by the fibroblast and other cells. Furthermore, changes in the fine structure of collagen have been demonstrated in amyloidosis. These later observations apply to all forms of amyloidosis, but, although important, fail to shed light on the basic alteration that occurs in FMF.

Genetics

The data collected by the Tel Hashomer group during their genetic analysis of 229 complete pedigrees (yielding 350 cases) supports an autosomal recessive mode of inheritance in FMF. However, in a few reported families FMF has occurred in more than 2 generations, which suggests genetic heterogeneity.

Among Jews, FMF occurs primarily in the North African Sephardi communities and with a very high gene frequency among Libyan Jews (Table 6.17). In this ethnic group 1 out of approximately 600 persons is affected, as compared to about 1:3,000–1:5,000 among the Ashkenazim. The overall gene frequency among the Sephardim is estimated to be about 0.022. The possibility that heterozygotic advantage balances the deleterious effect of the gene on reproduction in the Libyan Jewish community remains to be studied. Among the non-Jewish population of the countries in which most of the Sephardim with FMF were born (North Africa, Turkey, and the Balkans), FMF seems to be quite rare; however, it does occur in Turkey in individuals not of Armenian or Jewish ancestry and also in Arabs of the Middle East. On the other hand, it is known from the early reports of French physicians that only the Jewish communities of North Africa, and not the Arab population, developed the disease.

FMF occurs relatively frequently in Iraqi Jews and Armenians (Table 6.18). No satisfactory explanation has been given for this peculiar linking of the Sephardi Jews with the Armenians; however, clinically the manifestation of FMF in Armenians appears to be different (amyloidosis is apparently rare) from that in Sephardi Jews. Among the Ashkenazi Jews in Israel this disease is rare and in the Yemenite and Iranian Jewish communities it is virtually unknown. In his 1964 review of 50 cases of FMF from the United States, Siegal noted that 42 were Jews; 35 of these were of Ashkenazi origin, 3 of probable Ashkenazi descent, and 4 were Sephardi Jews. Of the more than 1,500 cases of FMF seen by the Tel Hashomer group, only 15 were Ashkenazi Jews. Why is there a discrepancy in the number of Ashkenazi cases seen in Israel and the United States? Differences in the Ashkenazi population structure of these two countries are not enough to account for this inconsistency.

Table 6.17. Country of origin of 470 FMF patients in the
Tel Hashomer series

Country of Origin	Jews		Non-Jews
	Sephardi	Ashkenazim	
Morocco, Tunis, Algeria	144	—	—
Libya	119	—	—
Iraq	64	—	—
Turkey	38	—	—
Other Mediterranean countries	32	—	—
Egypt	16	—	—
Kurdistan	9	—	—
Greece	9	—	—
Caucasia	8	—	—
Bulgaria	8	—	—
Syria, Lebanon	7	—	—
Italy	1	—	—
Romania	—	5	—
Poland	—	4	—
Germany	—	1	—
Israeli Arabs	—	—	5
Total	455	10	5

Source: E. Sohar et al. 1967, *Am. J. Med.* 43:227.

Table 6.18. Ethnic origin of 357 FMF patients reported as of 1967

Ethnic origin	Number		Percent[a]
Jews	200		57.5
Non-Ashkenazi		181	
Ashkenazi		3	
Not specified		16	
Armenians	87		27.0
Arabs	38		10.0
Levantine		36	
Algerian		1	
Not specified		1	
Other non-Jews[b]	22		6.0
Unknown	10		
Total	357		100.0

Source: E. Sohar et al., 1967, *Am. J. Med.* 43:227.

[a] Percentages calculated excluding unknowns.

[b] Ethnic origin presumed identical to country of origin: 16 from Mediterranean countries (France, 4; Spain, 3; Italy, 3; Turkey, 3; Greece, 2; Iran, 1), 4 from Sweden, and 1 from Holland.

Since the diagnosis of FMF is clinical, it is conceivable that part of the difference could be attributed to diagnostic opinion.

Many interesting genetic questions remain to be answered concerning the ethnic distribution of FMF and the possible role of heterogeneity in the disease (see Chapter 12).

Prognosis and treatment

No patient has ever been known to recover from FMF, and all autopsied cases from the Tel Hashomer series have shown amyloidosis to be the cause of death.

COLCHICINE

Numerous agents have been used to lessen the pain and severity of FMF attacks, but it was not until 1972 that Goldfinger demonstrated that the daily administration of colchicine aids in their prevention. The efficacy of colchicine in FMF has been proved in various studies, but one of the best was a well-designed, 4-month, double-blind, crossover study of 22 Israeli patients. The regimen consisted of either 0.5 mg of colchicine or a placebo taken twice daily for 2 months, followed by 2 additional months of the other treatment. Each patient served as his own control.

During the first 2 months of the study, the colchicine group experienced significantly fewer attacks (a mean of 1.15 per patient) than the placebo group (a mean of 5.25 per patient; $p < 0.01$). The patients who completed the crossover study had significantly fewer attacks while on colchicine than when they were on the placebo ($p < 0.01$). The mean decrease in the number of attacks experienced while taking colchicine was 3.85 for the 2-month period.

The use of colchicine to treat FMF raises a number of questions which in 1976 the Tel Hashomer group answered in part in their brief account of the response of 84 patients (13 with amyloid nephropathy) to colchicine treatment for 1–3 years. Because of the importance of this drug, an account of the Tel Hashomer findings follows.

Frequency of attacks. Fifty patients had no attacks, although many noted sensations usually premonitory of an attack; in 28 patients the frequency and severity of the attacks were markedly reduced. These results were achieved through a 1-mg daily dosage of 67 patients, while 11 patients required 1.5–2.0 mg daily. Development of drug tolerance was not noted. Six patients failed to respond to doses as high as 3 mg daily.

Effect on children. Children responded to an adult dosage of colchicine, but not to dosages calculated according to body weight. No untoward effect on growth and development was noted. Indeed, children who were underdeveloped, presumably because of frequent attacks, showed a spurt in growth and weight after colchicine-induced remission. Three girls experienced a normal menarche.

Effect on reproduction. Eleven unplanned pregnancies pre-empted the stopping of colchicine (as per instructions) 3 months before conception. Three male patients fathered normal children while on colchicine. Eight female patients conceived while on colchicine; 1 continued the drug through pregnancy and gave birth to a normal child. Of the 7 who stopped taking colchicine after pregnancy was detected, 1 (with nephrotic syndrome due to amyloidosis) aborted in the second month after a recurrence of the attacks, 1 gave birth to a child with Down syndrome, 2 continued their pregnancies, and 3 gave birth to healthy infants.

It is not possible to form any definite conclusions about the one child with Down syndrome born to a mother with FMF who took colchicine early in pregnancy; however, the Israeli group recommends the discontinuation of the drug 3 months before pregnancy is planned. Pregnancy does not seem to lessen the symptomatology in FMF.

Amyloid nephropathy. Urinary protein levels of 2+–3+ intensity diminished to traces or disappeared, and in 6 patients the decrease was quantitated (Table 6.19). Proteinuria did not increase in any patient, nor did it appear in any patients who had none at the beginning of treatment. Patients with renal insufficiency continued to deteriorate.

Table 6.19. Proteinuria measured at half-year intervals in colchicine-treated FMF patients

Case no.	Urinary protein level (mg/24 hr)	
	Study 1 (before treatment)	Study 2 (six months later)
1	360	100
2	3,000	850
3	3,000	260
4	450	240
5	575	280
6	240	0

Source: D. Zemer et al., 1976, *N. Engl. J. Med.* 294:170. Reprinted, by permission.

Side effects. Angioneurotic edema, in one patient and epistaxis (without laboratory evidence of disordered blood coagulation) in another prohibited continuation of colchicine when they recurred upon challenge by the drug. Diarrheal stools in 5 patients, muscle pains in 5, and rashes in 8, usually appearing early in treatment, subsided without necessitating interruption of treatment.

There is little doubt about the efficacy of colchicine in treating FMF, and as more patients are treated for a longer time our understanding of the effect of this drug will increase. Experimentally it has been shown that colchicine inhibits casein-induced amyloidosis in mice.

Other therapeutic measures that should be considered in the treatment of the renal phase of this disease are renal dialysis and renal transplantation.

References

Camatte, G.; Rouguette, M.; and Ruiz, M. 1953. Un cas de maladie périodique. *Bull. Mém. Soc. Méd. Hôp. Paris* 69:60.

Cattan, R. 1955. La maladie périodique. *Moroc. Méd.* 34:876.

Gafni, J.; Ravid, M.; and Sohar, E. 1968. The role of amyloidosis in familial Mediterranean fever: A population study. *Israel J. Med. Sci.* 4:995.

Gafni, J.; Sohar, E.; and Zemer, D. 1979. Amyloid nephropathy. In *Nephrology*, ed. J. Hamburger. Philadelphia: W. B. Saunders, forthcoming.

Gazit, E.; Orgad, S.; and Pras, M. 1977. HLA antigen in familial Mediterranean fever. *Tissue Antigens* 9:273.

Goldfinger, S. E. 1972. Colchicine for familial Mediterranean fever. *N. Engl. J. Med.* 287:1302.

Heller, H.; Gafni, J.; and Sohar, E. 1966. The inherited systemic amyloidoses. In *The metabolic basis of inherited disease,* ed. J. B. Stanbury, J. B. Wyngaarden, and D. S. Fredrickson, 2nd ed., p. 995. New York: McGraw-Hill.

Heller, H.; Sohar, E.; Kariv, I.; and Sherf, L. 1955. Familial Mediterranean fever. *Harefuah* 48:91.

Heller, H.; Sohar, E.; and Sherf, L. 1958. Familial Mediterranean fever. *Arch. Intern. Med.* 102:50.

Kedar, I.; Ravid, M.; Sohar, E.; and Gafni, J. 1974. Colchicine inhibition of casein-induced amyloidosis in mice. *Israel J. Med. Sci.* 10:787.

McKusick, V. A. 1975. *Mendelian inheritance in man,* 4th ed. p. 489. Baltimore: The Johns Hopkins University Press.

Mamou, H., and Cattan, R. 1952. La maladie périodique (sur 14 cas personnels dont 8 compliqués de néphropathies). *Semaine Hôp. Paris* 28:1062.

Pras, M., and Reshef, T. 1972. The acid-soluble fraction of amyloid: A fibril-forming protein. *Biocrim. Biophys. Acta* 271:193.

Reimann, H. A. 1948. Periodic disease: Probable syndrome including periodic fever, benign paroxysmal peritonitis, cyclic neutropenia, and intermittent arthralgia. *JAMA* 136:239.

Shamir, H.; Pras, M.; Sohar, E.; and Gafni, J. 1974. Cryofibrinogen in familial Mediterranean fever. *Arch. Intern. Med.* 134:125.

Sherf, L. 1953. Mamou-Cattan syndrome. M.D. Thesis, Hebrew University Medical School, Jerusalem.

Siegal, S. 1945. Benign paroxysmal peritonitis. *Ann. Intern. Med.* 22:1.

———. 1964. Familial paroxysmal polyserositis: Analysis of fifty cases. *Am. J. Med.* 36:893.

Siguier, F.; Welti, J. J.; Zara, M.; and Funck-Brentano, J. J. 1953. Maladie périodique à manifestations particulièrement aberrants. *Bull. Mém. Soc. Méd. Hôp. Paris* 69:422.

Sohar, E.; Gafni, J.; Pras, M.; and Heller, H. 1967. Familial Mediterranean fever: A survey of 470 cases and review of literature. *Am. J. Med.* 43:227.

Zemer, D., et al. 1974. A controlled trial of colchicine in preventing attacks of familial Mediterranean fever. *N. Engl. J. Med.* 291:932.

Zemer, D.; Pras, M.; Sohar, E.; and Gafni, J. 1976. Colchicine in familial Mediterranean fever. *N. Engl. J. Med.* 294:170.

Wolff, S. M.; Dinarello, C. A.; Dale, D. C.; Goldfinger, S. E.; and Alling, D. W. 1974. Colchicine therapy of familial Mediterranean fever. *Clin. Res.* 22:567A.

GLANZMANN THROMBASTHENIA

Historical note

In 1918 Glanzmann first described this rare genetic disorder, which is manifested by a severe, lifelong bleeding tendency. In 1973 Reichert and co-workers called attention to its occurrence mainly among Jews of Iraqi origin. In 1975 Reichert and co-workers reviewed their experience with 22 cases of this disease in Israel.

Clinical features

Table 6.20 lists the bleeding manifestations noted in 22 Israeli patients with thrombasthenia. Most of these patients gave a history of numerous bleeding episodes. All patients had had purpura; in 14 it was observed soon after delivery. Except for 3 patients, all had had epistaxis and gum bleeding. Menorrhagia was observed in all 7 females above the age of puberty; in 6 it had been excessive on many occasions. Anemia due to blood loss was observed in all patients at one time or another; in 18 it necessitated multiple blood transfusions.

Such bleeding usually begins in childhood, and examination of affected patients does not reveal any other characteristic physical findings.

Table 6.20. Glanzmann thrombasthenia: Bleeding manifestations in 22 Israeli patients

Bleeding	No. of cases studied	No. affected	Percent affected
Purpura	22	22	100
Following circumcision	9[a]	9	100
Menorrhagia	7	7	100
Epistaxis and gum bleeding	22	19	86
Gastrointestinal	22	15	68
Following tooth extraction	4[b]	2	50
Hematuria	22	7	32
Hemarthrosis	22	2	9
Umbilical cord	22	1	5

Source: N. Reichert et al., 1975, *Thrombos. Diathes. Haemorrh.* 34:806.

[a] Two additional patients underwent uneventful circumcisions following platelet transfusion.

[b] In 3 patients, teeth were extracted following platelet transfusion: 1 bled (10 teeth extracted); the others did not.

Diagnosis

The diagnosis of thrombasthenia is based on a prolonged bleeding time, impaired clot retraction, a normal platelet count, and defective ADP-induced platelet aggregation.

The hemostatic function tests performed on the 22 Israeli patients are summarized in Table 6.21. A normal Duke bleeding time was observed in 4 patients. A normal Ivy bleeding time was sometimes observed in 3 additional patients who had been examined repeatedly. All patients examined by either method of ADP aggregation showed a marked abnormality.

Prothrombin time was normal in all patients. The intrinsic clotting system was examined in all patients by means of at least 2 of the following tests: clotting time, partial thromboplastin time, thromboplastin generation, prothrombin consumption, and recalcification time. Normal results were obtained except in the test for prothrombin consumption, which was impaired in 8 of the 20 patients tested.

Basic defect

The basic defect in thrombasthenia remains obscure, although it has been suggested that the alteration is one of platelate glycolysis and abnormal platelet aggregation in the presence of ADP. The studies by Degos and co-workers raise the possibility that the antigenic determinant absent from thrombasthenic patients is borne by some specific molecule involved in platelet aggregation.

Genetics

Pedigree analysis in the Israeli study was possible for 21 of the patients, who belonged to 13 unrelated kindreds. Twelve kindreds were Jewish and 1 was Arab. Eleven of the 12 Jewish kindreds belonged to the Iraqi Jewish community. Autosomal recessive inheritance was confirmed on the basis of the high rate of consanguinity observed in 9 of 16 sibships, the absence of vertical transmission, ethnic distribution, and a calculated correction for the segregation ratio (0.20).

Although the gene frequency of this disorder in the Iraqi Jewish community is not known, it is thought to be quite high. The only other ethnic group or groups in which this disorder has been commonly observed are the gypsy tribes of France.

Some investigators have recorded mild bleeding and various abnormalities in hemostatic functions in parents and other allegedly normal members of thrombasthenic patients' families. However, none of the 30 obligatory carriers questioned by Reichert and co-workers showed any bleeding manifestations, and no impaired hemostatic functions were observed in the 12 who were studied intensively. Recently, using the quantitative complement-fixation test, Degos and co-workers have shown that healthy heterozygotes can be distinguished from normal or thrombasthenic individuals by their platelets, which carry an intermediate amount of reactive antigen.

A number of clinical and laboratory discrepancies have been observed in thrombasthenia patients and their families. As has been suggested, these discrepancies probably reflect the heterogeneity of expression of thrombasthenia.

Table 6.21. Hemostatic function tests in 22 thrombasthenic patients

Case no.	Platelets ($\times 1000/mm^3$)	Bleeding time (min): Duke (D), Ivy (I)	Clot retraction	Platelet appearance	ADP aggregation tests Visual (sec)[a]	ADP aggregation tests Fragiligraph	ADP aggregation tests Aggregometer
1	372	> 18 (I)	0	isolated	—	—	none
2	189	20 (I)	0	—	none	—	—
3	195	20 (I)	0	—	none	—	—
4	328	15 (I)	0	isolated	none (12)	none	—
5	334	4 (D)	0	isolated	none (19)	none	—
6	170	> 30 (I)	0	—	none (12)	—	—
7	190	> 18 (I)	0	isolated	—	—	—
8	274	> 15 (I)	0	isolated	none (17)	none	—
9	158	5 (D)	0	isolated	none (17)	none	—
10	210	> 12 (I)	0	isolated	—	—	—
11	180	> 13 (I)	0	isolated	none (4)	none	—
12	222	> 20 (D)	0	isolated	—	—	—
13	200	1 (D)	0	isolated	none (20)	—	—
14	195	> 20 (I)	0	isolated	none (15)	none	—
15	160	> 15 (D)	0	isolated	none	—	—
16	298	15 (D)	0	isolated	none (15)	none	—
17	348	> 18 (I)	0	isolated	none (17)	none	—
18	295	20 (I)	0	isolated	none (22)	none	—
19	224	41 (I)	0	isolated	none (20)	none	—
20	281	15 (D)	0	isolated	none (8)	none	—
21	280	3 (D)	0	isolated	none	—	none
22	248	12 (I)	0	isolated	none	—	—
No. impaired/ no. tested	0/22	19/22	22/22	19/19	18/18	11/11	2/2

Source: N. Reichert et al., 1975, *Thrombos. Diathes. Haemorrh.* 34:806.

Note: Numbers in parentheses denote control values; dashes indicate "not determined."

[a] In 50 normal subjects the mean result was 20.6 ± 14.4 sec (2 SD).

Prognosis and treatment

The prognosis in this disorder is generally good, since severe bleeding is uncommon. Transfusions of fresh, whole blood or platelets are helpful when bleeding is severe. When surgery is required, some physicians advise giving platelet transfusions before and after the surgical procedure, but one should always be concerned about the possible reaction of platelet antibodies. Some observers have noted an amelioration of bleeding manifestations with age.

References

Caen, J. 1972. Glanzmann's thrombasthenia. *Clin. Haematol.* 1:383.

Degos, L.; Dautigny, A.; Brouet, J. C.; Colombani, M.; Ardaillou, N.; Caen, J. P.; and Colombani, J. 1975. A molecular defect in thrombasthenic platelets.

Glanzmann, E. 1918. Hereditäre hämorragische Thrombasthenie. Ein Beitrag zur Pathologie der Blut Plättchen. *Jahrb. Kinderheilk.* 88: 113.

Levy, J. M.; Mayes, G.; Sacren, R.; Ruff, R.; Françfort, J. J.; and Rodier, L. 1971. Thrombasthenie de Glanzmann-Naegeli. Étude d'un groupe ethnique à forte endogamie. *Semaine Hôp. Paris* 47:129.

Reichert, N.; Seligsohn, U.; and Ramot, B. 1973. Thrombasthenia in Iraqi Jews. *Israel J. Med. Sci.* 9:1406.

————. 1975. Clinical and genetic aspects of Glanzmann's thrombasthenia in Israel: Report of 22 cases. *Thrombos. Diathes. Haemorrh.* 34:806.

GLUCOSE-6-PHOSPHATE DEHYDROGENASE DEFICIENCY

Historical note

An awareness of the toxic responses to certain substances by individuals known to be glucose-6-phosphate dehydrogenase (G6PD) deficient dates back to ancient times. In the 6th Century B.C.E. Pythagoras warned of the consequences of eating beans and in the 5th Century B.C.E. Herodotus mentioned favism. In modern times acute hemolytic anemia was reported by Cordes in 1926 in Panamanian plantation workers who had received plasmochin during treatment for malaria. The actual discovery of G6PD deficiency was a direct result of investigations of the hemolytic effect of the antimalarial drug primaquine carried out in the early 1950s. These studies by Dern and co-workers were conducted among prison volunteers in a malaria research unit in Joliet, Illinois, and from them a wealth of information has been acquired on the epidemiology, genetics, biochemistry, and pathophysiology of this disorder.

In 1958 Szeinberg and co-workers showed that the red cells of patients with a history of favism also exhibit glutathione instability. Later reports from Israel indicated that this condition is prevalent among Sephardi and Oriental Jews and that, among the latter, the Kurds have one of the highest frequencies of G6PD deficiency on record.

Several excellent reviews on G6PD deficiency are listed in the references.

Clinical features

The clinical manifestations of G6PD deficiency may be episodic, masked by complete clinical recovery in the intervening periods (as noted in most affected black patients exposed to primaquine), or they may be chronic, but often marked by periods of acceleration. In addition they may occur under conditions of stress associated with infection or drug administration, or they may appear in the neonatal period or after exposure to fava beans.

DRUG-INDUCED HEMOLYTIC ANEMIA

Table 6.22 lists the main drugs and chemicals that are capable of producing hemolytic reactions in G6PD-deficient individuals. The clinical manifestations begin to appear 1–3 days after the drug is administered. Acute hemolytic anemia of moderate severity is induced and is accompaned by the usual hematologic and pigmentry changes and the appearance of Heinz bodies. Abdominal or back pain may occur; the urine may turn dark, even black, with hemoglobinuria; and then signs of erythrocyte regeneration appear, during which the Heinz bodies disappear, presumably because of sequestration and removal in the spleen.

G6PD deficiency is most severe in the Mediterranean populations, and the hemolytic anemia may not clear spontaneously while drug therapy is continued, because the G6PD content of even the youngest cell is low.

HEMOLYTIC ANEMIA IN THE ABSENCE OF DRUG ADMINISTRATION

Hemolytic episodes have been noted in some G6PD deficient individuals when they have had bacterial or viral infections, diabetic ketoacidosis, acute or chronic hepatitis, or nephritis. These episodes have been attributed to the oxidative activity generated by naturally occurring substances such as ascorbic acid, cysteine, and pyruvic acid, to toxic products formed in the course of the disease, or to hydrogen peroxide production by phagocytosing leukocytes.

FAVISM

Favism is one of the most severe forms of G6PD deficiency and affects individuals with the Mediterranean phenotype. Hemolysis may occur within a few hours following inhalation of the plant's pollen or within one or two days after ingestion of either fresh or dry fava beans. The urine becomes red or very dark, and in severe cases shock may develop within a short time, followed by death in some instances.

NEONATAL JAUNDICE

This form of neonatal hyperbilirubinemia is relatively common in G6PD-deficient infants of Mediterranean, Chinese, or other origin, but is rare in newborn blacks. The jaundice may be severe and if untreated may result in kernicterus.

Table 6.22. Compounds known to produce hemolysis
in patients with G6PD deficiency

Acetanilid	Naphthalene	Quinidine
N-acetylsulfanilamide	Neoarsphenamine	Quinocide
2-amino-5-sulfanilythiazole	Nitrofurantoin	Salicylazosulfapyridine
Chloramphenicol	Nitrofurazone	Sulfamethoxypyridazine
Diaphenylsulfone	Pamaquine	Sulfanilamide
Furaltodone	Pentaquine phosphate	Sulfapyridine
Furazolidone	Phenylhydrazine hydrochloride	Trinitroluene
Furmethonol	Primaquine	

NONSPHEROCYTIC CONGENITAL HEMOLYTIC ANEMIA

This form of hemolytic anemia is usually recognized during infancy or childhood. Hemolysis is often exacerbated by febrile illnesses or by the administration of drugs. In most cases the anemia is not severe, but occasionally transfusions are necessary. Splenomegaly is common, but splenectomy is not indicated. Most patients with this disorder have one of the rare types of G6PD deficiency or are of the Mediterranean phenotype.

Diagnosis

The diagnosis of G6PD deficiency depends on the demonstration of decreased activity through either a quantitative enzyme assay or a screening test. Assay of the enzyme is generally done by measuring the rate of reduction of NADP to NADPH in an ultraviolet spectrophotometer. Various acceptable visual screening tests have been developed and the reagents for carrying out some of these procedures are commercially available.

After an episode of hemolysis it may be impossible to diagnose the deficiency state in the proband, and thus one may attempt family studies or wait until the circulating red cells have aged sufficiently to show their lack of enzyme.

Detection of the heterozygous enzyme deficiency state is often difficult, for the enzyme assays may be in the normal range for heterozygous females. Furthermore, females who are heterozygous for G6PD deficiency vary significantly from one another, not only in the activity of red cell G6PD but also in the percentage of G6PD-deficient red cells in their circulation. Some variation in the proportion of deficient cells is to be expected, given the X-inactivation that occurs at a stage in embryonic development when the number of red cell precursors is relatively small, but there is some evidence that the distribution of inactivated X chromosomes is itself subject to genetic modification.

Basic defect

Glucose-6-phosphate dehydrogenase catalyzes the initial step in the pentose phosphate or aerobic glycolytic pathway. Therefore, deficient G6PD activity is characterized by a decrease in glucose utilization and in oxygen consumption. The oxidative catabolism of glucose is the sole mechanism by which an erythrocyte can reduce NADP to NADPH, which is an important source of red cell-reducing power. The first step in reductive detoxification is the formation of increased amounts of NADPH, and in normal erythrocytes the rate-limiting factor in the pentose phosphate pathway appears to be the availability of NADP. Since G6PD interferes with NADPH regeneration, the G6PD-deficient red cell lacks this protective capacity; its ability to resist oxidative damage is contingent upon its G6PD content.

Because NADPH is the preferred hydrogen donor for the reduction of glutathione, the glutathione of G6PD-deficient erythrocytes is particularly susceptible to oxidation. The resultant deficiency of reduced glutathione permits the oxidative destruction of certain erythrocytic components. The sulfhydryl groups of the globin chains and the cell membrane are especially vulnerable. Oxidation of hemoglobin culminates in the precipitation of irreversibly denatured hemoglobin; these degradation products of hemoglobin are identifiable as Heinz bodies by special staining techniques. Cells containing Heinz bodies encounter difficulties in negotiating the microcirculation, especially in the spleen, and oxidation of the sulfhydryl groups of the membrane results in decreased red cell deformability. These mechanisms, among other as yet poorly understood pathophysiological effects, culminate in the premature destruction of the erythrocytes.

Although various theories have been proposed, the exact reason why the life span of G6PD-deficient red cells is shortened during drug administration, the neonatal period, or infections is not known. Immunologic factors have long been suspected of playing a role in the hemolytic anemia induced by fava beans, but this has not been proved. Furthermore, an additional factor seems to be required, for not even all G6PD-deficient persons in the same family are susceptible to favism.

For additional details concerning the basic defect and the chemical features of the enzyme G6PD the reader is referred to the 1971 review by Kirkman.

Genetics

G6PD deficiency is a heterogenous disorder transmitted in an X-linked recessive manner. When this condition occurs in blacks a different mutation is involved compared to the G6PD deficiency observed in Mediterranean and Middle Eastern populations. As a result of this different mutation there are certain characteristic differences between the 2 conditions. For example, the level of G6PD in the red cells of males with the Mediterranean type of G6PD deficiency is usually about 3 or 4 percent of the normal level, whereas in the type that affects blacks it is about 15 percent of normal. Also a significant reduction of the enzyme level may be demonstrated in white cells and other tissues in the Mediterranean type, whereas in the type seen in blacks such a reduction in G6PD either is not found or is very slight. Thus, in terms of the level of enzyme activity, the Mediterranean type is a more severe abnormality.

A further distinction between these 2 types has been noted in electrophoretic studies. G6PD in healthy black subjects separates into 2 forms: the slower form, B, and the faster form, A. Males may have A or B, but not both. Blacks who are G6PD deficient almost invariably show the A form.

In the Mediterranean type of G6PD deficiency the enzyme has the B electrophoretic mobility, as does the enzyme in normal individuals in these populations. Thus the allele causing the Mediterranean type is at the same locus as the common alleles occurring in the black population.

Four alleles—Gd^B, Gd^A, Gd^A− (enzyme activity 15 percent of normal with A mobility), and Gd^Mediterranean—appear to determine 4 structurally distinct forms of G6PD enzyme protein. Over the years a number of distinct variant forms (over 100; see Beutler and Yoshida, 1973) of the enzyme have been identified, each apparently determined by a different allele at the locus on the X-chromosome which codes for the structure of the enzyme. These variants differ from one another and from the 4 above in 1 or more of their qualitative characteristics. Among these numerous variants a few have been discovered in Israel (Tel Hashomer, Ramat Gan, Bat Yam, Ashdod, and Lifta) among Jewish patients and primarily in the Oriental communities. In general, no correlation has been found between the characteristics of these variant enzymes and the general clinical manifestations of the disease.

In the non-Ashkenazi Jewish community, G6PD deficiency varies from 1 percent to 2 percent among European Sephardim, 25 percent among Iraqi Jews, 28 percent among some Caucasus Jews, and as high as 60 percent among Kurdish Jews.

While most geneticists accept the idea that G6PD deficiency has persisted in some parts of the world because of the protective advantage of heterozygotes against *P. falciparum* malaria, the late Dr. Sheba suggested that the prevalence of this gene among the various Jewish ethnic groups could be explained by the origins of the communities now living in the Mediterranean and Near Eastern regions. Using G6PD deficiency as an example, Dr. Sheba quoted the different frequencies among Jewish communities, and between Jews and non-Jews, as support for his concept that this polymorphism is an excellent genetic marker, an indicator of ancient East Mediterranean or Phoenician origin. On that basis he argued that the rarity of the condition among the Sephardim and particularly among the Ashkenazim was due to their outbreeding rather than to their having moved into nonmalarial zones.

G6PD deficiency among Jews is similar to that found among other Mediterranean populations but differs from that observed in Africa and the American black. Enzyme activity is 0–8 percent of normal and there is increased susceptibility to hemolysis upon exposure to various drugs and agents that stress the oxidative reactions of the phosphate-pentose pathway. It is interesting to note that neonatal jaundice due to G6PD deficiency does not occur in Jews as it does in other Mediterranean peoples.

Table 6.23 lists the percentage of G6PD deficiency among various Jewish and non Jewish communities of the Middle East.

In 1961 Adam and co-workers were the first to show a linkage between G6PD and color blindness. It has been estimated that the G6PD locus may be at a re-combination fraction of only 0.03–0.04 from the deutan locus and 0.07 from the protan locus. The G6PD locus may be between these two loci for color blindness. Close linkage also exists between the loci for G6PD and hemophilia A and thus may prove useful in genetic counseling when hemophilia A involves populations having a relatively high gene frequency for G6PD abnormalities.

Prognosis and treatment

In contrast to the hemolytic episodes in type A G6PD deficiency, those occurring in the more severe, Mediterranean type (involving Jews) may not terminate rapidly, but in most cases recovery does take place. Gallstone formation may be a complica-tion if the hemolytic process is frequent or prolonged. The prognosis is unquestion-ably more serious in favism than in the other forms of G6PD deficiency, but little is known regarding the ultimate prognosis in individuals with this disorder.

Treatment includes avoidance of drugs and agents that might induce hemolytic episodes. Whole blood or packed red cells may be lifesaving in favism and may or may not be indicated in the milder forms.

The use of G6PD-deficient blood for transfusion is potentially harmful. Patients given such blood may receive drugs or suffer from illnesses that may lead to the hemolysis of G6PD-deficient cells. Especially inadvisable is the use of red cells from donors with the Mediterranean type of G6PD deficiency, since a large portion of such cells may be destroyed.

Table 6.23. G6PD deficiency among various Jewish and
non-Jewish communities of the Middle East

Community and Population	No. examined	% G6PD deficient males	Population	No. examined	% G6PD deficient males
Israel			Iraq		
Jews			Arabs	489	9.4
Ashkenazi	819	0.4	Kurds	211	7.5
Non-Ashkenazi from:			Turkomans	142	6.3
Turkey	256	1.9	Chaldeans	131	8.4
Greece and Bulgaria	152	0.7	Assyrians	70	11.4
Kurdistan	536	61.6	Iran		
Iraq	902	24.8	Moslems	221	9.1
Iran	557	15.1	Moslems	984	7.1
Caucasus	25	28.0	Zoroastrians	146	—
Afghanistan	29	10.3	Armenians	158	0.6
Yemen and Aden	415	5.3	Tribes		
(Habbanites)	284	1.4	Gasghai	133	11.3
Syria and Lebanon	80	6.3	Bassera	83	13.3
Bukhara	46	—	Mamassani	91	20.0
India (Cochin)	58	10.3	Moslems	?	9.9
India (Bnei Israel)	102	2.0	Armenians	?	13.3
Egypt	112	3.8	Jews	?	15.2
Morocco	219	0.5	Saudi Arabia		
Algeria and Tunisia	112	0.9	Adults	306	15.0
Libya	219	0.9	Children (in oasis villages)	351	50.0
Arabs	264	4.4	Kuwait	461	21.4
Druzes	92	4.4	Lebanon		
Circasians	57	—	Maronites	117	4.3
Karaites	18	—	Sunnites	97	6.2
Karaites	250	—	Shiites	101	4.9
Samaritans	69	—	Druzes	105	0
Israel and Jordan			Armenians	36	0
Samaritans	132	—	Egypt	500	26.4
Southern Sinai				388	2.3
Towara bedouins	197	2.0	Algeria	583	3.4
Jebeliya bedouins	81	—			
Turkey					
Turks	521	1.7			
Eti-Turks	105	11.4			
Armenians	44	—			

Source: A. Szeinberg, 1973, *Israel J. Med. Sci.* 9:1171.

References

Adam, A. 1961. Linkage between deficiency of glucose-6-phosphate dehydrogenase and colour-blindness. *Nature* 189:686.

———. 1973. Genetic diseases among Jews. *Israel J. Med. Sci.* 9:1383.

Beutler, E. 1957. The glutathione instability of drug-sensitive red cells: A new method for the *in vitro* detection of drug sensitivity. *J. Lab. Clin. Med.* 49:84.

———. 1966. A series of new screening procedures for pyruvate kinase deficiency, glucose-6-phosphate dehydrogenase deficiency, and glutatione reductase deficiency. *Blood* 28:553.

———. 1968. The genetics of glucose-6-phosphate dehydrogenase deficiency. In *Hereditary disorders of erythrocyte metabolism*, ed. E. Beutler, pp. 114–20. New York: Grune and Stratton.

————. 1978. *Hemolytic anemia in disorders of red cell metabolism.* New York: Plenum Medical Book Co.

Boyer, S. H., and Graham, J. B. 1965. Linkage between the X chromosome loci for glucose-6-phosphate dehydrogenase electrophoretic variation and hemophilia A. *Am. J. Hum. Genet.* 17:320.

Bottini, E.; Bottini, F. G.; and Maggioni, G. 1978. On the relation between malaria and G-6-PD deficiency. *J. Med. Genet.* 15:363.

Cohen, T. 1971. Genetic markers in migrants to Israel. *Israel J. Med. Sci.* 7:1509.

Cordes, W. 1926. Experiences with plasmochin in malaria (preliminary reports). *United Fruit Company Medical Department Annual Report* 15:66.

Davidson, R. G. 1968. The Lyon hypothesis. *Ann. N.Y. Acad. Sci.* 151:157.

Davidson, R. G.; Childs, B.; and Siniscalco, M. 1964. Genetic variation in the quantitative control of erythrocyte glucose-6-phosphate dehydrogenase activity. *Ann. Hum. Genet.* 28:61.

Davidson, R. G.; Nitowsky, H.; and Childs, B. 1963. Demonstration of two populations of cells in the human female heterozygous for glucose-6-phosphate dehydrogenase variants. *Proc. Natl. Acad. Sci. USA* 50:481.

Dern, R. J.; Weinstein, I. M.; LeRoy, G. V.; Talmage, D. W.; and Alving, A. S. 1954. The hemolytic effect of primaquine. I: The localization of the drug-induced hemolytic defect in primaquine-sensitive individuals. *J. Lab. Clin. Med.* 43:303.

Harris, H. 1975. *The principles of human biochemical genetics.* Amsterdam: North Holland.

Kirkman, H. N.: Characteristics of glucose-6-phosphate dehydrogenase from normal and primaquine-sensitive erythrocytes. *Nature* 184:1291.

————. 1966. Properties of X-linked alleles during selection. *Am. J. Hum. Genet.* 18:424.

————. 1968. Glucose-6-phosphate dehydrogenase variants and drug-induced hemolysis. *Ann. N.Y. Acad. Sci.* 151:753.

————. 1971. Glucose-6-phosphate dehydrogenase. In *Advances in human genetics,* ed. H. Harris and K. Hirschhorn, 2:1–60. New York: Plenum Press.

Kirkman, H. N.; Ramot, B.; and Lee, J. T. 1969. Altered aggregational properties in a genetic variant of human glucose-6-phosphate dehydrogenase. *Biochem. Genet.* 3:137.

Kirkman, H. N.; Riley, H. D.; and Crowell, B. B. 1960. Different enzymic expressions of mutants of human glucose-6-phosphate dehydrogenase. *Proc. Natl. Acad. Sci. USA* 46:938.

Ramot, B.; Ashkenazi, I.; Rimon, A.; Adam, A.; and Sheba, C. 1961. Activation of glucose-6-phosphate dehydrogenase of enzyme deficient subjects. II: Properties of the activator and the activation reaction. *J. Clin. Invest.* 40:611.

Ramot, B.; Bauminger, S.; Brok, F.; Gafni, D.; and Schwartz, J. 1964. Characterization of glucose-6-phosphate dehydrogenase in Jewish mutants. *J. Lab. Clin. Med.* 64:895.

Ramot, B.; Ben-Bassat, I.; and Shchory, M. 1969. New glucose-6-phosphate dehydrogenase variants observed in Israel and their association with congenital nonspherocytic hemolytic disease. *J. Lab. Clin. Med.* 74:895.

Ramot, B., and Brok, R. 1964. A new glucose-6-phosphate dehydrogenase mutant (Tel-Hashomer mutant). *Ann. Hum. Genet.* 28:167.

Ramot, B.; Fisher, S.; Szeinberg, A.; Adam, A.; Sheba, C.; and Gafni, D. 1959. A study of subjects with erythrocytic glucose-6-phosphate dehydrogenase deficiency. II: Investigation of leukocyte enzymes. *J. Clin. Invest.* 38:2234.

Szeinberg, A. 1973. Investigation of genetic polymorphic traits in Jews: A contribution to the study of population genetics. *Israel J. Med. Sci.* 9:1171.

Szeinberg, A.; Asher, Y.; and Sheba, C. 1958. Studies on glutathione stability in erythrocytes of cases with past history of favism or sulfa-induced hemolysis. *Blood* 13:348.

Szeinberg, A., and Marks, P. A. 1961. Substances stimulating glucose catabolism by the oxidative reactions of the pentose phosphate pathway in human erythrocytes. *J. Clin. Invest.* 40:914.

Szeinberg, A.; Sheba, C; and Adam, A. 1958. Enzymatic abnormality in erythrocytes of population sensitive to *Vicia faba* or haemolytic anemia induced by drugs. *Nature* 181:1256.

Szeinberg, A.; Sheba, C.; Hirschorn, N.; and Bodonyi, E. 1957. Studies on erythrocytes in cases with past history of favism and drug-induced acute hemolytic anemia. *Blood* 12:603.

Yoshida, A.; Beutler, E.; and Motulsky, A. G. 1971. Table of human glucose-6-phosphate dehydrogenase variants. *Bull. WHO* 45:243.

Yoshida, A.; Stamatoyannopoulos, G.; and Motulsky, A. G.; 1968. Biochemical genetics of glucose-6-phosphate dehydrogenase variation. *Ann. N.Y. Acad. Sci.* 155:868.

GLYCOGEN STORAGE DISEASE TYPE III
(DEBRANCHER ENZYME DEFICIENCY)

Historical note

In 1929 von Gierke was the first to describe the clinical and pathological findings in "hepatic" glycogen storage disease, which later became known as von Gierke's disease. In 1932 Pompe reported a more generalized form of glycogen storage disease with marked cardiac involvement. In 1952 the Coris first demonstrated a specific enzymatic defect in glycogen synthesis in a patient with the hepatic form of the disease. In 1953 Forbes described the features of this particular form of type III glycogen storage disease. Today we know there are several forms and subtypes of the glycogen storage diseases which primarily involve the liver, heart, and musculoskeletal system. In 1967 Levin and co-workers observed that type III glycogen storage disease occurs mainly in Sephardi Jews from North Africa and especially those from Morocco.

Clinical features

The age of onset of type III glycogen storage disease is any time between infancy and late childhood. Although type III is less severe than type I, the manifestations in both are so similar that the forms are often indistinguishable clinically. The outstanding features of this disease include hepatomegaly, rounded face, hypoglycemic convulsions, fasting ketosis, elevated free fatty acids, hyperlipidemia, xanthomatosis, nose bleeds, and growth retardation.

Glycogen may accumulate in the skeletal and cardiac muscles. Muscle flaccidity may be present, and some patients in adult life develop a debilitating myopathy. A moderate cardiomegaly is sometimes seen, as are nonspecific electrocardiographic changes, but cardiac symptoms usually are not present.

In some cases the manifestations of type III glycogen storage disease are severe during the first few years of life. Around puberty spontaneous improvement may occur, with some patients showing a normal liver size, improvement in linear growth, and subsidence of the hypoglycemia, ketonuria, and hyperlipidemia. Table 6.24 lists the clinical features noted in 22 cases from Israel.

Diagnosis

Diagnosis can be tentatively established on the basis of some of the clinical findings described previously. In addition, various function studies, using glucagon, galactose, or fructose administration, may be helpful. For example, one may obtain a normal glucagon response 2 hours after feeding and no response after a 14-hour fast. This has been interpreted as an indication of the availability of glucose from the elongated outer branches (after feeding) which could be degraded by phosphorylase, in the absence of debranching activity. Unfortunately, this is not a consistent finding in all patients.

A marked elevation in erythrocyte glycogen with abnormally shorter outer branches has been shown to be specific for this type of glycogen disease. This has been observed repeatedly but is not invariable.

Final evidence of the disorder depends upon direct enzyme assays showing a deficiency of amylo-1,6-glucosidase (the "debrancher" enzyme).

Basic defect

The basic defect involves a deficiency in the enzyme amylo-1,6-glucosidase. Recently, it has been shown that there are various subtypes, depending upon the presence of amylo-1,6-glucosidase or oligo-1,4→1,4-glucantransferase. A deficiency of either enzyme can result in "limit dextrinosis." In some cases both enzymes are deficient in liver and muscle tissues, while in other cases one of the enzymes is normal in one tissue, deficient in the other, and independently distributed in other tissues.

Genetics

The tendency for sibs to be affected, the equal occurrence in males and females, and a high rate of consanguineous marriages all support an autosomal recessive mode of inheritance for this disorder.

The enzyme deficiency in type III glycogen storage disease is manifested in many tissues, including leukocytes, cultured skin fibroblasts, and cultured amniotic fluid cells. Heterozygote detection is possible in some instances through enzyme assay in the previously mentioned tissues. However, heterozygote detection may be difficult due to the widespread variability in tissue enzyme activity noted within single affected families.

In Israel this form of glycogen storage disease accounts for 73 percent of the cases reported, as compared to rates of 20–56 percent noted in series from other countries. Furthermore, all the proven cases of glycogen storage disease in Israel have occurred in non-Ashkenazi Jews. Of the 14 affected Jewish families with type III studied by Levin and co-workers, 11 could trace their origin to Morocco (Table 6.25). Consanguinity was present in 64 percent of these 14 families. A minimal esti-

Table 6.24. Clinical features of glycogen storage disease type III in Israel

Case no.	Age	Sex	Country of origin	Age at diagnosis	Consanguinity in family	Psychomotor retardation
1	4 yr	F	Morocco		+	
2	8 yr	F	Morocco	3 yr	−	+
3	12 yr	M	Morocco		−	+
4	5 yr	M	Morocco	7 mo	+	+
5	4 yr	M	Morocco	18 mo	+	+
6	6 yr	M	Morocco	3 yr	−	+
7	3 mo	F	Morocco	3 mo	−	+
8[a]	5 yr	M	Morocco	7 mo		+
9[a]	4 yr	M	Morocco	8 mo		
10[b]	5 yr	M	Morocco	2 mo		+
11	11 yr	F	Morocco	15 yr	+	+
12	14 mo	F	Morocco	14 mo		
13	16 yr	F	Morocco	11 yr		
14	2 yr	M	Morocco			
15	3 yr	M	Iraq	8 mo		+
16	6 yr	F	Iraq			+
17	1 yr	F	Morocco			
18	18 yr	F	Morocco	17 yr	+	+
19	7 yr	F	Morocco	3 yr	+	
20	6 yr	M	Tunisia	14 mo	+	
21	4 yr	F	Morocco			
22	7 yr	M	Iraq	21 mo	−	+

Source: S. Levin et al., 1967, *Israel J. Med. Sci.* 3:397.
[a] Diagnosed on clinical, biochemical, and pathological grounds.
[b] Affected sibling, presumptive type III.

mation of the frequency of this type of disorder in the North African Jewish community is 1:5420. The calculated gene frequency is 0.0136.

Van-Hoof and Hers found that 75 percent of 45 European cases with amylo-1,6-glucosidase deficiency had neither hydrolase nor transferase activity. The other 25 percent showed a very heterogeneous picture.

The North African patients examined exhibited a pattern which differed markedly from that found in the European cases; 9 out of 10 cases, belonging to 4 unrelated families originating from the west coast of Morocco, exhibited an unusual type of enzyme defect which differed from the single case originating from a distant town near the northeast coast. Furthermore, the enzyme defect in all these cases differed markedly from that observed in a majority of the European cases and from other cases among Jews from Iraq or among Arabs from Israel (Table 6.26).

Prognosis and treatment

During infancy and childhood frequent feedings and a high-protein diet are indicated for patients presenting symptoms. As mentioned previously, many of these children will show a dramatic improvement in growth and a reduction in symptoms with the onset of puberty. Many adults are relatively asymptomatic, and the prognosis for a healthy life is good for the majority of patients.

Hypo-glycemic attacks	Recurrent infections	Rounded face	Hepa-tomegaly	Cardi-omegaly	Glycogen excess		No. of siblings
					Liver	Muscle	
			+				2
+		+	+	+	+	−	8
+		+	+		+	−	7
+	+	+	+		+		} 8
+			+		+	−	
+		+	+	+	+		} 3
+	+	+	+		+		
−	+	+	+		+		} 3
+			+		+		
+	+	+	+	+	+	−	} 3
+	+	+	+		+		
	+		+		+		} 2
+		+	+				} 3
+	+		+	+	+		4
			+	+	+		8
		+	+		−	−	3
+	+	+			+		2
					+		3
+	+	+	+		+	+	8
							67

References

Chayoth, R.; Moses, S. W.; and Steinitz, K. 1967. Debrancher enzyme activity in blood cells of families with type III glycogen storage disease: A method for diagnosis of heterozygotes. *Israel J. Med. Sci.* 3:422.

Cori, G. T., and Cori, C. F. 1952. Glucose-6-phosphatase of the the liver in glycogen storage disease. *J. Biol. Chem.* 199:661.

Field, J. B., and Drash, A. L. 1967. Studies in glycogen storage disease. II: Heterogeneity in the inheritance of glycogen storage diseases. *Trans. Assoc. Am. Physicians* 80:284.

Forbes, G. B. 1953. Glycogen storage disease. *J. Pediatr.* 42:645.

Howell, R. R. 1972. The glycogen storage diseases. In *The metabolic basis of inherited disease,* ed. J. B. Stanbury, J. B. Wyngaarden, and D. S. Fredrickson, 3rd ed. pp. 149–173. New York: McGraw-Hill.

Justice, P.; Tyan, C.; and Hsia, D. Y. 1970. Amylo-1,6-glucosidase in human fibroblasts: Studies in type III glycogen storage disease. *Biochem. Biophys. Res. Commun.* 39:301.

Levin, S.; Moses, S.; Chayoth, R.; Jadoga, N.; and Steinitz, K. 1967. Glycogen storage disease in Israel: A clinical, biochemical, and genetic study. *Israel J. Med. Sci.* 3:397.

Moses, S. W.; Bashan, N.; Skibin, A.; Biran, H.; and Gutman, A. 1973. Genetic traits and diseases in the North African Jewish Community. *Israel J. Med. Sci.* 9:1407.

Pompe, J. C. 1932. Over idiopatische hypertrophie van het hart. *Ned. Tijdschr. Geneeskd.* 76:304.

Table 6.25. Ethnic distribution of glycogen storage disease
type III among Israeli Jews

Origin	No. of cases	No. of families
Morocco	18	11
Iraq	3	2
Tunisia	1	1
Total	22	14

Note: As of 1973, 8 more cases of this disorder had been
diagnosed, all in the Sephardi Jewish community.

Table 6.26. Amylo-1,6-glucosidase activity in leukocytes of patients with
glycogen storage disease type III (means and ranges)

Origin of patients	No. of patients	^{14}C incorporation ($\%/hr \times 10^{10}$)	Glucose release (nmole/min $\times 10^7$)[a]	Transferase (% covering/ min $\times 10^7$)	Hydrolase (μmole/min $\times 10^7$)
Morocco					
Agadir, Marakesh	9	0	0	2.2 (0.0–5.5)[b]	1.5 (0.6–2.7)
Fez	1	0	0	0	0
Iraq	3	0	0	0	1.5
Arabs (Israel)	3	4.7 (3.0–7.0)	0	5.0	0.6
Normal subjects	20	8.2 (4.3–10.2)	8.0	5.2 (3.0–7.0)	2.4 (0.9–5.4)

Source: S. W. Moses et al., 1973, *Israel J. Med. Sci.* 9:1407.

[a] Glucose released from phosphorylase limit dextrin.

[b] One of these patients had no detectable transferase activity in leukocytes; however, findings in
other tissues and pedigree data place him in this group.

Van Creveld, S., and Huijing, F. 1965. Glycogen storage disease. *Am. J. Med.* 38:554.

Van-Hoof, F., and Hers, H. G. 1967. The subgroups of type III glycogenosis. *Eur. J. Biochem.* 2:265.

Von Gierke, E. 1929. Hepato-nephromegalia glykogenia (Glykogenspeicherkrankhei den Leber und Nieren). *Beitr. Pathol. Anat.* 82:497.

Williams, C., and Field, F. B. 1968. Studies in glycogen storage disease. III. Limit dextrinosis: A genetic study. *J. Pediatr.* 72:214.

ICHTHYOSIS VULGARIS

Historical note

Ichthyosis vulgaris has been known since ancient times and the name is derived
from the Greek word *ichthys*, meaning "fish." Since the 1930s this skin disorder
has been known to be transmitted as an autosomal dominant or X-linked recessive
disease. In 1966 Wells and Kerr delineated the clinical and histological differences
between the two forms. The studies of Ziprkowski, Adam, Feinstein, and co-workers
from 1966 to 1972 further contributed to our understanding of the clinical and
genetic features of the disease and revealed its unique distribution among the various

Table 6.27. Ichthyosis vulgaris: Age distribution of
Israeli patients, 1966–1972

Age (yr)	No. of patients with XLI	No. of patients with ADI
0–9	73	38
10–19	101	38
20–29	23	35
30–39	16	6
40–49	6	9
50–59	10	9
60–69	—	2
Total	229	137

Source: L. Ziprkowski and A. Feinstein, 1972, *Br. J. Dermatol.* 86:1.

Jewish ethnic groups. In 1978 Shapiro and co-workers discovered the basic defect in the X-linked form of ichthyosis.

Clinical features

From 1966 to 1972 Ziprkowski, Adam, Feinstein, and co-workers studied 366 patients with ichthyosis vulgaris. Of these, 229 had the X-linked recessive form (XLI); 137 had the autosomal dominant type (ADI). The age distribution of these patients is shown in Table 6.27. Skin changes in both forms of the disease usually begin before the age of 5 years. Generally the disease is most pronounced in those XLI patients who present with widespread, large, dark scales. These scales cover most of the trunk and limbs. In the ADI form the legs are mainly involved, with the upper extremities being affected to a lesser degree. The trunk is rarely affected in the ADI form, and then mildly. Follicular keratosis of the arms and hyperkeratosis with prominent creases of the palms and soles are observed only in the ADI type. Table 6.28 shows the areas and degree of involvement in both forms. Table 6.29 compares the scales in each form.

Table 6.28. Ichthyosis vulgaris: Area of body and degree of
involvement observed in XLI and ADI cases

Area of body	XLI	ADI
Face	+	—
Neck	++	—
Upper trunk	++	—
Lower trunk	++	+
Upper limbs	++	+
Lower limbs	+++	+++
Antecubital and popliteal fossae	±	—
Hands and feet	—	++

Source: L. Ziprkowski and A. Feinstein, 1972, *Br. J. Dermatol.* 86:1.
Note: — = no involvement; ± = minor involvement; + = mild involvement; ++ = moderate involvement; +++ = severe involvement.

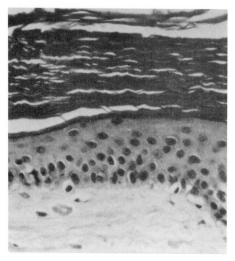 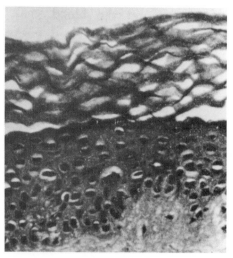

Figure 6.17. Compact, laminated hyper-keratosis and a granular zone 3 cells thick from a patient with X-linked ichthyosis. From L. Ziprkowski and A. Feinstein, 1972, *Br. J. Dermatol.* 86:1.

Figure 6.18. Basket-weave hyperkeratosis, without granular layer, from a patient with autosomal dominant ichthyosis. From L. Ziprkowski and A. Feinstein, 1972, *Br. J. Dermatol.* 86:1.

Diagnosis

Diagnosis of ichthyosis vulgaris can easily be confirmed by histological findings in those areas where the scaling is most pronounced (region of the anterior shin). The XLI form shows compact laminated hyperkeratosis with thickening of the granular layer, whereas in the ADI form the hyperkeratosis appears as a basket-weave configuration with a thin or no granular layer (Figures 6.17 and 6.18). The sweat glands are normal in number and structure in both forms. Sebaceous glands are absent only in ADI cases.

Since steroid-sulphatase activity is demonstrable in cultured amniotic-fluid cells and is deficient in cells from affected fetuses, prenatal diagnosis of XLI is now possible.

Basic defect

In 1978 Shapiro and co-workers showed that the basic defect in XLI is a deficiency of the enzyme 3-beta-hydroxysteroid-sulphate sulphatase. The basic defect in ADI is not known.

Table 6.29. Ichthyosis vulgaris: Comparison of scales in
XLI and ADI cases

Scales	XLI	ADI
Size	1–3 cm	1 mm–1 cm
Color	Gray-brown-black	gray-brown
Shape	Polygonal (4–5 edges)	"Powdery" or polygonal (4–5 edges)

Source: L. Ziprkowski and A. Feinstein, 1972, *Br. J. Dermatol.* 86:1.

Genetics

Although both forms of ichthyosis vulgaris have been seen in most of the Jewish ethnic groups, the XLI type has been observed mainly in Jews from Iraq, while the ADI type occurs predominantly among Jews from India. Neither of these major affected groups expresses both forms of the disorder. Table 6.30 shows the distribution of these two forms among the Jewish ethnic groups in Israel.

Adam and co-workers have shown that the gene for the XLI form is closely linked to the locus for the Xg^a blood groups. The best estimate of the recombination fraction is 0.105, and the 90 percent probability limits are 0.06 and 0.16. In addition, these studies have ruled out linkage of the XLI gene with the genes for color vision (deutan and protan) or G6PD.

The estimated prevalence of XLI ichthyosis in the Jewish communities of Israel is at least 1:9,500 males. Although there is no estimate for the prevalence of XLI among non-Jewish Israelis or for other forms of ichthyosis in Israelis, it is thought that XLI accounts for about 50 percent of all cases of ichthyosis vulgaris in the Israeli Jewish population. This is considerably higher than previously estimated for other populations.

The manifestations of XLI in heterozygous females vary widely, from dry skin to temporary mild ichthyosis. This partial and variable expressivity of the gene is similar to that described for other X-linked recessive genes in heterozygous females.

Prognosis and treatment

Table 6.31 provides information on the clinical course of ichthyosis vulgaris. Note that a family history of atopy was recorded for 30 percent of the patients with ADI, while such a history was not given by XLI patients. Treatment of both forms is symptomatic.

References

Adam, A.; Ziprkowski, L.; Feinstein, A.; Sanger, R.; and Race, R. R. 1966. Ichthyosis, Xg^a blood groups, and protan. *Lancet* 0:877.

Adam, A.; Ziprkowski, L.; Feinstein, A.; Sanger, R.; Tippett, P.; Gavin, J.; and Race, R. R. 1969. Linkage relations of X-borne ichthyosis to the Xg^a blood groups and to other markers of the X in Israelis. *Ann. Hum. Genet.* 32:323.

Shapiro, L. J., et al. 1978. Enzymatic basis of typical X-linked ichthyosis. *Lancet* 2:756.

Shapiro, L. J.; Weiss, R.; Webster, D.; and France, J. T. 1978. X-linked ichthyosis due to steroid-sulphatase deficiency. *Lancet* 1:70.

Ziprkowski, L., and Feinstein, A. 1972. A survey of ichthyosis vulgaris in Israel. *Br. J. Dermatol.* 86:1.

Ziprkowski, L.; Feinstein, A.; and Adam, A. 1968. A genetic study of X-linked ichthyosis in Israel. In *Congressus Internationalis Dermatologiae—München 1967*, p. 562. Berlin, Heidelberg, and New York: Springer-Verlag. 1968.

METACHROMATIC LEUKODYSTROPHY
(LATE INFANTILE TYPE AMONG THE HABBANITES)

In 1975 Elian and co-workers diagnosed a case of late infantile metachromatic leukodystrophy (MLD) in a Jewish Habbanite family. Upon questioning members of

Table 6.30. Ichthyosis vulgaris: Ethnic origin of
Israeli Jewish patients

Country of origin	No. of patients with XLI	No. of patients with ADI
Ashkenazim		
Germany	17	—
Russia	8	6
Poland	17	10
Hungary	6	4
Czechoslovakia	—	6
Romania	16	14
Sephardim		
Yugoslavia	3	—
Greece	9	14
Turkey	3	—
Morocco	29	18
Libya	6	6
Egypt	6	—
Oriental Jews		
Syria	17	2
Iraq	56	—
Yemen	16	6
Iran	20	2
India	—	49
Total	229	137

Source: L. Ziprkowski and A. Feinstein, 1972, *Br. J.
Dermatol.* 86:1.

this Jewish isolate they found that several children had died following illnesses with
a history similar to that of MLD. Recently this group has been screening various
members of the Habbanite community to detect heterozygous carriers. The screening method being used is the determination of aryl sulfatase A activity in peripheral
leukocytes. Out of 150 subjects examined, 30 individuals (including 3 married
couples) have been found to be carriers. Since this survey is far from complete, it is

Table 6.31. Ichthyosis vulgaris: Historical data on
XLI and ADI cases

Date	XLI (%)	ADI (%)
Age of patient at onset of the disease		
At birth	60	64
Up to 6 mo	15	15
6–12 mo	10	—
1–5 yr	10	15
More than 5 yr	5	6
Course of the disease		
Without change	45	50
Improvement with time	55	50
Improvement in summer		
Marked	56	56
Slight	39	24
No change	5	20
"Atopy" in the family	—	30

Source: L. Ziprkowski and A. Feinstein, 1972, *Br. J. Dermatol.*
86:1.

not possible to determine the gene frequency of this disorder among the Habbanites, but preliminary evidence suggests that it will be quite high, especially given the fact that this group numbers no more than 1,000–1,500 individuals.

Jews from Habban, South Arabia, emigrated to Israel en masse shortly after the state was formed in 1948 and have been living as a closed community within Israeli society. Their population consists of four lineages which now total approximately 1,250 people. The rate of consanguineous matings is high among the Habbanites (56 percent), and many of these are first-cousin marriages. In addition to MLD, an autosomal recessive form of macular degeneration is common in this Jewish isolate.

For additional information on MLD the reader is referred to page 262, where a new variant of MLD is described.

References

Austin, J. 1973. Metachromatic leukodystrophy (sulfatide lipidosis). In *Lysosomes and storage diseases,* ed. H. G. Hers and F. Van-Hoof, p. 411. New York: Academic Press.

Bonné, B.; Ashbel, S.; Modai, M.; Godber, M. J.; Mourant, A. E.; Tills, D.; and Wood-head, B. G. 1970. The Habbanite isolate. *Hum. Hered.* 20:609.

Elian, E.; Zlotogora, J.; Bach, G.; Cohen, M.; and Bonné-Tamir, B. Metachromatic leukodystrophy in Habbanite Jews (in preparation).

Percy, A. K., and Brady, R. O. 1968. Metachromatic leukodystrophy: Diagnosis with samples of venous blood. *Science* 161:594.

PHENYLKETONURIA

Historical note

In 1934 Følling first reported this disorder, describing several sibs with mental retardation who excreted phenylpyruvic acid. In 1937 Penrose and Quastel introduced the term *phenylketonuria* (PKU), which has generally been adopted. In 1939 Jervis showed that this condition is transmitted as an autosomal recessive trait. In 1947 he demonstrated the excess accumulation of phenylalanine in this disease and in 1953 showed that phenylalanine hydroxylase of the liver is inactive in these patients. From Jervis's studies came a rational approach to treatment consisting of a low-phenylalanine diet. In 1956 Hsia and his group showed that it is possible to detect heterozygotes. In 1963 Guthrie and Susi developed a simple neonatal screening test which ushered in a new era regarding the genetic distribution, detection, and treatment of PKU patients.

In the past PKU has been considered extremely rare among Jews. Beginning in 1963, a series of investigations in Israel showed that this disorder is not uncommon in the Yemenite Jewish community and other Oriental and Sephardi Jewish groups.

Clinical features

Patients with PKU tend to have a small head, the circumference of which does not increase at a normal rate during the first year of life. A few have blue eyes and fair hair and skin; however, most have the same but significantly lighter-colored eyes, skin, and hair than their unaffected sibs.

In general, infants with PKU are normal at birth. Some may have a musty odor due to the presence of phenylacetic acid in their excretions. After the first 2 months all developmental milestones become delayed, and by the end of the first year of life these infants show severe mental retardation. By the age of 2 years the characteristic IQ of < 30 has usually been attained and there is, with rare exception, only a slow deterioration thereafter. Other mental abnormalities can be noted, such as autistic behavior and hyperkinetic actions. In some children such behavior patterns are self-limiting.

Approximately a quarter of all children with PKU have epileptic seizures. Minor convulsions are more common than major seizures. These seizures usually appear toward the end of the first year and gradually disappear by the late teens or early twenties.

Other neurological findings in these patients include muscular hypertonicity, hyperactive tendon reflexes with ankle and patellar clonus, fine, rapid, and irregular tremors of the outstretched hands, and a variety of abnormal body movements. A small percentage of PKU patients show signs of severe brain disease in association with severe mental retardation. Whether or not the severe brain disease is a result of the phenylketonuria is not fully known, but is suggested by the occurrence of leukodystrophy in some of the cases.

Diagnosis

The biochemical diagnosis of phenylketonuria has been made easy by the development of various screening procedures. One of the simplest methods is testing the urine with 10 percent ferric chloride or reagent-impregnated strips (Phenistix-Ames Co.). Diagnosis should then be confirmed by quantitative determination of the level of phenylalanine in the plasma.

Mass screening surveys of newborns can be done using the method developed by Guthrie and Susi. Table 6.32 shows the findings from PKU screening among newborns in Israel from 1964 to 1972. This blood test depends on the inhibition of growth of *B. subtilis* by a phenylalanine analogue, β-2-thienyalanine.

Urine tests are of limited value in the first months of life, since phenylpyruvic

Table 6.32. Phenylketonuria: Screening program among newborns in Israel, 1964–1972

Screening data	1964–1967	1967–1972	Total
Total number of live births	197,225	354,070	551,295
Infants screened	110,535	264,986	375,521
Screening coverage	56%	74%	68%
PKU cases	7	21	28
Frequency of PKU in Ashkenazi Jewish communities	1:15,790	1:12,618	1:13,411
Frequency of PKU in other communities	1:11,000 (approx.)	1:8,500 (approx.)	1:9,000 (approx.)
Presumptive positives	42	491	539
Frequency of presumptive positives	1:2,663	1:540	1:693
Mild persistent hyperphenylalaninemia	2	47	49

Source: B. E. Cohen et al., 1973, *Israel J. Med. Sci.* 9:1393.

acid is not detected until plasma phenylalanine levels exceed 15–20 mg/100 ml. These levels may be absent from the urine for 1 or 2 months. Furthermore, it has been shown that some patients with PKU in whom there is early elevation of phenyl-alanine in the blood excrete phenylalanine metabolites in the urine so late that such a delay in diagnosis could result from insistence on the presence of metabolites in the urine. In most cases, testing fresh urine with ferric chloride reveals the presence of phenylpyruvic acid very early.

Although the renal threshold of phenylalanine is high, restricting losses in the urine, the blood level may be quite high. For example, phenylalanine in the blood can reach over 100 mg/100 ml in infants, but is usually 20–40 mg/100 ml in older, untreated children and adults.

Investigative studies over the past several years have shown that many variant forms manifest elevated levels of phenylalanine in the blood (see section on Persistent mild hyperphenylalaninemia, p. 396).

Basic defect

The primary defect in phenylketonuria is the alteration of the enzyme phenyl-alanine hydroxylase. This enzyme contains two distinct protein fractions—a labile fraction found only in the liver, and a stable fraction which is widely distributed in mammalian tissues. In PKU the defect lies in the labile fraction.

Although most of the clinical features of this disease can easily be explained by this enzymatic defect, the precise mechanism accounting for the mental retardation is not fully understood. In 1972 Bowden and McArthur found that phenylpyruvic acid inhibits pyruvate decarboxylase in the brain but not in the liver. They suggested that this accounts for the defect in formation of myelin and thus in the mental retardation.

Two isoenzymes of phenylalanine hydroxylase exist in human fetal liver. The hydroxylation of phenylalanine is highly complex. At least three enzymes are known to be involved, and mutation at two loci can affect at least two of these. Furthermore, multiple alleles probably exist at the locus (or loci) determining phenyl-alanine hydroxylase apoenzyme. Thus, there are various possibilities for the many varieties of phenylalaninemia.

Genetics

Extensive genetic studies of families of PKU patients show that this disorder is transmitted in an autosomal recessive manner. In most affected families the parents are normal, often consanguineous, and rarely have affected relatives. Table 6.33 shows the degree of consanguinity in the families of Israeli PKU patients.

The prevalence of classic PKU varies in different populations. For example, it is approximately 1:4,000 in southern Ireland and western Scotland; 1:9,000 in Poland; 1:20,000 in England, Wales, and the U.S.; 1:29,000 in southern Sweden; and 1:6,000 in Japan. Table 6.32 shows the frequency of PKU in Israel from 1964 to 1972.

Among Jews PKU is not uncommon in the Yemenite community and has occasionally been observed among the Oriental and Sephardi communities. Table 6.33 shows the distribution of PKU among the various non-Ashkenazi Jewish commun-

Table 6.33. PKU cases in Israel

Ethnic group	No. of sibships	Consanguinity		No. of cases	No. treated
		1st degree	Lesser		
Jews from					
North Africa	12 + 1[a]	6	1	18 + 1[a]	12
Iran	7 + 1[a]	4		10 + 1[a]	5
Iraq	5	3	1	9	
Yemen	19	6	6	30	11
Afghanistan	1	1		2	1
Turkey	2	1		4	2
Israeli Arabs	7	5	2	9	8
Total	55	26	10	84	39

Source: B. E. Cohen et al., 1973, *Israel J. Med. Sci.* 9:1393.

Note: PKU of the classical type: blood phenylalanine, 20 mg/100 ml; urine phenylpyruvic acid and o-hydroxyphenylacetic acid positive.

[a] One child of mixed ethnic group.

ities. The actual gene frequency in the Yemenite Jewish community may be as high as 0.015, which is the order of magnitude found in some West European populations. Its occurrence in the Ashkenazi population is almost unknown, with only an occasional case being reported.

The question has been raised in Israel as to whether the origin of most of the Yemenite PKU patients (30 cases) could be traced to a restricted subgroup of the population. In 1973 Adam attempted to answer this question by taking detailed histories from the families affected. He showed that there were some genetic links between patients which reduced the number of independent sources. However, 20 unrelated sources of PKU were identified as presumed heterozygotes. These 20 lived about 100 years ago in Yemen and were widely scattered geographically (Figure 6.19). Knowledge of the geographical conditions and poor means of transportation in Yemen 100 years ago led Adam to conclude: "It is hardly conceivable that all Israeli Yemenite cases of PKU have a recent common ancestor."

Individuals who are heterozygous for the PKU gene show an elevation of blood phenylalanine, but it is very slight, and on the average the levels in the fasting state are only about one and a half times those found in controls. It is not possible to detect all carriers using this method since 25 percent or more have blood phenylalanine levels that are in the range of normal homozygotes. The carrier state can be better demonstrated by giving the suspected heterozygotes a phenylalanine loading test. When the test is given orally, the blood phenylalanine rises to higher levels in the heterozygotes than in the controls and returns to the fasting level more slowly. While these and other findings suggest a partial deficiency of the enzyme phenylalanine hydroxylase in the liver of heterozygotes, no untoward clinical or developmental abnormality is associated with this metabolic disturbance.

Prognosis and treatment

The results of treatment of PKU patients are in complete accord with the view that the PKU infant is normal at birth but that in the first few months of life retardation begins and progresses to a severe state. Therapeutic findings indicate

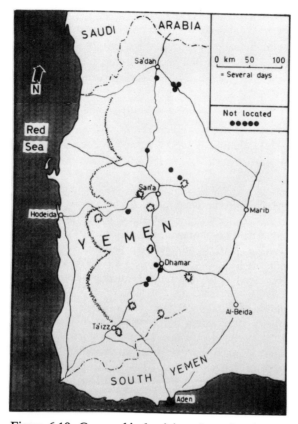

Figure 6.19. Geographical origins of unrelated, presumably heterozygous 19th-century ancestors of Yemenite Jews with phenylketonuria. From A. Adam, 1973, *Israel J. Med. Sci.* 9:1383.

that this retardation is largely irreversible but can be prevented or arrested by lowering the level of phenylalanine in the blood. This can be achieved by means of various dietary preparations that reduce the concentration of phenylalanine in the blood to almost the normal level. These commercial preparations all need to be supplemented with a carefully measured source of phenylalanine such as milk, the daily amount of which must be adjusted according to the individual child's blood phenylalanine level. Too low a pheynlalanine intake may lead to failure to thrive and to serious illness.

Treatment is usually started during the first few weeks of life and if well controlled can lead to generally normal intellectual development. The later in infancy treatment is started, the lower the intelligence quotient. In older children who already show intellectual deterioration and other features of PKU, dietary restriction usually results in an almost immediate improvement in behavior.

When treatment is started early in infancy and terminated after 2–6 years, there is no immediately obvious effect; however, over the years the IQ level may drop—the performance-scale IQ faster than the verbal.

A calculated loss of 5 intelligence quotient units for each 10 weeks that treatment is delayed provides a strong argument for early diagnosis and the early institution of therapy. However, in each suspected PKU infant the diagnosis must be confirmed by elevated plasma phenylalanine level, and subsequently the degree of control must be evaluated by periodically measuring phenylalanine levels.

References

Adam, A. 1973. Genetic diseases among Jews. *Israel J. Med. Sci.* 9:1383.

Bowden, J. A., and McArthur, C. L. III. 1972. Possible biochemical model phenylketonuria. *Nature* 235:230.

Cohen, B. E.; Szeinberg, A.; Pollak, S.; Peled, I.; Likverman, S.; and Crispin, M. 1973. The hyperphenylalaninemias in Israel. *Israel J. Med. Sci.* 9:1393.

Følling, A. 1934. Über Ausscheidung von Phenylbrenztraubensäure in den Harn als Stoffwechselanomalie in Verbindung mit Imbezillität. *Z. Physiol. Chem.* 227:169.

Guthrie, R., and Susi, A. 1963. A simple phenylketonuria screening method for newborn infants. *Pediatrics* 32:338.

Harris, H. 1971. *The principles of human biochemical genetics,* pp. 145–48. Amsterdam: North-Holand.

Hsia, D. Y.-Y.; Driscoll, K.; Troll, W.; and Knox, W. E. 1956. Detections by phenylalanine tolerance tests of heterozygous carriers of phenylketonuria. *Nature* 178:1239.

Jervis, G. A. 1939. The genetics of phenylpyruvic oligophrenia. *J. Ment. Sci.* 85:719.

———. 1947. Studies of phenylpyruvic oligophrenia: The position of the metabolic error. *J. Biol. Chem.* 169:651.

———. 1953. Phenylpyruvic oligophrenia: Deficiency of phenylalanine oxidizing system. *Proc. Soc. Exp. Biol. Med.* 82:514.

Knox, W. E. 1972. Phenylketonuria. In *The metabolic basis of inherited disease,* ed. J. B. Stanbury, J. B. Wyngaarden, and D. S. Fredrickson, 3rd ed., pp. 266–95. New York: McGraw-Hill.

Szeinberg, A. 1971. Neonatal screening for phenylketonuria and some other metabolic disorders. In *Proc. Int. Sympos. on Phenylketonuria and Allied Disorders,* ed. B. E. Cohen, M. I. Rubin, and A. Szeinberg, p. 23. Tel Aviv: Translator's Pool.

Szeinberg, A.; Cohen, B. E.; Boichis, H.; and Pollack, S. 1963. Phenylketonuria among Jews. In *Genetics of migrant and isolate populations,* ed. E. Goldschmidt, p. 296. Baltimore: Williams and Wilkins.

Woolf, L. I. 1973. Article in *Metabolic disorders in clinical genetics,* ed. Arnold Sorsby, pp. 82–88. London: Butterworths.

PITUITARY DWARFISM II
(LARON TYPE, HIGH IMMUNOREACTIVE HUMAN GROWTH HORMONE [IR-HGH])

Historical note

In 1966 Laron and co-workers described a patient from a Jewish Yemenite family with a new form of dwarfism characterized by a high serum concentration of growth hormone. Since that time other patients in Israel have been diagnosed as having this same metabolic defect and the majority of these individuals have been of Oriental Jewish ancestry. Pituitary dwarfism II is not limited to Jews, however, for it has been observed in other populations throughout the world. In 1971 Laron and co-workers reviewed their findings in 26 patients with this form of dwarfism.

Clinical features

The following description of the clinical features of pituitary dwarfism II is based on the 26 cases reviewed by Laron and co-workers. Pregnancy and delivery were normal in all cases. Birth weight was normal in all but one case. In 7 of the 13 cases in which birth length was known, it was 2 SD below the mean birth length for the respective ethnic groups. A variety of congenital malformations (strabismus, clinodactyly, partial syndactyly of toes 2 and 3, congenital dislocation of hip joints, and congenital heart disease) have been observed in these infants, but the significance of these defects has not been determined.

Motor development and skeletal maturation tended to be slow in the children studied. Many sat up only after the age of 1 year and started walking at 1.5 years or older. Teething was late in onset and fontanelle closure occurred between 3 and 7 years.

One of the earliest and most striking findings in pituitary dwarfism II is a small face and mandible, which give the false impression of a large head. The disproportion between face and calvarium produces a saddle nose appearance. Often the teeth are discolored and dentition is defective. Characteristically these children have a high-pitched voice.

From early infancy affected children grow slowly, their height being below the third percentile. In addition, their hands and feet are small. The body proportions are infantile, with a mean upper/lower segment ratio of 1.53. In normal boys over 10 years of age this ratio is 1 or below.

The subcutaneous fat tissue, measured by skinfold thickness, is well developed from early infancy and the patients are obese at all ages. The fat is mainly truncal and the degree of obesity is not always evident when calculating the weight age, for the bones are very thin and the muscle tissue underdeveloped. The genitalia are small from early childhood, a finding which is more easily recognized in males. The boys appear to mature more slowly than the girls. These patients do reach sexual maturity, however, and are able to reproduce.

Psychological evaluations were made of 17 of the 26 patients studied by Laron and co-workers. With the exception of 3, all showed some retardation and deficiency in visuomotor functioning.

Diagnosis

All patients had high growth hormone (HGH) concentrations in the acromegalic range. However, in these same patients fluctuations were detected that were unrelated to age and these are not fully understood (Figure 6.20). Most patients have a low blood sugar level at some time and, usually, the younger the patient, the more frequent the occurrence of low glucose levels. Twelve of the 26 patients had a history of hypoglycemic episodes during infancy. In about half the cases plasma FFA and 11-OHCS were higher than the normal range.

Infusion of arginine resulted in a rise of plasma HGH in all cases except one adult. It is noteworthy that despite the many high fasting values there was no paradoxical response—e.g. a decrease in plasma HGH like that often observed in normal females who start with an elevated HGH concentration. Three paradoxical decreases occurred during insulin hypoglycemia, a finding rarely observed.

The many low values of plasma insulin obtained in response to arginine infusion are a characteristic finding with this syndrome.

In 11 instances IR-HGH was measured during oral glucose tolerance tests and in 9 instances a significant suppression was observed; in 1 patient the starting value was low and in 21 patients there was no change.

For a discussion of other endocrinological studies of this disorder the reader is referred to the 1971 review by Laron and co-workers.

Basic defect

The basic defect in pituitary dwarfism II is not known. The central questions that must be answered are: Is the immunoreactive hormone in this disorder biologically inactive? Is there an inherited lack of synthesis of an intermediary substance such as sulfation factor? Or is there a primary end-organ defect?

Using a radioimmunoassay technique, no antibodies against HGH could be demonstrated.

Genetics

Family studies clearly suggest an autosomal recessive mode of transmission in this disorder (Figures 6.21 and 6.22). Consanguinity is common among the Israeli cases. When this disease does occur in Jews it is usually found in those of Asian ancestry (Table 6.34). Although this condition has now been reported in other ethnic groups, there is a clustering of cases in patients of Dutch and Arabic origin

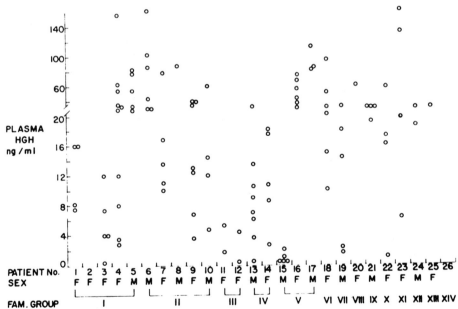

Figure 6.20. Fasting plasma HGH in patients with dwarfism and high plasma IR-HGH. From Z. Laron et al., 1971, *Excerpta Medica, Internat. Cong. Ser.*, no. 244, p. 458.

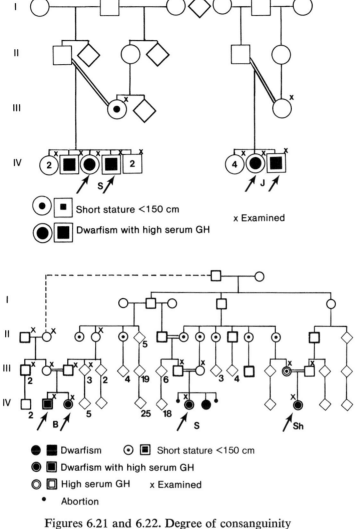

Figures 6.21 and 6.22. Degree of consanguinity in Jewish families with pituitary dwarfism II. From Z. Laron et al., 1971, *Excerpta Medica, Internat. Cong. Ser.*, no. 244, p. 458.

(Table 6.35). This may be due to some bias that only time will clarify. Detection of the heterozygous state is not possible at the present time.

Prognosis and treatment

All patients with pituitary dwarfism II are predestined to be dwarfed. However, intramuscular administration of HGH 3 times a week can give added height to these individuals. The effects of several years of this therapy on linear growth can be seen in Figure 6.23. The results are expressed as the ratio between the actual growth velocity found and that expected for the corresponding chronological age (50th

Table 6.34. Pertinent data on families of patients with familial dwarfism and
high plasma immunoreactive human growth hormone

No.	Sex	Family group	Country of origin	Hered-itary	No. of normal siblings	Consanguinity
1	F	I	Iraq	+	—	1 and 2 are sisters. Parents are first cousins.
2	F	I	Iraq	+	—	
3	F	I	Iraq	+	—	Parents are second cousins.
4	F	I	Iraq	+	—	4 and 5 are sibs. Parents are distant relatives.
5	M	I	Iraq	+	—	
6	M	II	Yemen	+	6	6, 7, and 8 are sibs. Parents are third cousins.
7	F	II	Yemen	+		
8	M	II	Yemen	+		
9	F	II	Yemen	+	4	9 and 10 are sibs. Father is half-brother of mother's grandmother.
10	M	II	Yemen	+		
11	F	III	Afghanistan	+	5	11 and 12 are sisters. Parents are first cousins. Grandparents are first cousins.
12	F	III	Afghanistan	+		
13	M	IV	Iraq	+	—	13 and 14 are sibs. Parents are first cousins.
14	F	IV	Iraq	+	—	
15	M	V	Iraq	+		Father of 16 and 17.
16	F	V	Iraq	+	1	16 and 17 are sibs, offspring of 15.
17	M	V	Iraq	+		Normal sib is from another mother.
18	F	VI	Algeria	+	4	Parents are first cousins.
19	M	VII	Iraq	+	5	Parents are first cousins.
20	M	VIII	Iran	+	2	Parents are first cousins.
21	M	IX	Iran	+	8	Parents are first cousins.
22	F	X	Iran	−	2	
23	F	XI	Iran	−	3	
24	M	XII	Iran	+	1	Mother is father's niece.
25	F	XIII	Iran	+	3	
26	F	XIV	South America			Parents are related. Father and maternal grandmother are first cousins.

Source: Z. Laron et al., 1971, *Excerpta Medica, Internat. Cong. Ser.*, no. 244, p. 458.

percentile for age). According to Laron and co-workers, this calculation helps to exclude the sex and age growth variability. It is evident that without treatment the ratio is low in all patients, but, whereas the patients lacking HGH show a marked increase in growth velocity ratio during HGH therapy, the patients with high IR-HGH show a minor response.

References

Laron, Z.; Karp, M.; Pertzelan, A.; Kauli, R.; Keret, R.; and Doron, M. 1971. The syndrome of familial dwarfism and high plasma immunoreactive human growth hormone (IR-HGH). *Excerpta Medica, Internat. Cong. Ser.*, no. 244, p. 458.

Laron, Z.; Pertzelan, A.; Karp, M.; Kowadlo-Sibergeld, A.; and Daughaday, W. A. 1971. Administration of growth hormone to patients with familial dwarfism with high plasma immunoreactive growth hormone: Measurement of sulfation factor, metabolic, and linear growth responses. *J. Clin. Endocrinol. Metab.* 33:332.

Table 6.35. Dwarfism with high plasma IR-HGH diagnosed in patients from various countries and not of Jewish origin

Patient	Sex	Country in which studied	Origin	No. of sibs	Con-sanguinity
1	M	Holland	Dutch		
2	M	Holland	Dutch	1–2	+
3	M	Holland	Dutch		
4	M	Canada	Dutch		
5	F	Canada	Dutch	4–5	+
6	M	Lebanon	Arabian		
7	F	Lebanon	Arabian	6–7	+
8	M	U.S.	Arabian		+
9	F	Iran	Persian		+
10	M	Spain	Spanish		
11	F	Spain	Spanish	10–11	
12	M	U.S.	Italian		
13	F	Germany	German		
14	F	Sweden	Swedish		
15	M	Canada			

Source: Z. Laron et al., 1971, *Excerpta Medica, Internat. Cong. Ser.*, no. 244, p. 458. For references pertaining to these cases the reader should consult this article.

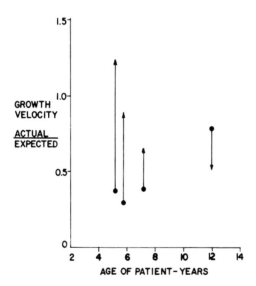

Figure 6.23. Effect of repeated courses of HGH therapy on a patient with familial dwarfism and high plasma IR-HGH. From Z. Laron et al., 1971, *Excerpta Medica, Internat. Cong. Ser.*, no. 244, p. 458.

Laron, Z.; Pertzelan, A.; and Mannheimer, S. 1966. Genetic pituitary dwarfism with high serum concentration of growth hormone: A new inborn error of metabolism? *Israel J. Med. Sci.* 2:152.

PSEUDOCHOLINESTERASE DEFICIENCY

As a result of the widespread use of the muscle relaxant suxamethonium, the polymorphic system of serum pseudocholinesterase was discovered. Under normal conditions the effects of this drug are quite short (3–5 minutes) because it is rapidly hydrolyzed into inactive products by serum cholinesterase. However, soon after its introduction by anesthesiologists some surgical patients developed prolonged muscular paralysis and respiratory apnea which often lasted two or more hours rather than the usual period of a few minutes. It was found that in these sensitive individuals the level of serum cholinesterase was consistently low. Family studies showed that a significant number of the immediate relatives of suxamethonium-sensitive individuals also had reduced levels of serum cholinesterase. This finding suggested that cholinesterase sensitivity was genetically determined and that suxamethonium-sensitive persons with low levels of serum cholinesterase were homozygous for the abnormal gene, while heterozygous individuals had a moderate reduction in the enzyme level.

Two different nomenclatures have been proposed for the various cholinesterase genes. The first, suggested by Motulsky, uses the symbol E for esterase; the second, proposed by Goedde and Baitsch, uses the symbol Ch. In the present text the symbol E will be used. The four allelic genes that are known to exist at the locus E_1 control the formation of different enzyme types. They are E_1^u for the usual type, E_1^a for the atypical (dibucaine-resistant) type, E_1^f for the fluoride-resistant type, and E_1^s for the "silent gene." Table 6.36 lists the genetic types of pseudocholinesterase.

Early population studies showed a remarkably uniform distribution of the gene E_1^a, resulting in a 2–5 percent frequency of the heterozygote type $E_1^u E_1^a$ (phenotype I) among people of European origin and certain regions of South America and Indonesia. More recent studies, however, have shown a significant deviation from this uniform distribution, with a relative rarity or absence of the E_1^a gene among blacks, East Asian populations, Eskimos, Icelanders, and Australian aborigines.

In 1966 Szeinberg and co-workers reported a significantly increased frequency of the E_1^a gene among Oriental Israeli Jews from Iraq and Iran. In 1972 they extended their survey of the Israeli Jewish population to include 9,506 subjects. Their findings are noted in Table 6.37. A very high frequency (the highest yet reported) of the E_1^a gene was observed among Jews from Iran and Iraq (frequency of

Table 6.36. Genetic types of pseudocholinesterase

Genotype	Phenotype	Suxamethonium sensitivity
$E_1^u E_1^u$ ...	U	Not sensitive
$E_1^u E_1^s$ ...		Probably not sensitive
$E_1^u E_1^a$ ...	I	Probably not sensitive
$E_1^u E_1^f$ ...	UF	Probably not sensitive
$E_1^f E_1^f$ ...	F	Moderately sensitive
$E_1^f E_1^s$ ...		Probably moderately sensitive
$E_1^a E_1^f$ ...	AF	Moderately sensitive
$E_1^a E_1^a$ ...	A	Markedly sensitive
$E_1^a E_1^s$ ...		Markedly sensitive
$E_1^s E_1^s$ ...	S	Markedly sensitive

Source: A. Szeinberg et al., 1966, *Acta Anaesthesiol. Scand.* [*Suppl.*] 24:199.

Table 6.37. Pseudocholinesterase: Frequency of variants among
various Jewish ethnic groups in Israel

Population and place of origin	No. examined	No. with phenotype A[a]	No. of heterozygotes for $E_1{}^a$ gene[b]	Frequency of $E_1{}^a$ heterozygotes (%)	$E_1{}^a$ gene frequency $\pm$ SE
Ashkenazim (Europe)	4196	—	146(3)	3.5	0.017 ± 0.001
Non-Ashkenazim					
Iraq	1057	3	94(2)	8.9	0.047 ± 0.004
Iran	159	3	18	11.3	0.075 ± 0.015
Yemen	459	—	18(1)	3.9	0.019 ± 0.004
North Africa	1106[c]	1	32(2)	2.9	0.015 ± 0.002
Balkans & Turkey	674	1	36	5.3	0.026 ± 0.004
Lebanon & Syria	203	—	7	3.4	0.017 ± 0.006
Unspecified	1652	—	69	4.2	
Total[d]	9506	8	420(8)		

Source: A. Szeinberg et al., 1972, *Clin. Genet.* 3:123. © 1972 Munksgaard International Publishers Ltd., Copenhagen, Denmark.

[a] In two cases the parents of the phenotype A subjects could not be examined and therefore their identity as $E_1{}^a E_1{}^a$ or $E_1{}^a E_1{}^s$ was not established. The calculation of the frequency of the $E_1{}^a$ gene was made on the assumption that all the subjects of phenotype A were of the genotype $E_1{}^a E_1{}^a$.

[b] In parentheses the number of subjects with $E_1{}^a E_1{}^f$ genotype (phenotype AF) is shown. All the other subjects were of $E_1{}^u E_1{}^a$ genotype (phenotype I).

[c] One subject homozygote for $E_1{}^s$ gene (phenotype S).

[d] Heterogeneity test for distribution of the $E_1{}^a$ gene in the investigated sample (without the unspecified group): $\chi^2_{6d.f.} = 117.95$; $p < 0.0005$.

heterozygotes 11.3 percent and 8.9 percent, respectively). These two communities differed significantly from all the other groups ($p < 0.005$). The lowest frequency of the gene was noted among Jews from North Africa (frequency of heterozygotes 2.9 percent). However, this was not significantly different from the frequency observed among Ashkenazi Jews or Jews from Syria, Lebanon, and Yemen.

In an exercise of preventive medicine, Szeinberg and co-workers examined 53 members of the families of subjects with phenotype A or AF. Among these, 6 with phenotype A, one with phenotype AF, and one with phenotype F (genotype $E_1{}^f E_1{}^f$) were identified. The propositi and suxamethonium-sensitive family members were given certificates stating their phenotype and recommending avoidance of the drug.

Rapid and easy screening tests for the detection of the mutant genotypes have been developed, thereby permitting examination of every patient to whom suxamethonium is to be administered. In a well-equipped operating room, under normal conditions, little danger exists if prolonged apnea develops in a sensitive patient. However, given the information now available, it would seem wise to test all Oriental Jews of Iraqi and Iranian ancestry for their sensitivity to this drug prior to its use.

References

Goedde, H. W., and Baitsch, H. 1964. Nomenclature of pseudocholinesterase polymorphism. *Br. Med. J.* 2:310.

Harris, H. 1970. *The principles of human biochemical genetics,* pp. 109–20. Amsterdam: North-Holland.

Lehmann, H., and Liddell, J. 1972. The cholinesterase variants. In *The metabolic basis of inherited disease,* ed. J. B. Stanbury, J. B. Wyngaarden, and D. S. Fredrickson, 3rd ed., pp. 1730–76. New York: McGraw-Hill.

Motulsky, A. G. 1964. Pharmacogenetics. In *Progress in medical genetics,* vol. 3, ed. A. G. Steinberg and A. G. Bearn. New York: Grune and Stratton.

Szeinberg, A.; Pipano, S.; Assa, M.; Medalie, J. H.; and Neufeld, H. N. 1972. High frequency of atypical pseudocholinesterase gene among Iraqi and Iranian Jews. *Clin. Genet.* 3:123.

Szeinberg, A.; Pipano, S.; and Ostfeld, E. 1966. Frequency of atypical pseudo-cholinesterase in different population groups in Israel. *Acta Anaesthesiol. Scand.* [*Suppl.*] 24:199.

SELECTIVE HYPOALDOSTERONISM
(CORTICOSTERONE METHYL OXIDASE DEFECT TYPE 2)

Historical note

In 1973 Rösler and co-workers first described a syndrome characterized by salt wastage, hyponatremia, and hyperkalemia associated with high levels of plasma renin activity and inappropriately low levels of aldosterone. In 1977 these investigators published their findings on the nature of the basic defect and mode of transmission of this inborn error of metabolism which seems to affect mainly Jews of Iranian ancestry.

Clinical features

The clinical features of selective hypoaldosteronism range from acute salt-wasting crisis in infancy to an asymptomatic state in adulthood that is detectable only by biochemical screening. Manifestations of intermediate degrees of severity include unexplained short stature, salt craving, and postural hypotension.

A total of 12 patients from 8 Israeli families have been diagnosed as having this disorder. Table 6.38 summarizes the clinical features observed in these cases.

Patients with the most severe defect became clinically dehydrated during the early weeks of life (patients 1–7 and 11), manifesting varying degrees of weakness, apathy sometimes alternating with irritability, loss of skin turgor, sunken eyes and fontanelles, and low-grade fever. Children who became severely dehydrated manifested peripheral vascular collapse marked by dusky-gray skin color, mottled cyanosis, tachycardia, and hypotension, a state which resembled the Addisonian crisis of salt-losing congenital adrenal hyperplasia. The course of the untreated severe form of the disorder in the early months of life is illustrated by the death of an undiagnosed sib of patients 3 and 4 at 3 months of age as a consequence of dehydration.

Children with less severe manifestations who survived the first 2 months of life without treatment tended to present the general symptom of failure to thrive. In the first recorded case of this disorder the patient was not diagnosed as having a salt-wasting disorder until the age of 6 months. His symptoms were lack of weight gain since birth and chronic constipation, but he had not suffered any acute hypovolemic episode. This somewhat delayed mode of presentation in infancy is illu-

Table 6.38. Selective hypoaldosteronism: Summary of clinical features in Israeli Jews of Iranian ancestry

Clinical feature	Patient no.											
	1	2	3	4	5	6	7	8	9	10	11	12
Age (wk) at onset of symptoms	4	5	2	2	2	1	4	?	4	?	3	?
Parental consanguinity	+	+	−	−	+	+	+	+	+	+	+	+
Failure to gain weight and grow	+	+	+	+	+	+	+	+	+	−	+	−
Severe dehydration[a]	+	+	+	−	−	+	−	−	+	−	−	−
Mild dehydration	+	+	+	−	−	+	−	−	+	−	−	−
Apathy or irritability, anorexia, or vomiting	+	+	+	+	+	+	+	−	+	−	+	−
Weakness or hypotonia	+	+	+	+	+	+	+	−	+	+	+	−
Postural hypotension							+	−		+		+
Low-grade fever	+	+	+	+	+	+	+	−	+	+	+	−
Constipation	+	+	+	−	+	+	+	+	+	+	−	−
Salt craving	+	+	+	−	+	−	+	+	−	+	+	+

Source: A. Rösler et al. 1977, *J. Clin. Endocrinol. Metab.* 44:279. Reprinted by permission of J. B. Lippincott Company.

[a] Severe dehydration indicates that hypovolemia is sufficiently severe to produce circulatory manifestations such as cyanosis, tachycardia, thready pulse, and hypotension. Mild dehydration refers to sunken eyes and fontanelles and diminished skin turgor.

strated by patient 9, who was hospitalized at 3 months of age for failure to thrive. Although hospital records show that he was suffering from mild dehydration, hyperkalemia, and metabolic acidosis at that time, these manifestations had not led to his admission to hospital. The predominance of growth retardation over hypovolemic manifestations was even more apparent in patient 8, who was first examined by a physician at 4:6 years of age because of short stature. At that time her bone age was retarded and her height and weight were that of a 1:8-year-old. The only electrolyte abnormality detected was reversible prerenal azotemia. The evolution of selective hypoaldosteronism is well illustrated by patient 7, who was hospitalized at 1 month of age for dehydration. At this time his serum Na and K concentrations were 125 mEq/l and 6.7 mEq/l, respectively. Sodium repletion therapy was begun and continued until he was 2:6 years old, at which time his serum electrolytes were normal and therapy was discontinued. He was next seen at the age of 7:2 years for severely retarded growth but showed no electrolyte abnormalities at that time.

A third category of severity consists of patients discovered in childhood or adult life through the screening of apparently asymptomatic relatives of patients by means of the urinary C-18 oxygenated steroid ratio. Patient 10, the 15-year-old sister of patient 7, was detected in this way. She was in the tenth percentile of her age group for height and weight and on closer questioning revealed that she had experienced episodes of postural hypotension and weakness, especially during hot weather, along with constipation and mild salt craving. The only electrolyte abnormalities detected were elevated plasma renin activity and an abnormal C-18 oxygenated steroid ratio. Patient 12, the mother of patients 1 and 2, also was found to have the defect after screening of apparently asymptomatic relatives. Her serum electrolytes were entirely normal, although she was somewhat short and had postural hypotension.

Diagnosis

All patients who presented with signs of dehydration showed the following electrolyte abnormalities: hyponatremia, hyperkalemia, acidosis, and prenatal azotemia.

The marked elevation in plasma renin activity detected in all patients with the biosynthetic defect was corrected after sodium repletion therapy. This elevation seems to be a more sensitive index of the presence of the defect than the plasma levels of aldosterone in the untreated state, which are generally in the range for normal children on a regular sodium intake, and in some instances in the range for normal children on a low sodium intake.

The best diagnostic index for selective hypoaldosteronism is the excretory ratio of 18-hydroxytetrahydro compound A relative to tetrahydroaldosterone. All patients who were studied in the untreated state showed a marked overproduction of the 18-hydroxy metabolite relative to that of aldosterone, with a mean excretory ratio of 189 ± 73, compared to the normal value of 2.1 ± 0.7.

Basic defect

The basic defect in this disorder is thought to lie in the second of a two-step, mixed-function oxidation reaction required to convert the angular methyl group of corticosterone to an aldehyde. The true intermediate in the reaction may not be 18-hydroxycorticosterone itself, but a reactive mono-oxygenated derivative from which 18-hydroxycorticosterone is derived by a side reaction. A less ambiguous nomenclature, *corticosterone methyl oxidase defect type 2*, has been suggested to distinguish this second-step defect from that which occurs in the first oxidation re-action, where corticosterone, not 18-hydroxycorticosterone, accumulates.

An important qualification in understanding the basic defect in this disorder is that the overproduced 18-hydroxycorticosterone must come from the glomerulosa zone rather than from the fasciculata zone, since increased secretion of 18-hydroxycorticosterone, 18-OH-DOC, and corticosterone also occurs in the 17-alpha-hydroxylase defect.

Genetics

All the affected families studied by Rösler and co-workers were Jewish and originated from Iran (Table 6.39). Their pedigrees are shown in Figure 6.24. Six of the 8 families came from the city of Isfahan, whose Jewish population has been documented for many centuries. In 7 of the 8 families various degrees of con-sanguinity were observed among the parents (Figure 6.24 and Table 6.39). The coefficient of inbreeding of the 8 sibships was found to be 0.043, as compared to 0.015 for a randomly ascertained Iranian Jewish population. This high coefficient of consanguinity, along with various other genetic analyses, strongly supports autosomal recessive inheritance of this rare disorder. At present it is not possible to detect the heterozygous state of the disease.

The factors probably responsible for the increased frequency of this disorder are the high rate of consanguinity among Iranian Jews and the likelihood of an elevated prevalence of the mutant gene among Jews from Iran, mainly from Isfahan.

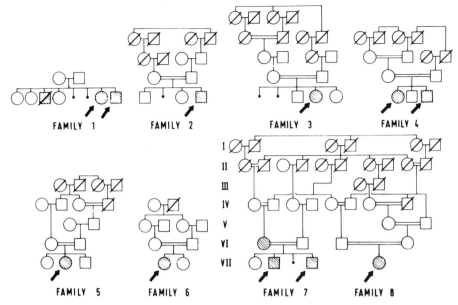

Figure 6.24. Selective hypoaldosteronism: Pedigrees of 8 affected families. From T. Cohen et al., 1977, *Clin. Genet.* 11:25. © 1977 Munksgaard International Publishers Ltd., Copenhagen, Denmark.

The frequency of this disorder in the general population is not known and would be difficult to determine, especially since cases with quantitatively milder defects are not readily detectable by clinical means.

Prognosis and treatment

The range of clinical manifestations in selective hypoaldosteronism and the degree of their expression vary greatly. The severity of symptoms is inversely correlated with age. Not only does the disorder tend to be milder in older children and adults, but severity decreases with age. It has been postulated that compensatory mechanisms serve to minimize the effects of this disease. Two possible mechanisms of compensation are glomerulosa zone hyperplasia under continued stimulation and increased salt intake exercised through salt craving. A major compensatory mechanism is very likely maturation of renal tubular transport mechanisms during the first year of life, with decreased requirement for aldosterone.

Treatment of acute dehydration consists of parental fluid therapy and intramuscularly administered DOCA. Some patients have received sodium supplements alone, while others have been given additional salt-retaining steroids. The supplements were given as NaCl alone or in association with $NaHCO_3$. The mineralocorticoid used was 9-alpha-fluorocortisol at a dose of 0.05–0.2 mg/day.

In all cases these forms of treatment corrected the electrolyte abnormalities and there was a rapid and sustained increase in weight and linear growth. This effect was seen in patients of all ages and was especially dramatic in infants, who improved more markedly and in a relatively shorter period of time than the older children.

Table 6.39. Genetic data on families with selective hypoaldosteronism

Family (no.)	Origin of 4 grandparents	Affected subjects		
		Sex	Year of birth	Coefficient of inbreeding (F)
1	Isfahan	M	1962	⎫
		F	1971	⎬ 0
		M	1972	⎭
2	Isfahan	M	1972	1/64 = 0.0156
3	Teheran	F	1971	1/64 = 0.0156
4	Isfahan	F	1959	
		M	1964	1/32 = 0.0312
5	Isfahan	F	1972	5/128 = 0.0391
6	Kermansha	F	1972	1/16 = 0.0625
7–1	Isfahan	F	1943	5/64 = 0.0781
7–2	Isfahan (3)	M	1970	
	Shiraz (1)	M	1972	5/256 = 0.0195
8	Isfahan	F	1969	65/512 = 0.1270

Source: T. Cohen et al., 1977, *Clin. Genet.* 11:25. © 1977 Munksgaard International Publishers Ltd., Copenhagen, Denmark.

References

Cohen, T.; Theodor, R.; and Rösler, A. 1977. Selective hypoaldosteronism in Iranian Jews: An autosomal recessive trait. *Clin. Genet.* 11:25.

Rösler, A.; Rabinowitz, D.; Theodor, R.; Raminez, L. C.; and Ulick, S. 1977. The nature of the defect in a salt-wasting disorder in Jews of Iran. *J. Clin. Endocrinol. Metab.* 44:279.

Rösler, A.; Theodor, R.; Boichis, H.; Rabinowitz, D.; and Ulick, S. 1974. Salt-wastage and a corticosterone methyl oxidase defect. In *56th Annual Meeting, Endocrine Society, Atlanta*, p. A-87.

Rösler, A.; Theodor, R.; Gazit, E.; Boichis, H.; and Rabinowitz, D. 1973. Salt wastage, raised plasma-renin activity, and normal or high plasma-aldosterone: A form of pseudohypoaldosteronism. *Lancet* 1:959.

SELECTIVE VITAMIN B_{12} MALABSORPTION

Historical note

Juvenile pernicious anemia can be divided into two types: (1) that which results from inadequate secretion of intrinsic factor (IF) and is characterized by normal absorption of B_{12} in the presence of exogenous IF; and (2) selective B_{12} malabsorption of intestinal origin, which is associated with normal IF secretion and is not corrected by administration of exogenous IF.

In 1960 Imerslund and Gräsbeck and co-workers independently described a familial syndrome in children which is characterized by isolated malabsorption of B_{12} without the IF deficiency usually associated with proteinuria. In 1968 Visakorpi and Furuhjelm reviewed the literature and collected data on 55 cases. Twelve of the 55 cases were from Norway, 21 from Finland, and the remainder were sporadic cases from several different countries. In 1969 Ben-Bassat and co-workers reported 18 cases of this disorder in 14 Jewish Israeli families. In 1973 Furuhjelm and

Nevanlinna reviewed the literature and reported family studies of 15 Finnish propositi.

Clinical features

The clinical features of selective vitamin B_{12} malabsorption are quite characteristic and in most cases present themselves during infancy. The most common presenting symptoms are pallor, weakness, and failure to thrive. Gastrointestinal symptoms such as anorexia, vomiting, and diarrhea also are frequently noted. If the disease progresses undetected, glossitis and mild hepatosplenomegaly develop in most cases. Some children show minor physical retardation, but neurological findings are not common.

Diagnosis

In addition to the above clinical findings, which are characteristic but non-specific, the following diagnostic criteria have been suggested by Spurling and co-workers: (1) the appearance of megaloblastic anemia within the first 5 years of life in response to parenteral B_{12}, and relapse after the cessation of therapy; (2) malabsorption of labeled B_{12} even after the addition of exogenous IF and normal absorption of other nutrients; and (3) the presence of proteinuria without evidence of kidney disease.

The anemia tends to be quite severe. In the 18 cases studied by Ben-Bassat and co-workers the following laboratory observations were made. Hemoglobin ranged between 4.9 g% and 8.8 g%, with a mean level of 6.7 g%. Moderate leukopenia, relative lymphocytosis, and thrombocytopenia were usually found. All patients had typical megaloblastic peripheral blood and bone marrow. Serum B_{12} levels were very low (< 100 pg/ml).

Response to parenteral therapy with B_{12} was dramatic, with a peak reticulocyte response occurring between the fourth and sixth days of therapy. A normal hemoglobin level was reached after 3 weeks in all cases.

Proteinuria was present in all patients and all had normal values for blood urea and creatinine. No amino aciduria was noted, although other investigators have reported it in a few cases. A renal biopsy was done in only 1 of the 18 patients and it was normal. All patients were subjected to an intravenous pyelographic study, but an abnormality (intraparenchymal pelvis) was noted in only 1.

The mean age of the patients at the time of diagnosis was 8:6 years; the youngest was 3 years old, the oldest 15.

Basic defect

The mechanism of defective vitamin B_{12} absorption is not known. However, recent studies have shown that it is not associated with a morphologically identifiable lesion and indicate that the absorptive defect does not result from lack of ileal receptors for intrinsic-factor-vitamin B_{12} complex (IF-B_{12}). It has been postulated that the defect appears at a stage of vitamin B_{12} absorption that occurs after IF-B_{12} attaches to the surface of the ileal cell and before the absorped vitamin binds to transcobalmin II.

Table 6.40. Selective B_{12} malabsorption: Ethnic distribution of
Israeli patients based on country of parental origin

Country of origin of parents	No. of cases	No. of families	Consanguinity
Tunisia[a]	11	9	4
Libya	5	3	1
Algeria	1	1	1
Central Europe	1	1	1

Source: I. Ben-Bassat et al., 1969, *Israel J. Med. Sci.* 5:62.

[a] Since this original report 2 more cases have been diagnosed, 1 in a Jewish child whose parents are from Tunisia and the other in another Sephardi Jewish child.

Genetics

Fewer than 100 cases of this rare disorder have appeared in the literature, with the majority of cases being of either Scandinavian (Finnish and Norwegian) or Sephardi Jewish origin.

Of the 18 cases of this disorder reported among Israeli Jews, 14 were males, 4 were females, and the 18 were distributed among 14 families. This distorted sex ratio has not been noted in other series reported in the literature and may reflect incomplete ascertainment in the Israeli survey. Thirteen of the 14 Sephardi families were of North African ancestry. In 7 of these families the patients' parents were first cousins. None of the parents suffered from a similar disorder, and a Schilling test was normal in each of 5 individual parents studied. Such information strongly supports an autosomal recessive form of inheritance, and other studies confirm this mode of transmission. Table 6.40 summarizes the distribution of the Jewish cases on the basis of parental origin.

The minimal prevalence of selective B_{12} malabsorption among Israeli Jews of Tunisian ancestry aged 3–15 years is estimated to be 1:1,200. The calculated gene frequency, taking into account the high rate of consanguinity in Tunisian Jews, is 0.025 and the frequency of heterozygotes is about 0.05.

Prognosis and treatment

For patients who have been recognized and treated, the prognosis is excellent. Relapses tend to occur from 7 months to 3 years after therapy is discontinued, so parenteral B_{12} should be considered a lifetime treatment. The proteinuria in this disorder is thought to carry a good prognosis.

References

Ben-Bassat, I.; Feinstein, A.; and Ramot, B. 1969. Selective vitamin B_{12} malabsorption with proteinuria in Israel: Clinical and genetic aspects. *Israel J. Med. Sci.* 5:62.

Furuhjelm, U., and Nevanlinna, H. R. 1973. Inheritance of selective malabsorption of vitamin B_{12}. *Scand. J. Haematol.* 11:27.

Gräsbeck, R. 1960. Familjar selektiv B_{12}-malabsorption with proteinuri eff perniciosaliknande syndrome. *Nord. Med.* 63:322.

Imerslund, O. 1960. Idiopathic chronic megoblastic amenia in children. *Acta Paediatr. Scand.* 49 (suppl. 119): 1.

Mackenzie, I. L.; Donaldson, R. M., Jr.; Trier, J. S.; and Mathan, V. I. 1972. Ileal mucosa in familial selective vitamin B_{12} malabsorption. *N. Engl. J. Med.* 286:1021.

Spurling, C. L.; Sacks, M. S.; and Jiji, R. M. 1964. Juvenile pernicious anemia. *N. Engl. J. Med.* 271:995.

Visakorpi, J. K., and Furuhjelm, U. 1968. Selective malasorption of vitamin B_{12}. *Mod. Probl. Paediatr.* 11:150.

THALASSEMIA

In 1945, twenty years after the original description of this disorder by Cooley and Lee in Detroit, Schieber first reported a form of this disease in two Palestinian Jewish sibs originating from the Bucharian area near the southeast bank of the Caspian Sea. Schieber was later better known by his Aramaic name, Sheba (one of the founders of medical genetics in Israel and former director of the Tel Hashomer Hospital, now the Chaim Sheba Medical Center), which he took in 1948 while serving as chief medical officer of the Israel Defence Forces.

Since 1940 it has become apparent that the thalassemia syndrome is remarkably heterogeneous, for some 50 combinations of different genetic disorders have been shown to produce the clinical picture of thalassemia. Furthermore, it has been realized that these disorders occur throughout the world and are not localized to the Mediterranean region.

In general, the thalassemias may be defined as a group of disorders of hemoglobin synthesis characterized by a partial or total reduction in the rate of synthesis of one or more of the globin chains leading to imbalanced globin chain synthesis. The disorders may be classified broadly as the *alpha*-thalassemias and the *beta*-thalassemias (Figure 6.25). However, it is evident that within both of these groups there is marked heterogeneity.

Most of the clinical features of thalassemia can be related to the deleterious effects on erythropoiesis caused by the precipitation of unpaired globin chains. Figure 6.26 is a schematic representation of the pathophysiology of beta-thalassemia.

In Israel most available estimates of the frequency of the beta-thalassemia gene are based on the screening of population samples for Hb-A_2 and Hb-F rather than on an analysis of the frequency of thalassemia patients. In 1964 Ramot and co-workers published their findings on the frequency of the beta-thalassemia gene in various Jewish ethnic groups arriving to settle in Israel. Table 6.41 indicates that the beta-thalassemia gene is common in Indian and Kurdish Jews, but low among Jews from Iran and Morocco.

In 1973 T. Cohen reviewed her experience with beta-thalassemia in Kurdish Jews over a 20-year period (1951–1970). Her study involved 50 patients, 33 living and 17 deceased. These patients were, or had been, members of 28 sibships living in Jerusalem and its surroundings. In 26 families 50 parents were from the Kurdish areas of Iraq, Turkey, and Iran. The fact that the overwhelming majority of thalassemia major patients originated from a relatively well-defined geographical area confirms that the genes for beta-thalassemia are highly concentrated in the Kurdish Jewish community of Israel. When Cohen analyzed her data she found that fewer affected children have been born in recent years (31 between 1951 and 1960 versus 17 between 1961 and 1970). The reasons for this decrease are: (1) a purposeful limitation of family size; and (2) more individuals of Kurdish origin are

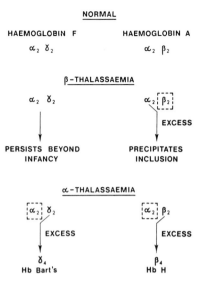

Figure 6.25. Alpha- and beta-thalassemia. From D. J. Weatherall,
1976, The thalassaemias: Genetic
and pathological aspects, in *Aspects
of genetics in paediatrics*, ed. D.
Barltrop. (London: Postgraduate
Medicine).

marrying into other ethnic groups. It has been estimated that 39 percent of Kurdish
Jewish matings are interethnic, which produces a dilution of beta-thalassemia genes
in the Kurdish community and a concomitant spread of these genes into the general
population of Israel.

Table 6.42 lists estimates of the frequency of the beta-thalassemia gene among
various Jewish ethnic groups.

There are two main clinical disorders which result from the interaction of the
different alpha-thalassemia genes found in Oriental and Mediterranean populations.
These are the Hb Bart's hydrops fetalis syndrome and Hb H disease. Infants with
hydrops fetalis are either stillborn or die within a few minutes of birth. Clinically
they appear pale and bloated and have massively enlarged livers and spleens. Eighty
to 90 percent of the hemoglobin in these cases is Hb Bart's (see Figure 6.26),
which releases so little oxygen to tissues that it is essentially useless as an oxygen-
transport protein. Hydrops fetalis is the most devastating of all the thalassemias. In
Hb H disease, which is particularly prevalent in Southeast Asia and the Middle
East, the clinical findings usually resemble those of thalassemia intermedia, but
the manifestations vary in severity from little disability to severe anemia. These two
conditions result from the interaction of 3 alpha-thalassemia genes: alpha-thalassemia 1, which results in complete abolition of alpha chain synthesis; alpha-
thalassemia 2, a gene which partially reduces alpha chain production, and Hb
Constant Spring, an abnormal alpha chain variant synthesized in low amounts. The
Hb Bart's hydrops fetalis syndrome results from the homozygous state for the

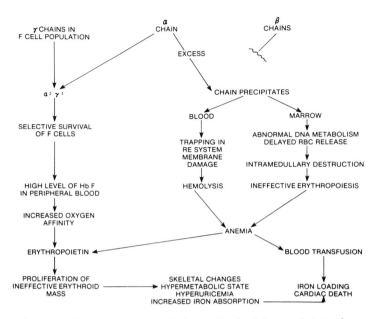

Figure 6.26. A summary of the pathophysiology of beta-tha-lassemia. From D. J. Weatherall, 1976, *Johns Hopkins Med. J.* 139:205.

alpha-thalassemia 1 gene. Hemoglobin H disease can result from the heterozygous states for both the alpha-thalassemia 1 and Hb Constant Spring genes.

A number of surveys have been carried out in Israel to determine the frequency of Hb Bart's and all have shown this form of alpha-thalassemia to be particularly frequent among the Yemenite Jews. Table 6.43 shows the results of a survey done by Halbrecht and Ben-Porat on cord blood from 3,247 newborn infants. In this series the concentration of Hb Bart's ranged from 4 percent to 17 percent. In a survey for alpha-thalassemia in the Yemenite and Iraqi Jewish communities, Zaizov and Matoth found 17 percent Hb Bart's in the cord blood of infants from Yemenite parents and 11 percent in infants from parents originating from Iraq.

Using the criterion of 4 percent or more of Hb Bart's in cord blood at birth, a group of Jerusalem investigators has shown that approximately 1 in 80 Kurdish Jews is affected, while for Yemenites and Ashkenazim the ratios are 1:25 and 1:500, respectively.

The alpha-thalassemia phenotype among Kurdish Jews seems to differ from that observed in Yemenite and Ashkenazi Jews. Among the latter, using the usual hematological methods, detection of carrier parents and sibs of newborns with elevated Hb Bart's is rarely possible. It has been postulated that in Yemenite and Ashkenazi Jews the gene behaves as a silent gene or recessive trait.

Within the Kurdish and Yemenite communities cases of Hb H disease have been recorded. Since the frequency of the alpha-thalassemia carrier among Yemenites is about 0.04, Kurdish-Yemenite matings may also produce Hb H disease. However,

Table 6.41. Frequency of beta-thalassemia in certain Israeli Jewish communities

Country or ethnic group	No. of subjects	No. of cases with elevated			Total no. of cases	%
		A₂ only	F only[a]	A₂ + F		
Persia	182	4	0	1	5	2.7
India						
Cochin	66	8	1	1	10	15.2
Beni-Israel	172	20	5	4	29	16.9
Morocco	147	2	2	0	4	2.7
Kurdistan	110	7	2	13	22	20.0

Source: B. Ramot et al., 1964, *Br. J. Haematol.* 10:155.

[a] The level of Hb-F ranged from 2.8 percent to 7.5 percent. All patients were over 2 years of age.

Table 6.42. Estimates of the frequency of the beta-thalassemia gene among various Israeli Jewish ethnic groups

Jewish ethnic group	Gene frequency
Kurdish	0.08
Iraqi	0.01
Iranian	0.01
Yemenite	Rare
Indian	
Beni-Israeli	0.08
Cochinian	0.07
Sephardi	Very rare
Ashkenazi	Absent

these marriages are rare, as noted in the finding of only 12 such couples among parents of 8,000 newborns examined for Hb Bart's.

Table 6.44 lists the frequencies of Hb Bart's in cord blood for a few of the Oriental Jewish communities. Despite these relatively high frequencies of Hb Bart's, no cases of hydorps fetalis have been reported in Israel. Zaizov and Matoth have postulated that the mutation present among the Jewish communities of Israel is different from that in Southeast Asians, where the condition is relatively common. This possibility has been tentatively corroborated by data from Saudi Arabia.

Unfortunately the treatment of thalassemia is still limited to the symptomatic control of the anemia and to efforts to counteract the main complication of treatment—transfusional siderosis.

References

Adam, A. 1973. Genetic diseases among Jews. *Israel J. Med. Sci.* 9:1383.

Chernoff, A. I. 1959. The distribution of the thalassemia gene: A historical review. *Blood* 14:899.

Clegg, J. B. 1975. The molecular defect in thalassaemia. In *Aspects of genetics in paediatrics,* ed. D. Barltrop, p. 97. London: Fellowship of Postgraduate Medicine.

Cohen, T. 1973. Thalassemia types among Kurdish Jews. *Israel J. Med. Sci.* 9:1461.

Cohen, T.; Horowitz, A.; Abrahamov, A.; and Levene, C. 1966. Hemoglobin H disease: alpha- and beta-thalassemia traits in a family of Kurdish Jews. *Israel J. Med. Sci.* 2:600.

Table 6.43. Incidence of hemoglobin Bart's in cord blood
of newborns from various Israeli ethnic groups

Ethnic group	No. of newborns examined	Incidence of Hb Bart's	
		No.	%
Jewish			
Yemenite	756	131	17.3
Iraqi-Iranian	597	26	4.3
Sephardi	396	7	1.9
North African	297	2	0.8
Ashkenazi	941	8	0.7
Arab (Israeli)	260	13	5.0
Total	3,247	187	

Source: I. Halbrecht and S. Ben-Porat, 1971, *Kupat Holim Yearbook*
1:90.

Table 6.44. Level and frequency of hemoglobin Bart's in
cord blood in certain Oriental Jewish groups

Group	Level of Hb Bart's	
	1–4%	4%
Yemenite	0.14	0.04
Iraqi	0.08	0.03
Kurdish	?	0.013

Source: A. Adam, 1973, *Israel J. Med. Sci.* 9:1383.

Cooley, T. B.; and Lee, P. 1925. Series of cases of splenomegaly in children with anemia and peculiar bone changes. *Trans. Am. Pediatr. Soc.* 37:29.

Goldschmidt, E.; Cohen, T.; Isacsohn, M.; and Freier, S. 1968. Incidence of hemoglobin Bart's in a sample of newborn from Israel. *Acta Genet.* 18:361.

Halbrecht, I., and Ben-Porat, S. 1971. Incidence of hemoglobin Bart's in the cord blood of Jewish and Arabic ethnic groups in Israel. *Kupat Holim Yearbook* 1:90.

Horowitz, A.; Cohen, T.; Goldschmidt, E.; and Levene, C. 1966. Thalassemia types among Kurdish Jews in Israel. *Br. J. Haematol.* 12:555.

Klibansky, Ch.; Djaldetti, M.; Joshua, A.; and de Vries, A. 1960. Haemoglobin H thalassemia disease in a Sephardic Jewish family from Turkey. *Israel Med. J.* 19:199.

Matoth, Y.; Shamir, Z.; and Freundlich, E. 1955. Thalassemia in Jews from Kurdistan. *Blood* 10:176.

Ramot, B.; Abrahamov, A.; Frayer, Z.; and Gafni, D. 1964. The incidence and types of thalassaemia-trait carriers in Israel. *Br. J. Haematol,* 10:155.

Ramot, B.; Sheba, C.; Fisher, S.; Ager, J. A. M.; and Lehmann, H. 1959. Haemoglobin H disease with persistent haemoglobin "Barts" in an oriental Jewess and her daughter: A dual alpha-chain deficiency of human haemoglobin. *Br. Med. J.* 2:1228.

Schieber, C. 1945. Target-cell anaemia: Two cases in Bucharan Jews. *Lancet* 2:851.

Wasi, P.; Na-Nakorn, S.; and Pootrakul, S. 1974. The alpha-thalassaemias. In *Clinics in haematology,* ed. D. J. Weatherall. London: W. B. Saunders.

Weatherall, D. J. 1975. The thalassaemias: Genetic and pathophysiological aspects. In *Aspects of genetics in paediatrics,* ed. D. Barltrop, p. 87. London: Fellowship of Post-graduate Medicine.

———. 1976. Thalassemia—Historical introduction. *Johns Hopkins Med. J.* 139:194.

———. 1976. The molecular basis of thalassemia. *Johns Hopkins Med. J.* 139:205.

Weatherall, D. J., and Clegg, J. B. 1972. *The thalassaemia syndromes,* 2nd ed. Oxford: Blackwell Scientific Publications.

Zaizov, R.; Kirschmann, C.; Matoth, Y.; and Adam, A. 1973. The genetics of alpha-thalassemia in Yemenite and Iraqi Jews. *Israel J. Med. Sci.* 9:1457.

Zaizov, R., and Matoth, Y. 1972. Alpha-thalassemia in Yemenite and Iraqi Jews. *Israel J. Med. Sci.* 8:11.

Zlotnik, A.; Ramot, B.; and Hamosh, P. 1964. Haemoglobin H disease with persistent haemoglobin "Barts" in a Jewish family of Aleppo-Urfalian ancestry. *Israel Med. J.* 23:57.

WERDNIG-HOFFMANN DISEASE
(SPINAL MUSCULAR ATROPHY TYPE I)

Historical note

Werdnig in 1894 and Hoffman in 1900 were the first to report this form of spinal muscular atrophy. In 1971 Emery reviewed the nosology of the spinal muscular atrophies (SMAs) and suggested that SMA characterized by proximal limb weakness may be divided into at least 4 types: infantile, intermediate, juvenile, and adult. In 1977 Fried and Mundel published a brief report on the high incidence of SMA type I (Werdnig-Hoffmann disease) in the Karaite community of Israel.

Clinical features

Onset of SMA type I usually occurs before the age of 9 months and often occurs *in utero.* The early findings are weakness and hypotonia of the proximal and distal limbs and intercostal and bulbar muscles. Patients tend to lie in a frog-leg position with hips and knees flexed. Mental development is normal and the bright look of these infants is a striking contrast to their lack of motor activity.

Diagnosis

The diagnosis of SMA type I is based mainly on clinical findings. In addition to the above clinical features, affected infants usually have visible fibrillations in the tongue, absent tendon reflexes, paradoxical breathing with inward movement of the chest on inspiration, and normal extraocular eye movements.

Electromyographic studies often show evidence of muscle denervation, including fibrillation potentials and fasciculations. A muscle biopsy shows groups of muscle fibers in varying stages of degeneration. Spinal fluid values, nerve conduction studies, and serum enzyme values are normal.

Basic defect

The basic defect in SMA type I is not known. The primary neuropathological change consists of atrophy of anterior horn cells in the spinal cord and of motor nuclei in the brain stem. Secondarily there is atrophy of motor nerve roots and muscles.

Table 6.45. Karaite patients with SMA type I (infantile Werdnig-Hoffmann disease) born during the period 1970–1975

Case no.	Sex	Age at onset (mo)	Age at death (mo)	Consanguinity of parents	No. of sibs older than 1 year
1	M	1	18	First cousins	4
2	M	5	15	None	0
3	F	7	28	None	0
4	M	1	6	None	2

Source K. Fried, Israel.

Genetics

SMA type I is known to be transmitted as an autosomal recessive disorder. In a large study involving 112 cases in 70 families, almost 6 percent of the parents were consanguineous, a value 8 times that in a control group.

While no adequate data exist on the incidence of SMA type I, Fried and Mundel believe it is reasonable to assume that between 1 in 5,000 and 1 in 50,000 infants will have the disease in most populations. In their study in Israel they found 4 unrelated cases (Table 6.45) among 1,600 Karaite infants (1:400), which suggests an incidence 1 or 2 orders of magnitude higher than that found in other populations. In 1 case the parents were first cousins.

These investigators admit that chance alone may account for their findings, but they prefer the more likely explanation that due to genetic drift the gene frequency of SMA type I in this Karaite isolate has reached 0.05 and that thus 1 in 10 persons in this community is a heterozygote carrier of the recessive gene.

For a historical account of the Karaites the reader is referred to Chapter 1.

Prognosis and treatment

SMA type I is a fatal disease. Death is usually caused by respiratory failure due to aspiration of food. Onset *in utero* usually results in death before the age of 2 years, while in cases of later onset (before the age of 9 months) death occurs by the fourth year of life.

References

Emery, A. E. H. 1971. The nosology of the spinal muscular atrophies. *J. Med. Genet.* 8:481.

Fried, K., and Mundel, G. 1977. High incidence of spinal muscular atrophy type I (Werdnig-Hoffmann disease) in the Karaite community in Israel. *Clin. Genet.* 12:250.

Hoffmann, J. 1900. Dritter Beitrag zur Lehre von der hereditären progressiven spinalen Muskelatrophie im Kindesalter. *Dtsch. Z. Nervenheilk.* 18:217.

Werdnig, G. 1894. Die frühinfantile progressive spinale Amyotrophie. *Arch. Psychiatr. Nervenkr.* 26:706.

7

Rare or isolated
genetic syndromes

THE MAJORITY of disorders presented in this chapter are autosomal recessive in nature, and appear in non-Ashkenazi Jewish communities where there is a significant rate of consanguineous marriages. Although some of these syndromes are quite rare, there are cogent reasons why they should be brought to the attention of clinicians and medical geneticists: (1) not all of these disorders are isolated to single families, and therefore their frequency among Jews and non-Jews can be determined only through the recognition of additional cases; (2) the study of rare genetic disorders frequently advances medical knowledge that is applicable to more common diseases; and (3) it is important for physicians to know of these conditions for purposes of treatment and genetic counseling.

ACUTE HEMOLYTIC ANEMIA WITH FAMILIAL ULTRASTRUCTURAL ABNORMALITY OF THE RED-CELL MEMBRANE

Historical note

In 1962 Danon and co-workers reported episodes of acute hemolytic anemia in a 39-year-old Ashkenazi Jewish woman who had a familial red-cell disorder characterized by spherocytosis, an ultrastructural abnormality of the red-cell membrane as revealed by electron microscopy, but with normal red-cell fragilities and, in the interval between attacks, a normal red-cell life span. Further clarification of this disorder has not been achieved nor has it been described in other patients.

Clinical features

In 1955 a 38-year-old Polish-born Jewish housewife was admitted to a hospital in Israel because of marked weakness and pallor. She had been admitted to the hospital 7 years before for treatment of an acute episode of hemolytic anemia that was possibly drug induced.

Two months before her 1955 admission, while she was in the fourth month of her tenth pregnancy (following three spontaneous and five artificial abortions), she began to bleed from the uterus. The bleeding continued for 3 weeks, and she then received an intravenous injection of neosalvarsan (although serology for lues was negative); this was followed within 24 hours by a high temperature and spontaneous abortion. The only additional drug she received was salicylate. After 3 days, marked pallor and a slight icteric tinge of the conjunctivae were noted, the urine became dark, and a red-cell count of 2.3 million/cu.mm was found. The serum bilirubin was 1.5 mg/100 ml and the E.S.R. 100 mm in the first hour (Westergren). She was admitted to another hospital, received one blood transfusion, and was discharged after 1 week without fever. Four days before the admission detailed here she became ill with an upper respiratory infection, her temperature rose, and she became markedly pale. She had not taken any drugs.

On admission, physical examination revealed a rather obese woman with marked pallor and slight jaundice. Her temperature was normal. The only additional abnormal finding was a firm, nontender spleen, which was palpable 1 cm below the costal margin.

All available family members were evaluated and these findings are summarized in Table 7.1. The evaluation showed that the same abnormality was present in the patient's son, both of her sisters, and in the 2 sons of 1 of her sisters. In the other children about half of the red cells were smooth and thin, but they were not unusually pitted, indicating a quantitatively less striking red-cell abnormality.

Diagnosis

The precise diagnosis of this disorder is not clear. Danon and co-workers postulated that they were dealing with a mild form of hereditary spherocytosis or of nonspherocytic congenital hemolytic anemia. However, they pointed out that in these disorders the red-cell life span is persistently decreased, in contrast to their patient's normal red-cell life span when she is not anemic.

Electron microscopy revealed that the majority of the patient's red-cell membranes were smooth, thin, and slightly pitted, in contrast to the majority of thicker and granular membranes found in normal subjects (Figures 7.1–7.3).

Basic defect

The basic defect in this disorder is not known, but it undoubtedly involves some alteration in the red blood cell membrane. Recently I discussed this case with the senior investigator and he mentioned that more advanced techniques are now available for studying the basic defect in this red-cell membrane abnormality, and that if a similar case were to be studied today an entirely different approach would be initiated.

Genetics

The observation that more than one generation is affected and that the condition is variably expressed strongly supports an autosomal dominant form of transmission. Because the condition shares some of the features of hereditary spherocytosis the possibility of a variant of that disorder should be considered.

The reason that other cases have not been reported may be that the methods of investigation described here have not been applied to similar cases.

Table 7.1. Acute hemolytic anemia: Hematological data on a patient and her relatives

Data	Proband		Son of proband	Sister (1) of proband
	During attack	In remission		
Hb (g/100 ml)	7.2	13.5	12.9	9.8
Red cells (mill./cu.mm)	2.3	4.5	4.3	3.2
White cells (thous./cu.mm)	7.6	—	5.7	4.6
Platelets (thous./cu.mm)	1.75	—	1.5	1.8
Reticulocytes (%)	16.4	0.8	0.7	0.8
Spherocytes[a]	++	+	+	+
E.S.R. (Westergren)				
(mm 1 hr/2 hr)	100/135	10/28	15/40	58/90
		35/60		
Red-cell fragilities				
Osmotic (% NaCl)				
post-incubation	0.50–0.20	0.48–0.30	0.46–0.30	0.46–0.30
	Normal	Normal	Normal	Normal
Autohemolysis	Normal	Normal	Normal	Normal
Mechanical	Normal	Normal	—	Normal
Acid serum test	Normal	Normal	—	Normal
Serology				
Antiglobulin test				
direct	+	—	—	—
indirect	+	—	—	—
Cold agglutinins	1 in 64	—	—	—
Electron microscopy of red-cell membranes	Majority smooth	Majority smooth	Majority smooth	Majority smooth

Source: D. Danon et al., 1962, *Br. J. Haematol.* 8:274.

[a] Darker cells of small diameter.

Prognosis and treatment

Presently available information suggests that this condition may be benign and that episodes of hemolytic anemia are probably drug or virus induced. Treatment consists of avoiding those agents that are known to precipitate a bout of anemia. If anemia occurs, therapy is one of symptomatic care.

Reference

Danon, D.; de Vries, A.; Djaldetti, M.; and Kirschmann, C. 1962. Episodes of acute haemolytic anemia in a patient with familial ultrastructural abnormality of the red-cell membrane. *Br. J. Haematol.* 8:274.

ACROCEPHALOPOLYSYNDACTYLY TYPE IV:
A NEW GENETIC SYNDROME

Historical note

In 1909 Carpenter described 3 sibs with multiple malformations that included the key features of acrocephalopolysyndactyly. In 1959 Noack reported a father and daughter who also exhibited acrocephalopolysyndactyly. Although affected mem-

Daughters of sister (1)			Sister (2) of proband	Sons of sister (2)	
A	B	C		1	2
13.0	12.3	13.2	11.4	12.7	11.9
3.8	4.3	4.6	3.8	4.6	4.4
5.4	6.2	7.4	5.0	—	—
—	—	—	1.8	—	—
0.6	0.8	0.6	0.8	0.1	0.1
?	?	?	+	?	?
13/35	—	—	29/64	5/15	7/20
0.46–0.30	—	—	0.48–0.30	0.48–0.30	0.46–0.20
Normal	—	—	Normal	Normal	Normal
Normal	—	—	Normal	Normal	Normal
—	—	—	—	—	—
—	—	—	—	—	—
—	—	—	—	—	—
Almost half smooth	Almost half smooth	Almost half smooth	Majority smooth	Majority smooth	Majority smooth

Note: ? indicates a few darker cells of somewhat smaller diameter that could not be classified as spherocytes.

bers in these two families shared certain physical features, they differed in others and in mode of genetic transmission. Currently the autosomal dominant form is referred to as acrocephalopolysyndactyly type I (ACPS I, or Noack syndrome) and the autosomal recessive form is called acrocephalopolysyndactyly type II (ACPS II, or Carpenter syndrome). In 1971 Sakati and co-workers reported a single case of what appeared to be type III ACPS (Sakati syndrome or ACPS with leg hypoplasia) possibly involving autosomal dominant transmission. In addition to acrocephalopolysyndactyly, their patient had distinctive defects of the ear, skin, and lower limbs. In 1979 Goodman and co-workers studied 2 of 3 affected sibs from a consanguineous Jewish Iranian family who presented with acrocephalopoly-syndactyly plus other features that had not previously been reported. This new constellation of findings is thought to represent a new genetic malformation syn-drome termed acrocephalopolysyndactyly type IV (ACPS IV).

Clinical features and diagnosis

Because ACPS IV is a new genetic syndrome a detailed account of clinical findings and diagnostic procedures will be given for the proband (III-7), a 17-year-old girl.

At birth the proband was noted to have bilateral polydactyly, the extra digits

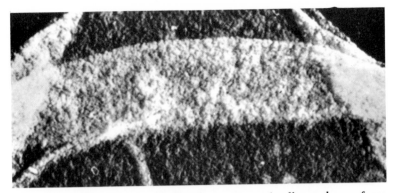

Figure 7.1. Electron micrograph of a young red-cell membrane from a normal donor. Note the thickness and granular appearance of the membrane; about 80 percent of the red-cell membranes present this structure. From D. Danon et al., 1962, *Br. J. Haematol.* 8:274.

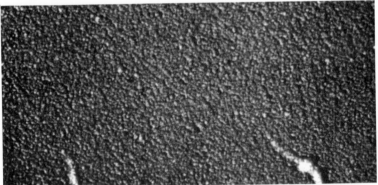

Figure 7.2. Electron micrograph of an old red-cell membrane from a normal donor. Note the thinner membrane and lack of granularity; about 20 percent of the membranes presented this structure. From D. Danon et al., 1962, *Br. J. Haematol.* 8:274.

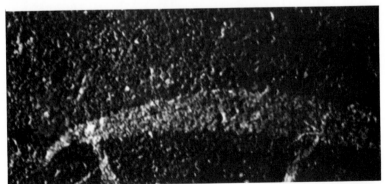

Figure 7.3. Electron micrograph of red-cell membrane of proband. Eighty percent of the patient's red-cell membranes were thin in appearance with tiny holes scattered across a relatively smooth surface; the other 20 percent were indistinguishable from the granular membranes of normal donors. From D. Danon et al., 1962, *Br. J. Haematol.* 8:274.

arising from both fifth fingers. These were removed soon after birth. At the age of 4 months she was diagnosed as having congenital heart disease. During her early childhood she suffered from multiple bouts of lower respiratory tract infections. Despite her multiple handicaps, however, she developed well and is considered to be a good student. At the age of 14 years she underwent several orthopedic corrections to her legs and feet. Soon thereafter she developed episodes of fainting with cyanosis which led to the decision to reevaluate her cardiac condition.

At the age of 16 years the patient was admitted to hospital for cardiac studies. Physical examination showed an apparently healthy girl with an obviously malformed skull and malformations of the hands and toes. All vital signs were normal. She measured 158.5 cm in height, arm span was 156 cm, head circumference was 56 cm, and her weight was 63 kg. There was marked acrocephaly. Her facial features were altered by highly arched eyebrows, micrognathia, prominent nose with moderate flaring of the nares, and moderate facial hirsutism. Her oral cavity showed a very highly arched palate with severe crowding of the teeth. The palpebral fissures had a mild mongoloid slant, while epicanthal folds were observed bilaterally. The ears were large, protruding, and the external pinnae were not well demarcated.

The patient's chest showed an increased A-P diameter, with mild thoracic scoliosis to the left. The right side of the chest appeared larger than the left and there was pectus carinatum.

Cardiac examination showed normal peripheral pulses. On palpation there was a right ventricular heave without a thrill. On auscultation the first heart sound was normal, followed by a systolic click. The second heart sound was single and very accentuated over the pulmonic area. No murmurs were heard and there were no signs of cardiac failure.

Examination of the upper extremities showed mildly cyanotic nail-beds and moderate clubbing. Bilateral scars were observed on the lateral aspect of the fifth digits (the former sites of polydactyly). There was severe bilateral clinodactyly with camptodactyly of the fifth digits with ulnar deviation of the second and third fingers. The second digit appeared short while the thumbs were long. Syndactyly involving only the skin was present between all fingers except the thumbs and forefingers (Figure 7.4). The lower extremities showed genu valgum, surgical scar about both knees, poor muscular development of the lower legs, bilateral pes cavus, equinovarus, and syndactyly involving the skin between all the toes.

The remainder of the physical examination was within normal limits.

An electrocardiogram showed left axis deviation with counterclockwise rotation in the frontal plane and right ventricular hypertrophy and strain. These findings were considered compatible with a persistent common atrioventricular canal malformation.

Right-heart catheterization with dye dilution and selective angiography showed pulmonary hypertension (160/60 in the main pulmonary artery, with a mean pulmonary wedge pressure of 10) and a persistent common atrioventricular canal with atrial and ventricular septal defects with reversed shunt (Eisenmenger syndrome).

Roentgenographic studies of the skeletal system confirmed the various skeletal malformations involving the skull (Figure 7.5) and extremities.

Chromosomal studies in the proband showed a normal female karyotype.

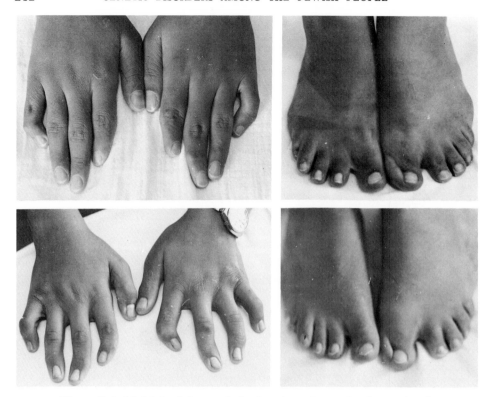

Figure 7.4. Multiple defects of the hands and toes in the proband (*top*) and her affected brother (*bottom*). Note the clinodactyly, camptodactyly, ulnar deviation of the fingers, and syndactyly of the fingers and toes. The extra digits (polydactyly) in the proband were removed during infancy.

The proband's 15-year-old brother (III-8) showed clinical findings (Figure 7.4) almost identical to those observed in his sister, except that he showed no signs of heart disease.

In 1958, III-6, an 8-month-old male sib of the proband, was admitted to another hospital for fever, diarrhea, and vomiting. Although he recovered from this episode of acute gastroenteritis, he died at the age of 2 years from heart failure. His hospital record in 1958 strongly suggests that he had exactly the same malformation syndrome. Positive physical findings recorded at that time included the following. His skull showed towering (acrocephaly), with a pointed, narrow frontal region. Cardiac examination showed peripheral cyanosis with a harsh systolic murmur. An electrocardiogram revealed right atrial enlargement. The cardiac diagnosis at that time was cyanotic congenital heart disease. His hands showed bilateral polydactyly involving the fifth digits, brachydactyly, and syndactyly. The toes all showed syndactyly. Roentgenographic studies of the extremities showed that fingers 2, 3, and 4 had only 2 phalanges while finger 5 had only 1. There was also a malformation of the left femur. However, these roentgenograms were not available for study. The consensus from the above studies was that this child was similarly affected.

The main clinical features in this syndrome are listed in Table 7.2.

Figure 7.5. Roentgenogram of the skull of the proband showing acrocephaly. The same finding was noted in her affected brother.

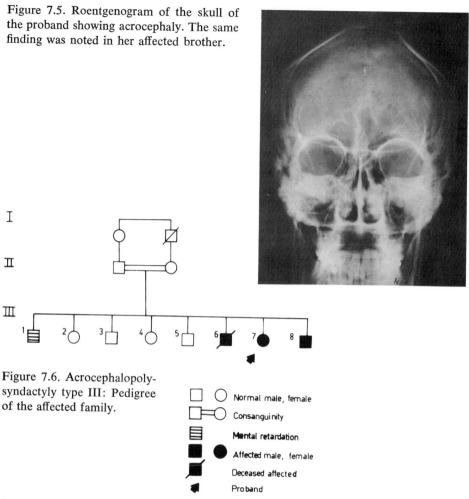

Figure 7.6. Acrocephalopoly-syndactyly type III: Pedigree of the affected family.

□ ○ Normal male, female
□—○ Consanguinity
▤ Mental retardation
■ ● Affected male, female
◪ Deceased affected
◀ Proband

Basic defect

The basic defect in ACPS IV is not known.

Genetics

The family pedigree of the proband (III-7) is shown in Figure 7.6. Note that the first sib (III-1) suffers from mental retardation. His parents stated that this 27-year-old man has had hemiplegia from birth. He presently resides in an institution for the mentally retarded. His parents deny that he in any way resembles the other 3 affected sibs.

The parents are first cousins of Jewish Iranian ancestry. The father is 57 years old and the mother 42 years old. Both are in good health and neither show any of the craniofacial or skeletal abnormalities observed in their affected offspring. It is thought that ACPS IV is transmitted as an autosomal recessive disorder.

It will be interesting to see whether this newly described type IV ACPS is an isolated syndrome or occurs in other ethnic groups. Several cases of ACPS type II have been reported with no special ethnic distribution, and ACPS type I (some-

Table 7.2. Acrocephalopolysyndactyly type IV: Clinical
features observed in 3 sibs

System and findings	III-6: 2-yr-old male (deceased, not examined)	III-7: 17-yr-old female	III-8: 15-yr-old male
Craniofacial			
Acrocephaly	+	+	+
Highly arched eyebrows		+	+
Mongoloid slant to palpebral fissures		+	+
Epicanthal folds		+	+
Prominent nose		+	+
Flared nares		+	+
Highly arched palate		+	+
Crowding of teeth		+	+
Micrognathia		+	+
Facial hirsutism		+	
Large, deformed, protruding ears		+	+
Chest			
Increased A-P diameter		+	+
Thoracic asymmetry		+	+
Pectus carinatum		+	+
Thoracic scoliosis		+	+
Congenital heart disease	+	+	
Eisenmenger syndrome		+	
Upper Extremities			
Polydactyly	+	+	+
Syndactyly	+	+	+
Brachydactyly	+	+	+
Clinodactyly		+	+
Camptodactyly		+	+
Ulnar deviation of fingers		+	+
Angulation of elbow		+	+
Lower Extremities			
Genu valgum		+	+
Muscular hypoplasia		+	+
Equinovarus		+	+
Pes cavus		+	+
Syndactyly of toes	+	+	+

times referred to as acrocephalosyndactyly type V, or Pfeiffer syndrome) is known to occur in various ethnic groups.

Prognosis and treatment

The degree of cardiac involvement in ACPS IV makes the prognosis a guarded one. Surgical correction of cardiac and skeletal malformations should be considered when indicated.

References

Carpenter, G. 1909. Case of acrocephaly with other malformations. *Proc. R. Soc. Med.* 2:45, 199.

Eaton, A. P.; Sommer, A.; Kontras, S. B.; and Sayers, M. P. 1974. Carpenter syndrome—acrocephalopolysyndactyly type II. *Birth Defects* 10:249.

Gnamey, D., and Farriaux, J. P. 1972. Syndrome dominant associant polysyndactylie, pouces en spatule, anomalies facials et retard mental (une forme particulière de l'acrocephalo-polysyndactylie de type Noack). *J. Genet. Hum.* 19:299.

Goodman, R. M., and Gorlin, R. J. 1977. *An atlas of the face in genetic disorders*, 2nd ed. St. Louis: C. V. Mosby.

Goodman, R. M.; Sternberg, M.; Shem-Tov, Y.; Bat-Miriam Katznelson, M.; Hertz, M.; and Rotem, Y. 1979. Acrocephalopolysyndactyly type IV: A new genetic syndrome in 3 sibs. *Clin. Genet.*, in press.

Noack, M. 1959. Ein Beitrag zum Krankheitsbild du Akrozephalosyndaktylie (Apert). *Arch. Kinderheilk.* 160:168.

Pfeiffer, R. A. 1969. Associated deformities of the head and hands. *Birth Defects* 5:18.

Sakati, N.; Nyhan, W. L.; and Tisdale, W. K. 1971. A new syndrome with acrocephalo-polydactyly, cardiac disease, and distinctive defects of the ear, skin, and lower limbs. *J. Pediatr.* 79:104–9.

Temtamy, S. A. 1966. Carpenter's syndrome: Acrocephalopolysyndactyly, an autosomal recessive syndrome. *J. Pediatr.* 69:111.

ALDOLASE A DEFICIENCY

Historical note

In 1973 Beutler and co-workers described a 5-year-old Ashkenazi Jewish boy who suffered from nonspherocytic hemolytic anemia, mental retardation, and increased hepatic glycogen apparently due to a deficiency of red-cell aldolase. In 1977 Lowry and Hanson noted many dysmorphic features in the same patient, some of which are observed in the Noonan syndrome. To date, no other cases of this syndrome have been reported.

Clinical features

At birth the child weighed 4 pounds 15 ounces. He had a flat nose, puffy eyes, a short neck, and dry, lax skin, his abdomen was distended, and his liver was palpable 2 cm below the costal margin. At the age of 6 weeks he was hospitalized with pallor, 5 cm hepatomegaly, a 7.5 percent hemoglobin count, and a 10 percent reticulocyte count. During the next three months the patient was transfused on 4 occasions and his hemoglobin ranged from 4 to 11 g percent. A peripheral smear was reported as being normal and his bone marrow was hypercellular. No blood was found in the patient's urine or stools. The bilirubin concentration of his blood was less than 1 mg percent.

At the age of 4 months a liver biopsy was done and only excess glycogen was noted in the liver; no well-defined enzymatic defect was detected.

The child's development was retarded. He sat only at 8 months and did not talk until 4:4 years of age. At 4:8 years his height was 83 cm, his weight was 9.94 kg, and peculiar facial features, including flat nose, epicanthic folds, strabismus, short neck without webbing, pallor, and lax skin, were noted. The abdomen was distended and the liver was 5.5 cm below the right costal margin. The spleen tip was palpable but there was no ascites.

When this patient was seen by Lowry and Hanson at the age of 8 years, they noted that some of his features (growth and mental retardation, ptosis, epicanthal folds, short neck, and low posterior hairline) were reminiscent of the Noonan syndrome; however, the hematologic situation was not.

Diagnosis

Because the course of this disorder in this child was atypical of a glycogen storage disease, Beutler and co-workers thought it worthwhile to survey the erythrocyte enzymes. The aldolase activity of cultured skin fibroblasts from the patient was 3.5 units per gram protein in contrast to control cultures that had a mean activity of 18 units of aldolase per gram protein. Further studies showed the child to be deficient in aldolase A, which is the principal type found in muscle and red cells. Beutler and co-workers were unable to detect any structural abnormality in the child's aldolase by isoelectric focusing, electrophoresis, heat stability studies, or kinetic examination.

Basic defect

Much remains to be learned about the basic defect in this syndrome. Beutler and co-workers point out that the occurrence of nonspherocytic congenital hemolytic anemia in patients with defects of the glycolytic pathway is well-known; thus, it is not surprising that their patient had such a hemolytic anemia. The mental retardation also could be explained on the basis of aldolase A deficiency, for aldolase A is the principal aldolase at work in the brain during early development, while aldolase C appears only later. The mild storage of glycogen in the liver could be explained as a diversion of dietary glucose and fructose from the peripheral tissues, which are aldolase deficient, to the liver, where aldolase is under separate control. No adequate explanation has been offered to account for the dysmorphic features of the child or the fact that both his parents show normal aldolase activity.

Genetics

Because the proband's parents are first cousins, it is postulated that this disorder is transmitted as an autosomal recessive condition. Theoretically, prenatal diagnosis should be possible in this syndrome. Currently this Ashkenazi Jewish boy is an isolated case of this disorder.

Prognosis and treatment

Experience with one patient does not provide adequate prognostic information. Treatment at this time is symptomatic.

References

Beutler, E., et al. 1973. Red cell aldolase deficiency and hemolytic anemia: A new syndrome. *Trans. Assoc. Am. Phys.* 86:154.

Lowry, R. B., and Hanson, J. W. 1977. Aldolase A deficiency with syndrome of growth and developmental retardation, midfacial hypoplasia, hepatomegaly, and consanguineous parents. *Birth Defects Orig. Art. Ser.* 13(3B): 223.

Figure 7.7. Lateral view of the eye showing the configuration of keratoglobus. From G. Greenfield et al., 1973, *Clin. Genet.* 4:8. © 1973 Munksgaard International Publishers Ltd., Copenhagen, Denmark.

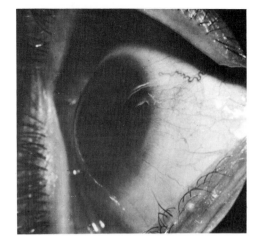

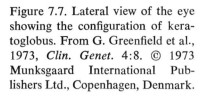

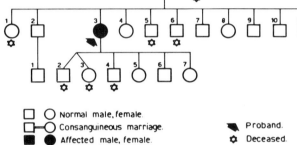

Normal male, female.
Consanguineous marriage.
Affected male, female.
Spontaneous abortion.

Proband.
Deceased.

Figure 7.8. Blue sclerae and keratoconus: Pedigree of the affected Jewish Iraqi family. From G. Greenfield et al., 1973, *Clin. Genet.* 4:8. © 1973 Munksgaard International Publishers Ltd., Copenhagen, Denmark.

BLUE SCLERAE AND KERATOCONUS

Historical note

Blue sclerae and keratoconus are findings commonly associated with a number of heritable disorders of connective tissue. In 1913 Behr first called attention to the possibility that these features might form a distinct syndrome. In 1968 and 1969, 4 cases from 2 Jewish families originating from Tunisia were reported. In 1973 Greenfield and co-workers reported 2 more affected Jewish sibs from a Jewish Iraqi family and reviewed the literature.

Clinical features

The main clinical features of this disorder are blue sclerae and keratoconus (Figure 7.7). A variety of other findings have been reported and include the following: hyperextensible joints in the majority of cases, corneal fragility, decrease in hearing, dry skin and hair, poor dental development, dislocated hips, red hair, umbilical hernia, arachnodactyly, spondylolisthesis, and mental retardation.

A history of fractures, the most conspicuous finding in osteogenesis imperfecta, has not been noted in any of the reported patients. Table 7.3 summarizes the main findings noted from a review of the literature.

Table 7.3. Blue sclerae and keratoconus: Review of the literature

Author	Year	Case no.	Age	Sex
Behr	1913	1		M
		2		M
Attiah, Sobhy Bay	1931	1	Few weeks	F
Badtke	1941	1		F
		2		F
Tucker	1959	1	Newborn	M
Stein (Jewish, Tunisia)	1968	1	3 yr	M
		2	13 yr	M
Hyams (Jewish, Tunisia)	1969	1	4 yr	F
Babel	1969	1	10 yr	M
Gregoratos	1971	1	4 yr	M
Greenfield (Jewish, Iraqi)	1972	1	32 yr	F
		2	19 yr	M

Source: G. Greenfield et al., 1973, *Clin. Genet.* 4:8. © 1973 Munksgaard International Publishers Ltd., Copenhagen, Denmark.

Diagnosis

Blue sclerae and keratoconus or keratoglobus, coupled with possible autosomal recessive inheritance, add certainty to the diagnosis of this syndrome. Present-day laboratory studies are not helpful in making the diagnosis.

Basic defect

The basic defect in this disorder is not known. Pathological and biochemical studies of keratoconus and blue sclerae suggest that these 2 alterations may be the consequence of a fundamental disorder of collagen synthesis. Biochemical studies on keratoconic corneas show a decreased production of collagen and an increased production of glycoprotein. Microscopic studies of specimens of blue sclerae have shown pathological changes similar to those in keratoconus. The collagen fibrils appear normal but their number is reduced. Increased amounts of glycoprotein and a greater number of reticular fibers are found in the interstitial spaces.

Genetics

Of the 9 families reported to have this syndrome, consanguinity was present in 7 (see Table 7.3). No parent-to-offspring transmission has been observed, so these findings would support autosomal recessive inheritance.

Of the 13 cases reported from the 9 families, 5 are Jews from 3 separate families. Two of these families are from Tunisia; the other is from Iraq. Figure 7.8 shows the pedigree of the Jewish Iraqi family.

The distinctiveness of this syndrome seems relatively certain, but to infer a higher frequency of this disorder among Jews of Sephardi or Oriental background would

		Clinical findings				
Blue sclerae	Kerato- conus or kerato- globus	Corneal fragility	Hyper- extensible joints	Fractures	Hearing defect	Consan- guinity
+	+	−	+	−	−	?
+	+		+	−	+	?
+	+	−	+	−	−	+
+	+	−	+	−	−	
+	+	−	+	−	−	+
+	+	−	+[a]	−	−	+
+	−	+	−	−	−	
+	−	+	+	−	−	+
+	+	+	+	−	+[b]	+
+	+	−	+	−	−	−
+	+	−	−	−	−	+
+	+	−	−	−	+	+
+	+	−	+	−	+	+

[a] Congenital dislocation of hips.
[b] Secondary to chronic otitis media, cholesteotoma.

be presumptuous at this time. Recognition of the disorder in other patients will aid in clarifying the ethnic distribution of this heritable disease of connective tissue.

Prognosis and treatment

Eye complications such as rupture of Descemet membrane and fragility of the cornea with rupture must be carefully assessed and properly treated. In keratoglobus the thinning of the cornea is generalized or peripheral, while in keratoconus it is mainly central.

References

Behr, C. 1913. Beitrag zur Aetiologie des keratokonus. *Klin. Monatsbl. Augenheilk.* 106:585.

Greenfield, G.; Romano, A.; Stein, R.; and Goodman, R. M. 1973. Blue sclerae and keratoconus: Key features of a distinct heritable disorder of connective tissue. *Clin. Genet.* 4:8.

Hyams, S. W.; Dar, H.; and Neumann, E. 1969. Blue sclerae and keratoglobus: Ocular signs of a systemic connective tissue disorder. *Br. J. Ophthalmol.* 53:53.

Stein, R.; Lazar, M.; and Adam, A. 1968. Brittle cornea: A familial trait associated with blue sclerae. *Am. J. Ophthalmol.* 66:67.

CAMPTODACTYLY WITH FIBROUS TISSUE HYPERPLASIA AND SKELETAL DYSPLASIA

Historical note

The term *camptodactyly* was coined by Landouzy in 1906 to describe a form of contractures of the fingers. The etiology of this malformation is variable; it may be genetic or it may occur as a sporadic event of unknown cause. A number of genetic

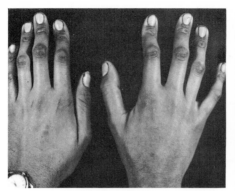 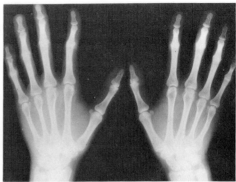

Figure 7.9. Hands of the proband showing arachnodactyly, camptodactyly, and knuckle pad formation.

Figure 7.10. Radiograph showing arachnodactyly and camptodactyly in the proband.

syndromes are associated with the finding of camptodactyly. In 1972 Goodman and co-workers reported a new camptodactyly syndrome affecting 3 sibs of Jewish Iranian ancestry.

Clinical features

The proband, a healthy appearing 17-year-old boy, was 175 cm tall with an arm span of 183 cm and an upper segment/lower segment ratio of 81 cm/94 cm or 0.86. Although his body habitus appeared Marfanoid, there was little else in the way of a family history or physical findings on which to make this diagnosis. The patient had a broad nose with flaring nostrils. His hands and feet were large and arachnodactylic. All digits of the hands except the thumbs showed the changes caused by of camptodactyly, the onset of which was said to have occurred at the age of 10 years (Figure 7.9). Knuckle pads were observed on the second, third, and fourth fingers bilaterally. Hammer toes were also present bilaterally. There was mild scoliosis of the thoracic spine. The patient had a surgical chest scar from a ligation of a patent ductus arteriosus at the age of 7 years. With the exception of a lower than normal intelligence, the remainder of the physical examination was normal.

The patient had 2 older sisters who, with the exception of the patent ductus, were identically affected. All 3 affected sibs stated that they first noted the changes of camptodactyly around the age of 10 years. The similar facial features of these sibs were quite distinct from those of their normal parents, sibs, and relatives. In general, broad facial features are not characteristic of the Jewish Iranian community.

Diagnosis

The diagnosis of this syndrome is mainly clinical. Table 7.4 shows the main features detected in affected sibs from one family. Roentgenographic studies of these 3 sibs showed scoliosis of the thoracic spine, camptodactyly and arachnodactyly of the hands (Figure 7.10), and a hammer toe deformity of the feet.

Table 7.4. Camptodactyly with fibrous tissue hyperplasia and skeletal dysplasia: Common clinical features and degree of severity noted in 3 affected sibs

Defect	Degree of severity		
	IV-5 (F aged 24)	IV-6 (F aged 21)	IV-7 (proband; M aged 19)
Facies			
Broad nose	+	+	+
Flaring nostrils	+	+	+
Dull expression with low normal intelligence	+	++[a]	++
Spine			
Thoracic scoliosis	+	+	+
Extremities			
Large hands and feet with archnodactyly	+	+	+
Camptodactyly	+	+	+
Knuckle pads	+	+	++
Hammer toes	+	+	+

Source: R. M. Goodman et al., 1972, *J. Med. Genet.* 9:203.

[a] ++ = more severe.

Laboratory tests, including screening for urinary amino acids and growth hormone assay, were not remarkable. Dermatoglyphic findings were not unusual.

Basic defect

The basic defect in this syndrome is not known. It is postulated that an abnormality in connective tissue synthesis is involved.

Genetics

Figure 7.11 shows the family pedigree of the above sibs. The parents are first cousins of Jewish Iranian ancestry. Because the parents are normal but closely consanguineous, it is thought that the mode of transmission of this syndrome is autosomal recessive. To date, no other reports of the disorder have been published.

Prognosis and treatment

This syndrome seems compatible with a normal life span, yet it may be too early to state a full prognosis. Patients do not suffer greatly from any of the clinical findings associated with this syndrome; however, they do have a limited ability to fully extend and flex their fingers.

Reference

Goodman, R. M.; Katznelson Bat-Miriam, M.; and Manor, E. 1972. Camptodactyly: Occurrence in two new genetic syndromes and its relationship to other syndromes. *J. Med. Genet.* 9:203.

222

222

222

222

222

222

222

CHRONIC AIRWAY DISEASE IN A SAMARITAN FAMILY

The present Samaritan community numbers about 500 individuals living in two cities: Holon in Israel, and Nablus on the West Bank in Samaria. From the extensive genetic studies of this ethnic group by Dr. Bonné-Tamir, we know that the rate of consanguinity is very high among these people. Approximately 34 percent of all marriages are consanguineous. In 1974 Khasis-Gerblich and co-workers reported chronic airway disease—consisting of recurrent spastic bronchitis, bronchiectasis, chronic bronchitis, and emphysema—in 9 of 16 members of 3 generations of one Samaritan family (Figure 7.12). Due to the lack of any known environmental agent, the investigators concluded that this multifaceted lung condition was probably genetically determined. Despite the presence of consanguinity, it would appear from the pedigree that this disorder is transmitted as an autosomal dominant disease. Tests for alpha-1-antitrypsin deficiency, including trypsin inhibitory capacity and proteinase inhibition, were normal. There was no apparent immunologic defect in 4 of the patients examined, nor did any findings suggest cystic fibrosis.

Reference

Bonné, B. 1966. The Samaritans: A demographic study. *Am. J. Hum. Genet.* 18:60.
Khasis-Gerblich, Y.; Marcus, J. H.; Shamrat, R.; and Legum, C. P. 1974. Chronic airway disease in a Samaritan family. *Harefuah* 86:455.

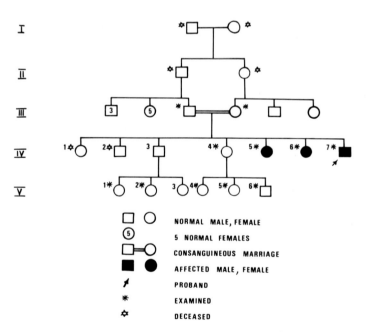

Figure 7.11. Camptodactyly: Pedigree of the affected family.

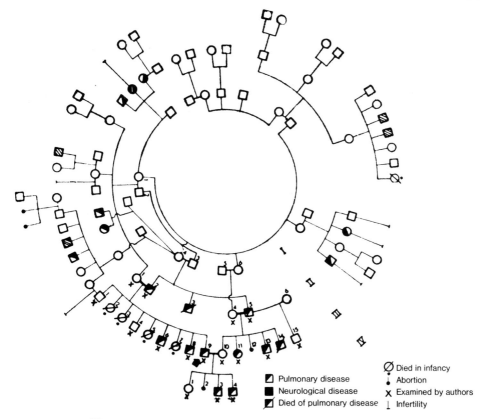

Figure 7.12. Pedigree of a Samaritan family showing pulmonary disease and Parkinson-like neurological disease. From Y. Khasis-Gerblich et al., 1974, *Harefuah* 86:455.

CLEIDOCRANIAL DYSPLASIA
(AUTOSOMAL RECESSIVE TYPE)

Historical note

In 1897 Marie and Sainton first described the characteristic clinical findings in cleidocranial dysplasia, which is now a well-recognized genetic disorder of connective tissue. Extensive genetic reviews on the subject substantiate the fact that the classic form of this disease is caused by an autosomal dominant gene with complete penetrance and an unusually high mutation rate.

In 1975 Goodman and co-workers reported 2 unrelated consanguineous Jewish Iraqi families with this disorder. Due to the severity of involvement and the genetic setting, it was postulated that there may be an autosomal recessive form of cleidocranial dysplasia.

Clinical features

Three cases were reported—2 male sibs aged 4 and 8 years, respectively, and a 38-year-old male from another family. A brief account of the physical findings in each case will be given in order to emphasize the severity of involvement.

FAMILY A

The proband, a 4-year-old boy, is presently institutionalized for severe mental retardation. He does not speak and is unable to walk. His height is 74 cm (< 3rd percentile) and his head circumference is 49 cm. His head is brachycephalic in shape with a wide-open anterior fontanelle. There is marked frontal and parietal bossing. The nose is depressed at the base and the nares are flared. Ocular hypertelorism can be noted. He has 6 permanent teeth which appear normal, but the deciduous teeth appear dysplastic. Macroglossia is present. Chest examination showed the patient to have bilateral absence of the clavicles and hypoplasia of the scapulae. The abdomen was protuberant, a finding which was accentuated in the sitting position by the smallness of the chest cage. Other pertinent physical findings consisted of bilateral clinodactyly and hypoplasia of all the nails.

The proband's 8-year-old brother also suffers from the same disorder but is of normal intelligence. He is also very short for his age, measuring 107 cm in height (< 3rd percentile). His skull is brachycephalic, measuring 36.5 cm in circumference. He has marked frontal and parietal bossing with nonclosure of the anterior fontanelle and sutures. Ocular hypertelorism was present. Examination of the oral cavity showed many dental caries. Chest examination showed bilateral absence of the clavicles, winging of the scapulae, and bilateral flaring of the rib cage. Other findings included a marked lumbar lordosis, coxa vara, and hypoplasia of the nails.

FAMILY B

The proband, aged 38 years, is of very short stature, measuring only 131 cm (< 3rd percentile). His height is below that of his parents and sister. Classic physical findings include a brachycephalic skull, measuring 54 cm in circumference, with a large, open anterior fontanelle. The frontal part of the skull is depressed. There is evidence of ocular hypertelorism with bilateral strabismus. Many teeth are missing and the patient gave a history of poor dentition over a long period of time. Chest examination showed bilateral absence of clavicles with a short and flared rib cage. Upon standing the patient displayed kyphoscoliosis with a marked lumbar lordosis. Other physical findings include brachydactyly of the hands and feet with bilateral stub thumbs and hypoplasia of all nails, particularly those of the toes.

Table 7.5 lists the roentgenographic findings noted in these 3 patients.

Diagnosis

Diagnosis of this disorder is made by noting the classic clinical findings and substantiating them with roentgenographic studies. There is no specific biochemical test for this abnormality, and chromosomal studies are normal.

Basic defect

The basic defect in this disorder is not known. However it is apparent from clinical features that this is a diffuse connective tissue disease involving primarily the formation and development of cartilage and bone. Viewing the 3 main anatomical sites of involvement (clavicles, skull, and pelvis) embryologically, the absence or hypoplasia of the clavicles could be explained by an alteration in

Table 7.5. Cleidocranial dysplasia: Roentgenographic findings observed in 3 patients

Location	Defect	Case 1 (4 yr)	Case 2 (8 yr)	Case 3 (38 yr)
Skull	Brachycephalic	+	+	+
	Frontal + parietal bossing	+	+	+
	Incomplete closure of fontanelle	+	+	+
	Wide, persistent sutures	+	+	+
	Persisting metopic suture	+	−	+
	Wormian bones	+	+	+
	Calvarial thickening (occipital)	+	+	+
	Narrow, short sphenoid	+	+	+
	Large foramen magnum (wide base)	+	+	+
	Small facial bones	+	+	+
	Absent paranasal sinuses	−	−	+
	Hypertelorism	+	+	+
	Mandibular prognatism	+	+	+
Dentition	Embedded teeth	−	−	+
	Supernumerary teeth	−	−	+
	Carious deciduous teeth	+	+	+
Chest	Cone-shaped thorax	+	+	+
	Small scapula	+	+	−
Clavicles	Complete absence	+	+	+
Pelvis	Hypoplasia of iliac wings	+	+	+
	Wide sacral iliac joint	0	0	+
	Failure of fusion of symphysis pubis	+	+	−
Spine	Kyphosis	+	+	+
	Scoliosis	+	+	+
	Lordosis	+	+	+
	Spina bifida (cervico-thoracic)	−	−	+
	Hemivertebrae	−	−	+
	Posterior wedging of thoracic segment	−	−	+
Long bones	Broad and short femoral neck	−	−	+
	Coxa vara	−	+	−
Extremities Hands	Short distal phalanges	+	+	+
	Accessory epiphyses at metacarpal base	+	+	−
Feet	Delay in development of terminal phalanges	+	+	−

Source: R. M. Goodman et al., 1975, *Clin. Genet.* 8:20 © 1975 Munksgaard International Publishers Ltd., Copenhagen, Denmark.
Note: + = present; − = absent; 0 = not yet developed.

embryonic induction, while failure of the skull sutures to close and delay in the development of the pelvic bones could be due to some missing or altered factor involving morphogenic movements. It is likely that the basic defect is capable of influencing a variety of stages in fetal development.

Genetics

Autosomal recessive inheritance is postulated for the following reasons: (1) the severity of the disease in all 3 cases, compared to the wide range of expressivity observed in the classic dominant form; (2) normal parents both clinically and radiographically; and (3) close parental consanguinity in both families (Figures 7.13 and 7.14). Autosomal dominant inheritance could be argued on the basis of undetected involvement in one of the parents of family A or a new mutation in the

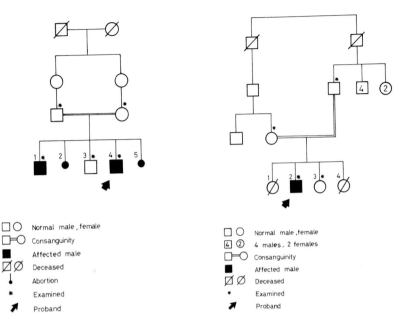

Figure 7.13 Cleidocranial dysplasia: Pedigree of family A.

Figure 7.14. Cleidocranial dysplasia: Pedigree of family B.

case of family B. Arguing along these lines, X-linked recessive transmission also could be proposed, since all affected are male, but it is the opinion of the author that autosomal recessive inheritance is most plausible.

The fact that these two unrelated families were of Jewish Iraqi ancestry may be just a coincidence. Further documentation of this form of cleidocranial dysplasia is needed before any definite genetic conclusions can be reached.

Unusual clustering of the dominant form has been recorded by Jackson in the family of an affected man of Chinese descent who embraced the Moslem religion and had 7 wives. Of his 356 descendants, 70 were affected with cleidocranial dysplasia.

Prognosis and treatment

The mental retardation observed in the proband of family A usually is not considered to be part of this disorder. At this time it is difficult to state whether or not there is a cause-and-effect relationship between the two. Treatment of this condition is symptomatic care. If a recessive form does indeed exist, the risk of recurrence drops from 50 percent in the dominant form to 25 percent in the recessive type.

References

Goodman, R. M., and Gorlin, R. J. 1977. *An atlas of the face in genetic disorders*, 2nd ed., pp. 92–93. St. Louis: C. V. Mosby.
Goodman, R. M.; Tadmor, R.; Zaritsky, A.; and Becker, S. A. 1975. Evidence for an autosomal recessive form of cleidocranial dysostosis. *Clin. Genet.* 8:20.

Jackson, W. P. U. 1951. Osteo-dental dysplasia (cleido-cranial dysostosis): The "Arnold head." *Acta Med. Scand.* 139:292.

Marie, P., and Sainton, P. 1897. Observation d'hydrocéphalié héréditarie (père et fils) par vice de developpement du crâne et du carveau. *Bull. Mém. Soc. Méd. Hôp. Paris* 14:706.

COMBINED FACTOR V AND FACTOR VIII DEFICIENCY

Historical note

Congenital hemorrhagic disorders characterized by a deficiency of 2 clotting factors are a disputed group; however, the combined deficiency of factors V and VIII is supported by relatively convincing genetic and laboratory data. These defects in coagulation were first described by Oeri and co-workers in 1954. In 1969 Seligsohn and Ramot called attention to the disorder in 5 patients from 2 non-Ashkenazi families.

Clinical features

Combined factor V and factor VIII deficiency is characterized by a severe bleeding tendency. It may be detected in males after circumcision or in females later in life with the onset of menarche associated with severe menorrhagia. Multiple bouts of epistaxis are common, as is severe and prolonged bleeding after trauma, extraction of teeth, or surgical procedures.

No unusual physical findings are associated with this disorder, although some observers have noted that their patients have psychopathological personalities. Mental retardation has been noted in one patient. However, these altered mental states are probably unrelated findings.

Diagnosis

The correct diagnosis of this disorder is based on the demonstration of a combined deficiency in factors V and VIII.

Basic defect

The basic defect in this disorder is the combined deficiency of factors V and VIII; however, the etiological relationship between these 2 factors has not been clarified.

Genetics

Most reports suggest that the mode of transmission for this disorder is autosomal recessive. Parental consanguinity has been noted in the majority of affected families. Findings in the family reported by Gobbi and co-workers in 1967 indicate that there may be a dominant form of the disease.

The heterozygous state may be characterized by a variety of clinical states: mild bleeding with normal levels of factor V and factor VIII; mild bleeding with mild deficiency of factors V and VIII; mild deficiency of factor V and/or factor VIII without bleeding; absence of bleeding or blood-clotting abnormalities.

Since the original report of this disorder in 1954, approximately 20 cases have been recorded in the literature. Of these 20 cases, 5 have come from 2 non-Ashkenazi Jewish communities. In 1 family the parents are normal first cousins from the Iraqi Jewish community. Of their 9 children, 4 are affected with this disorder. The other family, of Jewish Egyptian descent, has 1 affected child. Recent studies in Israel have turned up 3 more affected Jewish families, all originating from countries of the Middle East. Thus, there is evidence to suggest that this condition may occur more commonly among the non-Ashkenazi Jewish communities than among non-Jews.

Prognosis and treatment

In general the prognosis in this disorder is good. Treatment consists of the administration of fresh whole blood or plasma. Cryoprecipitate may be used to raise the level of factor VIII.

References

Cimo, P. L., et al. 1977. Inherited combined deficiency of factor V and factor VIII: Report of a case with normal factor VIII antigen and ristocetin-induced platelet aggregation. *Am. J. Pathology* 2:385.

Gobbi, F.; Ascari, E.; and Barbieri, U. 1967. Congenital combined deficiency of factor VIII (antihemophilic globulin) and factor V (proaccelerin) in two siblings: Clinical study and genetic speculations. *Thrombos. Diathes. Haemorrh.* 17:194.

Jones, J. H.; Rizza, C. R.; Hardisty, R. M.; Dormandy, K. M.; and MacPherson, J. C. 1962. Combined deficiency of factor V and factor VIII (antihemophilic globulin): A report of three cases. *Br. J. Haematol.* 8:120.

Oeri, J.; Matter, M.; Isenschmid, H.; Hauser, F.; and Koller, F. 1954. Angeborener Mangel an Faktor V (Parahaemophilie) verbunden mit echter Haemophilie A bei zwei Brüedern. *Mod. Probl. Paediatr.* 1:575.

Seibert, R. H.; Margolius, A., Jr.; and Ratnoff, O. D. 1958. Observations on hemophilia, parahemophilia, and coexistent hemophilia and parahemophilia: Alterations in the platelets and the thromboplastin generation test. *J. Lab. Clin. Med.* 52:449.

Seligsohn, U., and Ramot, B. 1969. Combined factor V and factor VIII deficiency: Report of four cases. *Br. J. Haematol.* 16:475.

CONGENITAL DEAFNESS AND ONYCHODYSTROPHY

Historical note

Familial deafness is known to be relatively common among Sephardi and Oriental Jews, as shown by Dar and Winter in 1969 (see page 149). Moreover, numerous syndromes are associated with various forms of deafness. In 1969 Feinmesser and Zelig reported the occurrence of congenital sensorineural deafness and onychodystrophy in a Sephardi Jewish family. At present the 2 affected sibs in this family are the only reported cases of this disorder.

Clinical features

At birth both affected female infants showed marked dystrophic changes involving the nails of all the fingers and toes. Although deafness also was present at

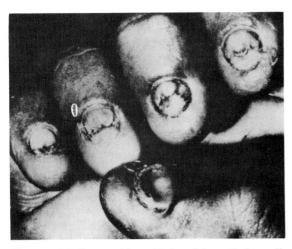

Figure 7.15. Dystrophic nails involving all the nails on the right hand of the proband. From M. Feinmesser and S. Zelig, 1961, *Arch. Otolaryngol.* 74: 507. Copyright 1961, American Medical Association.

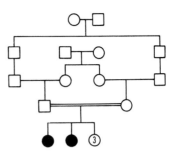

Figure 7.16. Congenital deafness and onychodystrophy: Family pedigree showing the 2 affected sisters. From M. Feinmesser and S. Zelig, 1961, *Arch. Otolaryngol.* 74:507. Copyright 1961, American Medical Association.

birth in these sisters, it was not evaluated until later in childhood. The only other malformation observed was convergent strabismus of the left eye in the older affected child.

Diagnosis

This disorder should be easily recognizable in infancy owing to the presence of severe dystrophic nail changes (Figure 7.15) coupled with congenital bilateral hearing impairment.

Otoscopic examination of the older sister showed a normal right ear with evidence of an old otitis media on the left side. In the younger sib both ears appeared normal upon otoscopic examination. Audiograms of both girls showed a 60–100 dB sensorineural hearing loss which was most marked in the higher frequencies. Caloric vestibular testing showed hypoactivity of the labyrinth in the older girl and normal vestibular reaction in the younger sister.

Roentgenograms of the skull and extremities were normal, as were various routine blood chemistry and urine tests.

Basic defect

The basic defect in this disorder is not known.

Genetics

The parents of these girls are consanguineous, being first cousins on the maternal side (Figure 7.16). Since both parents are completely normal and no other family members are known to be affected with either of these defects, autosomal recessive inheritance seems likely.

An almost identical condition has been described in a non-Jewish family in which the mode of transmission is autosomal dominant. Such an observation suggests the possibility of genetic heterogeneity in this syndrome.

Prognosis and treatment

There are too few cases on record to permit proper assessment of the prognosis for this disorder. One minor finding, however, is that there appears to be little change in the nail dystrophy over the years.

There is no specific therapy for nail dystrophy other than the use of artificial nails. The deafness associated with this disorder may be treated in the same manner as other severe sensorineural hearing losses.

References

Feinmesser, M., and Zelig, S. 1961. Congenital deafness associated with onychodystrophy. *Arch. Otolaryngol.* 74:507.

Goodman, R. M.; Lockareff, S.; and Gwinup, G. 1969. A new genetic form of congenital deafness with onychodystrophy. *Arch. Otolaryngol.* 90:96.

Konigsmark, B., and Gorlin, R. J. 1976. *Genetic and metabolic deafness,* pp. 272–73. Philadelphia: W. B. Saunders.

CONGENITAL HEPATIC FIBROSIS AND NEPHRONOPHTHISIS

Historical note

As noted by Kerr and co-workers in 1961, familial cases of congenital hepatic fibrosis (CHF) are known to be associated with cystic diseases of the kidney, and several distinct syndromes have now been adequately described. For example, cystic disease of the liver and pancreas, together with renal cysts and immature glomeruli, has been reported in infants. An adult form of polycystic kidneys with associated complications has been described in conjunction with CHF. Another renal disease frequently reported in association with CHF is medullary sponge kidney.

In 1973 Boichis and co-workers reported a new genetic entity consisting of congenital hepatic fibrosis associated with nephronophthisis, or cystic disease of the medulla. This disorder was observed in 3 sibs of consanguineous Jewish Iraqi parents.

Clinical features and diagnosis

Two of the 3 affected sibs have died of renal failure and the third is being maintained on chronic hemodialysis. The liver disease in this family is not severe, being limited to a firm hepatomegaly and only minor biochemical changes. The liver histology in the 2 deceased brothers showed congenital hepatic fibrosis. Renal symptoms in 3 of the sibs were initially insidious, with no findings in the urinary sediment, but they progressed rapidly in the later stages of the disease. A renal biopsy and post-mortem renal histology were compatible with the diagnosis of nephronophthisis.

The third son in this family was first seen at the age of 14 years because of weakness, enuresis, and polyuria. He had anemia, marked hepatosplenomegaly, and no ascites. Liver-function tests were within normal limits. Esophageal varices were not demonstrable by barium swallow. Intravenous urography showed contracted kidneys with poor excretion but no malformation of the urinary tract. Maximal urinary concentration was 250 mosmol/kg, and daily urinary output was 2.5 l. Blood-urea was 84 mg/100 ml, the level of creatinine was 3 mg/100 ml, and the sodium excretion rate was fixed at about 70 mEq/l. During the following 9 months uremia, anemia, and hypertension progressed and the patient died from pulmonary edema and hypertensive encephalopathy.

At autopsy the liver weighed 200 g and showed coarse nodularity (Figure 7.17). Histologically there was diffuse perilobular fibrosis and a few pseudolobules (Figure 7.18). No inflammatory changes were seen in the portal spaces or in the lobules. There was no bile-duct proliferation or dilatation, and the portal venules were normal. Hepatocytes throughout the lobules were filled with numerous granules. Their staining characteristics were consistent with those of lipofuscin pigment.

The kidneys were small and contracted and weighed 50 g each. Their external surface appeared smooth, but on examination with a hand lens numerous cysts were detected. Histological study revealed numerous glomerular cysts with collapsed tufts and some normal glomeruli (Figure 7.19). Bowman capsules were markedly thickened and stained positively with PAS. There was marked periglomerular fibrosis. No hypercellularity or hyalinization of the glomerular tufts was observed, nor was the basement membrane thickened. Amorphous eosinophilic material was present in the dilated Bowman spaces. Tubular dilatation was present in the cortex and the medulla. Atrophy of the tubules was noted, with peritubular fibrosis and irregular thickening of the tubular basement membrane. The epithelial lining of some tubules was hyperplastic, with hyperchromatic nuclei forming macula densa–like lesions. The tubular epithelium showed lipofuscin

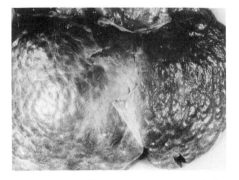

Figure 7.17. Gross appearance of the liver at autopsy showing coarse lobulation. From H. Boichis et al., 1973, *Quart. J. Med.* 42:221.

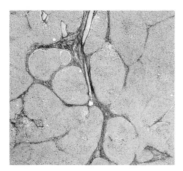

Figure 7.18. Photomicrograph showing enlarged fibrotic portal tracts with few portal vein radicles. Bile duct proliferation and bile duct dilatation are absent. From H. Boichis et al., 1973, *Quart. J. Med.* 42:221.

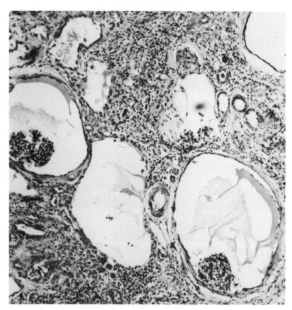

Figure 7.19. Photomicrograph showing glomerular and tubular cyst-like dilatations filled with proteinaceous material, atrophy of tubules, and lymphoid cell infiltration. From H. Boichis et al., 1973, *Quart. J. Med.* 42:221.

granules similar to those found in the liver cells. There was initial thickening of the renal arteries and arterioles. Marked lymphoid and plasma cell infiltration was seen in the interstitium. No cysts were seen in the pancreas or other organs. Left ventricular hypertrophy and signs of terminal heart failure were noted. The cardiac muscle also contained lipofuscin granules.

Basic defect

The basic defect in this disorder is not known.

Genetics

The presence of 3 affected sibs with normal consanguineous parents speaks for an autosomal recessive mode of transmission (Figure 7.20). At the present time no other cases of this syndrome have been reported. It is too early to state whether or not this will remain an isolated syndrome. When Boichis and co-workers were reviewing the literature on CHF associated with renal disease, they were impressed by the number of cases in which the renal lesion was not clearly defined functionally, radiographically, or histologically; thus this entity may have gone unrecognized or been diagnosed differently.

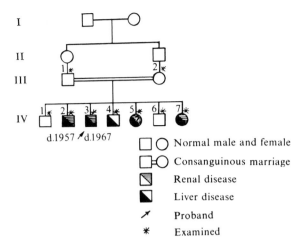

Figure 7.20. Congenital hepatic fibrosis and nephronophthisis: Pedigree of the affected family. From H.
Boichis et al., 1973, *Quart. J. Med.* 42:221.

Prognosis and treatment

The prognosis in CHF depends on the extent to which the kidney or liver is
involved. In the above family it appears that the kidney received the brunt of the
disease. Therapy at this time consists of symptomatic care. Organ transplantation
may be considered in future cases.

References

Boichis, H.; Passwell, J.; David, R.; and Miller, H. 1973. Congenital hepatic fibrosis and
  nephronophthisis. *Quart. J. Med.* 42:221.
Kerr, D. N. S.; Harrison, C. V.; Sherlock, S.; and Walter, R. M. 1961. Congenital
  hepatic fibrosis. *Quart. J. Med.* 30:91.

CONGENITAL ICHTHYOSIS WITH ATROPHY, MENTAL RETARDATION, DWARFISM, AND GENERALIZED AMINOACIDURIA

Historical note

A number of genetic syndromes are known in which ichthyosis erythrodermia
is a constant or variable finding. In 1973 Passwell and co-workers added a new
syndrome to this group—congenital ichthyosis with atrophy, mental retardation,
dwarfism, and generalized aminoaciduria. They reported this disorder in 3 of 5
children from consanguineous parents of Jewish Iraqi descent.

Clinical features

The proband was an 18-year-old girl 137 cm tall and weighing 40.5 kg. At birth
her skin was noted to be lighter than that of her parents and there was a distinct

erythrodermia of the face. A few bullae were present on both feet. Within a few months the skin over the entire body thickened and became scaly.

Upon examination, the classic features of ichthyosiform erythrodermia were observed. The erythrodermia was more marked on the lower part of the face. The skin, while showing the familiar appearance of ichthyosis with fine scaling, was also atrophic. The atrophic changes were particularly marked over the dorsum of the hands and feet, where the skin was wrinkled and parchment-like in appearance (Figure 7.21). A fine scale was constantly shed from all areas of the skin, especially the scalp. Bullae, usually not more than 5 mm in diameter, were visible on the exposed areas of the dorsum of the hands and the neck. There were several areas of hyperpigmentation, particularly on the trunk. All the flexural surfaces were involved.

The proband's hair was rough textured, but no abnormalities were noted upon microscopic examination. The teeth were dystrophic, several molars had not erupted, and marked caries and gingival inflammation were present. The nails were soft, but no excessive keratinization was noted.

Neurological examination showed weakness of both legs, spasticity, increased reflexes, and a negative Babinski sign. The proband's breasts were poorly developed and she had sparse pubic and axillary hair; however, she had had regular menstrual periods since the age of 16 years. Her IQ, as measured by the Binet test, was 38.

A 12-year-old female sib showed almost identical clinical findings and an IQ of 52. Her height was 121 cm and her weight 22.2 kg.

An 8-year-old brother of the proband also was similarly affected. His height was 110 cm and his weight 18.5 kg. In addition, he suffered from chronic constipation, and megacolon was demonstrated in radiographic studies. His IQ was 75.

Diagnosis

Clinically the diagnosis of this syndrome can be suspected in the presence of congenital ichthyosis with atrophy, mental retardation, and dwarfism.

Routine laboratory studies in the above cases were normal, while paper chromatography of the urine showed generalized aminoaciduria in the 3 affected sibs. They did not have abnormal aminoacidemia. Quantitative immundiffusion of gamma globulin showed marked hypergammaglobulinemia in all 3 cases.

Skin biopsy specimens taken from the dorsal surface of the forearms showed moderate hyperkeratosis, an atrophic epidermis, vacuolization, and increased melanization of the basal layer. The dermis showed lymphocytic and histiocytic infiltration and degenerating collagen (Figure 7.22).

Finger, palm, and sole imprints showed severe dermatoglyphic changes with obliteration of ridges and broad horizontal secondary creases in the palms probably secondary to the skin disease.

A somewhat puzzling finding was the increased excretion of uric acid along with renal glycosuria in the mother and in sibs IV-1, IV-3, IV-4, and IV-5 (see discussion under "Genetics").

Other investigative studies were done and all were within normal limits, including chromosomal studies.

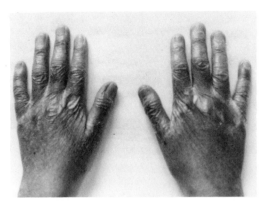

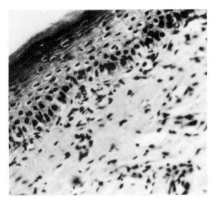

Figure 7.21. Hands of the proband showing wrinkled, parchment-like skin. From J. Passwell et al., 1973, *J. Pediatr.* 82:466.

Figure 7.22. Skin biopsy of forearm from the proband showing moderate keratosis and parakeratosis. The epidermis is atrophic; note the increased melanization of the basal layer and vacuolization of the cells. There is an inflammatory infiltrate of the dermis. From J. Passwell et al., 1973, *J. Pediatr.* 82:466.

Basic defect

The basic defect in this syndrome is not known. Absence of a specific aminoaciduria or group of similar amino acids in the urine of the 3 affected sibs indicates a nonspecific defect in proximal renal tubular transport rather than a specific transport defect.

Genetics

At the present time no other reports of this syndrome have been published. Close parental consanguinity, healthy parents, and the clustering of all affected members in one sibship strongly support an autosomal recessive form of transmission (Figure 7.23).

One could question whether the glycosuria and uricosuria are part of the disorder described in this family. Renal glycosuria is known to be an independent genetic entity transmitted as an autosomal dominant trait. However, the combination of renal glycosuria and uricosuria in the presence of a normal serum uric acid level, which was observed in the mother and in 2 unaffected sibs, but was absent in 1 affected sib, constitutes to the best of my knowledge a previously undescribed association. Administration of phloridzin, which selectively produces decreased reabsorption of glucose within the proximal convoluted tubule, has been shown to result in increased uric acid excretion, probably due to an interdependent mechanism of glucose and uric acid reabsorption in the proximal tubule. Perhaps the glycosuria and uricosuria in this sibship are caused by a similar defect in proximal tubular reabsorption.

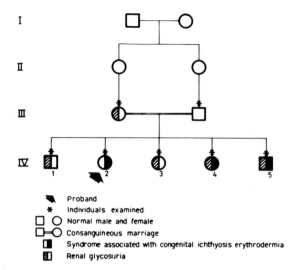

Figure 7.23. Congenital ichthyosis: Pedigree
of the affected family. From J. Passwell et al.,
1973, *J. Pediatr.* 82:466.

Passwell and co-workers have postulated that these two renal tubular reabsorption defects (glycosuria and uricosuria) are separate and independent from the
syndrome affecting the 3 sibs in generation IV.

Prognosis and treatment

Since all 3 affected family members showed mental retardation, it seems obvious
to conclude that this finding is part of the syndrome; nevertheless, variability in the
degree of mental retardation is likely. Follow-up studies are needed to properly
evaluate the prognosis in this disorder. Treatment at this time consists of
symptomatic care.

References

Passwell, J.; Ziprkowski, L.; Katznelson, D.; Szeinberg, A.; Crispin, M.; Pollak, S.;
Goodman, R. M.; Bat-Miriam, M.; and Cohen, B. E. 1973. A syndrome characterized
by congenital ichthyosis with atrophy, mental retardation, dwarfism, and generalized
aminociduria. *J. Pediatr.* 82:466.
Skeith, M. D.; Healey, L. A.; and Cutler, R. E. 1970. Effect of phloridzin on uric acid
excretion in man. *Am. J. Physiol.* 219:1080.
Steele, T. H. 1971. Control of uric acid excretion. *N. Engl. J. Med.* 284:1193.

CUTIS LAXA: A NEW VARIANT

Historical note

In 1888 Kopp first described a father and son with cutis laxa. In 1965 Goltz
and co-workers reported an autosomal recessive form and suggested the term

generalized elastolysis. In 1972 Beighton differentiated between the autosomal dominant and recessive forms of the disease. Through the years various rare syndromes have been reported in which cutis laxa is one of the main features. In 1976 Goodman and co-workers observed a "new" syndrome in a Jewish Iranian child in whom cutis laxa was one of the key findings.

Clinical features

A 1:6-year-old Jewish boy of Iranian birth was referred to the genetic clinic of the Sheba Medical Center for diagnostic evaluation. Upon physical examination the child appeared to have normal intelligence but looked much older than his stated age due to a marked wrinkling and laxity of the skin about the face and the entire body. Facial findings included a small mouth, long philtrum, micrognathia, antimongoloid slant of the palpebral fissures, blue sclerae, ocular hypertelorism, and highly arched eyebrows. Examination of the skull showed brachycephaly, a large, open anterior fontanelle, prominent veins about the forehead, and fine scalp hair. Other abnormal findings included marked hyperextensibility of the joints of the extremities, pectus excavatum, hypospadias, and bilateral cryptorchidism.

Diagnosis

During the above study the child could not be properly evaluated and only a limited amount of information was obtained. The main clinical diagnostic features were cutis laxa, joint hypermobility, multiple external eye findings, and a large anterior craniolacunia. Roentgenographic studies showed the large anterior craniolacunia, severe hypoplasia of the terminal phalanges of the foot, and excess wrinkling of the soft tissues (Figures 7.24 and 7.25). Dermatoglyphic studies showed multiple creases on the palms and soles. Chromosomal studies were normal.

This variant of cutis laxa should be distinguished from the syndrome reported by Debré and co-workers, which consisted of cutis laxa and bone dystrophy transmitted as an autosomal recessive trait. In 1968 de Barsy reported an autosomal dominant syndrome consisting of cutis laxa, corneal clouding, and mental retardation, and in 1974 Kaye and co-workers described a child with cutis laxa, short digits, absent phalanges, and ambiguous genitalia. Cutis laxa has also been reported with lamellar ichthyosis.

In some cases of cutis laxa investigators have described a reduced number of elastic fibers, which appear fragmented and granular in texture in the light microscope; however, these features have not been observed in all cases.

Basic defect

The basic defect in this heritable disorder of connective tissue is not known. It has been postulated that in some cases the alteration may be due to a deficiency in serum elastase inhibitor associated with a low level of serum copper.

Genetics

Figure 7.26 shows the family pedigree of the case studied by Goodman and co-workers. Normal but closely consanguineous parents suggest an autosomal

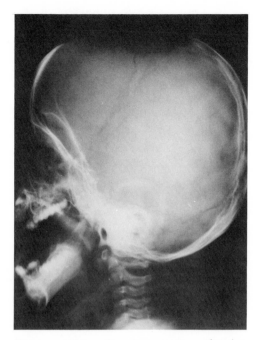

Figure 7.24. Roentgenogram showing marked absence of bone in the region of the anterior fontanel (anterior craniolacunia) and brachycephalic shape of the skull.

recessive mode of transmission. No other family members are known to be affected. It is apparent from the previously reported syndromes involving cutis laxa that heterogeneity plays a definite role in this disorder.

Prognosis and treatment

Not enough is known about this disorder to discuss its prognosis properly. Likewise, at this stage of our understanding, treatment is limited to symptomatic care. With regard to the anterior craniolacunia, it was decided to follow the child's development rather than attempt to close the opening at this time.

References

Beighton, P. 1972. The dominant and recessive forms of cutis laxa. *J. Med. Genet.* 9:216.

De Barsy, A. M.; Moens, E.; and Dierckx, L. 1968. Dwarfism, oligophrenia, and degeneration of the elastic tissue in skin and cornea: A new syndrome? *Helv. Paediatr. Acta* 23:305.

Debré, R.; Marie, J.; and Seringe, P. 1937. Cutis laxa avec dystrophies osseuses. *Bull. Mém. Soc. Méd. Hôp. Paris* 53:1038.

Goltz, R. W.; Hult, A. M.; Goldfarb, M.; and Gorlin, R. J. 1965. Cutis laxa, a manifestation of generalized elastolysis. *Arch. Dermatol.* 92:373.

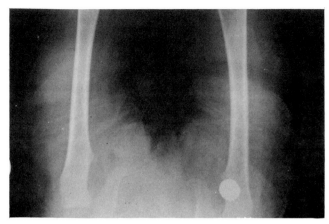

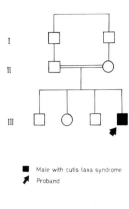

■ Male with cutis laxa syndrome
⤴ Proband

Figure 7.25. Roentgenogram showing multiple soft-tissue skin creases in the region of the upper thighs.

Figure 7.26. Cutis laxa: Pedigree of the affected family.

Goodman, R. M. 1976. Unpublished data.

Kaye, C. I.; Esterly, N. B.; and Booth, C. W. 1976. Cutis laxa and lamellar ichthyosis in siblings. *Clin. Genet.* 9:508.

Kaye, C. I.; Fisher, D. E.; and Esterly, N. B. 1974. Cutis laxa, skeletal anomalies, and ambiguous genitalia. *Am. J. Dis. Child.* 127:115.

Kopp, W. 1888. Demonstration zweier Fälle von "Cutis laxa". *Münch. Med. Wochenschr.* 35:259.

Lane, B. 1974. Erosions of the skull. In *The radiologic clinics of North America*, ed. N. E. Chase and I. I. Kricheff, pp. 257–82. Philadelphia: W. B. Saunders.

DEAF-MUTISM WITH TOTAL ALBINISM

Historical note

Albinism and deafness are known to be associated in several hereditary syndromes but in none of these has the albinism been described as total. In 1964 Ziprkowski and Adam first reported the simultaneous occurrence of autosomal recessive total albinism and congenital perceptive deafness in 4 children of 2 related consanguineous Jewish Moroccan sibships.

Clinical features

The albinism in the affected children was the classic type in which the skin is white with some pinkish-white areas. Skin turgor and elasticity were noted as normal. The hair was devoid of any pigmentation and thus completely white (Figure 7.27). The irides in the 2 children available for examination were translucent blue, the pupils pink, the fundi albinotic, and nystagmus and photophobia were very marked. According to the case reports there was some suggestion of ocular hypertelorism. In both sibs the medial portion of the eyebrows was absent.

Deafness was present in the 2 albinotic propositi and present alone in 3 of their sibs.

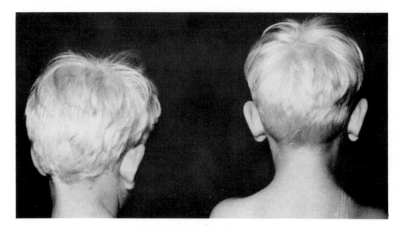

Figure 7.27. White hair of deaf-mute sibs with total albinism.

Intelligence appeared to be normal in all family members, but no measurements were made. No other abnormal findings were noted.

Diagnosis

The diagnosis of this syndrome tends to be clinical, although certain laboratory studies are indicated. A skin biopsy in one of the probands showed no pigment upon hematoxylin-eosin staining, but the dopa reaction was positive.

Audiometric studies showed marked variation in the degree of deafness among the affected children.

Urinary amino acid excretion and indican excretion were normal. Examination for phenolic and indolic compounds were positive in some family members, but the conditions were not well controlled and no conclusions were justifiable.

Basic defect

The basic defect in albinism is the absence of the enzyme tyrosinase or a deficient in its activity. No information is presently available regarding the basic alteration that produces perceptive deafness. The question remains whether the combination of albinism and perceptive deafness in the above family is in fact one disorder involving one locus.

Genetics

Figure 7.28 shows the family pedigree from the study by Ziprkowski and Adam. To date, this is the only family in which this combination of findings has been reported. Classic albinism and congenital perceptive deafness can be independently inherited traits. Moreover, each is known to be governed independently by more than one locus, but no clinical tools are available to discriminate between the different genotypes. The association of both traits in the same individuals may be explained either as double homozygosity for 2 independent loci or as homozygosity

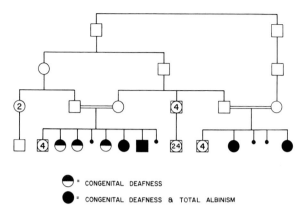

● = CONGENITAL DEAFNESS
● = CONGENITAL DEAFNESS & TOTAL ALBINISM

Figure 7.28. Deaf-mutism with total albinism:
Pedigree of the affected family.

for a single, as yet unknown, gene. Ziprkowski and Adam favor the second hypothesis, since it would account for the absence of nondeaf albino offspring and would restore the proportion of affected children to reasonable recessive ratios (3:9 for deafness only and 4:15 for deafness associated with albinism).

Prognosis and treatment

Throughout the life span of affected persons there is no apparent change in albinism or hearing loss. When diagnosed early, deafness can be helped considerably by the use of bilateral hearing aids. Protective skin care is of paramount importance to those suffering from albinism.

Reference

Ziprkowski, L., and Adam, A. 1964. Recessive total albinism and congenital deaf-mutism. *Arch. Dermatol.* 89:151.

FAMILIAL INFANTILE RENAL TUBULAR ACIDOSIS WITH CONGENITAL NERVE DEAFNESS

Historical note

In 1966 Konigsmark was the first to report renal tubular acidosis (RTA) associated with deafness. This is now a recognized genetic entity characterized by mild RTA and a slowly progressive, moderate nerve deafness. In 1973 Cohen and co-workers described a new allelic form in 4 children of a Jewish Kurdish family in whom the RTA was present in infancy in association with severe congenital nerve deafness and marked growth retardation.

Clinical features and diagnosis

The 4 affected children (Figure 7.29) presented similar clinical pictures and thus an account of only the proband will be given.

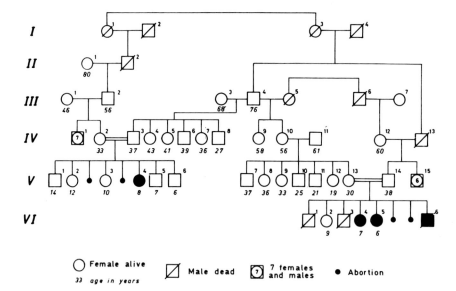

Figure 7.29. Pedigree of 4 children affected with renal tubular acidosis and nerve deafness. From T. Cohen et al., 1973, *Clin. Genet.* 4:275. © 1973 Munksgaard International Publishers Ltd., Copenhagen, Denmark.

Born in 1963, the female proband was admitted to hospital for severe vomiting initially at the age of 1 month and repeatedly thereafter for the same reason. At 9 months of age she weighed 6 kg and suffered from marked polyuria (1500–2200 ml/24 hr). Urinary osmolality was 100–250 mosmol/l. Pitressin administration did not alleviate the polyuria or increase the urinary osmolality. Metabolic acidosis was confirmed by pH of blood (7.24) and urine (7.20). Following an ammonium chloride loading test, the CO_2 content of the blood decreased from 23.4 mEq/1 to 16.8 mEq/1, while urinary pH remained at 7.20. Repetition of the test yielded similar results. Serum chloride and phosphorus levels were in the range of 111–121 mEq/1 and 2.4–2.7 mg%, respectively. Marked phosphaturia was present with a phosphor excretion index between +0.14 and +0.35 (normal range = 0.0 ± 0.09). Tubular phosphor reabsorption was diminished to 50 percent of normal. An intravenous pyelogram showed renal calcifications, and the diagnosis of RTA was made.

At 2 years of age the child showed marked growth retardation with clinical and radiological signs of rickets; an ammonium chloride loading test produced a decrease in blood pH from 7.29 to 7.18, while the urinary pH increased from 7.4 to 7.6. Hydrogen ion clearance was 0.11 (normal = 1.0 and over). A subtotal hearing loss due to nerve deafness was observed and later confirmed by audiogram (Figure 7.30). At 8 years of age the child showed marked growth retardation and was attending a special school for the deaf.

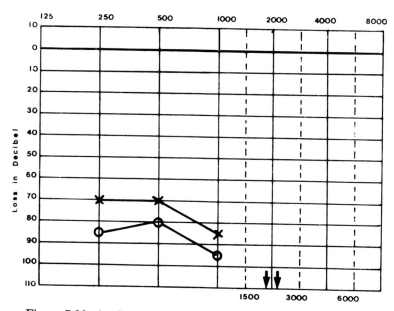

Figure 7.30. Audiogram of proband V-4 at the age of 7 years. From T. Cohen et al., 1973, *Clin. Genet.* 4:275. © 1973 Munksgaard International Publishers Ltd., Copenhagen, Denmark.

Basic defect

In 1974 Shapira and co-workers showed a specific enzymatic defect in red-cell carbonic anhydrase B in the 4 affected individuals. The mutant carbonic anhydrase B had 7 rather than 8 tyrosine residues.

Genetics

The above-mentioned family provides good evidence for a new variant of RTA with deafness transmitted as an autosomal recessive disorder (Figure 7.29). There now appear to be 2 distinct forms of RTA and deafness: (1) the slowly progressive form with onset in childhood; and (2) the severe infantile type mentioned in this report. It is not known at this time whether or not the latter form is found only among the Jewish Kurdish community. The mode of transmission of both forms of the disease is autosomal recessive.

Prognosis and treatment

Treatment with alkalyzing solutions should begin as soon as the diagnosis is made and continue throughout life. A hearing aid can be helpful in speech therapy. The early complication nephrocalcinosis makes the prognosis a guarded one.

References

Cohen, T.; Brand-Auraban, A.; Karshai, C.; Jacob, A.; Gay, I.; Tsitsianov, J.; Shapiro, T.; Jatziv, S.; and Ashkenazi, A. 1973. Familial infantile renal tubular acidosis and congenital nerve deafness: An autosomal recessive syndrome. *Clin. Genet.* 4:275.

Konigsmark, B. W. 1975. Renal tubular acidosis with progressive nerve deafness. Cited by V. A. McKusick in *Mendelian inheritance in man*, 4th ed., Baltimore: The Johns Hopkins University Press. p. 560.

Shapira, E.; Ben-Yoseph, Y.; Eyal, G.; and Russell, A. 1974. Enzymatically inactive red cell carbonic anhydrase B in a family with renal tubular acidosis. *J. Clin. Invest.* 53:59.

FAMILIAL SYNDROME OF THE CENTRAL NERVOUS SYSTEM AND OCULAR MALFORMATIONS

Historical note

In 1975 Chemke and co-workers described a new neurological syndrome in 3 infant sibs of Jewish Yemenite origin whose parents were third cousins.

Clinical features and diagnosis

Since the findings for all 3 affected sibs were almost identical, a detailed account will be presented of the one who was most thoroughly evaluated. VI-8 was a female infant who survived for 15 hours (Figure 7.31). She was markedly hypotonic and showed no response to external stimuli. Head circumference was 37 cm. A large occipital encephalocele was present, containing central nervous system tissue. The sagittal suture was widely separated in its posterior region. The ears were hairy

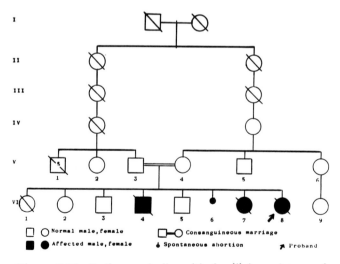

Figure 7.31. Pedigree of sibs with familial syndrome of central nervous system and ocular malformations. From J. Chemke et al., 1975, *Clin. Genet.* 7:1. © 1973 Munksgaard International Publishers Ltd., Copenhagen, Denmark.

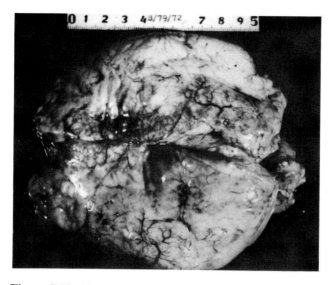

Figure 7.32. External surface of the lissencephalic brain showing almost complete lack of sulci. From J. Chemke et al., 1975, *Clin. Genet.* 7:1. © 1973 Munksgaard International Publishers Ltd., Copenhagen, Denmark.

and abnormally shaped. Both eyes were sunken, with an antimongoloid slant to the palpebral fissures; the left eye showed corneal opacity, the right a cataract. The mouth was small. The clitoris appeared hypertrophic, and there was marked pigmentation of the labia. A Sabin-Feldman complement fixation test of the infant's blood for toxoplasmosis was negative, and no cytomegalovirus fluorescent antibodies were found in maternal or infant serum. Chromosomal studies were normal.

Upon post-mortem examination the encephalocele was found to contain the larger part of the cerebellum. Examination of the brain revealed marked lissencephaly (Figure 7.32), a dysplastic cerebellum, moderate dilatation of all ventricles, and a hypoplastic corpus callosum. The cerebellar commissure was almost absent and the fourth ventricle was dilated, with a thin membrane covering it.

As seen in microscopic examination of the brain, the normal structure of the cerebral cortex was completely lost. Neurons were dispersed without any laminar structure. Large numbers of astrocytes, in a formation of glial whorls and bands, were localized in between groups of neurons. The normal architectural structure of the hippocampus was preserved. The centrum semiovale was poorly myelinated. Within the white matter, small groups of neurons were observed—neuronal heterotopia. The ependymal lining of the ventricles was destroyed and in only a few places were remnants of ependymal cells seen. The basal ganglia, brain stem, pons, and medulla appeared normal. The cerebellar cortex was completely disorganized. No sulci and gyri were detected. The cerebellar folia showed a mixture of the layers of the cerebellar cortex, with all layers intermingled. Only remnants of the external granular layer were present.

Examination of the eyes revealed totally detached retinas. The cataractous lens was displaced forward, and an oval choroidal coloboma was present posteriorly.

Histologically the eyes were similar. Anteriorly, the angle was incompletely opened, the iris was hypoplastic, and the pars plana was short. Posteriorly, the colobomatous area was covered by an atrophic retina that was dysplastic at the border, even penetrating deeply between the choroid and sclera, and adhered to the posterior face of the lens. Remnants of the primary vitreous were present between the detached retina and the cataractous lens, which showed numerous vacuoles and metaplastic fibrous tissue. The optic nerve showed marked gliosis.

Basic defect

The basic defect in this malformation syndrome is not known, but genetic factors are thought to be involved. It seems unlikely that some teratogenic or other environmental agent would have produced identical effects on 3 separate occasions.

The pathogenesis in this disorder seems to be related to the inhibition of normal neuron migration and normal brain differentiation at an early stage of embryonic development. It is possible that these 3 cases represent the maximal degree of expression of a genetic defect that is only partially expressed as lissencephaly or the Dandy-Walker anomaly.

Genetics

Autosomal recessive inheritance is most likely in patients from this family since both parents are normal and consanguineous (Figure 7.31).

Prognosis and treatment

The combination of malformations in this syndrome probably is not compatible with life beyond infancy.

Reference

Chemke, J.; Czernobilsky, B.; Mundel, G.; and Barishak, Y. R. 1975. A familial syndrome of central nervous system and ocular malformations. *Clin. Genet.* 7:1.

GLYCINURIA ASSOCIATED WITH NEPHROLITHIASIS

Historical note

In 1957 de Vries and co-workers described an Ashkenazi Jewish family in which 4 members had hyperglycinuria, 3 of whom had a history of renal colic or passage of urinary stones. This is apparently a unique family, for such a condition has not been reported elsewhere.

Clinical features

The clinical findings in this disorder are related to the obstructive symptoms produced by nephrolithiasis. The proband, a 22-year-old woman of Ashkenazi Jewish origin, had a long history of renal colic, beginning at the age of 4 years.

At the age of 6 a roentgenographic examination was performed and a calculus in the left kidney was demonstrated. The attacks of renal colic continued and at the age of 10 a roentgenographic examination showed several stones in the left kidney. Four stones were removed by pyelotomy and a nephrostomy was performed. When the proband was 11 years old the left kidney, which had been reduced to a sac of pus, was removed. She then remained well until the age of 19, when she had attacks of right lumbar pain with hematuria. Roentgenographic studies showed a peanut-sized stone in the right kidney. This stone gradually became larger and in 1956 it was removed surgically.

The patient gave a positive family history for renal colic and kidney stones. Table 7.6 shows the various clinical and biochemical findings noted in those members of her family who were studied.

Diagnosis

As noted in Table 7.6, the significant finding in the proband and other affected family members was glycinuria. Paper chromatographic studies showed no increase in other urinary amino acids in those affected. The renal stone that was removed in 1956 was analyzed and shown to be composed mainly of calcium oxalate. A rough estimation of the glycine content was 0.5 percent of the dry weight of the stone. The exact form in which the glycine was present in the stone was not determined.

Basic defect

The basic defect in this disorder is not known but probably involves some alteration in the renal tubular transport of glycine.

Genetics

The proband's family pedigree is shown in Figure 7.33. It would appear that this disorder is transmitted as an autosomal dominant condition. The fact that only

Table 7.6. Studies in a family with glycinuria

Family member	Age (yr)	Renal colic	Stones passed or diagnosed (X-ray)	Glycine in urine (mg/24 hr)[a]	Glycine in serum[b]
Proband	20	+	+	991	Normal
Mother	48	−	−	596	Normal
Father	52	−	−	195	
Sister	22	+	+	632	Normal
Daughter of affected sister	2	−	−	120	
Grandmother (maternal side)	75	+	−	593	
Uncle (maternal side)	55	−	−	Normal	

Source: A. De Vries et al., 1957, *Am. J. Med.* 23:408.

[a] Microbiological assay.

[b] Two-dimensional chromatography.

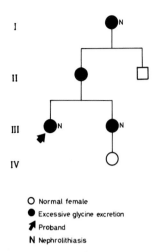

Figure 7.33. Glycinuria and nephrolithiasis:
Pedigree of the affected family.

females are affected cannot be fully evaluated; the family is quite small and the occurrence in females may reflect a chance happening. However, the possibility that this is a sex-influenced or X-linked dominant trait cannot be ruled out.

Scriver has suggested that the glycinuria trait observed in this family represents the heterozygous state of iminoglycinuria, a disorder that also has been found in Ashkenazi Jewish families (see section on iminoglycinuria, page 382).

Prognosis and treatment

If, as it appears from the family described here, one can have glycinuria without having nephrolithiasis, the prognosis for such an individual is excellent. In patients who are prone to renal stone formation, however, the prognosis is guarded because of the complications arising from nephrolithiasis.

Treatment consists of adequate fluid intake and periodic examinations for the presence of renal calculi.

References

De Vries, A.; Kochwa, S.; Lazebnik, J.; Frank, M.; and Djaldetti, M. 1957. Glyrinuria: A hereditary disorder associated with nephrolithiasis. *Am. J. Med.* 23:408.
Scriver, C. R. 1968. Renal tubular transport of proline, hydroxyproline, and glycine. III: Genetic basis for more than one mode of transport in human kidney. *J. Clin. Invest.* 47:823.

GLYCOPROTEINURIA, OSTEOPETROSIS, AND DWARFISM

Historical note

In 1974 Rosenthal and co-workers briefly described what may be a new syndrome consisting of glycoproteinuria, osteopetrosis, and dwarfism in a woman of Jewish Iraqi descent.

Clinical features

A 31-year-old married Jewish female of Iraqi origin was hospitalized for weakness and tiredness. At the age of 10 years she had been seen by a prominent physician and told that she had a bone disease. In 1966 she had suffered from a bout of peripheral edema. Three months prior to this hospitalization she had noted shortness of breath upon exertion.

The patient had completed 11 years of school, appeared to be of normal intelligence, and worked as a clerk in an office.

Physical examination showed a short, well-proportioned female in no acute distress. Her height was 145 cm, her arm span 145.5 cm. Her facial features tended to be coarse, with a square mandible, thick lips, and heavy eyebrows. Macroglossia was present. Slit lamp examination of the eyes revealed early bilateral opacities of the lens. She had pectus carinatum and small breasts. Bilateral clinodactyly involving the toes was noted. No joint immobility was observed.

The heart was considered to be moderately enlarged to percussion, while the heart tones were normal. There was 1 + pitting edema of the lower extremities. Although the abdomen was protuberant, no fluid wave or enlargement of the abdominal organs was noted.

The patient's primary medical problem was thought to be one of mild congestive heart failure due to myocarditis of unknown etiology. Although she responded well to treatment, she was again admitted to the hospital 4 months later in severe respiratory distress and died approximately 24 hours after admission. An autopsy was not performed, but it was thought that the cause of death was a massive pericardial effusion of unknown etiology.

Diagnosis

The main physical findings in this patient were short stature and coarse facial features. Roentgenographic and biochemical studies did not suggest one of the mucopolysaccharidoses or mucolipidoses. Tables 7.7 and 7.8 list the laboratory findings from glycoprotein studies in the proband and both of her parents. Increased glycoprotein content was also observed in the leukocyte membranes of the patient. These studies were done after the patient was free of edema. Other

Table 7.7. Glycoproteinuria: Analysis of mucopolysaccharides and protein-bound carbohydrates in urine after DEAE-Sephadex chromatography and pronase digestion

	Uronic acid		Amino sugars						
Patient	Carbazole	Orcinol	Galactosamine (mg/ 24 hr)	Glucosamine (mg/ 24 hr)	Sulfate	Neutral sugar	Sialic acid	Fructose	Protein
Normal[a]	2.6	2.0	1.6	0.6	1.1	1.9	0.9	0.4	8.9
Proband	5.9	6.8	4.3	4.8	4.5	8.4	5.3	2.7	35.8
Father	2.4	2.0	2.3	0.8	1.4	1.7	1.1	0.2	7.2
Mother	3.1	2.6	1.9	0.9	1.3	2.3	1.4	0.6	10.3

Source: T. Rosenthal et al., 1974, *Syndrome Identification* 2:15. Reprinted by permission of The National Foundation–March of Dimes, White Plains, New York.

[a] Average of 5 normal individuals.

Table 7.8. Glycoproteinuria: Protein-bound carbohydrate in serum

| Patient | Protein (g/100 ml) | Carbohydrate | | |
		Neutral sugar	Sialic acid (g/100 ml)	Amino sugar
Normal[a]	5.2–6.5	114–138	31.4–44.5	61–82
Proband	7.6	131	39.6	*102*
Father	5.6	130	46.5	82
Mother	5.3	145	37.8	74

Source: T. Rosenthal et al., 1974, *Syndrome Identification* 2:15.

[a] Range of values found in 5 individuals.

laboratory findings were within normal limits. Chromosomal analysis showed the patient to be a normal female 46 (XX). Roentgenographic studies showed osteopetrosis involving the spine, sternum, and skull (Figure 7.34).

Basic defect

The basic defect in this disorder is not known.

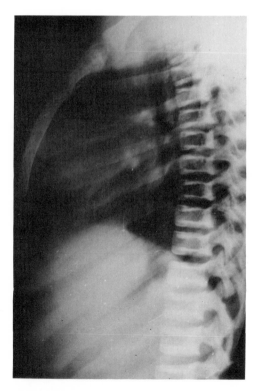

Figure 7.34. Roentgenogram showing osteopetrosis involving the sternum and spine.

Genetics

The patient's family history revealed that her parents are first cousins. She has a 21-year-old brother who is normal and well; another brother was killed at the age of 22 during the Six-Day War. Her parents were living and well and no other family members were known to be ill or malformed. It is postulated that this syndrome is transmitted as an autosomal recessive disorder.

No other cases of such a disorder have been reported.

Prognosis and treatment

Not enough is known about this disorder to properly discuss its prognosis or treatment. Because an autopsy was not performed, we have no knowledge of the cause of the pericardial effusion.

Reference

Rosenthal, T.; Berman, E.; Sheba, C.; and Goodman, R. M. 1974. Case report 24: Glycoproteinuria, osteopetrosis, and dwarfism—A new syndrome? *Syndrome Identification* 2:15.

HYDROTIC ECTODERMAL DYSPLASIA
(AUTOSOMAL RECESSIVE TYPE)

Historical note

In 1977 Fried described a new type of autosomal recessive hydrotic ectodermal dysplasia in a Karaite family from Israel.

Clinical features and diagnosis

The proband was born after a normal pregnancy in February 1972. His father and mother were 26 and 24 years of age, respectively, at the time of his birth. Right-sided cleft lip was noticed in the infant immediately. His birth weight was 3,350 g, and the placenta weighted 650 g. The Apgar score was 10, and other malformations were not noticed. At the age of 3 months the child underwent plastic surgery to repair the cleft lip. At this age his development was normal and he was considered healthy except for occasional breath-holding attacks and a tendency to sweat profusely. By the age of 3 years he had only 13 teeth and it was noted that his hair did not grow in length. Physical examination at that time showed the skin to be normal; the fingernails appeared somewhat thin while the toenails were small, thin, and slightly concave. The patient's scalp hair was fine, short, and dark brown in color. His eyebrows were scanty, but his eyelashes appeared normal. He had a prominent chin and his lips were everted. A postoperative scar from the cleft lip operation was noticeable. There was a groove between the lower lip and the chin. No other abnormal facial findings were observed.

Upon dermatoglyphic examination the patient's sweat pores appeared normal in number and size. His IQ was above average (129). Microscopic examination showed the hair was normal but of much less than average diameter. Dental examination revealed that both lateral incisors and the left canine were missing in the upper jaw. In the lower jaw all 4 incisors were missing. The teeth were conical in shape.

The second case in this family was a female double first and double second cousin of the proband who was born after a normal pregnancy in 1971. The findings in a general physical examination at the age of 4 years were similar to those noted in the proband but there was no cleft lip. The patient had a branchial cyst on the left side of her neck.

The cleft palate in the proband and the branchial cyst in his affected cousin may or may not be associated with this syndrome.

Basic defect

The basic defect in hydrotic ectodermal dysplasia is not known.

Genetics

Figure 7.35 shows the family pedigree of the 2 children. Both sets of parents were normal and there was no history of other affected family members. The above information, in conjunction with close parental consanguinity, strongly supports an autosomal recessive mode of transmission for this disorder. However, in 1965 Witkop described a similar condition involving nail dysplasia and hypodontia in a family in which the disorder was transmitted as an autosomal dominant trait.

Prognosis and treatment

The prognosis for this condition is favorable, but the absence of teeth and poor dentition require proper dental care.

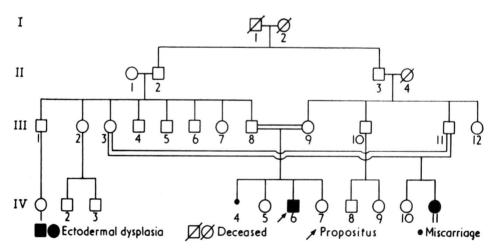

Figure 7.35. Hydrotic ectodermal dysplasia: Pedigree of the affected family. From K. Fried, 1977, *J. Med. Genet.* 14:137.

References

Fried, K. 1977. Case report: Autosomal recessive hydrotic ectodermal dysplasia. *J. Med. Genet.* 14:137.

Witkop, C. J., Jr. 1965. Autosomal dominant dysplasia of nails and hypodontia. In *Oral pathology,* ed. R. W. Tiecke, pp. 812–13. New York: McGraw-Hill.

HYPOURICEMIA, HYPERCALCIURIA, AND DECREASED BONE DENSITY

Historical note

In 1974 Sperling and co-workers reported a new metabolic syndrome in a Sephardi Jewish family which is characterized by hypouricemia, hypercalciuria, and decreased bone density.

Clinical features

The proband, a 53-year-old man, was admitted to the hospital for diagnostic evaluation of bone disease. In 1966 he gave up farming because of generalized pains that were theoretically attributed to bone disease radiographically interpreted as osteoporosis. He gave no history of bone fractures or kidney stones. Physical examination showed a relatively short man (height, 163 cm) with long arms (arm span, 172 cm). His upper segment/lower segment ratio was normal, 0.92. He had kyphosis and an increased A-P diameter of the chest. Only 3 upper and 3 lower teeth were present. No other abnormal physical findings were recorded.

Other affected family members included a 50-year-old brother, a 65-year-old sister, a 9-year-old grandson, and a 4-year-old granddaughter. No unusual physical findings were observed in any of these individuals. All were of normal stature and appeared to be healthy representatives of their age groups. The proband's brother complained of upper shoulder girdle pain and had at one time passed a renal stone.

Diagnosis

The diagnosis of this disorder is suggested by certain roentgenographic findings and by the presence of hypouricemia and hypercalciuria.

A survey of the proband's bones showed a generalized decrease in bone density. The spine showed accentuation of the vertical trabecular pattern, with loss of horizontal trabecular structure. The remaining vertebral trabeculae were thicker than usual. The vertebral plates, although thin, appeared dense. Compression fractures were observed in two vertebral bodies, while the other vetebrae were biconcave. In both hands the transverse trabeculae had completely disappeared, whereas the sparse longitudinal ones were thicker than normal. The proximal parts of the femurs showed identical changes. The calvarium appeared normal; disappearance of the upper portion of the sella was noted.

Examination of the proband's affected brother and sister revealed identical radiographic skeletal changes except that there were no compression fractures. Roentgenographic changes were also observed in the affected grandson. In his case there was diminished bone density in the hands with accentuated vertebral striation of the

Table 7.9. Hypouricemia, hypercalciuria, and decreased bone density:
Data on affected relatives

| Subject | Age (yr) | Sex | Weight (kg) | Uric Acid | | C_{ua} (ml/min/ 1.73 m^2 BSA) | Urine calcium (mg/24 hr) | De- creased bone density |
				Serum (mg/ 100 ml)	Urine (mg/ 24 hr)			
Proband (II-3)	53	M	83	0.8	580	46.2	332	+
Sister (II-2)	65	F	94	1.7	681	24.9	282	+
Brother (II-4)	50	M	53.5	1.05	680	49.1	500	+
Grandson (IV-1)	9	M	24	0.6	231	51.3	260	+
Grand- daughter (IV-4)	4	F	14	1.86	410	43.2	76	Not exam- ined

Source: O. Sperling et al., 1974, *Ann. Intern. Med.* 80:482.
Note: Numbers in parentheses refer to the pedigree assigned. C_{ua} = clearance of uric acid.
BSA = body surface area.

cancellous bone. The metaphyses and epiphyses had thin cortices without sub-periosteal resorption. Bone modeling was normal. The proband's granddaughter was not examined radiographically.

These bone changes were interpreted as being compatible with the diagnosis of osteoporosis rather than osteomalacia, although the distinction cannot be made with absolute certainty on the basis of radiographic evidence alone.

Biochemically the proband had hypouricemia (serum uric acid = 0.6–1.1 mg/100 ml) with an increased renal uric acid clearance (55 ml/min) and idio-pathic hypercalciuria (up to 460 mg/24 hr). Table 7.9 lists the abnormal bio-chemical findings in those family members who are known to be affected. Uric acid clearance was suppressed by pyrazinamide to 40.4 ml/min and increased by probenecid to 75 ml/min. No other metabolic abnormalities were detected and many other studies, including pulmonary function tests in the proband, were within normal limits.

Basic defect

The basic defect in this syndrome is not known, nor is the relationship between hypouricemia, hypercalciuria, and decreased bone density understood.

The hypercalciuria reported in the above kindred may be classified as idiopathic because in none of the examined hypercalciuric subjects was hypercalcemia or hypophosphatemia found, whereas the proband showed normal tubular phosphate reabsorption and a normal response to the calcium infusion test. It cannot be de-termined at this time whether the hypercalciuria is independent of the bone disease, a result of it, or the cause of it.

Genetics

Figure 7.36 shows the pedigree of this Sephardi Jewish family of North African origin. Although the parents of the proband are not known to be related, it can

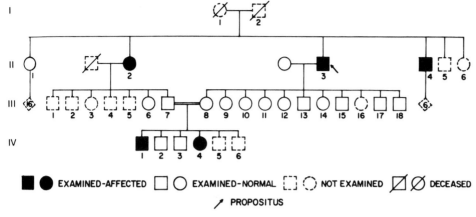

Figure 7.36. Hypouricemia, hypercalciuria, and decreased bone density:
Pedigree of the affected family. From O. Sperling et al., 1974, *Ann.
Intern. Med.* 80:428.

be assumed that they are heterozygous for the mutant gene since 3 of their 6
children are affected. The consanguineous mating in generation III with normal
parents and 2 known affected offspring suggests autosomal recessive transmission.
None of the biochemical abnormalities noted in those affected could be detected
in the obligate heterozygotes.

At the present time this is the only family known to have this disorder.

Prognosis and treatment

The age of the adults affected suggests that this disorder is compatible with a
normal life span. However, the complication of compression fracture of the
vertebral bodies observed in the proband does add a note of caution to this
prognosis.

It may be well to consider early treatment of the osteoporosis when young
children are affected, or at least to see if a therapeutic response can be achieved.

Reference

Sperling, O.; Weinberger, A.; Oliver, I.; Liberman, U. A.; and de Vries, A. 1974.
Hypouricemia, hypercalciuria, and decreased bone density: A hereditary syndrome.
Ann. Intern. Med. 80:482.

LEPRECHAUNISM

Historical note

In 1948 Donohue described a child with peculiar elfin facies, hirsutism, and
multiple endocrine abnormalities. In 1954 a second child with identical features
was born into the same family and Donohue selected the term *leprechaunism* for
this disorder. In 1977 David and Goodman reported leprechaunism in 4 sibs from a

Sephardi Jewish family and with electron micrographs documented for the first time important changes in various organ systems. Unpublished cases from Israel suggest that this disorder may be more common among Jews than among non-Jews.

Clinical features

Affected infants usually have a low birth weight and rather striking physical features. Their facies appears gaunt, with widely spaced eyes, large and low-set ears, abundant facial hair, broad nose with flaring nostrils, and large mouth with thick lips. In addition to facial hirsutism there is a generalized increase in body hair. Acanthosis nigricans has been observed in many cases. Enlargement of the breasts, clitoris, or penis is usually noted at birth. The hands and feet also appear large and there is generalized muscle wasting. A mild jaundice with slight hepatomegaly has been observed in some cases.

Diagnosis

No laboratory test is diagnostic for this disorder. However, the clinical features are so prominent at birth that they readily suggest the diagnosis. A number of abnormal endocrine functions have been observed: low fasting blood sugar, prolonged response to insulin, and hyperinsulinemia. Some affected infants also have hyperbilirubinemia, a low level of serum alkaline phosphatase, and nonspecific aminoaciduria.

All 4 sibs from the Sephardi Jewish family reported by David and Goodman expired between the ages of 7 days and 4 months. An autopsy was done in each case and several pertinent findings were noted. In all 4 cases light microscopy revealed acanthosis nigricans of the skin with diminished subcutaneous fat. The liver showed marked hemosiderosis and cholestasis with severe diminution in the number of portal intrahepatic bile ducts with formation of bile lakes and pseudoglandular structures in the hepatic lobules. There was hyperplasia of the beta cells of the Islet of Langerhans but no hyperplasia of the alpha cells. The renal collecting tubules and Henle loops were obstructed by basophilic material that in the electron microscope appeared to be calcium crystals. Further electron microscopic studies revealed many bundles of intracytoplasmic filamentous structures in the bile duct epithelium and numerous microtubules (Figures 7.37 and 7.38). Identical microfilamentous structures were present in the pericanalicular webs and in the luminal microvilli with bridging and sacular dilation of bile canaliculi. Prominent microfilaments were also present in the glomerular epithelial cells and in the skin fibroblasts. Nonspecific degenerative changes were noted in skeletal muscle.

David and Goodman have postulated that prenatal diagnosis may be possible by demonstrating increased numbers of microfilaments in electron micrographs of cultured fibroblasts obtained by amniocentesis.

Basic defect

The basic defect in leprechaunism is not known. Recent electron microscopic findings have led David and Goodman to propose that the basic alteration in this

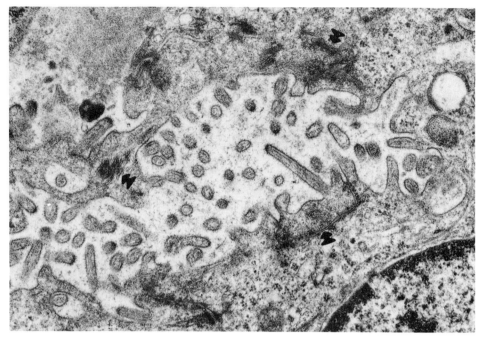

Figure 7.37. Electron micrograph of the liver of a patient with leprechaunism. Note the many bundles of intracytoplasmic filamentous structures (arrows), plus cholestasis with bridging and sacular dilation of the bile canaliculus and hypertrophy of the villi.

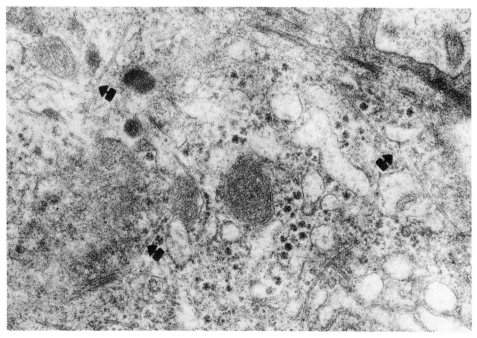

Figure 7.38. Electron micrograph of the liver of the same patient showing the large number of microtubules (arrows) in the cytoplasm.

disorder involves a defect in insulin-receptor binding sites. Evidence for this hypothesis is the abundance of microfilamentous material observed under the electron microscope; this material is now known to play a crucial role in the regulation of cell surface receptors. Such a hypothesis could explain the wasted appearance of affected infants, their altered glucose metabolism and hyperinsulinemia, and the various pathological changes described. Such a defect has been proposed for congenital lipodystrophy, which shares many clinical features with leprechaunism.

Genetics

No more than 25 well-documented cases of this disorder have been described in the literature since the original report by Donohue in 1948. Family studies strongly support an autosomal recessive mode of transmission. The pedigree of this Moroccan-Israeli Jewish family is shown in Figure 7.39. Four affected sibs is the largest number of reported cases in a single family. This in no way suggests that leprechaunism is unusually frequent among Jews, but in my search for additional cases in Israel, 4 other unrelated Jewish families, each having 1 affected child, were found. Three of these families have not been reported, and further documentation must be obtained before any conclusions can be drawn.

These preliminary observations warrant a more thorough study of leprechaunism among the various Jewish ethnic groups in Israel.

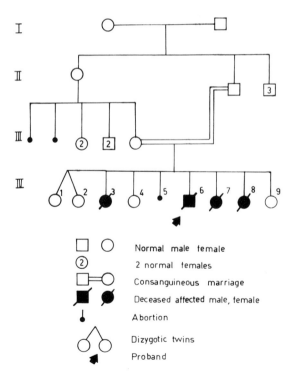

Figure 7.39. Leprechaunism: Pedigree of the affected family.

Prognosis and treatment

Leprechaunism is invariably fatal and most infants die between the ages of 6 months and 1 year.

References

David, R., and Goodman, R. M. 1977. Leprechaunism in 4 sibs: New pathologic and electron microscopic observations. *Hum. Hered.* 27:172.

Der Kaloustian, V. M.; Kronfol, N. M.; Takla, R.; Habash, A.; Khazin, A.; and Najjar, S. S. 1971. Leprechaunism: A report of two new cases. *Am. J. Dis. Child.* 122:442.

Donohue, W. L. 1948. Dyendocrinism. *J. Pediatr.* 32:739.

Donohue, W. L., and Uchida, I. 1954. Leprechaunism: A euphemism for a rare familial disorder. *J. Pediatr.* 45:505.

Evans, P. R. 1955. Leprechaunism. *Arch. Dis. Child.* 30:479.

Kahn, C. R.; Flier, J. S.; Bar, R. S.; Archer, J. A.; Gorden, P.; Martin, M. M.; and Roth, J. 1976. The syndromes of insulin resistance and acanthosis nigricans: Insulin-receptor disorders in man. *N. Engl. J. Med.* 294:739.

Kuhlkamp, F., and Helwig, H. 1970. Das Krankheitsbild des kongenitalen Dysendokrinismus oder Leprechaunismus. *Z. Kinderheilk.* 109:50.

Lakatos, I.; Kallo, A.; and Szijarto, L. 1963. Leprechaunism (Donohue syndrome). *Orv. Hetil.* 104:1075.

Oseid, S.; Beck-Nielsen, N.; Pedersen, O.; and Søvik, O. 1977. Decreased binding of insulin to its receptors in patients with congenital generalized lipodystrophy. *N. Engl. J. Med.* 296:245.

Patterson, J. H., and Watkins, W. L. 1962. Leprechaunism in a male infant. *J. Pediatr.* 60:730.

Salmon, M. A., and Webb, J. N. 1963. Dystrophic changes associated with leprechaunism in male infant. *Arch. Dis. Child.* 38:530.

Summitt, R. L., and Fovara, B. E. 1969. Leprechaunism (Donohue's syndrome): A case report. *J. Pediatr.* 74:601.

MECKEL SYNDROME

Historical note

In 1882 Meckel first described this syndrome in 2 sibs. In 1934 Gruber coined the term *dysencephalia splanchnocystica* to describe the malformation defects. It was not until 1969 that Opitz and Howe reported the first case in the English literature and suggested the term *Meckel syndrome*. In 1971 Fried and co-workers first called attention to the relatively high frequency of this syndrome among Jews. In 1977 Chemke and co-workers established the prenatal diagnosis of this disorder on the basis of elevated alpha-fetoprotein levels and positive beta–trace protein in the amniotic fluid.

Clinical features

Affected infants are stillborn or die shortly after birth from their multiple malformations. The characteristic malformations are occipital encephalocele, polycystic kidneys, polydactyly, and cleft lip/palate. In addition, these infants usually have severe microcephaly and occasionally have anencephaly, micrognathia, multiple eye malformations such as microphthalmia, anophthalmia, and colobomas, and malformed ears. The polydactyly tends to be postaxial, involving both the hands and the feet. Simian creases, camptodactyly, clinodactyly, and talipes equinovarus have been observed in the extremities. Male infants commonly have a hypoplastic phallus with hypospadias and cryptorchidism.

Diagnosis

The diagnosis of Meckel syndrome is a clinical one based on the main features mentioned above. Chromosomal studies have been normal. Clinically this syndrome should be differentiated from trisomy 13, the Smith-Lemli-Opitz syndrome, and a condition referred to as a Meckel-like syndrome. Recently Chemke and co-workers have made the prenatal diagnosis of this disorder by measuring levels of alpha-fetoprotein and beta–trace protein in amniotic fluid. Excessive synthesis of these fetal proteins by the dysplastic kidneys is postulated.

Basic defect

The basic defect in Meckel syndrome is not known. Pathological studies have showed multiple malformations involving the central nervous system: absence of the pituitary gland, cerebral and cerebellar dysgenesis, absent olfactory bulbs and optic nerves, microgyria, malformations of the brain stem and basal ganglia. Nearly all patients exhibit polycystic kidneys, and renal hypoplasia and horseshoe kidneys may be noted. Cardiac malformations and hepatic fibrosis also have been observed.

Genetics

The numerous reports of affected sibs of consanguineous parents strongly suggest an autosomal recessive mode of transmission. As of 1974 approximately 70 cases had been reported in the literature (excluding those from Israel). Of these 70 cases, 7 were from 2 Jewish families. In 1973 Fried reported 24 affected individuals from 7 Israeli Jewish families. The majority of these Jewish families were of Yemenite and Iraqi origin (Figure 7.40). This report spanned the period 1948–1972. Fried estimated the minimal prevalence of this syndrome among Jews in Israel to be 1:50,000. This is a minimal estimate because a systematic search for all cases was not possible, and only those cases in which diagnosis was confirmed by autopsy were included.

Prognosis and treatment

Meckel syndrome is not compatible with life. All affected infants die shortly after birth or are stillborn.

References

Chemke, J.; Miskin, A.; Rav-Acha, Z.; Porath, A.; Sagiv, M.; and Katz, Z. 1977. Prenatal diagnosis of Meckel syndrome: Alpha-fetoprotein and beta-trace protein in amniotic fluid. *Clin. Genet.* 11:285.

Fried, K. 1973. Relatively high prevalence of Meckel syndrome among Jews. *Israel J. Med. Sci.* 9:1399.

Fried, K.; Liban, E.; Lurie, M.; Friedman, S.; and Reisner, S. H. 1971. Polycystic kidneys associated with malformations of the brain, polydactyly, and other birth defects in newborn sibs. *J. Med. Genet.* 8:285.

Fried, K.; Mundel, G.; Reif, A.; and Bukovsky, J. 1974. A Meckel-like syndrome? *Clin. Genet.* 5:46.

Goodman, R. M., and Gorlin, R. J. 1977. *An atlas of the face in genetic disorders,* 2nd ed., pp. 300–301. St. Louis: C. V. Mosby.

Hsia, Y. E.; Bratu, M.; and Herbordt, A. 1971. Genetics of Meckel syndrome (dysencephalia splanchnocystica). *Pediatrics* 48:237.

Meckel, J. F. 1822. Beschreibung zweier durch sehr ähnliche Bildungsabweichungen entstellter Geschwister. *Dtsch. Arch. Physiol.* 7:99.

Opitz, J. M., and How, J. J. 1969. The Meckel syndrome (dysencephalia splanchnocystica, the Gruber syndrome). *Birth Defects* 5(2):167.

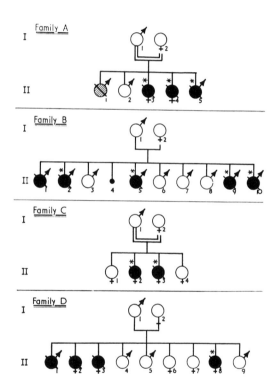

Figure 7.40. Pedigrees of Jewish families with Meckel syndrome. Family A is of Iraqi origin; families B, C, and D are of Yemenite ancestry. From K. Fried et al., 1971, *J. Med. Genet.* 8:285.

METACHROMATIC LEUKODYSTROPHY: A NEW VARIANT

Historical note

Metachromatic leukodystrophy (MLD) of the late infantile type was first described by Greenfield in 1933. At present MLD is thought to embody several apparently closely related and progressive neuropathic entities. These clinical entities are classified mainly according to the predominant age of onset: infantile, late infantile, juvenile, and adult. The adult and late infantile forms are considered to be allelic disorders. In 1964 Austin and co-workers showed that the basic defect in this group of disorders is a deficiency of the enzyme aryl sulfatase A, and it is now known that this deficiency is sometimes combined with defects of one or more of its isoenzymes. In 1979 Russell and Yatziv described a new variant in 3 Jewish sibs whose parents were consanguineous and of Iranian origin.

Clinical features

Since this is a new variant of MLD, a detailed account of the clinical findings follows.

The 3 sibs studied by Russell and Yatziv were 21, 19, and 13 years old.

Pregnancy and delivery had been normal in all 3 cases. There was no history of previous abortions or prenatal drug administration. The sibs' birth weights ranged between 3.0 kg and 3.5 kg.

The earliest manifestation of the disorder in the oldest child was an apparent delay in motor development, with late standing (14–15 months) and walking (18–24 months). As soon as unsupported walking was achieved, however, an unusual clumsiness or unsteadiness of gait became apparent, as did involuntary movements, which were intensified by effort.

By the age of 3–4 years, speech difficulties had become conspicuous, the dysarthria being accompanied by contortion of the lips. In spite of such problems this child was never bedridden, and in play she made relatively good contact with other children, although with recurrent difficulties of adjustment. Intellectual development appeared to be within the normal range. Vision and hearing were considered good. Until the age of 21 years an exceedingly slow progression of clinical manifestations was expressed in this patient in a very gradual intensification of the dysarthria and the intermittent movements simulating athetosis. The patient attended a special school and in her community remained an isolated figure. Nonetheless, during her twentieth year she effectively managed a children's clothes shop.

The age of 6 years marked the onset of signs and symptoms in each of the other 2 sibs. The evolution of clinical manifestations in these 2 sibs was very similar to that in the oldest sib, although more insidious and as yet less advanced. The youngest sib still attends a special school, and both of the younger sibs experience considerable difficulties in making and keeping friends.

The predominant physical finding in the 3 sibs was varying degrees of intention dystonia, with special strain and difficulty in walking in a straight line or in performing fine movements. Only minor movements of choreiform character were manifest, and were largely confined to the fingers and toes in the 2 younger sibs.

In all 3 sibs, but especially in the oldest, now the most severely affected, the tensions associated with such minor flickering involuntary movements swiftly spread in a torsion, spasm-like process to simulate athetosis. Dystonia in terms of facial musculature and tongue produced dysarthria and contorted grimacing. No abnormal pyramidal reflexes were noted, although ankle clonus was elicited. The severity of the above signs appeared to be generally related to the age of the 3 sibs.

Diagnosis

These affected individuals and their parents were studied extensively, but only the main laboratory findings will be noted.

Peripheral nerve conduction velocity was markedly reduced in all 3 sibs but was normal in their mother.

Sural nerve biopsies were done in the 3 sibs and both parents. In all 3 sibs brown metachromatic granules were seen in Schwann cells and myelin layers. Demyelinization was evident in the sibs, but in the mother the results were negative and in the father only a thin undeveloped or residually degenerate sural nerve was detected.

Aryl sulfatase A (AS-A) activity was determined in the urine, leukocytes of venous blood, and cultured skin fibroblasts of all 3 sibs and both parents. These findings are noted in Table 7.10. The specific activity of AS-A in urine was significantly low in the mother and the 3 sibs, whereas in the father it was about 50 percent of that in normal controls. In leukocytes and fibroblasts, on the other hand, depression of AS-A activity was profound only in the 3 sibs; in the parents the deficiency was no more than 50 percent. In addition, the leukocyte activity of AS-B and AS-C isoenzymes in the 3 sibs was found to be about 50 percent of that in normal controls: AS-B specific activity was 20–25 μmoles/hr/mg of protein (normal range = 40–60); AS-C specific activity was 17–22 μmoles/hr/mg of protein (normal range = 30–45).

The specific activity of N-Ac glucosaminidase, -glucosidase, β-galactosidase, -fucosidase, β-fucosidase, -mannosidase, β-mannosidase, β-glucoronidase, and acid phosphatase in leukocytes all proved to be within the normal range.

No effect on AS-A activity could be demonstrated by adding the children's

Table 7.10. Metachromatic leukodystrophy: AS-A specific activity in the urine, WBC, and cultured skin fibroblasts of an affected family

Patient	Urine[a]	WBC[b]	Fibroblasts[c]
Father	5.1	65.8	145.2
Mother	1.06	55.5	100.4
Affected sib 1	1.4	12.7	26.4
Affected sib 2	1.66	8.3	20.5
Affected sib 3	0.87	11.0	21.8
Controls	10 ± 2.5 (30)	120 ± 35.2 (20)	450 ± 205 (15)

Source: A. Russell, Israel.

Note: Figures in parentheses indicate number of samples.

[a] Specific activity expressed as μg of p-nitrocatechol released/hr/ml of urine.

[b] Specific activity expressed as nmoles of p-nitrocatechol released/hr/mg of protein.

[c] Specific activity expressed as nmoles of p-nitrocatechol released/hr/mg of protein.

plasma to normal leukocyte homogenates, or by mixing leukocyte homogenates of the 3 children with those of normal individuals.

Urinary mucopolysaccharides were normal in all 3 sibs.

Basic defect

The basic defect in this variant of MLD appears to be a deficiency in aryl sulfatase A and in its isoenzymes B and C. Russell and Yatziv postulate that the main foci of disposition of excessive cerebroside sulfate in these sibs are (1) the oligodendrocytes of the basal ganglia and their intercommunication to induce some extrapyramidal symptomatology and (2) the Schwann cells or myelin sheaths of peripheral motor nerves.

Genetics

The basis for calling this a new variant of MLD is the distinct clinical picture noted in the above-mentioned sibs and not the biochemical alterations involved, which are clearly compatible with MLD syndrome.

The age of onset of this variant in the 3 sibs overlaps that in the late infantile and juvenile forms, but the disorder becomes distinct in its clinical manifestations insofar as the gait is awkward and unsteady and intermittent spontaneous torsion movements simulating choreoathetosis are precipitated or intensified by voluntary effort. There is no trace of the paralysis, weakness, hypotonia, or mental or visual disturbance so characteristic of the infantile and juvenile forms of MLD.

The fact that the parents of these sibs were first cousins and showed an intermediate level of AS-A activity in their urine and various cells supports autosomal recessive transmission of this variant. The 3 affected children are the only offspring of this couple.

At present this is the only family known to have this form of MLD and it will be interesting to learn if this will remain an isolated variant, a variant more common to Oriental (Iranian) Jews, or a variant with no special ethnic distribution.

Prenatal diagnosis is possible in this disorder.

Prognosis and treatment

Despite its early onset, this new variant of MLD obviously progresses more slowly than the infantile and juvenile forms. Furthermore, it is less severe, in that it is not associated with the mental retardation, hypotonia, paralysis, and dementia that are so common in the previously mentioned types. Nevertheless, this is a progressive disorder which markedly incapacitates the individual. A follow-up report on these patients would be helpful in order to better understand the prognosis of this form of MLD. Treatment is symptomatic.

References

Austin, J. 1973. Metachromatic leukodystrophy (sulfatide lipidosis). In *Lysosomes and storage diseases*, ed. H. G. Hers and F. Van-Hoof, p. 411. New York: Academic Press.

Austin, J.; McAfee, O.; Armstrong, D.; et al. 1964. Abnormal sulphatase activities in two human diseases (metachromatic leukodystrophy and gargoylism). *Biochem. J.* 93:15C.

Greenfield, J. G. 1933. Form of progressive cerebral sclerosis in infants associated with primary degeneration of interfascicular glia. *Proc. R. Soc. Med.* 26:690.

Russell, A., and Yatziv, S. 1979. A variant of metachromatic leukodystrophy as expressed in one family. *J. Pediatr.,* in press.

NEUROLOGICAL SYNDROME SIMULATING FAMILIAL DYSAUTONOMIA

Historical note

Although Engel and Aring reported the first case of familial dysautonomia in 1945, the classical description of this genetic disorder belongs to Riley, Day, and co-workers, who published their findings in 5 cases in 1949. It is now known that this disorder afflicts mainly Ashkenazi Jews (see section on familial dysautonomia). In 1970 Schmidt and co-workers described 2 sibs of Sephardi Jewish origin with features similar to, but not identical with, familial dysautonomia. Evidence suggests that the disorder they described is a new one and not a variant of familial dysautonomia.

Clinical features and diagnosis

Because of the importance of this disorder, a detailed clinical and diagnostic account follows.

The proband, a 16-year-old Jewish girl of Moroccan origin, was admitted to the hospital in 1967 with abdominal pain, fever, and vomiting. The mother's pregnancy, delivery, and neonatal course in Morocco were reported to have been uneventful; the infant's birth weight had been 4.5 kg. Vomiting after almost every meal was observed in the proband after the age of 6 months. She walked at 5 years of age and spoke some words at 6 years. She never cried with tears. At the age of 8, a laparotomy was performed. No details of this operation are known; however, the vomiting continued. One year later she was operated on again. A hiatus hernia with marked dilatation of the esophagus and a stricture with fibrosis and mucosal ulceration at the cardioesophageal junction were found. Heller's operation was performed, but vomiting continued until her hospitalization in 1967.

Physical examination upon admission showed a slender girl 144 cm tall (50th percentile for 8:6 years) with a head circumference of 49 cm (50th percentile for 3 years). When she became excited, blotching appeared over her whole body. Except for minimal breast development and sparse pubic hair, no signs of sexual maturation were present. Although she was short in stature, her extremities were relatively long. Her hands and feet were cold and cyanotic, with webbing between the second and third toes. Her speech was dysarthric and her vocabulary was limited. The radial pulse was felt with some difficulty. Her blood pressure ranged from 150/80 mm Hg to 80/60 mm Hg, with lower values occurring when she was erect. Muscular hypotonia and an ataxic gait were evident. Tendon reflexes were normal. Pain sensation was decreased. Fungiform papillae and apparently normal taste sensation were present. Incoordination of eye movements on lateral gaze and slight corneal ulceration were noted. Pupillary margins were irregular and the reaction to light was similar to that of Adie pupil; eyegrounds were normal. There was almost complete absence of tearing, even while crying; only 3–5 mm of humidity were obtained within 5 minutes from both eyes (Schirmer test; normal = 15 mm or more). Neostigmine (0.25 mg administered subcutaneously) produced no visible tears, but when repeated the Schirmer test showed an increase in lacrimation to 7 mm and 10 mm in the right and left eyes, respectively. Instillation of 2 percent methacholine into the conjunctival sac was followed, after 2 minutes, by miosis of pin-point size. Gonioscopy revealed open angles with marked pigmentation. On a revised Stanford-Binet Scale, Terman form L and M, the proband scored an IQ of 30.

Results of routine laboratory tests were normal. A chest roentgenogram revealed a nonhomogeneous shadow at the base of the left lung (apparently caused by aspiration) which subsequently disappeared. A skull roentgenogram was normal. The child's bone age corresponded to her chronological age. Upon radiological examination of the upper gastrointestinal tract, proximal dilatation and relative constriction of the distal third of the esophagus with a niche were seen. The proband's electroencephalogram was interpreted as dysrhythmic, with dyssynchronous background activity and an excess of slow waves. Her electrocardiogram was interpreted as normal. Chromosomal analysis and dermatoglyphics were normal. Urinary excretion of VMA was 3.5–5.9 μg/mg of creatinine (normal); catecholamine excretion was 18.2–25.5 mg/24 hr (normal). Response to intracutaneous injection of histamine (1:1,000) was normal. Intravenous injection of 0.1 unit of insulin per kilogram was followed by a drop in blood sugar to 50 percent of the fasting level after 15 minutes and a gradual increase to the fasting level after 90 minutes. Motor velocity along the median nerve was normal, but sensory conduction time was prolonged.

After treatment with antibiotics, the proband's temperature returned to normal and the pulmonary infiltration disappeared. The abdominal pain subsided after intensive treatment with antacids, but vomiting continued.

The younger sister of the proband resembled her sib in many respects. She was born in Morocco in 1959. The pregnancy was uneventful, delivery was by breech extraction, and birth weight was 3.5 kg. Cyanosis was noted after birth. She sat up at the age of 18 months, walked at 3 years, spoke words at 4 years, and spoke in sentences at 5.

At present she attends a day school for retarded children. Physical examination when she was 8 years old showed a thin girl who was 121 cm tall (50th percentile for 5:6 years), weighed 20 kg (50th percentile for 6 years), and whose head circumference was 54 cm. Like her sister she had elongated features and cold, cyanotic hands and feet. She also cried without tears, but did not vomit. When she was excited her skin blotched, although less frequently than her sister's. Her speech was dysarthric, her gait ataxic, and a fine tremor was observed. She had general muscular hypotonia, incoordination of the hands, and nystagmus on lateral gaze. Her tendon reflexes were hypoactive and no gag reflex could be elicited. Her blood pressure ranged between 120/80 and 50/0. The radial pulse was regular but could be felt only with some difficulty; the rate did not increase under stress. Fungiform papillae were present on the tongue; taste sensation was normal.

Ophthalmological examination showed irregular pupils and anisocoria; the right pupil was dilated and fixed at a diameter of 8 mm. The left pupil reacted normally to light and accommodation, but an irregular outline was seen on constriction. The fundi were normal and showed some fine pigmentation. There were no corneal ulcerations. Gonioscopy revealed open angles with pigmentation. There was no lacrimation; the patient's reaction to methacholine and response to neostigmine were similar to those of her sister, although no contraction of the right pupil could be elicited. On a revised Stanford-Binet Scale, Terman form L and M, she scored an IQ of 50.

Routine laboratory tests, similar to those given to her sister, were normal. Roentgenograms of the chest, skull, wrists, and esophagus were normal. Urinary excretion of VMA was 4.2–5.4 μg/mg of creatinine. Intracutaneous injection of histamine (1:1,000) evoked a normal response. No exaggerated hypoglycemic response to injection of insulin (0.1 mg/kg) could be elicited.

Table 7.11 shows the similar and differing features of familial dysautonomia in these two sibs. There is little to suggest that these children had a form of congenital analgesia and neuropathy or congenital sensory neuropathy with anhidrosis.

Basic defect

The basic defect in this disorder is not known.

Table 7.11. Diagnostic findings in 2 sibs afflicted with neurological syndrome simulating familial dysautonomia

Diagnostic finding	Familial dysautonomia	Sib I	Sib II
Familial occurrence	+	+	+
History of feeding problems and vomiting	+	+	−
Aspiration pneumonia	+	+	−
Hypoactive deep-tendon reflexes	+	−	+
Tremor, dysarthria, hypotonia	+	+	+
Labile blood pressure	+	+	+
Postural hypotension	+	+	+
Hypesthesis	+	+	+
Blotching of skin	+	+	+
Abnormal temperature control	+	+	+
Decreased lacrimation	+	+	+
Pupillary constriction upon instillation of methacholine	+	+	+
Irregular pupillary margins	−	+	+
Corneal ulcerations	+	+	−
Psychomotor retardation	+	+	+
Absence of fungiform papillae on tongue	+	−	−
Impairment of taste	+	−	−
Abnormal histamine response	+	−	−
Decreased excretion of VMA	+	−	−
Abnormal response to insulin	+	−	−
Ashkenazi Jewish extraction	+	−	−

Source: R. Schmidt et al., 1970, *J. Pediatr.* 76:283.

Genetics

The family pedigree of the affected sibs is shown in Figure 7.41. Originally from Morocco, the family migrated to Israel in 1961. Of the mother's 14 pregnancies, 4 ended in early miscarriages, 4 children died in infancy of various infections, and 4 sibs are well and reported to be of normal intelligence. In the larger family many miscarriages and infant deaths have occurred; however, none of the children have been mentally retarded or have had absence of lacrimation. Urinary VMA excretion rates in both parents are normal.

Normal consanguineous parents suggest autosomal recessive transmission of this disorder.

Prognosis and treatment

It is difficult to state the prognosis of a disease that has not been clearly defined, and such is the situation with these 2 affected sibs. However, it is obvious that both children suffer from profound mental retardation and thus require special, long-lasting care, in addition to symptomatic treatment. This entity awaits further documentation and clarification.

References

Engel, G. L., and Aring, C. D. 1945. Hypothalamic attacks with thalamic lesion. I: Physiologic and psychologic considerations. *Arch. Neurol. Psychiatr.* 54:37.

Riley, C. M.; Day, R. L.; Greeky, D. M.; and Langford, W. S. 1949. Central autonomic dysfunction with defective lacrimation. Part I: Report of five cases. *Pediatrics* 3:468.

Schmidt, R.; Alkan, W. J.; Moses, S. W.; Mundel, G.; and Roizen, S. 1970. A clinical entity simulating familial dysautonomia in a North African Jewish family. *J. Pediatr.* 76:283.

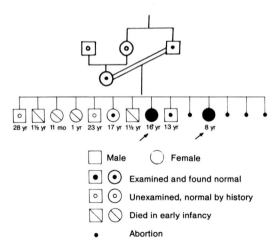

Figure 7.41. Neurological syndrome simulating familial dysautonomia: Pedigree of the affected family. From R. Schmidt et al., 1970, *Pediatrics* 76:283.

OCULOPHARYNGEAL MUSCULAR DYSTROPHY
(AUTOSOMAL RECESSIVE TYPE)

Historical note

In 1915 Taylor was the first to report the combination of ptosis and pharyngeal palsy; he also commented on the familial nature of these findings. In 1962 Victor and co-workers described a family with late onset of dysphagia and progressive ptosis of the eyelids. They recognized the autosomal dominant mode of transmission of this disorder and gave it the name oculopharyngeal muscular dystrophy. Since then several families with this genetic disease have been reported and all have shown autosomal dominant inheritance. In 1975 Fried and co-workers reported two affected Ashkenazi Jewish sibs whose parents were normal and consanguineous, which suggested there may be an autosomal recessive form of the disease.

Clinical features and diagnosis

A clinical and diagnostic account of these 2 sibs follows.

The proband (VI-10) is a 37-year-old mother of 3 healthy children. Since the age of 34 she has noticed mild bilateral ptosis, and gradually she developed difficulty in looking forward. There were no other complaints. She used to wrinkle her forehead and extend her neck in an attempt to look forward. She had never experienced double vision. Neurological examination revealed bilateral symmetrical ptosis down to the midpupillary level. The facies was expressionless. Eye movements were limited in all directions, but especially upward. The patient was not able to raise her eyes above the level of the horizon, but there was no limitation in their convergence. The neurological examination also revealed bilateral drop foot, and ankle reflexes could not be elicited. There was no myotonia or muscle fibrillation. The gag reflex was reduced on both sides. The chest roentgenogram was normal and the thymus was not enlarged. EEC and ECG were normal. CPK and LDH levels were normal. EMG of the lateral recti of both eyes showed potentials of low amplitude and short duration and no fibrillation was observed, indicating a primary muscle disease. EMG of the orbicularis oculi and of the frontalis muscle showed a severe myopathic pattern. The right gastrocnemius and left deltoid muscles had normal potentials. Nerve conduction (right common peroneal) was normal (52 m/s). The Tensilon (edrophonium chloride) test for myasthenia gravis was negative.

The older sister of the proband, VI-9, is a 40-year-old mother of a healthy son. Since the age of 35 she has noticed mild bilateral ptosis. She gave birth to her only son at the age of 39 and since has noticed that her voice has become weak and that she has difficulty in pronouncing lingual letters. She has some difficulty in swallowing and while drinking she sometimes coughs. She also has difficulty climbing stairs. Physical examination showed a thin woman with bilateral ptosis down to the midpupillary level. The facies was expressionless. Symmetrical limitation in elevation of the eyes to the level of the horizon was observed, as was a limitation of lateral gaze movement.

Depression of the eyes and convergence were found to be normal. A bilateral weakness of the orbicularis oculi was noticed. Her speech had a nasal quality with a monotonous melody and low volume. Her tongue movements were clumsy. A paresis of the right vocal cord was observed.

The gag reflex was reduced on both sides. Standing up from the recumbent position was impossible without support from the arms. Bilateral knee and ankle jerks could not be elicited. The ECG was normal. There was no myotonia or muscle fibrillation.

EMGs of the frontalis, orbicularis oculi, and left lateral rectus muscles showed a severe myopathic pattern.

Basic defect

The basic defect in this myopathy is not known.

Genetics

Prior to the cases reported by Fried and co-workers in 1975, all cases with this disorder have conformed to autosomal dominant inheritance. It is known that many of these patients are of French-Canadian descent, and it has been shown that the majority of these patients can be traced back to a single ancestor who emigrated from France in the 1600s.

The pedigree of the Ashkenazi family studied by Fried and co-workers is shown in Figure 7.42. The parents of the affected sibs are both first cousins once removed and third cousins. Except for a distant relative (V-5) who is said to have a disease similar to that of the 2 sisters, the rest of the family is reported to be without

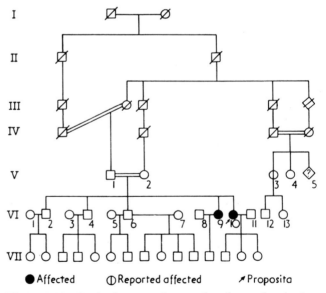

Figure 7.42. Oculopharyngeal muscular dystrophy (autosomal recessive type): Pedigree of the affected family. From K. Fried et al., 1975, *J. Med. Genet.* 12:416.

muscle disease. This relative is herself the product of a first-cousin marriage. She lives abroad, and details of her condition are not available. Both of the parents and the eldest brother of the proposita were examined personally. The father and mother were found to be in good health and without muscle weakness at the age of 75 and 70, respectively. The 3 brothers—aged 47, 46, and 40 years—were healthy. The presence of consanguinity in this family supports the proposed autosomal recessive mode of transmission for this form of oculopharyngeal muscular dystrophy.

Prognosis and treatment

In the classic form of this disorder the age of onset is between 45 and 60 years. The disease generally begins with ptosis of the eyelids and is followed after a brief interval by dysphagia. The clinical picture in the 2 patients described here is similar except that the onset is earlier, in the mid-30s.

Other muscle systems, such as the face, neck, distal limbs, and those of the anal and vesical sphincters, have been reported to be involved. This is a slowly progressive disease and the main problem is dysphagia. Treatment is symptomatic.

References

Barbeau, A. 1966. The syndrome of hereditary late onset ptosis and dysphagia in French-Canada. In *Symposium über progressive Muskeldystrophie, Myotonie, Myasthenie*, ed. E. Kuhn, pp. 102–9. Berlin: Springer-Verlag.

Fried, K.; Arlozorov, A.; and Spira, R. 1975. Case report: Autosomal recessive oculopharyngeal muscular dystrophy. *J. Med. Genet.* 12:416.

Taylor, E. W. 1915. Progressive vagus-glossopharyngeal paralysis with ptosis: Contribution to group of family diseases. *J. Nerv. Ment. Dis.* 42:129.

Victor, M.; Hayes, R.; and Adams, R. D. 1962. Oculopharyngeal muscular dystrophy: A familial disease of late life characterized by dysphagia and progressive ptosis of the eyelids. *N. Engl. J. Med.* 267:1267.

PARTIAL ALBINISM AND DEAF-MUTISM
(ZIPRKOWSKI SYNDROME)

Historical note

In 1962 Ziprkowski and co-workers described an X-linked syndrome consisting of deaf-mutism and partial albinism without ocular albinism in a Sephardi Jewish family of Moroccan origin. In 1965 Woolf and co-workers reported the same syndrome in two Hopi Indian brothers.

Clinical features

The characteristic clinical findings in this disorder are conspicuous and involve the skin and vestibuloacustic apparatus. Ziprkowski and co-workers described the skin as partly achromic and partly hyperpigmented. Each of the regions was sharply delineated. The distribution of the pigmented areas was mainly symmetrical and consisted of round or oval, polycyclic or geographical, spots and patches. The

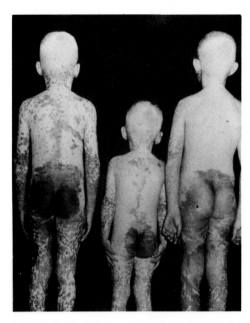

Figure 7.43. Three male sibs with partial albinism and deaf mutism showing the characteristic pigmentary pattern in the gluteal region. Scalp hair is albinoid. From L. Ziprkowski et al., 1962, *Arch. Dermatol.* 86:530. Copyright 1962, American Medical Association.

diameter of these areas varied from a few millimeters to several centimeters. The color ranged from light yellow-brown to deep brown-black. The gluteal region and parts of the scrotum and shaft of the penis were light to dark gray-brown in color (Figure 7.43). The achromic areas had a uniform whitish-pink appearance.

The hair was straight, somewhat coarse, and totally white in all patients except one, in whom it was straw-colored. The eyebrows and eyelashes were achromic, but in 2 affected individuals isolated darkly pigmented lashes were observed.

Upon examination the patients' eyes were normal in all respects except for a few cases of heterochromia of the iris. From a clinical viewpoint all family members were totally deaf, and audiometric studies revealed total perceptive deafness and a marked vestibular hypofunction. Physical examination of the external ears did not show any obvious pathological lesions. No other abnormal findings were noted.

Diagnosis

Partial albinism and deaf-mutism can be diagnosed in a male infant at birth on the basis of light to dark gray-brown pigmentation in the gluteal and scrotal regions combined with evidence of deafness.

A skin biopsy shows the hyperpigmented area to be strongly DOPA positive while the hypopigmented region is weakly positive. There is no increase in the number of melanocytes in the hyperpigmented area and no obvious decrease or abnormal distribution of melanocytes in the hypopigmented region.

A caloric test generally shows a severe hypofunction of the vestibular organ.

Basic defect

The basic defect in this syndrome is not known. It is postulated that the ear lesion involves the organ of Corti or its central tracts—most probably the former. Levels of melanin precursors have been shown to be within normal limits.

Genetics

To date, this X-linked recessive disorder has been reported in only 2 different ethnic groups, the largest being 14 affected members from 6 generations of a Sephardi Jewish family of Moroccan origin (Figure 7.44). The other group consists of 2 Hopi brothers.

In the large Sephardi Jewish family a search for X-chromosome markers was negative; no segregation was found with the genes for color blindness, glucose-6-phosphate dehydrogenase deficiency, or Xg^a blood groups.

In 1969 Fried and co-workers demonstrated a hearing impairment in the heterozygous female carriers of this Jewish family.

Prognosis and treatment

Some evidence from the affected Jewish family indicates the association of a sublethal effect with this syndrome (increased infant mortality rate and a shorter life span among affected individuals and carriers). Only through the recognition of this syndrome in other families, however, will this observation be documented. Treatment at this time is symptomatic.

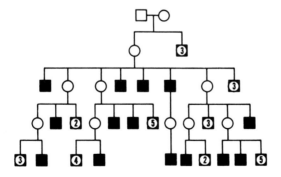

Figure 7.44. Partial albinism and deaf mutism: Family pedigree showing 14 affected males in 3 generations. From L. Ziprkowski et al., 1962, *Arch. Dermatol.* 86:530. Copyright 1962, American Medical Association.

References

Fried, K.; Feinmesser, M.; and Tsitsanov, J. 1969. Hearing impairment in female carriers of the sex-linked syndrome of deafness with albinism. *J. Med. Genet.* 6:132.
Woolf, C. M.; Dolowitz, D. A.; and Aldous, H. E. 1965. Congenital deafness associated
with piebaldness. *Arch. Otolaryngol.* 82:244.
Ziprkowski, L.; Krakowski, A.; Adam, A.; Costeff, H.; and Sade, J. 1962. Partial
albinism and deaf-mutism due to a recessive sex-linked gene. *Arch. Dermatol.* 86:530.

PYLORIC ATRESIA

Historical note

Pyloric atresia is a rare congenital malformation and, to date, only 36 newborns
with this defect have been reported. Although familial occurrence of this anomaly
has been noted on a few occasions, it was Bar-Maor and co-workers' 1972 report
of 5 cases from 2 unrelated Jewish Iraqi families that stressed the autosomal recessive nature of this abnormality.

Clinical features

Nonbilious vomiting in a newborn with a history of maternal hydramnios is
characteristic of pyloric atresia. The upper abdomen is distended and a small
amount of meconium may be passed.

Diagnosis

A plain film of the abdomen shows a typical "single bubble" in the stomach
with no air distally. The use of contrast media is not necessary to establish the
diagnosis. Delay in diagnosing this rare anomaly may be due in part to the absence
of bile in the vomit. Differentiation from hypertrophic pyloric stenosis, which
resembles pyloric atresia clinically, is based on the time of onset of symptoms.

Basic defect

The basic defect in pyloric atresia is not known. Some have considered it to be
failure of the gut to recanalize; others have suggested a mechanical and vascular
injury as the causative factor. Two anatomical types of pyloric atresia have been
observed. Complete membranous obstruction of the gastric outlet is the more
common; absence of continuity of the pyloric wall occurs about half as frequently.

Genetics

In 1972 Bar-Maor and co-workers reviewed the literature and found that of the
34 cases reported 9 were familial, including the 2 families they had studied (Figure
7.45). An autosomal recessive mode of transmission was postulated on the basis
of the following findings: (1) no known parent-to-child transmission; (2) parental
consanguinity; (3) an equal representation of the sexes among affected patients;
and (4) a 1:3 ratio of affected to nonaffected patients. In 1973 Tan and Murugasu

reported this defect in 2 infant sibs in whom a thick membrane completely obstructed the pylorus, but the parents were not consanguineous.

The two different anatomical variants of this anomaly have been observed twice
in the same sibships. The fact that the 2 Israeli families were unrelated (one was
consanguineous, the other was not) but of Jewish Iraqi ancestry makes it tempting
to speculate that this gene may be more common among Iraqi Jews. To date, no
other familial cases have been reported in this ethnic group.

Prognosis and treatment

Early diagnosis and surgical correction are essential if life is to be maintained.
Although the two anatomical types present an identical picture, the surgical treatments differ; a diaphragm can be excised through a gastrostomy, but a fibrotic band
should be by-passed by means of gastroduodenostomy or gastrojejunostomy. Delay
in diagnosis and such complications as aspiration pneumonia, the presence of other
congenital anomalies, or hyaline membrane disease may account for poor surgical
results.

References

Bar-Maor, J. A.; Nissan, S.; and Nevo, S. 1972. Pyloric atresia: a hereditary congenital
anomaly with autosomal recessive transmission. *J. Med. Genet.* 9:70.

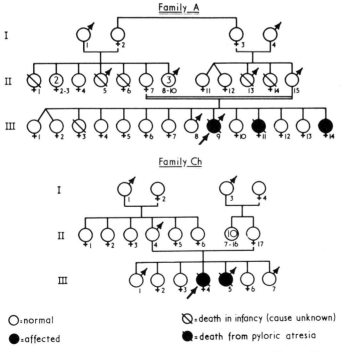

Figure 7.45. Pedigrees of 2 Jewish Iraqi families with
pyloric atresia.

Bronsther, B.; Nadeau, M. R.; and Abrams, M. W. 1971. Congenital pyloric atresia: A report of three cases and a review of the literature. *Surgery* 69:130.

Tan, K. L., and Murugasu, J. J. 1973. Congenital pyloric atresia in siblings. *Arch. Surg.* 106:100.

RADIOULNAR SYNOSTOSIS AND CRANIOSYNOSTOSIS

Historical note

Many genetic syndromes involve craniosynostosis, and in 1973 Berant and Berant added another to this expanding list. They described an affected Sephardi Jewish mother of Moroccan origin who had 4 children affected with various combinations of radioulnar synostosis and craniosynostosis.

Clinical features

The proband, a 9-month-old girl, was referred to the hospital because of scaphocephaly. In addition, her left forearm had an extra crease, appeared "twisted," and supination was limited. The saggital cranial suture was closed. Roentgenograms showed a typical midline ridge (Figure 7.46) and left radioulnar synostosis (Figure 7.47). The mother had right radioulnar synostosis. There were 3 other children, all boys. The oldest son, 16 years of age, had no limb abnormalities; the 12-year-olds, apparently identical twins, had bilateral radioulnar synostosis. All 3 of the boys had elongated skulls. Roentgenograms of their skulls revealed signs of fusion of a portion of the saggital suture and the typical bony ridge. Neither parent showed any evidence of craniosynostosis. Radioulnar synostosis was unilateral in the mother and her daughter and bilateral in the twins. Saggital synostosis was found in all 4 children with varying degrees of severity. No other malformations were noted. The father was of Polish extraction, but no details about his family were available.

Diagnosis

Diagnosis of this syndrome can be made clinically on the basis of the scaphocephalic appearance of the skull and limitation in pronation and supination of the forearm. Confirmation of the diagnosis is made by radiographic examination of the skull and forearm. Chromosomal studies of the mother and her 4 affected children were normal.

Basic defect

The basic defect in this disorder is not known.

Genetics

The combination of radioulnar synostosis and craniosynostosis appears to be transmitted in the above-mentioned family as an autosomal dominant trait. Since no other cases have been reported, it cannot be established at this time whether or

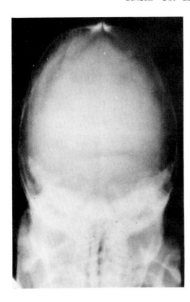

Figure 7.46. Radioulnar synostosis and craniosynostosis: Roentgenogram (Towne projection) of the skull of the proband, a 9-month-old girl, showing the midline ridge. From M. Berant and N. Berant, 1973, *J. Pediatr.* 83:88.

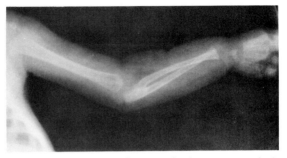

Figure 7.47. Left proximal radioulnar synostosis in the proband. From M. Berant and N. Berant, 1973, *J. Pediatr.* 83:88.

not this is a "private" syndrome. An autosomal recessive syndrome consisting of acrocephaly and radial aplasia has been described in a few non-Jewish families.

Prognosis and treatment

This disorder does not appear to be life threatening. Surgical evaluation of the radioulnar synostosis should be considered if the defect is severely limiting.

References

Berant, M., and Berant, N. 1973. Radioulnar synostosis and craniosynostosis in one family. *J. Pediatr.* 83:88.

Goodman, R. M., and Gorlin, R. J. 1977. *An atlas of the face in genetic disorders*, 2nd ed., p. 541. St. Louis: C. V. Mosby.

Greitzer, L. J.; Jones, K. L.; Schnall, B. S.; and Smith, D. W. 1974. Craniosynostosis–radial aplasia syndrome. *J. Pediatr.* 84:723.

SPONDYLOENCHONDRODYSPLASIA

Historical note

Osteochondromatosis (enchondromatosis, dyschondroplasia), or Ollier disease, was first described by Ollier in 1900. When hemangiomata are associated, the condition is known as Maffucci syndrome. Neither of these disorders is known to be genetically transmitted. In 1976 Schorr and co-workers described a consanguineous Jewish Iraqi family in which 2 sibs had osteochondromatosis with marked involvement of the spine. Since vetebral involvement is very rare in this disorder and the 2 affected brothers were from consanguineous parents, they postulated that the disease in this family may be due to autosomal recessive inheritance. The combination of the above findings led them to coin the term *spondyloenchondrodysplasia.*

Clinical features

The older brother, aged 11:9 years, appeared to be of normal intelligence, well nourished, and in good health. His measurements were as follows: height, 120 cm (50th percentile at 7 years); crown-pubis to pubis-heel, 1.07 (the average ratio at 7 years); arm span, 113 cm; head circumference, 51 cm (3rd percentile at 11:7 years). His head and neck were normal, but his upper limbs were rhizomelic and there was considerable shortening of the limbs and trunk. He had a marked genu valgum deformity. His chest was increased in the anterioposterior diameter and there was thoracic kyphosis and lumbar lordosis. His costochondral joints and the metaphyses of the elbow, wrist, and knee joints were more prominent than usual. His liver was palpable 1.5 cm below the right costal margin.

At 8:8 years the younger affected brother also appeared to be in good health and his measurements were as follows: height, 113 cm (50th percentile at 5:6 years); crown-pubis to pubis-heel ratio, 1.03 (the average ratio at 10 years); arm span, 100 cm; head circumference, 51 cm (above the 3rd percentile at 8:8 years). Like his brother he had rhizomelic shortening of the upper limbs, shortening of the lower limbs and trunk, an increased anterioposterior thoracic diameter, thoracic kyphosis, lumbar lordosis, genu valgum, and thickening of the costochondral joints and metaphyses adjacent to wrist, elbow, and knee joints. His liver was not palpable.

Diagnosis

The diagnosis of spondyloenchondrodysplasia is primarily roentgenographic. The 2 brothers showed multiple sites of enchondromatosis characterized by proliferation of cartilaginous masses within the bone shafts (Figure 7.48). These appear as intramedullary radiolucent areas separated by bony septa and sometimes as linear lucent streaks of cartilage paralleling one long axis of the bone. Radiographs of their hands showed abnormal thickening of the cartilaginous epiphyseal plates. Characteristically, the hand lesions are ovoid or round and usually devoid of septation. Frequently these enchondromas may expand, erode, and destroy the bony cortex. Stippled or mottled calcification is frequently seen within a lesion.

In addition to the previously described lesions, both brothers showed extensive involvement of the spine. Figure 7.49 demonstrates the platyspondyly, irregularity of the superior and inferior end plates, radiolucent islands, and increased density of the anterior end of the laminae noted in the proband at different ages.

Basic defect

The basic defect in spondyloenchondrodysplasia is not known. The enchondromatosis is characterized by an excess of hypertrophic cartilage at the growing ends of bones which has not been reabsorbed and ossified in a normal fashion. The disordered and irregular expansion of columnar areas of cartilage commonly pro-

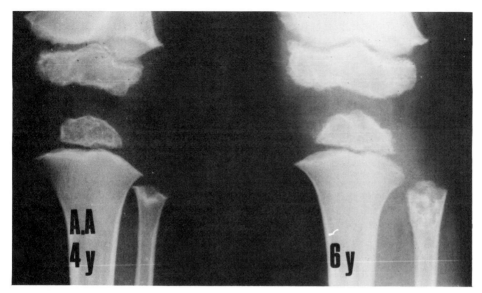

Figure 7.48. Spondyloenchondrodysplasia: Knee bones of the proband at the age of 4 and 6 years. Metaphyseal irregularity is seen in the small "cystic" radiolucent islands in the shaft at the proximal end of the fibula. Similar areas are present in the femur. Note the nonhomogeneous, irregular architecture of the epiphyseal centers involving the tibia and femur. The external distal femoral cartilaginous masses seem to be less extensive. From S. Schorr et al., 1976, *Radiology* 118:133.

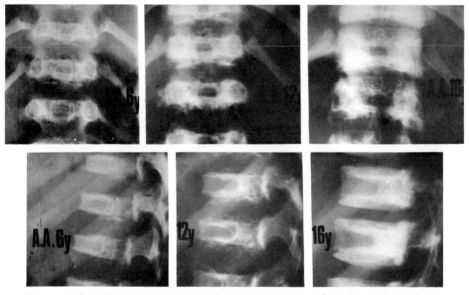

Figure 7.49. AP and lateral views of the 12th dorsal and 1st lumbar vertebrae. Note the abnormal development of the end plates and posterior portion of the vertebral body as observed in the proband over a period of natural growth from the age of 6 to 16 years. From S. Schorr et al., 1976, *Radiology* 118:133.

duces a longitudinally striped appearance in the radiograph. Multiple enchondromatosis may be unilateral or bilateral, localized or generalized, or predominantly
peripheral involving mainly the hands and feet.

Genetics

As mentioned in the historical note, enchondromatosis by itself is not considered
to be a genetic disorder. In this particular family normal consanguineous parents
(they were examined radiographically) with 2 identically affected sons indicate
autosomal recessive transmission of the disorder (Figure 7.50). This condition
has not been reported in any other family.

Prognosis and treatment

The short stature of these 2 affected brothers is undoubtedly related to the
marked vertebral involvement. Therapy in this disease consists of symptomatic
care. Cartilaginous malignancy (chondrosarcoma) may develop in 5–10 percent
of the patients with enchondromatosis.

References

Anderson, I. F. 1965. Maffucci's syndrome: Report of a case with a review of the
    literature. *S. Afr. Med. J.* 39:1066.
Carbonnel Juanico, M., and Vineta Teixido, J. 1962. Otro caso de discondroteosis
    generalizada congenita, tipo Ollier. *Rev. Esp. Pediatr.* 18:91.
Ollier, L. 1900. De la dyschondroplasie. *Bull. Soc. Chir. Lyon* 3:22.
Rossberg, A. 1959. Zur Erblichkeit dei Knochenchondromatose. *Fortschr. Roentgenstr.*
    90:138.
Schorr, S.; Legum, C.; and Ochshorn, M. 1976. Spondyloenchondrodysplasia: Enchondro-
    matosis with severe platyspondyly in two brothers. *Radiology* 118:133.

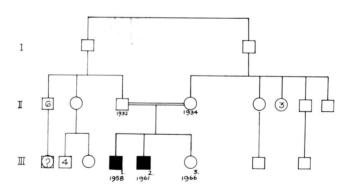

Figure 7:50. Spondyloenchondrodysplasia: Pedigree of the
affected family. From S. Schorr et al., 1976, *Radiology*
118:133.

TEL HASHOMER CAMPTODACTYLY SYNDROME

Historical note

In 1972 Goodman and co-workers described a new syndrome associated with camptodactyly in 2 sibs of Jewish Moroccan ancestry. In 1976 these investigators detected the same disorder in 2 Bedouin sisters. The name for this syndrome had been *camptodactyly with muscular hypoplasia, skeletal dysplasia, and abnormal palmar creases,* but Goodman and co-workers decided to shorten the name to the *Tel Hashomer camptodactyly syndrome,* referring to the place where it was first described.

Clinical features

Table 7.12 lists the various clinical findings observed in these 2 families. Figure 7.51 shows the characteristic hand abnormalities observed in all 4 patients.

Table 7.12. Tel Hashomer camptodactyly syndrome: Clinical findings in 2 sibships

	Jewish patients		Bedouin patients	
Defect	III-7 (F aged 17)	III-3 (M aged 13)	III-6 (F aged 20)	III-7 (F aged 19)
Stature				
Short	+	+	+ (152 cm)	+ (150 cm)
Skull				
Brachycephaly	+	++	+	+
Prominent forehead	+	++	+	+
Facies				
Asymmetry	++	+	±	+
Ocular hypertelorism	+	+	+	+
Small mouth	+	+	+	+
Highly arched palate	+	+	+	+
Increased philtrum length	+	+	+	+
Dental crowding	+	+	+	+
Chest				
Thoracic scoliosis	+	++	+	+
Winging of scapulae	+	++	+	+
Extremities				
Camptodactyly	+	++	+	+
Syndactyly	+	++	+	+
Clinodactyly	−	−	+	+
Brachydactyly thumbs	−	−	+	+
Spindle-shaped fingers	+	+	+	+
Abnormal hand prints	+	+	+	+
Dislocated radii	−	−	+	+
Clubfeet	+	+	−	−
Pes planus	−	−	+	+
Malformed toes	+	+	+	+
Muscular system				
Hypoplasia of chest	+	++	+	+
Hypoplasia of pelvis	+	++	+	+
Hypoplasia of limb and hand muscles	+	++	+	+

Sources: R. M. Goodman et al., 1972 and 1976, *J. Med. Genet.* 9:203 and 13:136.

Note: − = absent; ± = mild; + = present; ++ = severe.

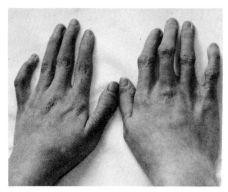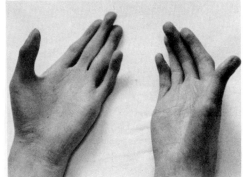

Figure 7.51. Tel Hashomer camptodactyly syndrome: Spindle-shaped fingers with camptodactyly, brachydactyly of the terminal phalanx of the right thumb, mild syndactyly, and hypoplasia of the palmar muscles of the hand—findings observed in all 4 patients.

Diagnosis

In addition to the distinct clinical findings involving the face and musculoskeletal system, a number of skeletal malformations were observed during roentgenographic studies. The last 2 cases reported were studied more intensively from a roentgenographic standpoint and thus these findings (which were very similar to those in the first 2 patients) are listed in Table 7.13.

Dermatoglyphic findings in this syndrome have been shown to be unique and thus characteristic of this disorder. Figure 7.52 shows these changes, and the accompanying legend describes the main features.

Various laboratory tests, including chromosomal examination, were within normal limits.

Basic defect

The basic defect in this syndrome is not known but is postulated to involve some abnormality in connective tissue synthesis.

Genetics

To date, only 2 families—one Sephardi Jewish and one Bedouin—have been reported to have this syndrome, so it is impossible to draw conclusions concerning the possible ethnic distribution of this syndrome, be it Jewish or Arab. The family studies noted in the pedigrees shown in Figures 7.53 and 7.54 strongly suggest autosomal recessive inheritance. It is hoped that further recognition of this syndrome will aid in clarifying its ethnic distribution.

Prognosis and treatment

Of the many abnormalities noted in this syndrome none is known to be life threatening. Orthopedic correction is recommended when some of the bone malformations make walking difficult.

Table 7.13. Tel Hashomer camptodactyly syndrome: Radiographic findings in 2 sibs

Area X-rayed	III-6 (F aged 20)	III-7 (F aged 19)
Skull	Brachycephalic; prominent maxilla on A-P; broad mandible	Same as for III-6
Spine		
Cervical	Spina bifida C_1; enlarged vertebral foramina C_3	Spina bifida C_1; enlarged vertebral foramina C_3; high vertebral bodies
Thoracic	Mild rotational deformities of dorsal vertebrae	Vertebral annular epiphyses present in all vertebrae; mild scoliosis centered at thoracic 9–10
Lumbar	Agenesis of left pedicle; L_4 with secondary scoliosis	Mild scoliosis of lumbar vertebrae to right
Pelvis	Normal	Normal
Thorax	Mild lateral retraction of chest wall	Same as for III-6
Upper extremities		
Humerus	Hypoplasia of trochlea and capitellum	Same as for III-6
Ulnar-radius	Posterior dislocation of radial head	Deformed and enlarged radial head
Hands	Clinodactyly; syndactyly of skin only; brachydactyly of 1st metacarpal right; narrow distal phalanges	Same as for III-6
Lower extremities		
Femur	Normal	Normal
Tibia, fibula	Elongated fibula; subluxation of tibiotalar joint	Normal
Feet	Vertical talus right with deformity of left talus; subluxation of subtalar joints; deformed navicular; deformed and flattened calcaneous; hallux valgus of both big toes; subluxation of interphalangeal joints of big toes, bilateral; severe deformity of terminal digits of feet, bilateral	Talus flat and deformed; subluxation of subtalar joint; deformed navicular; deformed and flattened calcaneous; brachydactyly of right metatarsals; hallux valgus of right big toe; subluxation of interphalangeal joints of great toes, bilateral; severe deformity of terminal digits of feet, bilateral

Source: R. M. Goodman et al., 1976, *J. Med. Genet.* 13:136.

References

Goodman, R. M.; Bat-Miriam Katznelson, M.; Hertz, M.; and Katznelson, A. 1976. Camptodactyly with muscular hypoplasia, skeletal dysplasia, and abnormal palmal creases: Tel Hashomer camptodactyly syndrome. *J. Med. Genet.* 13:136.

Goodman, R. M.; Bat-Miriam Katznelson, M.; and Manor, E. 1972. Camptodactyly: Occurrence in two new genetic syndromes and its relationship to other syndromes. *J. Med. Genet.* 9:203.

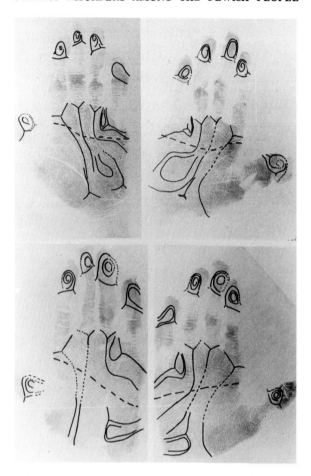

Figure 7.52. Dermatoglyphic prints from the Bedouin sisters affected with Tel Hashomer camptodactyly syndrome. Almost identical changes were observed in the affected Jewish sibs. Four outstanding identical features are noted, the first 3 of which also were observed in the previous 2 cases: (1) numerous palmar creases obliterating the normal structure of the ridges and openings of the sweat pores; (2) many digital whorls extending beyond the first interphalangeal creases; (3) the strikingly abnormal vertical orientation of the radiants; and (4) the presence of simian creases (horizontal dashed lines).

UPPER LIMB–CARDIOVASCULAR SYNDROMES

Historical note

A number of genetic malformation syndromes have been described in which the main physical findings involve the upper extremities and the heart. In 1974 Tamari and Goodman added 2 new syndromes to this list, each of which involves an individual from an Ashkenazi Jewish family.

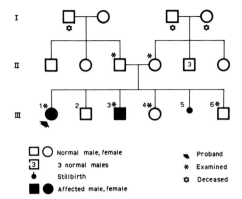

Figure 7.53. Tel Hashomer camptodactyly syndrome: Pedigree of the
affected Sephardi Jewish family. Although there was no history of consanguinity, the parents were from
small neighboring Moroccan communities.

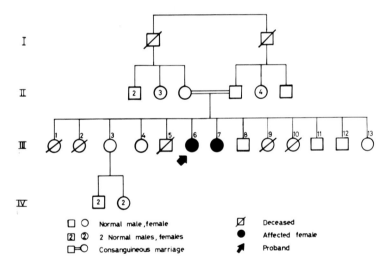

Figure 7.54. Tel Hashomer camptodactyly syndrome:
Pedigree of the Bedouin family.

Clinical features and diagnosis

Because the clinical features of these syndromes are distinct they will be discussed separately.

UPPER LIMB–CARDIOVASCULAR SYNDROME I

A 7-year-old Jewish boy of Ashkenazi origin was noted at birth to have a
malformed right thumb (Figure 7.55) and an anal stricture which responded well

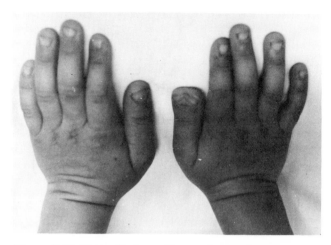

Figure 7.55. Upper limb–cardiovascular syndrome, Case 1. Note the broadness of the right thumb caused by a bifid distal phalanx.

to dilatations. His prenatal history was not remarkable. When he was 2 years old he was found to have a cardiac murmur and a malformation of the external ears.

At the age of 5 years, audiometric studies revealed bilateral hearing loss due to a severe (50–60 dB) conduction defect. Soon thereafter the boy underwent an ossiculoplasty on his left ear. During the operation he was found to have a normal malleus, but the long process of the incus ended without the lenticular process, and the incus touched the stapes tangentially rather than at the normal perpendicular position. The stapes was short and immobile, with a very thick crura and a thickened footplate.

Physical examination at the age of 7 showed a hyperactive boy. His height was 108 cm (3rd percentile for 7 years) and his head circumference, 53.5 cm, was normal. The circumference of his chest was 56 cm. Ocular hypertelorism was noted along with a left divergent strabismus. Examination of the external ears showed bilateral preauricular ear pits and tags. There was an obvious decrease in bilateral hearing. The tongue showed a geographical pattern. Skeletal abnormalities included a bifid right thumb and bilateral pes planus.

Cardiac catheterization and a left heart angiogram showed a ventricular septal defect (VSD) with a significant left-to-right shunt. A small atrial septal defect (ASD) of the foramen ovale type with a left-to-right shunt also was detected.

Because of the patient's multiple malformations, a chromosomal study was done (see Table 7.14). He had normal sex chromosomes (XY) but an extra small autosomal chromosome (total chromosome number, 47) which did not fit into any of the normal karyotype groups. This additional small chromosome was observed in both blood and skin cultures. Routine chromosomal studies of both parents and all sibs were normal. Banding studies were not done at this time.

Dermatoglyphic studies performed on the entire family were within normal limits except for the proband, who showed 7 whorls on the fingers and 6 whorls on the toes. The boy's total ridge count was high (176) but was in proportion to the high

Table 7.14. Key features in 2 new upper limb–cardiovascular syndromes

Feature	Syndrome I (M aged 7)	Syndrome II (F aged 16)
Stature	Short	Short
Intelligence	Normal	Moderate mental retardation
Head	Normal	Microcephaly
Face	Deafness, with ear pits and tags; malformation of middle ear bones; hypertelorism plus strabismus	Highly arched palate; hypoplasia of mandible; low-set ears; hypertelorism plus strabismus
Thorax	Normal	"Winging" of scapulae
Heart	VSD; ASD (foramen ovale)	Pulmonary hypertension; ASD (foramen ovale); PS
Limbs	Bifid thumb; abnormal dermatoglyphics	Radioulnar synostosis; genu varum; right lower limb smaller than left
Basic defect	Genetic (extra small chromosome)	Unknown

Source: I. Tamari and R. M. Goodman, 1974, *Chest* 65:632.

number of whorls. His hands and soles showed an increase in the number of patterns present. An unusual feature was a whorl in the fourth interdigital area of the soles.

The Wechsler intelligence test for children showed that the proband had a verbal scale of 82 (lower limit of normal), with a performance scale of 104. His full-scale IQ was 92 (normal).

UPPER LIMB–CARDIOVASCULAR SYNDROME II

At birth the patient was cyanotic; a cardiac murmur and many other physical abnormalities were noted. During her early years she suffered from recurrent pneumonia. From late infancy on it was obvious to her parents that her physical and mental development were retarded.

Physical examination showed an obviously mentally retarded 16-year-old Ashkenazi Jewish girl of short stature without secondary sex characteristics. Her height was 154 cm (below the 3rd percentile for her age), her head circumference 45.5 cm (also below the 3rd percentile). Facial findings included a dull expression, highly arched palate, mild acne, ocular hypertelorism, strabismus, and hypoplasia of the mandible. Other physical abnormalities included mildly low-set ears, short neck, and a shorter left arm than right, with deformity and limitation in movement of the left elbow and "winging" of the scapulae. The right leg was smaller than the left and showed genu varum; the left displayed pes cavus. There was bilateral clinodactyly of the fifth toes.

On auscultation of the heart the pulmonic second sound was accentuated and a grade 3/6 systolic murmur was heard best over the pulmonary valve. The remainder of the physical examination revealed no other abnormalities except mental retardation. Upon testing, the patient's mental age was 10 years and her IQ was 75.

Roentgenographic studies at the age of 13 years had revealed a bone age of 11 years in this proband. The left forearm showed radial ulnar synostosis, with posterior dislocation of the head of the radius (Figure 7.56). At this time a roentgenogram of the chest showed enlargement of the left ventricle and atrium. An ECG showed a mean QRS axis of $-90°$, left ventricular hypertrophy, tall, prominent P waves in leads $V_{1,2}$, and inverted T waves in all the precordial leads. At 7 years of age the patient underwent cardiac catheterization, which showed

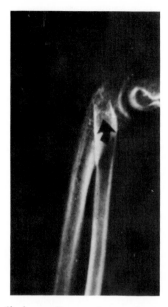

Figure 7.56. Upper limb–cardiovascular syndrome, Case 2. Note the abnormal left forearm with radial ulnar synostosis (arrow) and posterior dislocation of the head of the radius.

moderate pulmonary hypertension, pulmonic stenosis, and pulmonary venous obstruction. There was also a small ASD of the foramen ovale type, with a left-to-right shunt.

Chromosomal analysis showed the patient to have a normal female karyotype.

Table 7.14 summarizes the main clinical and laboratory findings observed in these two patients. Since syndrome II shares some abnormalities with ventricular-radial-dysplasia syndrome (VRD), it is important to distinguish between the two. The cardiac defect observed in the latter syndrome is VSD with or without pulmonary hypertension. ASD may be noted occasionally. The upper-limb malformations consist of hypoplasia or aplasia of the radius and a residual or absent thumb. Other frequently noted malformations involve the lungs, gastrointestinal and renal systems, and the cervical spine. This case resembles that of the VRD syndrome in that the patient has ASD with pulmonary hypertension. However, the upper-limb malformation differs somewhat because this patient has radial-ulnar synostosis. The absence of VSD plus multiple skeletal defects, including microcephaly with mental retardation and short stature, distinguish this case from the VRD syndrome.

Basic defect

The basic defect in syndrome I is probably due to the genetic imbalance produced by the extra small chromosome. The basis defect in syndrome II is not known. From an embryological viewpoint the relationship between the upper limb and heart deformities may be partially understood since these two anatomic structures undergo simultaneous differentiation. The period of development for both structures lasts from the fourth to the seventh week. Thus, some alteration in embryogenesis during this interval may produce a combined defect in both the limbs and heart. The fact that the upper limbs begin and complete their differentiation before the lower limbs may account for greater involvement of the upper extremities in such syndromes.

To further substantiate the developmental relationship between the upper limbs and heart, Birch-Jensen has shown that congenital heart defects occur frequently with radial defects. Furthermore, he stresses that the more serious the radial defect, the higher the frequency of congenital heart disease. This relationship is thought to represent a disturbance in embryogenesis occurring around the seventh week.

Genetics

At present these two cases represent isolated syndromes and to infer that they exist only among Ashkenazi Jews would be misleading. Case 1 belongs to that everexpanding group of malformation syndromes caused by some chromosomal abnormality while case 2 represents a malformation syndrome of unknown etiology, possibly genetic.

Prognosis and treatment

The prognosis in these two syndromes is related to the number and severity of the malformations involved. Decreased hearing seems to be part of syndrome I while mild mental retardation is most probably associated with syndrome II. Surgical intervention has improved the hearing of the patient with syndrome I. Cardiac surgery should be considered in both cases, depending on the severity of the complications that may arise from the malformed hearts.

References

Birch-Jensen, A. 1949. *Congenital deformities of the upper extremities.* Copenhagen: Ejnar Munksgaard.
Tamari, I., and Goodman, R. M. 1974. Upper limb–cardiovascular syndromes: A description of two new disorders with a classification. *Chest* 65:632.

WERNER SYNDROME

Historical note

In 1904 Werner first described this premature aging syndrome in his doctoral thesis. Oppenheimer and Kugel in 1934 and Thannhauser in 1945 clearly delineated this disorder from the one described by Rothmund. In 1966 Epstein and co-workers reviewed the literature and found 125 cases in 94 families. Seven of these families were Jewish. In 1976 Goldstein and Niewiarowski observed an increased procoagulant activity in cultured fibroblasts from patients with Werner syndrome and progeria and suggested that this factor may predispose patients to an increased risk of thrombosis, atherogenesis, and premature death.

Clinical features

The earliest manifestation of this syndrome is a symmetrical retardation of growth and absence of the adolescent spurt. By the age of 20 years obvious premature graying of the hair occurs, followed by atrophy and hyperkeratosis of the skin, generalized loss of hair, alterations of the voice (becoming high-pitched), cataracts (subcapsular and cortical, usually posterior), ulcerations of the skin of the feet, and in about half the cases mild diabetes mellitus. Other atrophic changes can be noted in the muscle, fat, and bone of the extremities. Vascular and soft-tissue calcification are common, as is generalized osteoporosis. Hypogonadism—manifested by small genitalia, female hair distribution, and decreased libido and impotency in males, and by oligomenorrhea or early menopause, small genitalia and breasts, and decreased libido in females—has frequently been observed. The fertility of both sexes is reduced.

Werner syndrome patients tend to have a typical facial appearance marked by a beaked nose and tight atrophic skin about the face and ears. By the age of 30 many have lost much of their scalp hair, and their eyebrows and eyelashes have become sparse.

Diagnosis

The diagnosis of Werner syndrome can usually be made in early adult life on the basis of characteristic clinical findings such as premature aging in a relatively short, thin adult with atrophic skin changes, cataracts, and mild diabetes mellitus.

Roentgenographic changes commonly show vascular calcification of the Monckeberg type, soft-tissue calcification, and patchy or generalized osteoporosis.

Many patients show evidence of coronary artery disease, as indicated by an abnormal ECG, myocardial infarction, or congestive heart failure.

Epstein and co-workers have shown that the effects of glucose and tolbutamide on circulating insulin levels in these patients are similar to those obtained in patients with the mild adult form of diabetes mellitus (delayed and prolonged response with elevated fasting levels of serum insulin).

Goldstein and Niewiarowski have demonstrated that skin fibroblasts from patients with Werner syndrome have markedly (fivefold increase) elevated levels of "tissue factor" (see discussion of the basic defect). In terms of the aging process, it has been shown that *in vitro* cultured fibroblasts from patients with this disorder undergo significantly fewer doublings than their age-matched controls.

Basic defect

The basic defect in Werner syndrome is not known. Many investigators have studied this disease (and other similar conditions) from the viewpoint of better understanding the aging process. The most recent observation of Goldstein and Niewiarowski is that "tissue factor" has the capacity to activate the extrinsic clotting mechanism through fibrinogen. It remains to be seen whether or not this is an explanation for the premature thrombosis and atherogenesis of Werner syndrome patients.

Genetics

Family studies show that Werner syndrome is transmitted as a rare autosomal recessive disease. In their extensive review of the literature in 1966 Epstein and co-workers collected data on 125 cases in 94 families. Seven, or 7.4 percent, of the families were Jewish (5 presumably Ashkenazi and 2 Oriental). Although the percentage of Jewish patients with this disorder may seem small, it is important to keep in mind the rarity of this disorder and the small size of the Jewish population. The percentage of affected Jewish families appears to warrant a more careful evaluation of the occurrence of this condition among the various Jewish ethnic groups. Nevertheless, it is conceivable that the reporting of these cases reflects the bias of Jewish physicians, who see Jewish patients from large Jewish population centers. In Israel only one Ashkenazi Jew is known to have this disorder. His parents were first cousins.

Werner syndrome has been observed in many ethnic groups throughout the world.

Prognosis and treatment

The life span of patients with this disorder is shortened due to their proneness to coronary artery disease at a young age. In addition, 10–15 percent of these patients develop sarcomas and meningiomas.

Cataract formation, leg ulcers, and diabetes mellitus all require close observation and proper management.

References

Epstein, C. J.; Martin, G. M.; Schultz, A. L.; and Motulsky, A. G. 1966. Werner's syndrome: A review of its symptomatology, natural history, pathologic features, genetics, and relationship to the natural aging process. *Medicine* 45:177.

Goldstein, S. 1971. The biology of aging. *N. Engl. J. Med.* 285:1120.

Goldstein, S., and Niewiarowski, S. 1976. Increased procoagulant activity in cultured fibroblasts from progeria and Werner's syndromes of premature aging. *Nature* 260:711.

Hayflick, L. 1973. The biology of human aging. *Am. J. Med. Sci.* 265:432.

Tri, T. B., and Combs, D. T. 1978. Congestive cardiomyopathy in Werner's syndrome. *Lancet* 1:1052.

Werner, O. 1904. *Über Katarakt in Verbindung mit Sklerodermie.* Kiel: Schmidt and Klaunig.

WRINKLY SKIN SYNDROME

Historical note

In 1973 Gazit and co-workers described a new heritable disorder of connective tissue in 3 sibs of consanguineous Jewish parents originating from Iraq.

Clinical features

A brief account of the physical findings in the affected members of this family (Figure 7.57) follows.

In 1972 the proband (IV-1), a 9-year-old girl, was admitted to the hospital with Sydenham chorea. In addition to her coreiform movements, she appeared thin, had poor posture, and seemed mentally retarded. Her weight was 19 kg, height 126 cm, and head circumference 47.5 cm (microcephalic). All the above measurements were at or below the 3rd percentile for her age group.

Her general muscle tone was poor, as exemplified by a bent posture, kyphosis, "winging" of both scapulae, and poor muscle development.

Her facial appearance was altered due to the presence of thick-lensed glasses for myopia, the smallness of her head, and a dull expression. Both fundi showed evidence of myopic changes with old chorioretinitis and partial optic atrophy.

The most striking physical finding pertained to the skin. Over most of the proband's body except for the face, the skin tended to be dry and easily formed wrinkles, as noted about the abdomen when she was in a sitting position (Figure 7.58). The skin on the anterior surface of the chest and the dorsal surface of the hands and feet showed a prominent venous pattern. Numerous skin wrinkles were observed on the dorsal surfaces of the hands (Figure 7.59) and feet and the ventral surfaces showed many creases. It was learned from the patient's mother that this wrinkly skin on the hands and feet was noticed at birth in the proband and in her sister (IV-2). When the skin over the proband's hand was stretched, the normal degree of elasticity was markedly reduced. No abnormal creases were observed about the face. There was no abnormal scar tissue and no history of easy bruisability. The patient could not perform any unusual feats of contortion, and her joints were not extremely hyperextensible for her age. In general her body musculature was hypotonic and poorly developed. The remainder of the physical examination was within normal limits.

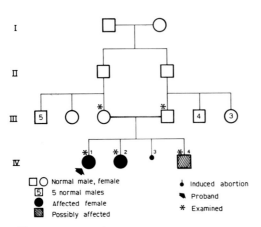

Normal male, female
5   5 normal males
●   Affected female
▨   Possibly affected

◆   Induced abortion
◣   Proband
*   Examined

Figure 7.57. Wrinkly skin syndrome: Pedigree of the affected family. The child noted as possibly affected is now considered to be definitely affected.

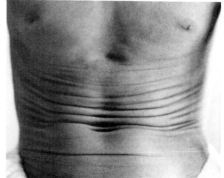

Figure 7.58. Multiple abdominal-skin wrinkles in the proband.

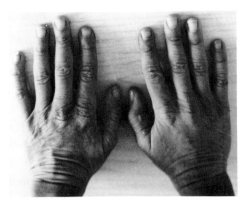

Figure 7.59. Wrinkled appearance of the dorsum of the hand in the proband, a 9-year-old girl.

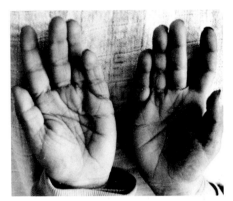

Figure 7.60. Many palmar creases in the proband's 5:6-year-old sister.

Through the family history it was learned that the proband's 5:6-year-old sister (IV-2) had identical skin changes (Figure 7.60) but was of normal intelligence. This sister displayed exactly the same clinical features of the skin and musculature, shared a facial appearance similar to that of the proband, but was not mentally retarded. She was also small for her age: height, 105 cm; weight, 16.5 kg; and head circumference, 47 cm.

Both parents (mother aged 30 and father aged 39) were of normal intelligence and upon physical examination showed none of the abnormalities observed in their 2 affected daughters. At the time of the initial examination the mother was in the last trimester of her third pregnancy. Five months later a home visit was made to examine her infant son. This 3-month-old boy (IV-4) also had excessive wrinkling of the skin about the dorsal surfaces of the hands and feet, with prominent creases on the ventral surfaces. No other findings were observed, but it was thought that this child was affected.

Diagnosis

At present the diagnosis of wrinkly skin syndrome is based on the clinical findings noted above. No distinct histopathological changes were observed in biopsied skin tissue studied under the light microscope. Electron microscopic studies have not been done. Dermatoglyphic findings show a marked increase in the number of palmar creases.

This disorder must be differentiated from the various forms of Ehlers-Danlos syndrome and cutis laxa.

Basic defect

The basic defect in this syndrome is not known. It is thought that biochemical studies utilizing fibroblasts from patients might shed more light on the problem.

Genetics

Three affected sibs of closely consanguineous parents, both of whom are normal, strongly indicates autosomal recessive inheritance.

Recently this same syndrome was observed in 2 children of Jewish Iranian ancestry whose parents are normal first cousins. Although members of 2 Oriental Jewish families are now known to have this disorder, it is too early to form any conclusions about the ethnic distribution of the syndrome; however, autosomal recessive transmission now seems certain.

Prognosis and treatment

Not enough is known about wrinkly skin syndrome to access all possible prognostic features of the disorder. Furthermore, one cannot be certain that the mental retardation seen in the proband is part of the syndrome. No special treatment other than symptomatic care is indicated.

Reference

Gazit, E.; Goodman, R. M.; Bat-Miriam Katznelson, M.; and Rotem, Y. 1973. Wrinkly skin syndrome: A new heritable disorder of connective tissue. *Clin. Genet.* 4:186.

X-LINKED GOUT CAUSED BY MUTANT FEEDBACK-RESISTANT PHOSPHORIBOSYLPYROPHOSPHATE SYNTHETASE

Historical note

In 1970 Sperling and co-workers described in an Ashkenazi Jewish family a new inborn error of metabolism characterized by gout and uric acid lithiasis associated with excessive purine production. This error has now been shown to be transmitted as an X-linked recessive trait caused by mutant feedback-resistant phosphoribosylpyrophosphate (PRPP) synthetase.

Clinical features

The proband, a 38-year-old man, reported a history of recurrent bilateral uric acid lithiasis since the age of 14 and severe gouty arthritis since the age of 20. At the age of 29 he began receiving Allopurinol and his response was excellent. When temporarily off treatment his serum uric acid excretion increased to 2,400 mg. The excessive rate of purine production in this patient was verified by measuring the incorporation of [^{15}N] glycine into his urinary uric acid; in 7 days it amounted to 3.32 percent of the administered dose, as compared to the 0.12, 0.13, and 0.17 percent observed in 3 normal subjects.

The proband has a similarly affected brother. There is no history of urolithiasis or gout in other family members, and abnormality in serum level or urinary excretion of uric acid was noted only in the proband's mother, who is hyperuricosuric.

Diagnosis

Table 7.15 shows the serum level and urinary excretion of uric acid in the proband and his family. To characterize the defect in this family, Sperling and co-workers studied PRPP and purine metabolism in cultured fibroblasts from various members. PRPP synthetase in dialyzed lysates of fibroblasts from the proband and his mother exhibited increased specific activity, more markedly at low inorganic phosphate concentration and decreased levels of sensitivity to inhibition by ADP and GDP. PRPP content and availability and the rate of *de novo* purine nucleotide synthesis were markedly higher in the fibroblasts of the proband and, to a lesser extent, were higher in the fibroblasts of his mother, but were normal in the fibroblasts of unaffected family members. The fibroblast studies demonstrated the following sequence of abnormalities: feedback-resistance of PRPP synthetase; superactivity of this enzyme in a normal physiological milieu; increased availability of PRPP; and increased *de novo* synthesis of purine nucleotides.

In a recent set of experiments measuring purine synthesis *de novo* in cultured fibroblasts following exposure to selective conditions, Sperling and co-workers detected 2 cell types in the fibroblast cultures from the mother—one with normal PRPP synthetase and the other with a mutant PRPP synthetase. Based on the Lyon hypothesis, this finding permits the conclusion that the mother is a carrier for this X-linked recessive disorder.

Table 7.15. X-linked gout: Serum level and urinary excretion of uric acid in an affected family

Subject	Age (yr)	Weight (kg)	Uric acid[a]	
			Serum level (mg/100 ml)	Urinary excretion (mg/24 hr)
Control subjects[b]	20–45		< 7.0	< 800
Family members				
Proband	38	95	13.5	2,400
Father	68	78	6.7	880
Mother	68	70	5.3	1,100
Healthy brother	23	80	6.0	
Affected brother	35	70	13.6	2,250
Sons				
A	16	61	5.2	361
B	9	26	3.7	330
C	10	26	3.7	300
D	4	16	—	220

Source: E. Zoref et al., 1978, *Proc. 2nd Int. Sympos. on Purine Metabolism in Man* (New York: Plenum).

[a] Values in the patients were obtained after 10 days cessation of treatment on low purine diet. Uric acid was determined by an enzymatic spectrophotometric method. The uric acid values given for the control subjects are the upper normal limits for normal subjects on normal home diet in our laboratory (colorimetric autoanalyzer method).

[b] The group consisted of 3 females and 2 males.

Basic defect

The enzymatic defect in X-linked gout has not yet been identified but is thought to involve control of a mutant feedback-resistant PRPP synthetase.

Genetics

This recently described inborn error of metabolism is transmitted as an X-linked recessive disease and the carrier state can be identified. Theoretically, prenatal diagnosis of the disorder could be done on cultured fibroblasts obtained from amniocentesis.

According to Sperling, 5 non-Jewish families are now known to have this disease. Only the initial family is of Ashkenazi origin, so it is possible that the condition will not prove to be characteristic of the Ashkenazi community.

In 1973 Becker and co-workers described 2 brothers with marked purine over-production and clinical gout in whom the activity of PRPP synthetase in red blood lysates was 2.5–3.0 times greater than that in normal persons or in other patients with gout. A daughter of one of the brothers showed equally increased enzyme activity. Increased activity was thought to be a property of the mutant enzyme molecule. Transmission of the disorder in this non-Jewish family was postulated to be autosomal dominant.

Prognosis and treatment

This disorder is a genetic variant of gout and thus has all the prognostic features of that disease. For treatment the reader is referred to any standard textbook of medicine.

References

Becker, M. A.; Kostel, P. J.; Meyer, L. J.; and Seegmiller, J. E. 1973. Human phosphoribyloprophosphate synthetase: Increased enzyme specific activity in a family with gout and excessive purine synthesis. *Proc. Natl. Acad. Sci. USA* 70:2749.

Sperling, O.; Boer, P.; Brosh, S.; Zoref, E.; and de Vries, A. 1978. Overproduction disease in man due to enzyme feedback-resistant mutation. *Enzyme* 23:1.

Sperling, O.; Eliam, G.; Persky-Brosh, S.; and de Vries, A. 1972. Accelerated erythrocyte 5-phosphoribosyl-1-pyrophosphate synthesis: A familial abnormality associated with excessive uric acid production and gout. *Biochem. Med.* 6: 310.

Sperling, O.; Frank, M. ; Ophir, R.; Liberman, U.A.; Adam, A.; and de Vries, A. 1970. Partial deficiency of hypoxanthine-guanine phosphoribosyl-transferase associated with gout and uric acid lithiasis. *Eur. J. Clin. Biol. Res.* 15:942.

Zoref, E.; de Vries, A.; and Sperling, O. 1975. Mutant feedback-resistant phosphor-ibosylpyrophosphate synthetase associated with purine overproduction and gout. *J. Clin. Invest.* 56:1093.

———. 1976. Metabolic cooperation between human fibroblasts with normal and with mutant superactive phosphoribosylpyrophosphate synthetase. *Nature* 260:786.

———. 1978. X-linked pattern of inheritance of gout due to mutant feedback-resistant phosphoribosylpyrophosphate synthetase. *Proc. 2nd Int. Sympos. on Purine Metabolism in Man.* New York: Plenum.

X-LINKED RECESSIVE RETINAL DYSPLASIA

Historical note

Sporadic cases of retinal dysplasia have been reported in the literature. Among these, a few familial cases suggest a recessive mode of transmission. In 1938 Weve noted a preponderance of affected male children and suggested that one form of retinal dysplasia may be inherited as an X-linked recessive disorder. In 1978 Godel and co-workers presented excellent documentation for an X-linked recessive form of retinal dysplasia in a Jewish Iraqi family in which 5 male offspring of 5 sisters were affected.

Clinical features and diagnosis

Figure 7.61 shows the family pedigree. All 5 sons suffered from severe loss of vision.

The characteristic ophthalmoscopic finding was an elevated retinal fold emanating from the optic disc, covering the macular region, and widening toward the temporal fundus (Figure 7.62). These retinal folds were vascularized and extended to the orra serrata and in some instances even to the ciliary body, being at times bordered by heavy clumps of pigment. It is not possible to localize the most common site of involvement, for in these 5 patients various areas of the retina were affected. In severely affected patients the fundal picture was that of a whitish mass protruding in the vitreous and destroying the normal retinal structure. Although retrolental fibroplasia can produce similar findings, the absence of a history of prematurity or of oxygen administration in this family makes such a diagnosis unlikely. Table 7.16 lists the various ophthalmoscopic findings in the affected sons and 2 of the carrier mothers.

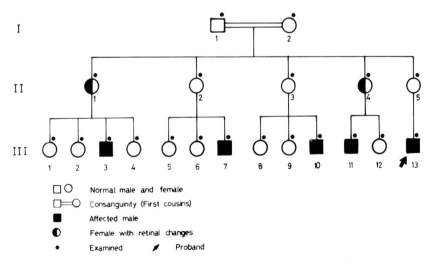

Figure 7.61. X-linked recessive dysplasia: Pedigree of the affected family. Courtesy of V. Godel, Israel.

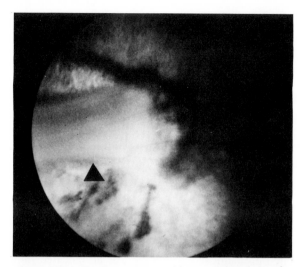

Figure 7.62. Typical retinal fold emanating from the optic disc (pointer) and extending toward the retinal periphery in case III-3. Courtesy of V. Godel, Israel.

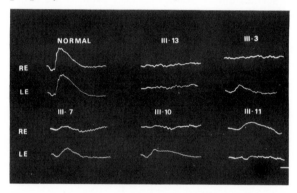

Figure 7.63. Electroretinograms of the 5 male children with retinal dysplasia compared with that of a normal patient of the same age. Note the various patterns ranging from unrecordable responses to potentials with subnormal amplitudes typical of photopic damage. Calibration: 200 μV, 40 msec. Courtesy of V. Godel, Israel.

Electroretinographic results coordinated well with the ophthalmoscopic observations. The typical pattern of the responses—a less steep slope of the ascending limb of the positive wave—and the delay in their implicit time suggested an impairment of the photopic mechanism. Because the ERG is a summary potential reflecting mainly the electrical activity of the nonmacular area, the electroretinograms obtained provided a reliable assessment that the retina outside the macular region remained functional in some patients. In cases where the structural alteration appeared severe, the electrical responses were completely absent (Figure 7.63).

Table 7.16. X-linked recessive retinal dysplasia: Ophthalmological findings in
5 hemizygous sons and 2 heterozygous carrier mothers

Pedigree no.	Age	Sex	External ocular findings	Ophthalmoscopic findings	ERG
			Hemizygous affected sons		
III-13	6 mo	M	Esotropia; nystagmus	BE: Whitish tumor-like protrusions in the vitreous	BE: Extinct
III-3	2:6 yr	M	Esotropia; nystagmus; head posture	RE: Whitish mass in vitreous	RE: Extinct
				LE: Retinal fold covering optic disc and macula widening temporarily	LE: Photopic involvement
III-7	1 yr	M	Esotropia; nystagmus; head posture	RE: Dysplastic fibrous tissue covering the posterior pole	RE: Extinct
				LE: Retinal fold running from the disc to the ciliary body	LE: Photopic involvement
III-10	1 yr	M	Esotropia; nystagmus head posture	RE: Hypoplastic disc; narrow vessels; retinal pigmentation	RE: Extinct
				LE: Retinal fold running from the disc to the temporal periphery	LE: Photopic involvement
III-11	2 yr	M	Esotropia; nystagmus; head posture; LE: megalocornea	RE: Dysplastic tissue covering the posterior pole	RE: Photopic involvement
				LE: Congenital glaucoma	LE: Extinct
			Heterozygous carrier mothers		
II-1	29 yr	F	Normal	LE: Paramacular small retinal fold	Normal
II-4	26 yr	F	Normal	RE: Peripheral retinal rossette	Normal

Source: V. Godel, Israel.

Basic defect

The basic defect in retinal dysplasia is not known.

Genetics

The pattern of inheritance of retinal dysplasia that emerges from study of the above family strongly supports X-linked recessive transmission. It is interesting to note that 2 of the heterozygous female carriers had mild manifestations of the disorder (see Table 7.16).

Linkage studies were done on the family using the blood group antigen Xg^a and G6PD as markers, but no linkage was detected. Color vision in the affected males could not be evaluated due to their ages and the severe loss of vision.

At present this Jewish Iraqi family represents the only well-documented family with this form of retinal dysplasia.

Prognosis and treatment

Although knowledge of this disorder is incomplete, the degree of retinal changes observed in the above-mentioned boys suggests that the visual prognosis is very poor. Unfortunately, no treatment other than symptomatic care is presently available.

References

Godel, V.; Romano, A.; Stein, R.; Adam, A.; and Goodman, R. M. 1978. Primary retinal dysplasia transmitted as X-chromosome-linked recessive disorder. *Am. J. Ophthalmol.* 86:221.

Weve, H. J. M. 1938. Ablatio falciformis congenita (retinal fold). *Br. J. Ophthalmol.* 22:456.

8

Disorders with complex or unproven inheritance

ALTHOUGH MOST of the disorders in this chapter do not conform to patterns of Mendelian inheritance, several can be characterized by familial aggregation. Since environmental factors are closely interwoven with genetic factors in the development of these diseases, most investigators consider their etiology to be multifactorial. Until more specific factors can be identified for these conditions, investigative studies must rely on an epidemiological approach. Much effort has been devoted to evaluating many of these disorders in exactly this manner, but in most instances such studies have not been properly designed to answer questions pertaining to the frequency and distribution of these diseases among the various Jewish communities. It is hoped that future investigations will be better planned to answer such questions.

In most instances the discussion of each disease in this chapter centers on its epidemiological and genetic features as they pertain to Jews. For information on other aspects of these disorders the reader is referred to the standard textbooks of medicine and specific subspecialties.

ALCOHOLISM

Alcoholic beverages are widely consumed by Jews, but it has long been known that rates of alcoholism and other drinking pathologies are very low among Jews. This observation has generated much interest, and various theories have been proposed to explain the phenomenon.

A commonly accepted theory is that of Bales, who proposes that group rates of extreme drinking pathologies are due to the interaction of three major sets of contributing factors. The first he calls *dynamic factors*, referring to the group incidence of acute psychic tensions or needs for adjustment sufficient to provide the driving force in drinking pathologies. The second is *alternative factors*, or

301

culturally defined possibilities of adopting behavior patterns other than excessive drinking which are nonetheless functional equivalents in channeling and relieving acute psychic tensions. The third is *orienting factors*, or the kinds of normative attitudes toward drinking which are carried in the cultures of different groups. Although these factors are difficult to weigh in a given empirical situation, Bales believes that the *orienting factors*—the customs of Orthodox Judaism—account for the differences between rates of drinking pathologies among Jews and the rates for other groups. He contends that early Jewish training and continued participation in the religious consumption of alcohol help to build stable drinking attitudes, which are reinforced by strong religious ideas and group sentiments. Synder agrees with Bales and summarizes his views as follows: "Through the ceremonial use of beverage alcohol, religious Jews learn how to drink in a controlled manner; but through constant reference to the hedonism of outsiders, in association with a broader pattern of religious and ethnocentric ideas and sentiments, Jews also learn how not to drink."

Another theory, the *ingroup-outgroup situation*, suggests that Jews purposely restrict their alcoholic intake because they have been the outgroup in society and would be subject to censure and greater discriminatory measures if they were to overindulge in alcohol. However, experience with alcoholics does not support the assumption that knowledge of the dangers and undesirable consequences of excessive drinking enables the exercise of good judgment sufficient to prevent alcoholism, and thus this theory is considered an inadequate explanation.

Tolerance to alcohol is considered by some to be an ethnically related variable. Eskimos and Indians, for example, are thought to take longer than whites to "sober up" after an alcoholic debauch. Fenna and co-workers have observed that Canadian Eskimos and Indians metabolize a standard dose of ethanol less rapidly than whites, as indicated by a decrease in blood concentrations. In 1972 Wolff noted that Japanese, Taiwanese, and Koreans, after drinking amounts of alcohol that produced no detectable effects on whites, showed marked facial flushing and symptoms of intoxication. These differences in response to alcohol were present from birth. Therefore, it has been suggested that the low frequency of alcoholism and other alcohol-related pathologies in Ashkenazi Jews may be related to some genetically determined physiological factor. Such a hypothesis awaits rigorous scientific documentation.

From studies done in the United States, Synder has shown that as religious affiliation shifts from orthodox, to conservative, to reform, to secular, signs of drinking pathologies tend to increase. This has suggested to some sociologists that alcoholism among Jews may increase as acculturation proceeds. However, it has been noted that Jews who drink in the acculturated style consider themselves to have overindulged or "been drunk" after drinking substantially smaller quantities than non-Jews. Furthermore, the accultural drinking style tends to be abandoned once the individual weds and begins his family. Only in the United States have Jewish drinking customs been studied extensively and systematically, but reports from other countries continue to note the sobriety of Jews.

In Israel in 1966 only 2 percent of all admissions to mental hospitals were for alcoholism. During a 6-year period only 23 deaths were attributed to alcoholism or its complications. There is some evidence of greater alcoholic indulgence by Asian-born Jews in Israel (but not by Israelis of Oriental descent). The rate of first admissions to mental hospitals for alcoholism is twice as high among Asian- and North African–born male Jews than among European-born male Jews; the rate among Israeli-born Jews, irrespective of descent, is only a third as great as that among European-born Jews. The rates for Jewish women of all ethnic groups are negligible.

In terms of alcohol consumption, Israel ranks 20th in a tabulation of 20 countries which provide adequate statistics.

In the United States, in the New Haven psychiatric census of 1950, no alcoholic Jews were found among the patients at any treatment site. In 1961, in his New York State studies, Malzberg found that the average annual rate of alcoholic psychosis among Jews was 0.6/100,000, as compared to 12.4/100,000 among non-Jews. These and other reports indicate the incidence of alcoholism and its complications is low among Jews. Recently, however, Dr. Blume, chief of the alcoholism rehabilitation unit of Long Island Central Islip Psychiatric Hospital in New York, presented preliminary evidence that alcoholism may not be as rare among Jews as previously considered. Because her study dealt with only 100 Jewish alcoholics, further studies are needed to better assess the question.

Despite factors of acculturation, Jews generally continue to be a people for whom alcoholism is not a major problem. The reason for this is not totally understood, but is probably related to the religious and cultural milieu of the Jewish people.

References

Bales, R. F. 1944. The fixation factor in alcohol addiction: An hypothesis derived from a comparative study of Irish and Jewish social norms. Ph.D. diss. Harvard University.

————. 1946. Cultural differences in rates of alcoholism. *Quart. J. Stud. Alcohol* 6:480.

Editorial. 1978. Jews and alcoholism: No cultural immunity found. *Medical World News,* June 26, pp. 20–21.

Fenna, D.; Mix, L.; Schaefer, O.; and Gilbert, J. A. L. 1971. Ethanol metabolism in various racial groups. *Can. Med. Assoc. J.* 105:472.

Fishberg, M. 1911. *The Jews: A study of race and environment.* New York: Charles Scribner's.

Glad, D. D. 1947. Attitudes and experiences of American-Jewish and American-Irish male youth as related to differences in adult rates of inebriety. *Quart. J. Stud. Alcohol* 8:406.

Glatt, M. M. 1970. Alcoholism and drug dependence amongst Jews. *Br. J. Addict.* 64:297.

Glazer, N. 1952. Why Jews stay sober: Social scientists examine Jewish abstemiousness. *Commentary* 13:181.

Goodwin, D. 1976. *Is alcoholism hereditary?* New York: Oxford University Press.

Hes, J. P. 1970. Drinking in a Yemenite rural settlement in Israel. *Br. J. Addict.* 65:293.

Jellinek, E. M. 1941. Immanuel Kant on drinking. *Quart. J. Stud. Alcohol* 1:777.

Jews and alcoholism: No cultural immunity found. *Medical World News,* June 26, 1978, pp. 20–21.

Keller, M. 1970. The great Jewish drink mystery. *Br. J. Addict.* 64:287.

Krasilowsky, D.; Halpern, B.; and Gutman, I. 1964. A study of hospitalized male alcoholics. *Israel Ann. Psychiatr.* 1:277.

————. 1965. The problem of alcoholism in Israel. *Israel Ann. Psychiatr.* 3:249.

McKusick, V. A. 1973. Ethnic distribution of disease in non-Jews. *Israel J. Med. Sci.* 9:1375.

Malzberg, B. 1973. Mental disease among Jews in New York State, 1960–1961. *Acta Psychiatr. Scand.* 49:479.

Mandel, M.; Gampel, J.; and Miller, L. 1971. *Admission to mental hospital in Israel— 1966.* Jerusalem: Government Printing Press.

Rolleston, H. 1928. Some diseases in the Jewish race. *Bull. Johns Hopkins Hospital* 43:117.

Schmidt, W., and Popham, R. 1976. Impressions of Jewish alcoholics. *J. Stud. Alcohol* 37:931.

Synder, C. R. 1958. *Alcohol and the Jews.* Glencoe, Ill.: The Free Press.

———. 1962. Culture and Jewish sobriety: An ingroup-outgroup factor. In *Society, culture, and drinking patterns*, ed. D. J. Pittman and C. R. Synder, pp. 188–225. Carbondale, Ill.: Southern Illinois University Press.

Synder, C. R.; and Landman, R. H. 1951. Studies of drinking in Jewish culture. II: Prospectus for sociological research on Jewish drinking patterns. *Quart. J. Stud. Alcohol* 12:451.

Wolff, P. H. 1972. Ethnic differences in alcohol sensitivity. *Science* 1975:449.

BRONCHIAL ASTHMA

It is well recognized that a familial predisposition operates in the development of bronchial asthma. Furthermore, in asthmatic patients there is an increased frequency of other IgE-mediated allergic disorders, such as hay fever, allergic rhinitis and nasal polyps, urticaria, angioneurotic edema, and infantile eczema. Knowing this, a number of investigators have looked for HLA association in patients with bronchial asthma, but no definite linkage has been found. More recently, Rachelefsky and co-workers have shown that those who succumb to asthma usually have B-lymphocyte group-2 specificity. This specificity is genetically determined and is not an acquired characteristic of the disease, as shown by family studies. This observation may be a useful new "tool" for the study of genetic susceptibility to asthma.

With the influx of Jewish immigrants to Israel in the early 1950s, it became apparent that the rate of occurrence of bronchial asthma was high in the Iraqi Jewish community. In 1964 Glazer and co-workers published a study of 200 consecutive cases of bronchial asthma seen at the allergy clinic of the Tel Hashomer Hospital. This hospital treats about equal numbers of Ashkenazi and non-Ashkenazi patients. Of the group of 200, 108 patients were Ashkenazi and 85 non-Ashkenazi. The latter group included 43 Jews of Iraqi origin, or about 21 percent of all cases. This was a significantly high percentage, considering that the Iraqi Jewish community at that time made up only about 7.5 percent of the Jewish population of Israel.

Glazer and co-workers also learned that two-thirds of the Ashkenazi patients were native-born, while less than one-third of the non-Ashkenazi Jews were. The group of 200 included 75 male draftee soldiers, of whom 19 (25 percent) were of Iraqi origin and only 2 were born in Israel.

In 1977 Brook screened 846 school children (aged 6–16) from Tel Aviv to estimate the prevalence of bronchial asthma. He noted that 6 percent of the children had suffered from recurrent episodes of wheezing during the preceding year; 17 percent had suffered from recurrent wheezing throughout their lives, but, of these, 11 percent had become free of respiratory symptoms by the age of 16.

Among the asthmatics, boys predominated by a ratio of 2 to 1. The prevalence of the disease decreased with age, and only 2 percent of the cases began after puberty.

Allergic rhinitis was noted in 9 percent of the affected children, while 11 percent suffered from skin allergy. Family studies showed that 23 percent of the sibs of these children also had bronchospastic crises, while 11 percent of the parents were affected. Bronchial asthma was observed to be more frequent among children whose parents originated from Iraq, Iran, Morocco, and Romania.

Although both of these studies suggest that the Iraqi Jewish community of Israel has a high rate of bronchial asthma, a note of caution is warranted. Unfortunately, the design of the studies does not provide adequate answers regarding the frequency of this disorder among the various Jewish communities.

In Israel today, fewer cases of bronchial asthma are observed in the Iraqi Jewish community than were recorded in the past. The early disproportion in numbers could well be accounted for by environmental factors. The Iraqi Jews did not have a history of an exceptionally high rate of asthma while living in Iraq. Their early years of settlement in Israel were quite difficult and this, combined with other environmental and climatic changes, could have created a situation in which bronchial asthma became a reaction to these circumstances.

Given present-day immunologic and genetic methods, it would seem that a well-designed study could further clarify the roles of heredity and environment in bronchial asthma and also better define its distribution and frequency among the various Jewish communities.

References

Baum, G. L., and Kleinerman, J. 1970. The respiratory system. In *Genetic disorders of man*, ed. R. M. Goodman, pp. 406–9. Boston: Little, Brown.

Blumenthal, M. N.; Amos, D. B.; Noreen, H.; Mendell, N. R.; and Yunis, E. J. 1974. Linkage to second locus of HL-A. *Science* 184:1301.

Brook, U. 1977. The prevalence of bronchial asthma among Tel Aviv children. *Harefuah* 93:400.

Glazer, I.; Racz, I.; and Baum, G. L. 1966. Bronchial asthma among various ethnic groups in Israel. *Dapim Refuiim (Folia Medica)* 25:2.

Lubs, M. L. E. 1972. Empiric risks for genetic counselling in families with allergy. *J. Pediatr.* 80:26.

Morris, M. J.; Vaughan, H.; Lane, D. J.; and Morris, P. J. 1977. HLA in asthma. *Monogr. Allergy* 11:30.

Rachelefsky, G., et al. 1977. Strong association between B-lymphocyte group-2 specificity and asthma. *Lancet* 2:1042.

Schwartz, M. 1952. *Heredity in bronchial asthma*. Copenhagen: Munksgaard.

Tips, R. L. 1954. A study of the inheritance of atopic hypersensitivity in man. *Am. J. Hum. Genet.* 6:328.

BUERGER DISEASE
(THROMBOANGIITIS OBLITERANS)

Historical note

In 1908 Buerger described inflammatory and occlusive changes in the arteries and veins of amputated lower extremities and referred to the process responsible for these findings as thromboangiitis obliterans (TAO). In 1879 Von Winiwarter had described similar occlusive changes in peripheral arteries and termed the process endarteritis obliterans.

Buerger disease was initially thought to occur primarily in Ashkenazi Jews, but this concept was fostered by the fact that Buerger performed his studies in a hospital in New York City that served predominantly Jews. Further studies have shown that the disease is not restricted to Jews; it has been described in many ethnic groups throughout the world.

In 1960 Wessler and co-workers created a flurry in the medical world by concluding from their studies that "the disease originally described by Buerger is indistinguishable from atherosclerosis, systemic embolism, or peripheral arterial or venous thrombosis, singly or in combination." Few physicians accepted their conclusion, however, and the entity Buerger disease today remains a distinct disorder. In 1965 Goodman and co-workers reported a clinical study of 80 patients with TAO. This study, along with the investigations of McKusick and colleagues published in 1961–1962, aided in clarifying the clinical distinctiveness of this disease and put into perspective its distributon among Jews and non-Jews. In 1974 Ohtawa and his group first noted the association of HLA-A9 with TAO in Japanese patients, and in 1976 McLoughlin and co-workers reported from England a significantly increased association of HLA-A9 and HLA-B5 in patients with Buerger disease.

Clinical features

For the most part the clinical features of Buerger disease are the same in Jews and non-Jews. The clinical findings presented here are based on a 1965 study from Israel and a more recent review of this disease among Israeli patients. The original Israeli study was designed to compare the clinical features of Buerger disease with those of arteriosclerosis obliterans and also to compare certain features with a control group matched for age, sex, and ethnic background. For further details concerning the design of and findings in this investigation the reader is referred to the original publication. In 1977 Elian and Goodman reviewed all the cases of TAO that had been seen at the Sheba Medical Center in Israel between 1965 and 1976. The primary purpose of this retrospective study was to evaluate the number of patients diagnosed and their ethnic distribution among the various Jewish communities.

TAO is known to affect far greater numbers of men than women. Of the 80 patients studied in Israel through 1964, 78 were men and 2 were women. The average age of onset of the disease was 29.9 years, with a range of 16–38 years and a standard deviation of ± 5.8 years. From 1965 to 1976, 92 patients were diagnosed as having TAO and, of these, 4 were women. Because that was a retrospective study it was not possible to obtain accurate information regarding age of onset. A rough estimate of the average age at the time of first hospitalization was 32 years.

The most frequent clinical symptom involving an extremity in these patients (based on the original 1965 study of 80 patients) was migrating thrombophlebitis, which was present in 60 percent of the cases. Although this occurred more frequently in the lower limbs, 10 patients stated that at one time or another their upper extremities also had been involved. Of the 47 patients with migrating thrombophlebitis, 43 gave a history of more than one episode and many stated they had had numerous bouts. This clinical finding served as the presenting symptom in 27 percent of the cases.

The next most common symptoms were Raynaud-like phenomena (57 percent), which usually occurred in the upper extremities, followed by hyperhidrosis, which was noted in 34 percent of the patients.

Table 8.1 lists in order of frequency the *initial* symptom and extremity involved in cases with TAO and arteriosclerosis obliterans. Although the number of patients with arteriosclerosis obliterans is only a little more than half that of those with Buerger disease, claudication was the initial symptom in 77 percent of the former as compared to 37 percent of the latter. In 4 patients with Buerger disease the initial symptom occurred in the upper extremities, while in the group with arteriosclerosis obliterans this finding was never observed.

Obvious clinical findings, such as amputation of a digit or extremity, atrophic changes in the nail pads of the fingers and toes, and ulcerations of the digits, were in all cases accompanied by symptoms and the absence or decrease in one or more of the peripheral pulses. Figure 8.1 shows some of the clinical manifestations noted in the upper extremities of these patients. Table 8.2 shows the frequency of involvement of the extremities in TAO and arteriosclerosis obliterans.

Almost identical clinical findings were recorded for the group of 92 Israeli patients with TAO seen between 1965 and 1976.

Table 8.1. Initial symptom and extremity involved in cases of
Buerger disease and arteriosclerosis obliterans

Data	Buerger disease (no. of cases)	Arteriosclerosis obliterans (no. of cases)
Initial symptom		
Claudication	29	33
Migrating thrombophlebitis	21	0
Pain in toes	8	1
Burning sensation in soles	8	4
Infection and ulceration in toes	6	3
Numbness in toes	3	2
Pain in fingers (hands)	3	0
Weakness in leg	1	0
Total	79[a]	43
Initial extremity involved		
Right leg	37	17
Left leg	35	16
Both legs	3	10
Right arm	3	0
Left arm	0	0
Both arms	1	0
Total	79[a]	43

Source: R. M. Goodman et al., 1965, *Am. J. Med.* 39:601.

[a] One patient was not able to communicate because of language difficulty.

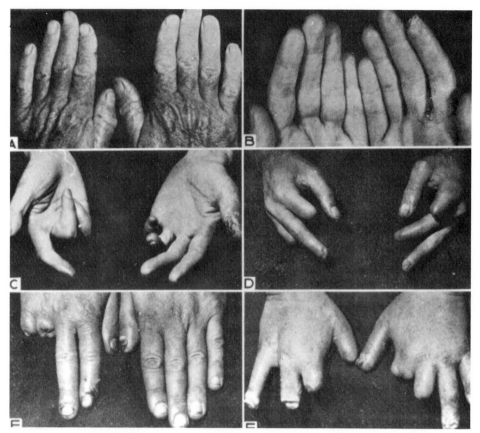

Figure 8.1. Various stages of hand involvement in Buerger disease. (A) Pallor of the distal fingers after exposure to cold (Raynaud's phenomenon). (B) Pallor of the fingers and a healing ulcer on the right index finger. (C) Gangrene of the left thumb and tip of the right index finger and amputation of the distal part of the fourth left finger with Dupuytren's contracture bilaterally. (D) Multiple finger amputations and chronic ulceration. (E) Chronic infection (paronychia) of fingers and amputation of the fourth and fifth right digits. (F) Acute infection involving the stumps on both hands. From R. M. Goodman et al., 1965, *Am. J. Med.* 39:601.

Diagnosis

The initial diagnosis of TAO is usually based on the above clinical features noted in a patient who has a history of heavy cigarette smoking. Figure 8.2 shows the average number of cigarettes smoked per day in 79 patients with TAO and the comparative number smoked in the control group and by those with arteriosclerosis obliterans. One patient in whom TAO developed at the age of 25 years had never smoked and 2 stated they had begun smoking after the onset of the disease. The difference between the smoking habits of those with TAO and arteriosclerosis obliterans, as compared to those in the control group without peripheral vascular disease, was highly significant ($\chi^2 = 50.9$; $p < 0.001$).

To date, no specific biochemical abnormalities have been detected in the blood, serum, or urine of TAO patients. However, recent studies suggest that there may

Table 8.2. Involvement of extremities in cases of Buerger disease
and arteriosclerosis obliterans

	Clinical findings		Amputation	
Extremity involved	Buerger disease (no. of cases)	Arteriosclerosis obliterans (no. of cases)	Buerger disease (no. of cases)	Arteriosclerosis obliterans (no. of cases)
Right leg	0	3	9	5
Left leg	4	3	8	4
Both legs	23	35	9	1
Right arm	0	0	1	0
Left arm	0	0	0	0
Both arms	0	0	0	0
Three extremities	10	0	3	0
Four extremities	43	2	5	0
Total	80	43	35	10

Source: R. M. Goodman et al., 1965, *Am. J. Med.* 39:601.

be an association between Buerger disease and certain HLA antigens. In a study
from England the incidence of HLA-A9 and HLA-B5 was much greater among
those with Buerger disease than among controls ($p < 0.001$). HLA-A9 and
HLA-1B5 occurred together in 7 (39 percent) of the 18 patients with TAO but in
only 9 (1.5 percent) of the 616 healthy controls. In Japan, Ohtawa and co-workers
found an increase not only in HLA-A9 and HLA-W10 but also in a particular
second sublocus group HL-A antigen termed J-1-1 ($p < 0.001$). Compared to a

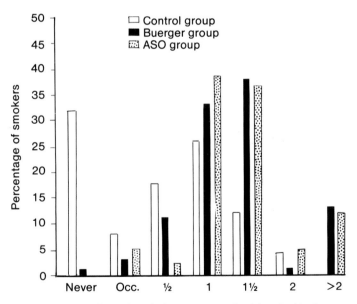

Figure 8.2. Comparative studies of the number of cigarettes
smoked per day in patients with Buerger disease, arteriosclerosis
obliterans, and a control group. From R. M. Goodman et al.,
1965, *Am. J. Med.* 39:601.

normal population occurrence of 18 percent, antigen J-1-1 was found in 46 percent of the TAO patients. Further documentation of these observations could aid in the diagnosis of this disorder.

Arteriographic studies in TAO patients tend to show rather distinct occlusive changes compared to those in patients with arteriosclerosis obliterans. Table 8.3 lists some of these distinguishing features. In general it may be stated that arteriosclerosis obliterans usually does not produce occlusive changes in the upper extremities, whereas this is a common feature of TAO. Arteriography of the upper extremities in the cases of Buerger disease showed that the most common site of arterial occlusion (21 of 34 cases) was the digital arteries, while the next most common site was the ulnar artery (15 of 34 cases). Other sites of arterial occlusion were the palmar and radial arteries, respectively. In no case was occlusion of the interosseus artery observed. Figure 8.3 shows a relatively advanced stage of upper extremity occlusive changes as noted upon brachial arteriography in TAO patients.

There are specific histological features in the vessels of TAO patients, but the difficulty in obtaining pathological material from such patients in the early diagnostic stages of the disease is well appreciated. The late vascular findings are often indistinguishable from arteriosclerosis obliterans.

The acute vascular lesion in this disease is that which Buerger described and which he considered to be the acute specific histological lesion of thromboangiitis obliterans. This lesion is characterized by peculiar, small, usually multiple microabscesses in a fresh or an organizing thrombus. The microabscesses consist of a central focus of polymorphonuclear leukocytes usually surrounded by macronuclear epithelioid cells. Multinucleated giant cells are present in or about these abscesses. The small abscesses are always seen in relatively fresh thrombi but never in completely organized thrombi (Figure 8.4). Appropriate stains have failed to demonstrate the presence of microorganisms. There is a chronic inflammatory infiltrate in the wall of the vessels that contain these lesions, but there is rarely any suggestion of necrosis of the vessel wall as seen in polyarteritis. In some vessels, healing or subacute lesions are demonstrated. Here the purulent foci have disappeared, but small epithelioid cell nodules remain, along with a few giant cells (Figure 8.5). At this stage there is only a slight residue of inflammatory infiltrate in the vessel wall and no scar that suggests healed necrosis.

Table 8.3. Arteriographic distinctions between Buerger disease and atherosclerosis

Aspect	Buerger disease	Atherosclerosis
Size of arteries involved in the disease process	Small and medium	Small, medium, and large
Upper versus lower extremity involvement	Both upper and lower extremities	Lower extremity predominantly
Extent of occlusive changes	Segmental	Diffuse
Character of artery proximal to site of occlusion	Smooth-lined vessel of even caliber	Irregularities in the intima and caliber of vessel
Appearance of collateral circulation	Tree roots configuration of vessels around point of abrupt occlusion	Not specific
Evidence suggesting atheroma in larger vessels	Absent	Present

Source: V. A. McKusick et al., 1962, *JAMA* 181:5. Copyright 1962, American Medical Association.

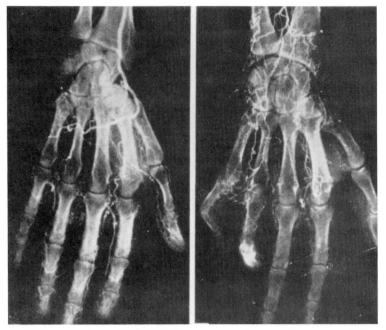

Figure 8.3. (Left) Hand of a 43-year-old man with Buerger disease showing advanced occlusive changes in the digital arteries and lack of visualization of the ulnar artery due to an obstruction higher in the forearm. (Right) Severe arterial occlusive changes in the radial, ulnar, palmar, and digital arteries in the hand of a 56-year-old man with Buerger disease. From R. M. Goodman et al., 1965, *Am. J. Med.* 39:601.

Occasionally the vessels of an amputated part illustrate the entire spectrum of lesions from the acute to the healing or subacute stage to the nonspecific picture of the organized thrombus.

Basic defect

The basic defect in TAO is not known. Numerous theories have been proposed, but none has withstood the rigor of scientific investigation. Exposure to cold, trauma to the extremities, and cigarette smoking can serve as initiating factors in those predisposed to the disease. Recent studies suggesting an association with HLA antigens may open up new avenues of thought and research regarding a possible immunologic alteration in TAO.

Genetics

There is little evidence to suggest that TAO is a genetic disease. However, there are scattered reports in the literature of familial occurrences of this disorder. From the Israeli group of 80 cases studied by Goodman and co-workers, familial aggregation was observed in 4 families, 2 of which were of Ashkenazi origin and

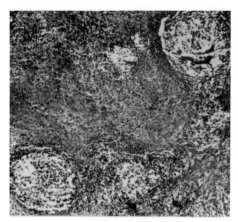

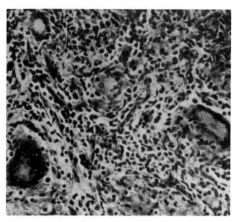

Figure 8.4. Fresh thrombus with micro-abscesses in a medium-sized artery of the epididymis of a patient with Buerger disease. From V. A. McKusick et al., 1962, *JAMA* 181:5. Copyright 1962, American Medical Association.

Figure 8.5. Subacute lesion of Buerger disease in organized arterial thrombus. Note the persistence of epithelioid cell nodules on giant cells. From V. A. Mc-Kusick et al., 1962, *JAMA* 181:5. Copyright 1962, American Medical Association.

2 of which were Sephardi. In 3 of the families 2 generations were affected, and in 1 family 2 male sibs had the disease. In the same investigators' recent review of 92 Israeli cases from 1965–1976, only 1 patient gave a history of having a brother affected with TAO. Additional family studies are needed to clarify this point.

For many years Buerger disease was considered to be a disease that afflicted mainly Ashkenazi Jews. It is now known that this disorder occurs in many populations of the world and it is questionable whether Jews are more affected than other ethnic groups. In our recent survey of the literature on TAO from 1965 to 1977 we found that a great number of papers were published during this period in Italy (86 publications), Germany (66), Poland (44), the U.S.S.R. (43), France (34), and Japan (29). We found fewer publications in the English-speaking countries (30 in the U.S., 18 in Great Britain, and in the others very few). Why? Does the number of publications from the various countries merely reflect interest or lack of interest in the disease? Of course, the answer to that question cannot be known, but it is possible that this disease is being seen more in European populations—perhaps even more in the East European countries—than in the English-speaking world. If this is true, the fact that few Jews remain in Western and Eastern Europe (with the exception of the U.S.S.R.) may indicate that TAO does not primarily afflict Jews. Only a properly designed epidemiological study can clarify this point.

Table 8.4 shows the distribution of TAO among the various Jewish ethnic groups in Israel in 1965. Of the 79 Jewish patients, 63 were Ashkenazi. This is a significant finding, for if a random distribution of TAO were assumed among the main Jewish groups, only 41 Ashkenazi would be expected in a group containing 79 Jewish patients ($\chi^2 = 37.47$; $p < 0.001$). Although the number of non-Ashkenazi cases was small, it is important to note that TAO is not isolated to the Ashkenazi Jewish community.

Table 8.4. Ethnic origin and number of patients
with Buerger disease in Israel, 1965

Ethnic origin	Male	Female	Total
Jewish			
Ashkenazi	62	1	63
Non-Ashkenazi			
Sephardi	12	1	13
Iraqi	2	0	2
Syrian	1	0	1
Arab	1	0	1
Total	78	2	80

Source: R. M. Goodman et al., 1965, *Am. J. Med.*
39:601.

Of the 63 Ashkenazi patients, 37, or 59 percent, were born in Poland, as were their parents. The exact location of the family residence was determined in each patient with TAO who came from Poland; no clustering of cases could be established other than the fact that most came from Eastern Poland, which was the great reservoir of European Jewry.

Table 8.5 shows the ethnic distribution of cases from a recent survey carried out at only one hospital in Israel. Again Ashkenazi Jews predominate, but TAO has also been observed in the Sephardi and Oriental Jewish communities. To the best of my knowledge this disease has not been diagnosed in a Yemenite Jew.

Many more males than females are affected with TAO, as substantiated by the fact that in a total of 172 cases from Israel only 6 were in women (3.5 percent).

Prognosis and treatment

If TAO patients continue to smoke, progression of the disease can be predicted with a certitude rare in medical prognosis. Contrariwise, if TAO patients stop smoking, the disease usually does not progress significantly. Some clinical evidence suggests that patients with TAO are prone to coronary artery disease.

Sympathectomy (both cervical and lumbar) has been used with some success in these patients. Vasodilating drugs seem to be of little help. Migrating thrombophlebitis usually responds well to rest and the use of indomethacin.

The later the age of onset, usually the better the prognosis. Good hygienic care of the toenails and keeping the extremities warm during cold are important health aids in this disease.

Table 8.5. Number of patients with Buerger disease treated
at the Sheba Medical Center, Israel, 1965–1976

Ethnic group	Male	Female	Total
Jewish			
Ashkenazi	53	3	56
Non-Ashkenazi			
Sephardi	25	1	26
Oriental	7	0	7
Arab	3	0	3
Total	88	4	92

References

Biddlestone, W. R., and Lefevre, F. A. 1954. Thromboangiitis obliterans: Occurrence in brother and a sister. *Cleve. Clin. Quart.* 21:226.

Buerger, L. 1908. Thrombo-angiitis obliterans: Study of vascular lesions leading to presenile gangrene. *Am. J. Med. Sci.* 136:567.

———. 1924. *The circulatory disturbances of the extremities, including gangrene, vasomotor, and trophic disorders.* Philadelphia: W. B. Saunders.

Elian, B., and Goodman, R. M. 1977. Unpublished data.

Goodman, R. M.; Elian, B.; Mozes, M.; and Deutsch, V. 1965. Buerger's disease in Israel. *Am. J. Med.* 39:601.

Hill, G. L. 1973. The Buerger syndrome in Java: A description of the clinical syndrome and some aspects of its aetiology. *Br. J. Surg.* 60:606.

McKusick, V. A., and Harris, W. S. 1961. The Buerger syndrome in the Orient. *Bull. Johns Hopkins Hospital* 109: 241.

McKusick, V. A.; Harris, W. S.; Otteson, O. E.; Goodman, R. M.; Shelley, W. M.; and Bloodwell, R. D. 1962. Buerger's disease: A distinct clinical and pathologic entity. *JAMA* 181:5.

McLoughlin, G. A.; Helsby, C. R.; Evans, C. C.; and Chapman, D. M. 1976. Association of HLA-A9 and HLA-B5 with Buerger's disease. *Br. Med. J.* 2:1165.

Martorell, F. 1952. Thromboangiitis obliterans in two brothers. *Angiology* 3:271.

Noble, T. P. 1931. Thromboangiitis obliterans in Siam. *Lancet* 1:288.

Ohtawa, T.; Juji, T.; Kawano, N.; Mishima, Y.; Tohyama, H.; and Ishikawa, K. 1974. HL-A antigens in thromboangiitis obliterans. *JAMA* 230:1128.

Richards, R. L. 1972. TAO (Buerger's disease) in the west of Scotland. *Scott. Med. J.* 17:50.

Samuels, S. S. 1932. The incidence of thromboangiitis obliterans in brothers. *Am. J. Med. Sci.* 183:465.

Weber, F. P. 1937. Thromboangiitis obliterans in father and son. *Lancet* 2:72.

Wessler, S. 1969. Buerger's disease revisited. *Surg. Clin. North Am.* 49:703.

Wessler, S.; Ming, S.; Gurewich, V.; and Freiman, D. A. 1960. A critical evaluation of thromboangiitis obliterans: The case against Buerger's disease. *N. Engl. J. Med.* 262:1149.

Wilensky, N. D., and Collens, W. S. 1938. Thromboangiitis obliterans in sisters. *JAMA* 110:1746.

CELIAC DISEASE

In 1968 Lasch and co-workers reported several epidemiological aspects of childhood celiac disease in Israel. Their main purpose was to evaluate the concept of a causal relationship between celiac disease and intestinal lymphomata associated with malabsorption.

Their survey reviewed all cases that had been diagnosed as celiac disease, idiopathic steatorrhea, nontropical sprue, or malabsorption syndrome in all the general hospitals in Israel from 1950 through 1965. They set the following as minimal criteria for the diagnosis of probable celiac disease: (1) diarrhea, continuous or intermittent for 6 months or longer; (2) onset after 6 months of age; (3) in patients under 18 years of age, evidence of malnutrition, growth retardation, or both; (4) at least one of the following laboratory manifestations of malabsorption—(a) steatorrhea (chemical or microscopic), (b) reduced absorption of lipiodol or of radioiodinated triolein or oleic acid, and (c) sideropenic anemia; (5) absence of a more likely alternative explanation for the clinical picture on the basis of the recorded data. Confirmation of the diagnosis of celiac disease was based on characteristic histological changes observed upon intestinal biopsy.

Lasch and co-workers reviewed 134 cases of probable and 34 cases of confirmed celiac disease. These included 139 children and 29 adults.

Table 8.6 shows the ethnic distribution and incidence of celiac disease among the various Jewish communities in Israel and also among the Israeli Arab population. Because of the reluctance of the Arab population to seek or accept hospitalization unless severely ill, the incidence among Arabs may be underestimated.

The overall incidence in Israel of 17.9/100,000 live births is of the same order of magnitude as that in 2 estimates reported from Great Britain (33.3/100,000 and 12.5/100,000 live births, respectively).

Although there is evidence to suggest that celiac disease is a genetic disorder, the exact mode of transmission is not clear. In the study undertaken by Lasch and co-workers, 4 families were discovered with 2 affected sibs. These case histories were obtained from hospital records, and further family and genetic studies were not done. Familial aggregation is well recognized in celiac disease. In 1965 McDonald and co-workers suggested that the mechanism of inheritance is autosomal dominant with incomplete penetrance. In 1970 Frézal and Rey reviewed the question of the genetics of the disease extensively and concluded that Mendelism is unlikely. In 1971 Robinson and co-workers proposed that celiac disease is multifactorial, its genetic component being polygenic and interacting with environmental factors.

During recent years the association of HLA-B8 with celiac disease in children and adults has been well established. In 1977 Gazit and co-workers confirmed this association in a group of 33 Israeli children with the disorder.

Lasch and co-workers showed that the apparent distribution of celiac disease among the various Jewish ethnic groups in Israel is somewhat similar to the distribution of small intestinal lymphomata. These lymphomata occur almost exclusively in Jews of North African and West Asian origin and in Arabs. Celiac disease also seems to be much more frequent in Jews of North African origin (46.3/100,000 live births) and in those from at least one West Asian country, namely Yemen (54.8/100,000 live births).

Table 8.6. Ethnic distribution of childhood celiac disease in Israel, 1950–1965

Ethnic origin of parents	No. of patients			Rate/100,000 live births	95% confidence limits
	Male	Female	Total		
Eastern and Central Europe	8	11	19	7.6	4.5–11.9
North Africa	32	24	56	46.3	35.1–60.1
Yemen	17	17	34	54.8	37.9–76.7
Iraq	5	4	9	6.6	3.0–12.5
Other Asian countries	3	3	6	8.6	3.2–18.7
Israeli Arabs	6	9	15	10.1	5.7–16.7
Total and average	71	68	139	17.9	15.1–21.2

Source: E. E. Lasch et al., 1968, *Israel J. Med. Sci.* 4:1260.

In addition to questions concerning the ethnic distribution of celiac disease in Israel and its possible relationship with intestinal lymphomata, other problems remain to be clarified, such as the precise role of genetics in the disease and the importance of its association with HLA-B8.

References

Carter, C.; Sheldon, W.; and Walker, C. 1958. The inheritance of celiac disease. *Ann. Hum. Genet.* 23:266.

Davidson, L. S. P., and Fountain, J. R. 1950. Incidence of the sprue syndrome. *Br. Med. J.* 1:1157.

Dennis, N. R., and Stokes, C. R. 1978. Risk of coeliac disease in children of patients and effect of HLA genotype. *J. Med. Genet.* 15:20.

Frézal, J., and Rey, J. 1970. Genetics of disorders of intestinal digestion and absorption. In *Advances in human genetics,* ed. H. Harris and K. Hirschhorn, 1:275. New York: Plenum.

Gazit, E.; Avigad, S.; Zfat, Z.; Efter, T.; Mizrachi, Y.; and Rotem, Y. 1977. The association of HL-A-B8 and childhood celiac disease in an Israeli population. *Israel J. Med. Sci.* 13:400.

Lasch, E. E.; Ramot, B.; and Neumann, G. 1968. Childhood celiac disease in Israel: Epidemiological aspects. *Israel J. Med. Sci.* 4:1260.

MacDonald, W. C.; Dobbins, W. O.; and Rubin, C. E. 1965. Studies on the familial nature of celiac sprue using biopsy of the small intestine. *N. Engl. J. Med.* 279:448.

Robinson, D. C.; Watson, A. J.; Wyatt, E. H.; Marks, J. M.; and Roberts, D. F. 1971. Incidence of small-intestinal mucosal abnormalities and of clinical coeliac disease in the relatives of children with coeliac disease. *Gut* 12:789.

Stokes, P. L.; Ferguson, R.; Holmer, G. K. T.; and Cooke, W. T. 1976. Familial aspects of coeliac disease. *Quart. J. Med.* 45:567.

CONGENITAL MALFORMATIONS

Descriptions of various congenital malformations from the Bible and Talmud can be found in Chapter 4. Most recent reports pertaining to congenital malformations in Jews have come from Israel, where the various Jewish ethnic groups that make up the Israeli population provide a unique means of evaluating and comparing a number of causative factors concerned with these defects. Various medical centers have been interested in epidemiological studies of congenital malformations, but the main reports have come from 2 groups, 1 in Jerusalem, the other in Ness Ziona-Rehovot. Unfortunately these groups have designed their studies in different ways and their observations are difficult to compare. Each will be presented separately.

First, however, a few general remarks about congenital malformations are in order. Gross structural malformations have been reported to occur in up to 8 percent of all newborns. Their prevalence is many times higher in early miscarriages and stillbirths, while other malformations may come to light later, during the first few years of life or in adulthood. A few malformations are known to be genetically determined, while others are thought to be produced by environmental causes such as drugs, chemicals, infections, and radiation. For the vast majority of such defects the etiology is not clear, and multiple factors, genetic and environmental, probably interact to cause these alterations.

In 1971 Harlap and co-workers reported their findings in 18,017 live births in Jerusalem during 1966–1968; 675 infants had 1 or more major malformations (37.5/1,000). An additional 195 infants were stillborn; of these, 17, or 87.2/1,000, had 1 or more major malformations.

Single or multiple minor malformations were found among 745 live-born infants, a rate of 41.5/1,000. Infants with a minor malformation were more than twice as likely to have a major malformation as those without—79.2/1,000 as opposed to 35.7/1,000.

Ethnic group differences in total malformations are listed in Table 8.7. Harlap and his group found significantly more malformed infants among Arabs (66.7/1,000) and Jews of Asian origin (48.3/1,000) than among the 3 remaining groups of Jews, for which the rates were very similar. Tables 8.8 and 8.9 pertain to the individual malformations and give crude rates for each.

The following points are emphasized by the investigators in this Jerusalem study.

(a) Comparisons of overall rates of malformations are of limited value, for they include a heterogeneous group of conditions. They do, however, provide a useful, if crude, check on the validity of the data. The 2 groups showing the highest rates of total malformations—Arabs and Jews of Asian origin—tend to represent the lower socioeconomic levels, and such status is often associated with lower rates of utilization of medical services and apparently low rates of reported malformations. This was not the case in the Jerusalem study, however, for the poor in Israel use organized medical services as often as their well-off counterparts.

Comparisons of ethnic differences between major and minor malformations show that while Arabs and Jews of Asian origin have higher rates for major malformations, there are no significant differences for minor abnormalities. These data

Table 8.7. Major and minor congenital malformations by ethnic group, 1966–1968

Ethnic group	No. of live births	Major malformations (rate/1,000 live births)	Minor malformations (rate/1,000 live births)
Arabs	465	66.7	45.2
Jews	17,552	36.7[a]	37.9
Birthplace of mother			
Israel	6,577	33.3	37.4
Asia	4,274	48.7[b]	41.9
North Africa	4,261	32.4	36.1
West	2,431	32.5	35.4
Birthplace of maternal grandfather			
Israel	2,231	32.7	37.2
Asia	5,978	48.3[b]	42.5
North Africa	4,404	32.0	35.6
West	4,927	28.6	34.7
Total (including unknowns) and average	18,017	37.5	38.1

Source: S. Harlap et al., 1971, *Israel J. Med. Sci.* 7:1520.

[a] Difference between Arabs and Jews significant at the 0.1 percent level.

[b] Difference between Asians and other Jews significant at the 0.1 percent level.

Table 8.8. Major congenital malformations among live-born children, 1966–1968

Malformation	No. of cases	Rate/1,000 live births
Down syndrome	70[a]	2.3[a]
Anencephaly and spina bifida	31[a]	1.0[a]
Total neural tube	33	1.8
Other central nervous system anomalies	27	1.5
Heart and great vessels	107	5.9
Tracheoesophageal fistula	2	0.1
Anus (imperforate, ectopic)	10	0.6
Pyloric stenosis	11	0.6
Other gut anomalies	20	1.1
Cleft lip and/or palate	47[a]	1.6[a]
Talipes	65	3.6
Hip (dislocation and dysplasia)	104	5.8
Polydactyly	19	1.1
Syndactyly	13	0.7
Other limb deformities (including absence of part)	12	0.7
Other skeletal deformities	34	1.9
Metabolic diseases	18	1.0
G6PD deficiency	60	3.3
Thalassemia (major or minor)	13	0.7
Other hereditary anemias	27	1.5
Other and "multiple" malformations	74	4.1
Infants with one or more major malformations	675	37.5

Source: S. Harlap et al., 1971, *Israel J. Med. Sci.* 7:1520.
[a] Based on number of live births and stillbirths, 1964–1968.

strongly suggest that the ethnic differences in major malformations are real, and not merely a consequence of differential reporting. Harlap and co-workers postulate that the higher rates of consanguineous marriage among the Arabs and Asian Jewish immigrants may be an important etiological factor.

(b) No exceptional rate of congenital heart malformations was observed when compared to other studies with a similar degree of follow-up. The authors suggest, however, that their data indicate a trend for such malformations to be most common among Arabs and Jews of Asian ancestry.

(c) The overall incidence of cleft lip and palate, 1.6/1,000, is in the upper part of the range reported for white populations but is more than 3 times the rate reported by another group from Israel in 1967. This large difference is thought to

Table 8.9. Minor malformations among live-born children, 1966–1968

Malformation	No. of cases	Rate/1,000 live births
Inguinal hernia	248	13.8
Umbilical hernia	98	5.4
Hypo- and epispadias	61	3.4
Cryptorchidism	68	3.8
Other abnormalities of genitalia (including hydrocoele)	87	4.8
Abnormal external ear	82	4.6
Abnormalities of skin	55	3.1
Other minor malformations	69	3.8
Infants with one or more minor malformations	745	41.5

Source: S. Harlap et al., 1971, *Israel J. Med. Sci.* 7:1520.

reflect differences in method and incompleteness of some hospital records. Few comparisons can be made, for the rates are based on very small numbers.

(d) Harlap and co-workers comment on the high rate of Down syndrome in Jerusalem but offer no explanation. For a more detailed discussion of this disorder in Jews the reader is referred to page 138.

e) Anencephaly and spina bifida are not common among Jews, and the observed rate of 1.0/1,000 was about the same as Naggan found in his survey of Israel during the same period. Previous studies of anencephaly and spina bifida in the United States also showed very low rates among Jews.

(f) The conclusion reached in this study was that none of the ethnic differences noted among the Jewish communities (cardiac malformations most prevalent in Asian Jewish immigrants, cleft lip and palate observed most often in offspring of Jewish mothers of Western origin, and Down syndrome most frequent in those born to Jewish mothers of North African and Asian ancestry) was significant when adjustment was made for differences in other demographic variables.

The Ness Ziona–Rehovot study, also published in 1971, covers the period from January 1, 1966, to October 31, 1970, and deals with 11,854 births, including 146 (1.2 percent) stillbirths. The male:female ratio for all births was 1.03 and for stillbirths was 1.32. Among the newborns 501 infants were identified as being malformed—447 with single deformities and 54 with multiple ones.

Table 8.10 divides infants with congenital malformations into 8 groups by anatomical system in descending order of rate. Malformations of the bone and joint system were the most frequent (13.8/1,000), followed by anomalies of the genitourinary tract (8.6/1,000). The largest group of newborns classified under the bone and joint category was diagnosed as having talipes (Table 8.11).

On the basis of their data, the Ness Ziona–Rehovot group reached the following conclusions: (a) There may be an association between talipes and ethnic origin on the one hand, and between bone and joint malformations and socioeconomic status (independent of ethnic origin) on the other. (b) Bone and joint malformations are most common among the low socioeconomic classes. (c) Talipes is observed most frequently in Oriental Jews. (d) A significant increase in talipes and congenital dislocation of the hip (CDH) occurred during the second phase of the study. In 1976 the same group reported a steady rise in the incidence of CDH from

Table 8.10. Frequency of congenitally malformed newborns, by anatomical system, among 11,854 births

Anatomical systems	No. of cases	Rate/1,000 births	Rank
Bone and joint	163	13.8	1
Genitourinary system	102	8.6	2
Central nervous system	54	4.6	3
Circulatory system	46	3.9	4
Alimentary and respiratory systems	32	2.7	5
Abdominal cavity	14	1.2	6
Special sense organs	12	1.0	7
Other or unspecified anomalies	78	6.6	—

Source: M. A. Klingberg et al., 1971, *Israel J. Med. Sci.* 7:1529.

Table 8.11. Malformations of the bone and joint system among 11,854 newborns

Malformation	Total No.	Total Rate/1,000 births	1966–1968 No.	1966–1968 Rate/1,000 births	1969–1970 No.	1969–1970 Rate/1,000 births
Syndactyly	9	0.8	6	0.9	3	0.6
Polydactyly	10	0.8	7	1.0	3	0.6
Talipes	83	7.0	30	4.4	53	10.6
Dislocation of hip	30	2.5	9	1.3	21	4.2
Missing extremity in whole or in part	2	0.2	2	0.3	0	—
Other and unspecified defects of the extremities	19	1.6	13	1.9	6	1.2
Other musculoskeletal defects of the head and trunk	7	0.6	7	1.0	—	—
Achondroplasia	2	0.2	0	—	2	0.4
Osseous or cartilaginous dystrophies	1	0.08	0	—	1	0.2

Source: M. A. Klingberg et al., 1971, *Israel J. Med. Sci.* 7:1529.

1966 to a peak in 1975, followed by a sharp decline to levels recorded in the 1960s. (e) Congenital heart disease may be most common among those belonging to the mixed Jewish ethnic group, but this possibility needs to be investigated further.

In 1973 the Ness Ziona–Rehovot group used their earlier data to evaluate the role of genetic factors in various congenital malformations. They found significant differences in the rates of CNS malformations among offspring of related parents as compared to those of unrelated parents (Table 8.12). No differences were noted among the ethnic groups. However, malformations of bone and joints did appear to be associated with ethnic groups. This tendency was noted in 1971, when they first analyzed their data. Ashkenazi Jews consistently showed fewer malformations in this category (Table 8.13).

High rates of consanguinity and distinct ethnic distribution suggested to the Ness Ziona–Rehovot group that genetic factors may be operating in the CNS and bone and joint categories of malformations.

Table 8.12. Effect of parental consanguinity on rate of congenital malformations of the central nervous system (excluding Down syndrome)

Parental consan- guinity[a]	Set 1[b] No.	Set 1[b] %	Set 2[c] No.	Set 2[c] %	Set 3[d] No.	Set 3[d] %	Total No.	Total %
Yes	7/759	9.2	3/445	6.7	5/361	13.9	15/1,565	9.6
No	12/6,118	2.0	15/4,615	3.3	13/4,316	3.0	45/15,049	2.7
Total	19/6,877	2.8	18/5,060	3.6	18/4,677	3.8	60/16,614	3.3
χ^2 (1 d.f.)	10.7 Significant		0.7 Insignificant		7.8 Significant		20.5 Significant	

Source: J. Chemke et al., 1973, *Israel J. Med. Sci.* 9:1400.

[a] At least second-degree cousins.

[b] Data collected January 1966–December 1968.

[c] Data collected January 1969–October 1970.

[d] Data collected November 1970–July 1972.

Table 8.13. Rate of malformations of the bone and joint system by ethnic group

Ethnic group	Set 1[a] No.	%	Set 2[b] No.	%	Set 3[c] No.	%	Total No.	%
Asian Jews	30/1,774	16.9	25/1,180	21.2	14/1,083	12.9	69/4,037	17.1
African Jews	35/2,614	13.4	39/1,876	20.8	24/1,623	14.8	98/6,113	16.0
Ashkenazi Jews	11/1,678	6.6	24/1,493	16.1	12/1,423	8.4	47/4,594	10.2
Total	76/6,066	12.5	88/4,549	19.3	50/4,129	12.1	214/14,744	14.5
χ^2 (2 D.F.)	7.7 Significant		1.3 Insignificant		2.7 Insignificant		8.7 Significant	

Source: J. Chemke et al., 1973, *Israel J. Med. Sci.* 9:1400.
[a] Data collected January 1966–December 1968.
[b] Data collected January 1969–October 1970.
[c] Data collected November 1970–July 1972.

What conclusions can be drawn from these 2 studies of congenital malformations in the various Jewish communities of Israel?

(1) Ethnic differences can be a factor in determining the rates of congenital malformations among Jews, but it is difficult to determine whether the influence is at the genetic or the environmental level.

(2) Close parental consanguinity most probably plays a role in certain congenital malformations of the CNS.

(3) Although sufficient data are lacking, it would seem from the material available that Jews in general are not exceptionally prone to any particular type(s) of congenital malformation(s).

References

Azaz, B., and Koyoumdjisky-Kaye, E. 1967. Incidence of clefts in Israel. *Cleft Palate J.* 4:227.

Chemke, J.; Chen, R.; Klingberg, M. A.; and Levin, S. 1973. Some indications for genetic factors in congenital malformations. *Israel J. Med. Sci.* 9:1400.

Davies, A. M.; Prywes, R.; Tzur, B.; Weiskopf, P.; and Sterk, V. V. 1969. The Jerusalem perinatal study. 1: Design and organization of a continuing, community-based, record-linked survey. *Israel J. Med. Sci.* 5:1095.

Halevy, H. S. 1967. Congenital malformations in Israel. *Br. J. Prev. Soc. Med.* 21:66.

Harlap, S.; Davies, A. M.; Haber, M.; Rossman, H.; Prywes, R.; and Samueloff, N. 1971. Congenital malformations in the Jerusalem perinatal study. *Israel J. Med. Sci.* 7:1520.

Klingberg, M. A.; Chemke, J.; Chen, R.; and Levin, S. 1971. A survey of congenital malformations in Israel. *Israel J. Med. Sci.* 7:1529.

Klingberg, M. A.; Chen, R.; Chemke, J.; and Levin, S. 1976. Rising rates of congenital dislocation of the hip. *Lancet* 1:298.

Legg, S.; Davies, A. M.; Prywes, R.; Sterk, V. V.; and Weiskope, P. 1969. The Jerusalem perinatal study. 2: A cohort study of socioethnic factors in deaths from congenital malformations and from environmental and other causes. *Israel J. Med. Sci.* 5:1107.

MacMahon, B.; Pugh, T. F.; and Ingalls, T. H. 1953. Anencephaly, spina bifida, and hydrocephalus: Incidence related to sex, race, and season of birth, and incidence in siblings. *Br. J. Prev. Soc. Med.* 7:211.

Naggan, L. 1971. Anencephaly and spina bifida in Israel. *Pediatrics* 45:577.

Naggan, L.; and MacMahon, B. 1967. Ethnic differences in the prevalence of anencephaly and spina bifida in Boston, Massachusetts. *N. Engl. J. Med.* 277:1119.
Wahrman, J., and Fried, K. 1970. The Jerusalem prospective newborn survey of
mongolism. *Ann. N.Y. Acad. Sci.* 171:341.

CORONARY HEART DISEASE

Coronary heart disease (CHD) is the most common cause of death in most countries of North America and Europe. For example, in the United States in 1975, of the approximately two million deaths, more than two-thirds were due to CHD. Although it is commonly thought that Ashkenazi Jews are more prone to CHD than non-Jews, relatively few well-designed studies have been undertaken to assess this problem.

In 1957 Epstein's comparison of rates among Italian and Jewish clothing workers in New York City revealed a higher rate among Jews (Ashkenazim), but the author preferred not to ascribe the difference to hereditary factors. In 1969 a study conducted in New York City by Shapiro using over 100,000 members of HIP (Health Insurance Plan) as subjects also showed higher rates for Jews (Ashkenazim) than for either white Protestants or Catholics (Table 8.14). The incidence of myocardial infarction (MI) was somewhat higher among European-born Jews than among Jews born in the U.S. In addition, Ross and Thomas found higher rates of CHD among fathers of Jewish (Ashkenazi) medical students at The Johns Hopkins University Medical School than among fathers of Catholic or Protestant students. An interesting report by Hrubec and Zukel on the epidemiology of CHD in young army men during World War II showed a significantly higher relative risk of CHD among men of the Jewish religion than among age-matched army

Table 8.14. Average annual incidence of specified manifestations of CHD in men and women by color and religion, New York, 1969 (age-adjusted rates per 1,000 population)

Sex, color, and religion	Myocardial infarction			Angina	Possible MI
	Total	Died within 48 hr	Other		
Males					
White	5.39**	1.66	3.73**	2.14**	1.22
Jewish	6.56**	1.54	5.02**	2.61‡	1.47
Catholic	4.54	1.71	2.83	1.97	1.13
Protestant	5.03	1.64	3.39	1.45	0.55#
Nonwhite	2.66	1.31	1.35	1.36	1.19
Females					
White	1.01	0.35	0.66	0.95	0.66
Jewish	1.05	0.20	0.85‡	1.19	0.53
Catholic	0.92	0.39	0.53	0.86	0.86
Protestant	0.93	0.65#	0.28#	0.38#	0.48#
Nonwhite	0.61#	0.09#	0.52#	0.85#	0.48#

Source: S. Shapiro et al., 1969, *Am. J. Public Health* 59 (suppl. 6):1. Reprinted by permission of the American Public Health Association.
Note: Confidence levels in the statistical significance of differences between rates are designated as ** for 0.99, * for 0.95, and ‡ for 0.90. # indicates that numerator frequency was less than 10.

Table 8.15. Myocardial infarction: Average annual
age-adjusted incidence per 1,000 population by area of birth

Area of birth	Rate/1,000 pop.
Israel	9.0
Eastern Europe	9.8
Central Europe	10.0
Southeastern Europe	9.0
Middle East	7.4
North Africa	8.0
Overall average	8.7

Source: J. H. Medalie et al., 1973, *J. Chronic Dis.* 26:329.
Reprinted by permission of Pergamon Press, Ltd.

controls. This risk factor held up even under strict stepwise multiple regression analysis for coronary insufficiency and angina pectoris, although not for myocardial infarction.

Studies of CHD among the various Jewish ethnic groups in Israel have consistently revealed higher rates among European-born (Ashkenazi) than among Asian-African-born (Sephardi) Jews (Table 8.15). Yemenite Jews are known to exhibit exceedingly low rates of heart disease. In 1960 Toor and co-workers' study of Yemenite immigrants (those living in Israel for 5 years or less) revealed rates of 0.1/1,000 for men and 0/1,000 for women. The rates for immigrants who had lived in Israel for 20 or more years were slightly higher—1.6/1,000 for men and 0.2/1,000 for women. Comparable rates for immigrants from Western countries were 17.7/1,000 for men and 4.4/1,000 for women (Table 8.16).

The reasons for such low rates of CHD among Yemenites are not known. It has been suggested that dietary factors are the key—in particular the level of saturated fat in the diet—since Yemenite immigrants who live in Israel for a long time are thought to change their eating habits to a more Westernized (higher fat) diet. In a recent survey, Medalie and co-workers found that Yemenites differed from the rest of the study population with respect to the following: ABO blood type (higher frequency of O); low educational level, high crowding index, high degree of religiosity; low hematocrit; and low consumption of linoleic acid, carbohydrates, and proteins. However, even when these differences, as well as differences in coronary risk profiles (i.e. the risk of developing CHD based on expected in-

Table 8.16. Myocardial infarction: Average annual incidence
per 1,000 population by area of birth and sex

Area of birth	Men	Women
Recent Yemenites[a]	0.1	0
Early Yemenites[b]	1.6	0.2
Eastern countries	5.2	1.4
Western countries	17.7	4.4

Source: M. Toor et al., 1960, *Circulation* 22:265. Reprinted by permission of the American Heart Association, Inc.

[a] $\leqslant$ 5 years in Israel.

[b] $\geqslant$ 20 years in Israel.

cidence derived from known risk factors), are taken into account, the observed rates of CHD among Yemenites remain surprisingly low.

The five-year incidence of CHD among Yemenites in Israel (1963–1968) was only 9/1,000, compared to 55/1,000 for the rest of the study population. After a multivariate analysis, Goldbourt and co-workers could not attribute the differences in rates to differences in coronary risk factors. Mortality rates are similarly much lower than expected among Yemenites, not only for CHD but also for certain malignant neoplasms. These findings suggest the operation of a genetic mechanism in the pathogenesis of coronary heart disease, rather than diet or some other habitual difference in life style.

In international comparisons of the rate of first MIs among males, Israel ranks among the highest in the world if all infarcts (including clinically unrecognized infarcts) are included (8.7/1,000). If only known infarcts are included, Israel assumes an intermediate position (5.3/1,000) (Table 8.17). In terms of intergenerational differences in the incidence of MI among the various Jewish ethnic groups in Israel, Medalie and co-workers have shown that second-generation Israelis have a lower incidence than either immigrants or first-generation Israelis, irrespective of their geographical origin (Table 8.18).

An interesting finding of the Israel Ischemic Heart Disease Project is that, despite the relatively high incidence of MIs in Israel, there is an extremely low case fatality rate. Case fatality rate = number of deaths of new MI subjects ÷ number of new MI subjects.

The epidemiology of coronary heart disease has been studied extensively and the major risk factors have been confirmed repeatedly. Those which are generally agreed upon are: age; sex; cholesterol and hyperlipidemia; smoking; hypertension; glucose intolerance; ECG abnormalities; positive family history of premature heart disease, diabetes mellitus, xanthoma, or hyperlipidemia; physical inactivity; obesity; and hyperuricemia. Personality type, psychological factors, anxiety, ABO blood phenotype, and degree of religiosity also are thought by some to play important roles in the etiology of CHD. Only a few of these risk factors will be discussed, primarily those emphasized in the recent studies from Israel.

Smoking has repeatedly been found to be strongly associated with CHD. There is an excess morbidity ratio of nearly 200 percent among smokers compared to nonsmokers, and a 70 percent increased mortality rate. Some have suggested that it is not smoking per se that results in these increased rates, but rather certain characteristics of smokers as a group which make them more prone to the disease. This hypothesis was tested in the Israel Ischemic Heart Disease population (composed of 10,000 adult Jewish males from various ethnic groups) and reported by Goldbourt and Medalie. A variety of sociodemographic, behavioral, physiological, biochemical, and genetic characteristics were compared among smokers, nonsmokers and ex-smokers. Although the authors took into consideration the methodological pitfalls of single variate analysis—the possibility of "chance" significant results—and the interrelationships among some variables, significant differences were found. More smokers were born in the Middle East (outside Israel) and Africa, had larger families (more people per room), had a low educational level, participated in little physical activity during leisure time, were nonreligious, and had blue-collar occupations. However, only small differences were found in constitutional factors such as height, weight, skinfold thickness, blood pressure, hemoglobin and hemato-

Table 8.17. International comparison of rates of first myocardial infarctions among males

Investigator	Year	Country	No. at risk	No. of MI cases	Years of obser-vation	Age range (yr)	Average annual incidence/ 1,000 pop.[a]
Djordjevic et at.	(1970)	Yugoslavia	1,545	8	5	40–59	1.1
Aravanis et al.	(1970)	Greece	1,207	10	5	40–59	1.6
Kozarević et al.	(1976)	Yugoslavia	11,034	164	7	35–62	2.1
Johnson et al.	(1968)	Japan	2,267	21	3.9 (avg.)	40–70+	2.8
Taylor et al.	(1970b)	Italy	758	9	5	40–59	3.0
Fidanza et al.	(1970)	Italy	1,695	28	5	40–59	4.4
Paul et al.	(1963)	U.S.–Chicago (W-E)	1,989	41	4.5	40–55	4.6
Zukel et al.	(1959)	U.S.–North Dakota	19,830	94	1	35–75	4.7
Medalie et al.	(1973)	Israel–IHD project (known infarcts)	9,764	257	5	40–70	5.3
Karvonen et al.	(1970)	Finland	1,620	44	5	40–59	5.7
Van Buchem	(1970)	Netherlands	864	28	5	40–59	6.0
Eisenberg et al.	(1961)	U.S.–Middlesex Co.	11,559	74	1	35–64	6.4
Taylor et al.	(1970a)	U.S.–Railway	2,454	77	5	40–59	6.5
Shapiro et al.	(1969)	U.S.–New York (HIP)	±100,000	613	3	35–64	6.6
Stamler et al.	(1960)	U.S.–Chicago	665	40	4	50–59	7.0
Morris et al.	(1969)	England–Med. Prac.	7,000	48	5	40–64	7.0
Medalie et al.	(1973)	Israel–IHD project (all infarcts)	9,764	427	5	40–70	8.7
Feinleib	(1968)	U.S.–Framingham	12,824	234	14	40–69	9.2
Rosenman et al.	(1975)	U.S.–Western Collab.	3,154	257	85	39–59	9.6
Kannel et al.	(1961)	U.S.–Framingham	1,037	62	6	45–62	10.0
Morris et al.	(1966)	England–Busmen	667	40	5	30–69	12.0

Source: Modified from J. H. Medalie et al., 1973, *J. Chronic Dis.* 26:329.

Note: Myocardial infarction = myocardial infarction and sudden death as defined in each study, except for U.S.–Chicago (W-E), which excluded sudden deaths. Some of the studies— e.g. U.S.–North Dakota—were not based on population examinations and therefore do not include "silent infarctions."

[a] These figures are taken from the studies or were calculated from them. However, owing to the ambiguity of some reports, some of the figures may be inaccurate.

crit, and cholesterol. The authors concluded that there is an overall similarity in major coronary risk factors between smokers and nonsmokers and that, therefore, "constitutional differences do not account for the increased mortality and morbidity among smokers."

An excess of blood group A and a corresponding deficit of O have been found by many investigators among CHD patients as compared to controls. In the Israel Ischemic Heart Disease population elevated MI rates were found in men with blood types A_1, B, A_1B, and Jk^{a-} (Kidd negative), and a tremendously inflated rate was

Table 8.18. Intergenerational variation in incidence
of MI, Israel, 1963–1968

Generation	Rate/1,000 pop.[a]
Immigrants	
Born in Europe	9.4
Born in Asia or Africa	7.7
All immigrants	8.7
First-generation Israeli[b]	
Fathers born in Europe	11.6
Fathers born in Asia or Africa	9.1
All first generation	10.4
Second-generation Israeli[b]	
Fathers born in Israel	7.5

Source: J. H. Medalie et al., 1973, *J. Chronic Dis.* 26:329.
Reprinted by permission of Pergamon Press, Ltd.

[a] Annual age-adjusted rates per 1,000 population.

[b] Excludes 117 patients whose fathers' birthplaces were
unknown or whose fathers were born outside Europe,
Asia, or Africa. Of these 177, 5 developed infarcts.

found among those with blood type A_1BJk^{a-} (Table 8.19). The highest mean
cholesterol level in that study occurred among men with blood types A_1 (212
mg/100 ml) and K+ (Kell positive, 212 mg/100 ml). The combination of A_1K+
further elevated the mean cholesterol level to 216.4 mg/100 ml. Consistent with
the data on the incidence of MI, Ashkenazi Jews were found to have the highest
cholesterol values, while non-Ashkenazi Jews had the lowest.

In 1969 Vlodaver and co-workers reported coronary artery findings in full-term
fetuses, infants, and children of 211 consecutive necropsy specimens from
Ashkenazi Jewish, Yemenite Jewish, and Bedouin groups. They found that the
intima and musculoelastic layers were more developed in Ashkenazi male children
than in Ashkenazi females or in Yemenite Jews or Bedouins of either sex. These
structural findings in the coronary arteries of children under 10 years of age

Table 8.19. Myocardial infarction: Incidence by combined
ABO-Kidd blood groups

Blood group	Rate/1,000 pop.[a]
A_1Jk^{a+}	47
A_1Jk^{a-}	51
A_2Jk^{a+}	37
A_2Jk^{a-}	28
A_1BJk^{a+}	45
A_1BJk^{a-}	125
A_2BJk^{a+}	31
A_2BJk^{a-}	(19)[b]
BJk^{a+}	47
BJk^{a-}	65
OJk^{a+}	41
OJk^{a-}	34

Source: J. H. Medalie et al., 1971, *N. Engl. J. Med.* 285:1348.
Reprinted, by permission.

[a] Five-year age-adjusted rates per 1,000 population.

[b] Fewer than 10 cases and fewer than 50 persons at risk.

parallel the epidemiological observations that the occurrence of CHD tends to be high among male Ashkenazi Jews and low among Yemenite Jews. If these observations were independently confirmed, they would strongly suggest an intrinsic mechanism of prime importance.

Concerning the hereditary aspects of coronary heart disease, studies have been conducted on familial aggregation of the disease, its occurrence in twins, and its association with varying genetic markers. In some cases the tendency has been to equate the genetic aspects of hypertension or hypercholesterolemia with those of coronary heart disease. It is thought that since both blood pressure and serum cholesterol are related to the incidence of CHD and are to some extent genetically determined, it should follow that familial aggregation of the disease would occur. Among male siblings it has been estimated that two-thirds of the aggregation can be accounted for by familial blood pressure and cholesterol levels. There is a definite tendency for members of the families of people with hypercholesterolemia or xanthomatosis to develop heart disease. One genetic study of MI survivors showed that 20 percent of those under 60 years of age had some form of simply inherited hyperlipidemia.

Førde and Thelle's population survey of risk factors associated with MI in Norway revealed a significantly higher risk of contracting the disease for men having first-degree relatives with MI than for healthy controls of the same age. For men below the age of 50, the relative risk was 12.8 if the subject had a female relative with MI and 5.5 if the relative was male. The small differences in cholesterol and blood pressure levels found between subjects with positive family histories of MI and those with negative histories were thought to contribute only slightly to the increased risk observed.

Using death from CHD as the endpoint, life insurance statistics collected over a 15-year period on 18,000 persons show a 75 percent increased risk among those with 2 or more cases of early cardiovascular-renal disease in their families. A two-fold increase in risk of CHD death was found in England among first-degree relatives of male cases aged 55 or below, as compared to age-matched controls in the general population. However, among 3,100 pairs of twins analyzed in Denmark, no differences in CHD death rate were found between monozygotic and dizygotic pairs, a finding which tends to diminish the role of heredity.

Proper family studies in CHD have not been carried out in the various Jewish communities in Israel or in other parts of the world. It is therefore difficult to unravel the threads of heredity and environment in this disease. In 1964 Epstein wrote on the hereditary factors in CHD:

It cannot be concluded in any way that familial factors are of relatively minor importance in the genesis of coronary heart disease. It seems more likely that the error lies in using as an index of genetic predisposition the end result, i.e. clinically manifest disease, rather than the underlying biologic disturbances in terms of metabolic or other defects. If one could identify and measure all of these predisposing traits, it would probably emerge that they are even more widespread than the prevalence of the disease would suggest and show more clear-cut distributions within kindreds. Prevention of coronary heart disease demands that the carriers of these traits be identified so that prophylactic measures can be instituted at an early age among genetically susceptible individuals.

Evidence suggests that the etiology of CHD is most probably multifactorial. However, further studies are needed to better understand the frequency of CHD among Jews as well as the interplay between heredity and environment.

References

Allan, T. M., and Dawson, A. A. 1968. ABO blood groups and ischaemic heart disease in men. *Br. Heart J.* 30:377.

Aravanis, C.; Corcondilas, A.; Dontas, A. S.; Lekos, D.; and Keys, A. 1970. The Greek islands of Crete and Corfu. In *Coronary heart disease in seven countries*, ed. A. Keys. *Circulation* 41 (suppl.): 88.

Brönte-Stewart, B.; Botha, M. C.; and Krut, L. H. 1962. ABO blood groups in relation to ischaemic heart disease. *Br. Med. J.* 1:1646.

Buzina, R.; Keys, A.; Mohacek, I.; Marinkovic, M.; Hahn, A.; and Blackburn, H. 1970. Five year follow-up in Dalmatia and Slavonia (Yugoslavia). In *Coronary heart disease in seven countries,* ed. A. Keys. *Circulation* 41 (suppl.): 40.

Dick, W.; Schneider, W.; Brockmüller, K.; et at. 1963. Interrelations of thromboembolic diseases and blood-group distribution. *Thrombas. Diathes. Haemorrh.* 9:472.

Djordjevic, B. S.; Balog, B.; Božinovic, L. J.; Josipovic, V.; Nedeljkovic, S.; Lambic, I.; Sekulic, S.; Slavkovic, V.; Stojanovic, G.; Simic, A.; Simic, B.; Strasser, T.; Blackburn, H.; and Keys, A. 1970. Three cohorts of men followed five years in Serbia. In *Coronary heart disease in seven countries*, ed. A. Keys. *Circulation* 41 (suppl.): 123.

Eisenberg, H.; Feltner, W. R.; Payne, G. H.; et al. 1961. The epidemiology of coronary heart disease in Middlesex County. *Conn. J. Chronic Dis.* 14:221.

Epstein, F. H. 1964. Hereditary aspects of coronary heart disease. *Am. Heart J.* 67:445.

Epstein, F. H.; Boas, E. P.; and Simpson, R. 1957. The epidemiology of atherosclerosis among a random sample of clothing workers of different ethnic origins in New York City. I: Prevalence of atherosclerosis and some associated characteristics. *J. Chronic Dis.* 5:300.

―――. 1957. The epidemiology of atherosclerosis among a random sample of clothing workers of different ethnic origins in New York City. II: Associations between manifest atherosclerosis, serum lipid levels, blood pressure, overweight, and some other variables. *J. Chronic Dis.* 5:329.

Feinleib, M. 1968. The Framingham Study: An epidemiological investigation of cardiovascular disease. Section 7, The National Heart Institute, The National Institutes of Health, Bethesda, Md.

Førde, O. H., and Thelle, D. S. 1977. The Tromsø heart study: Risk factors for coronary heart disease related to the occurrence of myocardial infarction in first degree relatives. *Am. J. Epidemiol.* 105:192.

Fidanza, F.; Pudda, V.; Imbimbo, B.; Menotti, A.; and Keys, A. 1970. Five-year experience in rural Italy. In *Coronary heart disease in seven countries,* ed. A. Keys. *Circulation* 41 (suppl.): 63.

Fredrickson, D. S. 1970. Atherosclerosis and other forms of arteriosclerosis. In *Harrison's principles of internal medicine*, ed. M. M. Wintrobe, G. W. Thorn, R. D. Adams, I. L. Bennett, Jr., E. Braunwald, K. J. Isselbacher, and R. G. Petersdorf, 6th ed. pp. 1239–52. New York: McGraw-Hill.

Friedberg, C. K. 1966. *Diseases of the heart*, 3rd ed. Philadelphia: W. B. Saunders.

Gertler, M. M., and White, P. D. 1954. *Coronary heart disease in young adults: A multidisciplinary study*. Cambridge, Mass.: Harvard University Press.

Goldbourt, U., and Medalie, J. H. 1975. Characteristics of smokers, nonsmokers, and ex-smokers among 10,000 adult males in Israel. I: Distribution of selected sociodemographic and behavioral variables and the prevalence of disease. *Israel J. Med. Sci.* 11:1079.

————. 1977. Characteristics of smokers, nonsmokers, and ex-smokers among 10,000 adult males in Israel. II: Physiologic biochemical, and genetic characteristics. *Am. J. Epidemiol.* 105:75.

Goldbourt, U., et al. 1978. Disappearing differences in coronary heart disease incidence between immigrants from Yemen and other Israelis: Fact or fancy? *Harefuah* 44:1.

Goldstein, J. L. 1973. Genetic aspects of hyperlipidemia in coronary heart disease. *Hosp. Pract.* 8:53.

Harvald, B., and Hauge, M. 1958. A catamnestic investigation of Danish twins. *Acta Genet. Stat. Med.* 8:287.

Hrubec, Z., and Zukel, W. J. 1974. Epidemiology of coronary heart disease among young army males of World War II. *Am. Heart J.* 87:722.

Johnson, K. G.; Yano, K.; and Kato, H. 1968. Coronary heart disease in Hiroshima, Japan: A report of a six-year period of surveillance, 1958–1964. *Am. J. Public Health* 58:1355.

Kahn, H. A.; Medalie, J. H.; Neufeld, H. N.; Riss, E.; Balogh, M.; and Groen, J. J. 1969. Serum cholesterol: Its distribution and association with dietary and other variables in a survey of 10,000 men. *Israel J. Med. Sci.* 5:1117.

Kannel, W. B.; Dawber, T. R.; Kagan, A.; Revotskie, N.; and Stokes, J., III. 1961. Factors at risk in the development of coronary heart disease—Six years of follow-up experience. *Ann. Intern. Med.* 55:33.

Karvonen, M. J.; Orma, E.; Punsar, S.; Kallio, V.; Arstita, M.; Luomanmäki, K.; and Takkunnens, J. 1970. Five year experience in Finland. In *Coronary heart disease in seven countries*, ed. A. Keys. *Circulation* 41 (suppl.) : 52.

Keys, A.; Taylor, H. L.; Blackburn, H.; Brozek, J.; Anderson, J. T.; and Simonson, F. 1963. Coronary heart disease among Minnesota business and professional men followed 15 years. *Circulation* 28:381.

Kozarević, D.; Pirc, B.; Dawber, T. R.; Gordon, S.; Zukel, W. J.; and Vojvodić, N. 1976. The Yugoslavia cardiovascular disease study—1. The incidence of coronary heart disease by area. *J. Chronic Dis.* 29:405.

Medalie, J. H.; Kahn, H. A.; Neufeld, H. N.; Riss, E.; and Goldbourt, U. 1973. Five-year myocardial infarction incidence. II: Association of single variables to age and birthplace. *J. Chronic Dis.* 26:329.

Medalie, J. H.; Kahn, H. A.; Neufeld, H. N.; Riss, E.; Goldbourt, U.; Perlstein, T.; and Oron, D. 1973. Myocardial infarction over a five-year period. I: Prevalence, incidence, and mortality experience. *J. Chronic Dis.* 26:63.

Medalie, J. H.; Kahn, H. A.; Neufeld, H. N.; Riss, E.; and Groen, J. J. 1968. *Physicians' fact book: Selected measurements on 10,000 Israeli males.* Jerusalem: Central Press.

Medalie, J. H.; Levene, C.; Papier, C.; Goldbourt, U.; Dreyfuss, F.; Oron. D.; Neufeld, H.; and Riss, E. 1971. Blood groups and serum cholesterol among 10,000 adult males. *J. Atherosclerosis Res.* 14:219.

————. 1971. Blood groups, myocardial infarction, and angina pectoris among 10,000 adult males. *N. Engl. J. Med.* 285:1348.

Morris, J. N., and Gardner, M. J. 1969. Epidemiology of ischemic heart disease. *Am. J. Med.* 46:674.

Morris, J. N.; Kagan, A.; Pattison, D. C.; Gardner, M. J.; and Raffle, P. A. B. 1966. Incidence and prediction of ischemic heart disease in London busmen. *Lancet* 2:553.

Morton, N. E. 1976. Genetic markers in atherosclerosis: A review. *J. Med. Genet.* 13:81.

Paul, O.; Lepper, M. H.; Phelan, W. H.; Dupertius, G. W.; MacMillan, A.; McKean, H.; and Park, H. 1963. A longitudinal study of coronary heart disease. *Circulation* 28:20.

Rosenman, R. H.; Brand, R. J.; Jenkins, C. D.; Friedman, M.; Straus, R.; and Wurm, M. 1975. Coronary heart disease in the Western Collaborative Group Study. *JAMA* 233:872.

Ross, D. C., and Thomas, C. B. 1965. Precursors of hypertension and coronary heart disease among healthy medical students: Discriminant function analysis. III. Using ethnic origin as the criterion, with observations on parental hypertension and coronary disease and on religion. *Bull. Johns Hopkins Hospital* 117:37.

Shapiro, S.; Weinblatt, E.; Frank, C. W.; and Sager, R. U. 1969. Incidence of coronary heart disease in a population insured for medical care (HIP): Myocardial infarction, angina pectoris, and possible myocardial infarction. *Am. J. Public Health* 59 (suppl. 6): 1.

Slack, J. 1969. Risks of ischaemic heart disease in familial hyperlipoproteinemic states. *Lancet* 2: 1380.

Stamler, J.; Lindberg, H. A.; Berkson, D. M.; et al. 1960. Prevalence and incidence of coronary heart disease in strata of the labor force of a Chicago industrial population. *J. Chronic Dis.* 11:405.

Taylor, H. L.; Blackburn, H.; Keys, A.; Parlin, W.; Vasquez, C.; and Puchners, T. 1970. Five year follow-up of employees of selected U.S. railroad companies. In *Coronary heart disease in seven countries*, ed. A. Keys. *Circulation* 41 (suppl.): 20.

Taylor, H. L.; Menotti, A.; Pudda, V.; Monti, M.; and Keys, A. 1970. Five years of follow-up of railroad men in Italy. In *Coronary heart disease in seven countries*, ed. A. Keys. *Circulation* 41 (suppl.): 113.

Toor, M.; Katchalsky, A.; Agnon, J.; and Allalouf, D. 1960. Atherosclerosis and related factors in immigrants to Israel. *Circulation* 22:265.

Van Buchem, F. S. 1970. Zutphen, a town in the Netherlands. In *Coronary heart disease in seven countries*, ed. A. Keys. *Circulation* 41 (suppl.): 76.

Vlodaver, Z.; Kahn, H. A.; and Neufeld, H. N. 1969. The coronary arteries in early life in three different ethnic groups. *Circulation* 39:541.

Zukel, W. J.; Lewis, R. H.; Enterline, P. E.; Painter, R. C.; Ralston, L. S.; Fawcett, R. M.; Meredith, B. S.; and Peterson, B. 1959. A short-term community study of the epidemiology of coronary heart disease: A preliminary report on the North Dakota study. *Am. J. Public Health* 49:1630.

Table 8.20. Cystic lung disease: Age, sex, and ethnic distribution of 88 patients at Tel Hashomer Hospital

| Ethnic origin | Age in years | | | | | | | |
| | <1 | | 1–10 | | 11–20 | | 21–30 | |
	M	F	M	F	M	F	M	F
Yemen	1				5		5	5
Iraq				1	2	1	4	4
Iran			1		1			1
Syria								
North Africa			1	1	5		1	
Miscellaneous non-Ashkenazi			1			1	3	
Sephardi			1					
Arab	1				1			2
Ashkenazi								1
Total	2	0	4	2	14	2	13	13
	2		6		16		26	

Source: I. Racz and G. L. Baum, 1965, *Am. Rev. Respir. Dis.* 91:552.

CYSTIC LUNG DISEASE

In 1953 Lichtenstein was the first to note ring shadows in the chest films of new immigrants to Israel, especially those from Yemen and Iraq. In 1954 Finkler reported similar roentgenographic changes and summarized his clinical experience with such cases. In 1965 and 1966 Baum and co-workers reported the prevalence of cystic lung disease in Israel based on a survey of 255 cases from 1952 to 1963.

Of the 255 cases, 88 patients were studied intensively at the Tel Hashomer Hospital. Table 8.20 lists the age, sex, and ethnic distribution of these patients while Table 8.21 shows the ethnic distribution of all the cases observed in Israel. Baum and co-workers are aware that their study does not fully explain the causative factors involved. Although there is a trend in the direction of familial aggregation, proper family studies have not been done to evaluate a possible genetic component. Nevertheless, much information can be gleaned from their report. Their survey clearly indicates the predominance of cystic lung disease among Oriental Jews. Of the 255 cases observed, only 22 (8.6 percent) were Ashkenazi Jews, whereas 139 (54.5 percent) were from one community of the non-Ashkenazi group, the Yemenites.

From the series of 88 patients intensively studied at Tel Hashomer Hospital a clinical picture evolved showing a difference between the Ashkenazi and non-Ashkenazi groups (Table 8.22). The former included 6 of 9 patients with predominant dyspnea, whereas in the latter group more than two-thirds of the patients demonstrated some manifestation of infection without disabling dyspnea.

Although the etiology of these cystic changes remains unknown, a congenital basis is suggested by the following clinical observations: (1) nonsymptomatic cases in young people with no history of infectious episodes; (2) a definite relationship between the disease and ethnic background; (3) pathological changes in the bronchi, vessels, and alveoli, beyond what would be expected as the sequel of infection alone; and (4) strikingly sparse parenchyma in cystic areas for no ob-

31–40		41–50		51–60		61–70		>70		Total		Combined total
M	F	M	F	M	F	M	F	M	F	M	F	
2	3	1	3	1		1				16	11	27
1	2	4		1						12	8	20
	2									2	3	5
	1									0	1	1
1	2									8	3	11
										4	1	5
		1								2	0	2
2	1				1					4	4	8
1	1		1	1		2	1	1		5	4	9
7	12	6	4	3	1	3	1	1	0	53	35	88
19		10		4		4		1		88		

Table 8.21. Cystic lung disease: Combined distribution of Israeli patients by ethnic origin

Patients observed at	Ethnic Origin				Total
	Iraqi	Yemenite	Other non-Ashkenazi	Ashkenazi	
Outpatient clinics	21	112	21	13	167
Tel Hashomer Hospital	20	27	32	9	88
Total	41	139	53	22	255

Source: I. Racz and G. L. Baum, 1965, *Am. Rev. Respir. Dis.* 91:522.

Table 8.22. Cystic lung disease: Relationship of ethnic origin to infection and dyspnea as major clinical manifestations

Ethnic origin	Infection		Dyspnea		No symptoms	
	No.	%	No.	%	No.	%
Ashkenazi	3	33.3	6	66.7		
Non-Ashkenazi	55	70.6	14	17.9	9	11.5
Yemenite	21	80.8	4	15.4	1	3.8
Iraqi	15	75.0	3	15.0	2	10.0
Sephardi						
North African	5	45.4	2	18.2	4	36.4
European	2					
Miscellaneous						
(Syrian and Persian)	7	63.6	2	18.2	2	18.2
Arab	5	62.5	3	37.5	—	—
Total and average %	58	66.7	20	22.9	9	10.4

Source: G. L. Baum et al., 1966, *Am. J. Med.* 40:578.

vious reason such as the fibrosis or collapse commonly seen in bronchiectasis. Figures 8.6–8.8 show the various clinical features of this disorder.

Baum and co-workers have pointed out that the significance of their study lies in the fact that 255 cases were uncovered in only a 12-year period in a country whose population at that time was 2.5 million, 2 million of whom were Jews. This is to be compared to a survey of the literature from 1859 to 1964 in which only 700 cases were recorded, a report that included the populations of North America and Europe and embraced any case involving cystic lung changes. In only one other instance has such an ethnic distribution been noted. In 1958 Hinds reported a fivefold greater incidence of bronchiectasis in Maori tribesmen of New Zealand as compared with the European population of the island. In at least 3 of Hinds's patients the cystic changes recorded on roentgenograms were similar to those of the Israeli patients.

Detailed family and genetic studies must be done to answer some of the important questions raised by Baum and co-workers' survey of cystic lung disease in Israel.

References

Baum, G. L.; Racz, I.; Bubis, J. J.; Molho, M.; and Shapiro, B. L. 1966. Cystic disease of the lung: Report of eighty-eight cases with an ethnologic relationship. *Am. J. Med.* 40:578.

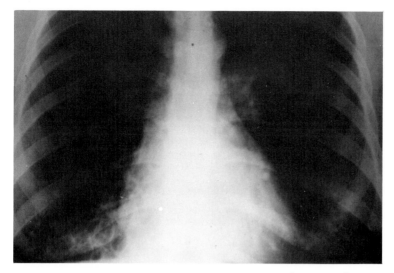

Figure 8.6. Posteroanterior chest film showing multiple-ring shadows typical of cystic lung disease. Courtesy of G. Baum, Israel.

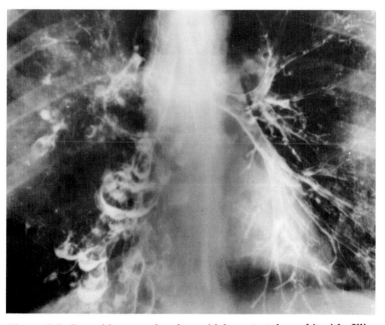

Figure 8.7. Branchiogram showing widely patent bronchi with filling of multiple cysts in the lower- and mid-lung field. Courtesy of G. Baum, Israel.

Finkler, E. 1954. Cystic disease. *Dapim Refuiim* 13:25.

Hinds, J. R. 1958. Bronchiectasis in the Maori. *N. Z. Med. J.* 57:328.

Lichtenstein, H. 1953. Congenital multiple cysts of the lung. *Dis. Chest* 24:646.

Racz, I., and Baum, G. L. 1965. The relationship of ethnic origin to the prevalence of cystic lung disease in Israel: A preliminary report. *Am. Rev. Respir. Dis.* 91:552.

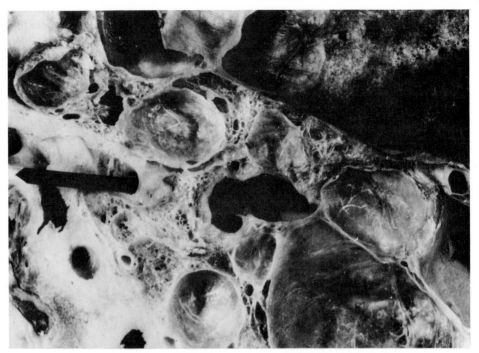

Figure 8.8. Gross slice of cystic lung area. Courtesy of G. Baum, Israel.

DIABETES MELLITUS

The first description of diabetes (from the Greek, meaning "to pass through") was written in the first century C.E. by Aretaeus of Cappadocia (Asia Minor). Because of the symptoms of parched mouth and skin, constant thirst and need to urinate, and weight loss, he envisaged the disease as "a melting down of the flesh into the urine." Centuries before Aretaeus, reference was made in the Indian Vedas to the sweet urine of diabetics.

Despite its long history and the vast amount of knowledge acquired, much remains to be learned about the etiology of diabetes mellitus and the interplay between genetic and environmental factors in this disease. Most authorities agree that the disorder is heterogeneous in nature, and this further challenges our ability to comprehend the condition.

A few introductory remarks will be made about the role of genetics in diabetes mellitus and then the discussion will center on the frequency of this disorder among the various Jewish communities.

Studies of twins and relatives of diabetics have led to the general belief that the potential for developing diabetes is hereditary. The disease occurs approximately three times more frequently among relatives of diabetics than among nondiabetic controls. Numerous reports have confirmed the familial aggregation of the disease. In Simpson's 1968 survey of Canadian diabetics the risk of first-degree relatives developing the disease was computed as an aid in genetic counseling. Simpson pointed out that although the relative risk of developing diabetes is about 22 times higher in the offspring of diabetics (compared to the general population), the absolute risk is quite low due to the rare occurrence of juvenile onset diabetes. The risk in a child whose father and mother are diabetic is estimated to be 2.9 times greater than if only one parent is diabetic. The degree of concordance among identical twins based on studies in Boston, Denmark, and the United Kingdom approached 50 percent (75 of 154 pairs). Among dissimilar twins, the concordance rate was approximately 8 percent (24 of 301 pairs). Other studies show higher concordance rates among both monozygotic and dizygotic twins. Since total concordance does not exist even among identical twins, it is thought that incomplete or variable penetrance of the diabetic trait may delay the onset of the disease in the unaffected twin. Other associated genetic factors or perhaps environmental stimuli trigger its onset in the predisposed member.

Diabetes mellitus is more common in married women over the age of 40 than in men. It is twice as common in those with 3 or more children than in the nonparous, and among single persons it is more frequent in men than in women.

Every possible mode of inheritance has been postulated in diabetes mellitus, and adherents can be found for each. Current thinking, however, favors multifactorial inheritance. According to Renold, "in its most general form this hypothesis states that there are alleles at an unspecified number of different loci which by their combined action produce a diabetic predisposition, and that the precise combination of alleles responsible for the disposition may vary from one diabetic to the next." Neel, on the other hand, thinks the main problem is the "near-impossibility of deciding whether a relatively common trait is due to a recessive gene with incomplete penetrance or to multifactorial inheritance."

New evidence suggests that susceptibility to pancreatic damage resulting from viral infections may be associated with certain histocompatibility antigens that may be linked with some genes controlling immune responses. The histocompatibility antigens HLA-B8 and BW-15 have been found in a greater percentage of juvenile diabetics than in normal subjects or in maturity-onset diabetics. In addition, the association of juvenile-onset diabetes with certain diseases known to be of autoimmune etiology suggests that an autoimmune process might also be involved in the etiology of insulin-dependent diabetes mellitus.

Islet-cell antibodies and antibodies to cultured human insulinoma cells have been identified in a significant proportion of patients with insulin-dependent diabetes. These findings provide direct evidence that autoimmune activity is involved in diabetes, although it still is not known whether this is a primary etiological factor.

It is conceivable that just as diabetes mellitus is composed of a spectrum of different phenotypes, likewise there may be a spectrum of varying genotypes—some multifactorial, some governing immune responses, and others of a varying nature.

Concerning the question of diabetes in Jews, much of the older literature published in Europe and the United States deals with the Ashkenazi community. In 1911 Fishberg wrote the following: "The testimony of many physicians who have had a large experience with this disease [diabetes mellitus] goes to show that it occurs from two to six times as frequently [in Jews] as it does among the people around them. Indeed, diabetes has been called by some German physicians, a *Judenkranheit,* a Jewish disease." Interestingly enough, Fishberg concluded with this statement: "On the whole there is no justification for considering diabetes a racial disease of the Jews. It has not been observed to be more frequent among the Jews in every country than among their non-Jewish neighbours." Unfortunately, few physicians have paid attention to Fishberg's concluding remarks, and most have chosen to think of this disorder as being quite common in the Ashkenazi Jewish community. As Sir Humphry Rolleston wrote in 1928: "The incidence of diabetes mellitus in the Hebrew race is notorious and the statistics of Joslin, Wallach, von Noorden, and Morrison, and of the records of the Metropolitan Life Assurance Company of New York support this impression. The incidence in Jews has been variously estimated as being from twice to six times as high as in other races."

Fishberg was not the only one to question the tremendous bias in ascertainment of this disease. In 1932 Sorsby and Sorsby wrote: "Most clinicians hold that it [diabetes mellitus] is undoubtedly more frequent among Jews, though a negative view is held by good authorities."

Surveys of diabetics conducted in Israel do not indicate extremely high rates of this disease among Jews. Whether or not this holds true for Jews in the Diaspora as well can be shown only through surveys outside Israel. It must be borne in mind that most studies have not been designed to answer the specific question of whether or not diabetes is more common among Jews than among non-Jews. Therefore, current comparative information from other studies is at best speculative.

In 1958–1959, in an effort to evaluate the occurrence of diabetes within the Jewish communities, A. M. Cohen compared rates of occurrence in 4 Jewish ethnic groups in Israel (based on father's place of birth). These were (1) Sephardi, (2) Ashkenazi, (3) Yemenite, and (4) Kurdish. Both the Yemenite and Kurdish groups were divided into recent ($<$ 10 years in Israel) and old settlers ($>$ 25 years in Israel). The study sample was composed of nearly 16,000 people, approximately half males and half females. Their age distribution resembled that of the general population of Israel. Rates of occurrence for these groups are listed in Table 8.23. The lowest rates were exhibited among the Yemenite newcomers (0.06 percent), followed by the Sephardi (1.0 percent). Interestingly enough, the old Yemenite settlers had the highest rate (2.9 percent), even higher than that of Ashkenazi Jews (2.5 percent). Cohen concluded that diabetes was not more prevalent among Jews in Israel than among non-Jews, although he gave no comparative figures from other studies.

Table 8.23. Prevalence of diabetes mellitus among various Jewish groups in Israel

Ethnic group	Prevalence M	(%) F	Total
Sephardi	0.8	1.1	1.0
Ashkenazi	1.7	3.0	2.5
Yemenite newcomers	0.12	0.0	0.06
Kurdish newcomers	(similar to Yemenite newcomers)		
Yemenite old settlers	4.6	0.9	2.9
Kurdish old settlers	1.0	3.2	2.0

Sources: A. M. Cohen, 1961, *Metabolism* 10:50; A. M. Cohen, 1960, *Israel J. Med. Sci.* 19:137.

In 1951, in a survey of city dwellers in Israel (Tel Aviv–Jaffa, Haifa, and Jerusalem), Zaide reported a prevalence of 0.81 percent (8.1/1,000) and concluded that "nothing confirms the opinion that the tendency of Jews to diabetes is 2–4 times higher than in other races, as often stated in various textbooks."

One of the few long-term prospective epidemiological studies on diabetes mellitus was conducted in Israel by Medalie and co-workers from 1963 to 1968 as part of a larger investigation of cardiovascular disease. The study population included 10,000 adult male government employees (aged 40 years and over) from 6 major areas of birth: Asia, North Africa, Israel, Eastern Europe, Central Europe, and Southeastern Europe. Contrary to previous studies in Israel, which had shown higher rates of diabetes among Ashkenazi Jews than among Sephardi Jews, this study revealed the opposite with regard to both incidence and prevalence, as seen in Table 8.24. The reason for this disparity may be a selection factor—i.e. because all study subjects were male government employees the sample may not have been representative of the general population; or perhaps the European workers were more "fit" in the Darwinian sense, having survived the hardships of war and persecution. Table 8.25 (from the same study) shows an interesting pattern of generational differences in diabetes mellitus among immigrants and first- and second-generation Israelis. The rate increased among Israelis of European origin from 31/1,000 in immigrants to 45/1,000 in first-generation Israelis, while it decreased in those of Asian or African origin from 51/1,000 in immigrants to 26/1,000 in first-generation Israelis. Second-generation Israelis exhibited a higher rate than either immigrant or first-generation Israelis—53/1,000. (Note that the rates are 5-year age-adjusted rates.)

In 1964, in an animal experiment, Schmidt-Nielsen and co-workers transferred sand rats from their natural desert habitat to a laboratory environment. The rats that were transferred and their first-generation offspring exhibited inappropriate hyperglycemia associated with obesity and diabetes. Subsequent generations tended to adapt to laboratory conditions and displayed mild or no hyperglycemia. In man, however, these adaptations do not occur as readily, as evidenced by the higher rate of diabetes among second-generation Israelis.

According to Neel's "thrifty genotype" hypothesis, obesity and diabetes may indicate failure to adapt to rapid changes in life style. (This hypothesis may apply to humans as well as sand rats.) For example, the Kurds and Yemenites who

Table 8.24. Prevalence and incidence of diabetes mellitus among Israelis by area of birth

Area of birth	Prevalence/ 1,000 pop.	Average annual incidence/ 1,000 pop.
Asia	57	11.2
North Africa	60	8.4
Israel	62	8.4
Southeastern Europe	42	7.0
Eastern Europe	40	5.6
Central Europe	38	5.6
Average	50	8.0

Sources: J. B. Herman et al., 1967, *Diabetes* 16:858; J. H. Medalie et al., 1974, *Israel J. Med. Sci.* 10:681.

Table 8.25. Five-year incidence of diabetes mellitus among immigrants and first- and second-generation Israeli male subjects, 1963–1968

Place of birth	No. of subjects	No. of cases	Simple rate/1,000 pop.	Age-adjusted rate/1,000 pop.
Immigrants				
Born in Europe	4,745	154	33	31
Born in Asia or Africa	3,415	163	48	51
Total no. and average rate	8,160	317	39	
First-generation Israelis				
Parents born in Europe	379	17	45	45
Parents born in Asia or Africa	307	7	23	26
Parent born elsewhere or unknown	114	4	35	32
Total no. and average rate	800	28	35	
Second-generation Israelis	534	28	52	53
Total no. and average rate for study population	9,494	373	39	40

Source: J. H. Medalie et al., 1974, *Israel J. Med. Sci.* 10:681.

came to Israel had extremely low rates of diabetes—as low as the Eskimos of Iceland and Greenland (0.3/1,000). These groups are similar in their history of community geographical isolation and little or no contact with the Western life style. However, after settlement in areas where Western habits prevail, there was a sharp rise in the prevalence of diabetes. This hypothesis may also help to explain the higher rates among Asians and Africans in the Israeli study by Medalie and co-workers.

In a multivariate analysis of their study variables, Medalie and co-workers found the following factors to be significantly associated with the incidence of diabetes: weight, presence of peripheral vascular disease, serum cholesterol level, blood pressure, uric acid level, and education (negative association). According to their data, the probability of developing diabetes increases from 17:1,000 (with none or few of these variables present) to 450:1,000 (with most or all factors present). One unusual feature of this study was that no dietary variables were found to be associated with the incidence of diabetes.

A study by T. Cohen and co-workers on the prevalence of juvenile diabetes in Israel in 1963 revealed an overall rate of 1:6,000 (0.16/1,000). As in the previous study, higher rates were found among children of Ashkenazi parents (0.24/1,000) than among children of Sephardi parents (0.09/1,000). A similar study conducted by Brand in 1950 revealed a prevalence of juvenile diabetes in Israel of 0.12/1,000. The results of a survey conducted by T. Cohen in 1968 reaffirmed this trend of increasing morbidity rates in Israeli children (see Table 8.26). However, even these rates are lower than the comparable rates for juvenile diabetes in England (1:1,200 or 0.83/1,000), in Erie County, N.Y. (1:1,750 or 0.57/1,000), and in the Philadelphia public school system (1:1,600 or 0.63/1,000).

The sex distribution in the above studies was found to be about equal in juvenile diabetics, whereas among adults, females tended to have diabetes more frequently than males. The number of consanguineous marriages among parents of diabetic

Table 8.26. Diabetes mellitus among children in Israel
in 1963 and 1968 (preliminary results)

Birthplace of father	Population size	No. of diabetics	Rate/ 100,000 pop.
1963 survey			
Europe or America	257,900	62	24
Asia or Africa	325,500	29	9
Israel	61,200	14	23
1968 survey			
Europe or America	215,000	100	46
Asia or Africa	433,000	56	13
Israel	95,000	25	26

Source: T. Cohen, 1973, *Israel J. Med. Sci.* 9:1404.

children was not excessive. A detailed study of insulin-dependent juvenile diabetics in Israel is in progress to establish whether or not there are associations with HLA determinants in both Ashkenazi and non-Ashkenazi Jews.

As noted initially, few investigators outside Israel have properly addressed themselves to the question of the prevalence of diabetes mellitus among Jews. However, considerable data show that certain ethnic groups (various American Indian tribes and certain tribes in South Africa) do have a distinctly high rate of diabetes mellitus. On the basis of available information it is not possible to place any of the Jewish communities into such a category. For a truer assessment of the prevalence of diabetes in Jews, further studies of Jewish communities outside Israel must be awaited. Such information would also be of aid in evaluating environmental factors contributing to the expression of the disease.

References

Barbosa, J. 1977. HLA and diabetes mellitus. *Lancet* 1:906.

Barrai, I., and Cann, H. M. 1965. Segregation analysis of juvenile diabetes mellitus. *J. Med. Genet.* 2:8.

Bondy, P. K. 1969. Diabetes mellitus. In *Duncan's diseases of metabolism*, ed. P. K. Bondy, 6th ed. pp. 226–67. Philadelphia: W. B. Saunders.

Brand-Auraban, A. 1956. Juvenile diabetes in Israel. *Harefuah* 50:108.

Cammidge, P. J. 1934. Heredity as a factor in the aetiology of diabetes mellitus. *Lancet* 1:393.

Cohen, A. M. 1960. Effect of change in environment on the prevalence of diabetes among Yemenite and Kurdish communities. *Israel J. Med. Sci.* 19:137.

———. 1961. Prevalence of diabetes among different ethnic Jewish groups in Israel. *Metabolism* 10:50.

Cohen, T. 1971. Juvenile diabetes in Israel. *Israel J. Med. Sci.* 12:1558.

———. 1973. Diabetes mellitus among children in Israel. *Israel J. Med. Sci.* 9:1404.

Cohen, T.; Nelken, L.; and Wolfsohn, H. 1970. Juvenile diabetes in immigrant populations in Israel. *Diabetes* 19:585.

Fishberg, M. 1911. *The Jews: A study of race and environment*. New York: Charles Scribner's.

Frank, L. L. 1957. Diabetes mellitus in the texts of old Hindu medicine (Charaka, Susruta, Vagbhata). *Am. J. Gastroenterol.* 27:76.

Garcia, M. J.; Gordon, T.; McNamara, P. M.; and Kannel, W. B. 1970. Morbidity and mortality in diabetes in a general population: Sixteen-year follow-up experience in the Framingham study. *Diabetes* 19:375.

Gazit, E.; Sartani, A.; Mizrachi, Y.; and Ravid, M. 1977. HLA antigen in Jewish patients with juvenile diabetes mellitus. *Diabete Metab.* 3:55.

Gottlieb, M. S., and Root, H. F. 1968. Diabetes mellitus in twins. *Diabetes* 17:693.

Hackell, J. M.; Lee, P. A.; and Plotnick, L. P. 1977. Current concepts in diabetes mellitus. *Johns Hopkins Med. J.* 140:331.

Harris, H. 1950. The familial distribution of diabetes mellitus: A study of the relatives of 1,241 diabetic propositi. *Ann. Eugen.* 15:95.

Harvald, B., and Hange, M. 1965. Hereditary factors elucidated by twin studies. In *Genetics and the epidemiology of chronic diseases*, ed. J. V. Need, M. W. Shaw, and W. J. Schull. U.S. Public Health Service Publication no. 1163. Washington, D. C.: Government Printing Office.

Hermann, J. B.; Mount, F. W.; Medalie, J. H.; Groen, J. J.; Dublin, T. D.; Neufeld, H. N.; and Riss, E. 1967. Diabetes prevalence and serum uric acid: Observations among 10,000 men in a survey of ischemic heart disease in Israel. *Diabetes* 16:858.

Joslin, E. P.; Root, H. F.; White, P.; and Marble, A. 1959. *The treatment of diabetes mellitus*, 10th ed. Philadelphia: Lea and Febiger.

Krikler, D. M. 1969. Diabetes in Rhodesian Sephardic Jews. *S. Afr. Med. J.* 43:931.

Lendrum, R.; Walker, G.; and Gamble, D. R. 1971. Islet-cell antibodies in juvenile diabetes mellitus of recent onset. *Lancet* 2:332.

McDonald, G. W. 1970. The epidemiology of diabetes. In *Diabetes mellitus: Theory and practice*, ed. M. Ellenberg and H. Rifkin. New York: McGraw-Hill.

MacLaren, N. K.; Huang, S. W.; and Fogh, J. 1975. Antibody to cultured human insulinoma cells in insulin-dependent diabetes. *Lancet* 1:997.

Marine, N.; Vinik, A. I.; Edelstein, I.; and Jackson, W. P. U. 1969. Diabetes, hyperglycemia, and glycosuria among Indians, Malays, and Africans (Bantu) in Cape Town, South Africa. *Diabetes* 18:840.

Medalie, J. H.; Levene, C.; Papier, C.; Goldbourt, U.; Dreyfuss, F.; Oron, D.; Neufeld, H.; and Riss, E. 1971. Blood groups, myocardial infarction, and angina pectoris among 10,000 adult males. *N. Engl. J. Med.* 285:1348.

Medalie, J. H.; Papier, C. M.; Goldbourt, U.; and Herman, J. B.; 1975. Major factors in the development of diabetes mellitus in 10,000 men. *Arch. Intern. Med.* 135:811.

Medalie, J. H.; Papier, C.; Herman, J. B.; Goldbourt, U.; Tamir, S.; Neufeld, H. N.; and Riss, E. 1974. Diabetes mellitus among 10,000 adult men. I: Five-year incidence and associated variables. *Israel J. Med. Sci.* 10:681.

Neel, J. V. 1969. Current concepts of the genetic basis of diabetes mellitus and the biological significance of the diabetic predisposition. In *Diabetes International Congress Series*, vol. 72S, p. 68. Amsterdam: Excerpta Medica Foundation.

Neel, J. V.; Fajans, S. S.; Conn, J. W.; and Davidson, R. T. 1965. Diabetes mellitus. In *Genetics and the Epidemiology of Chronic Diseases*, ed. J. V. Neel, M. W. Shaw, and W. J. Schull. U.S. Public Service Publication no. 1163. Washington, D. C.: Government Printing Office.

Nerup, J., et al. 1974. HLA antigens and diabetes mellitus. *Lancet* 2:864.

Oakley, W. G.; Pyke, D. A.; and Taylor, K. W. 1968. *Clinical diabetes and its biochemical basis*. Oxford: Blackwell Scientific Publications.

Pincus, G., and White, P. 1933. On the inheritance of diabetes mellitus. I: An analysis of 675 family histories. *Am. J. Med. Sci.* 186:1.

Post, R. H. 1962. An approach to the question, does all diabetes depend upon a single genetic locus? *Diabetes* 11:56.

Pyke, D. A.; Theophanides, C. G.; and Tattersall, R. B. 1976. Genetic origin of diabetes: Re-evaluation of twin data. *Lancet* 2:464.

Renold, A. E.; Stauffacher, W.; and Cahill, G. F., Jr. 1972. Diabetes mellitus. In *The metabolic basis of inherited disease*, ed. J. B. Stanbury, J. B. Wyngaarden, and D. S. Fredrickson, 3rd ed., pp. 83–118. New York: McGraw-Hill.

Rimoin, D. L. 1967. Genetics of diabetes mellitus. *Diabetes* 16:346.

Rimoin, D. L., and Schimke, R. N. 1971. *Genetic disorders of the endocrine glands*, pp. 151–207. St. Louis: C. V. Mosby.

Rolleston, H. 1928. Some diseases in the Jewish race. *Bull. Johns Hopkins Hospital* 43:117.

Schmidt-Nielsen, K.; Haines, H. B.; and Hackel, D. B. 1964. Diabetes mellitus in the sand rat induced by standard laboratory diets. *Science* 143:689.

Sievers, M. L. 1966. Disease patterns among Southeastern Indians. *Public Health Rep.* 81:1075.

Simpson, N. E. 1964. Multifactorial inheritance: A possible hypothesis for diabetes. *Diabetes* 13:462.

———. 1968. Diabetes in the families of diabetics. *Can. Med. Assoc. J.* 98:427.

Singel, D. P., and Blajchman, M. A. 1973. Histocompatibility (HLA) antigens, lymphocytotoxic antibodies, and tissue antibodies in patients with diabetes mellitus. *Diabetes* 22:429.

Sorsby, A., and Sorsby, M. 1932. Racial diseases of Jews. *Jewish Rev.* 1:59.

Stein, J. H.; West, K. M.; Robey, J. M.; Tirador, D. F.; and McDonald, G. W. 1965. The high prevalence of abnormal glucose tolerance in the Cherokee Indians of North Carolina. *Arch. Intern. Med.* 116:842.

Steinitz, H. 1956. The incidence of diabetes in Israel. *Harefuah* 50:106.

Sukenik, S. 1953. The incidence of diabetes among Kupat Holim members in Tel Aviv area. *Dapim Refuiim* 12:151.

Sultz, H. A.; Hart, B. A.; and Zielezny, M. 1975. Is mumps virus an etiologic factor in juvenile diabetes mellitus? *J. Pediatr.* 86:654.

Thompson, M. W., and Watson, E. M. 1952. The inheritance of diabetes mellitus: An analysis of the family history of 1,631 diabetics. *Diabetes* 1:268.

Zaide, J. 1951. The incidence of diabetes mellitus in our population. *Dapim Refuiim* 10:232.

GILLES DE LA TOURETTE SYNDROME

Historical note

Gilles de la Tourette syndrome is characterized by multiple motor tics and an irresistible compulsion to swear. It was first described by Itard in 1825. Later, at the Salpêtrière, under the tutelage of Charcot and Brissaud, George Gilles de la Tourette studied 9 cases, including Itard's original patient, and in 1885 published his account of the disease. Recently, a genetic etiology has been suggested on the basis of the finding of a family history of the disease in 10 percent of the cases reported. Numerous reports describe both parent and offspring with the disorder. In addition, it is thought that the syndrome is most common among Ashkenazi Jews.

Clinical features

The symptoms begin in childhood, usually in children between the ages of 2 and 12 years. These patients exhibit an expanding repertoire of motor tics that

include not only spasmodic grimacing but also violent, stereotyped tics such as hop-
ping, skipping, jumping, grinding of the teeth, and other sudden, spontaneous motor
outbursts requiring a certain amount of coordination. A compulsive coprolalia, in
which the patient is compelled to utter swear words or obscenities, is sometimes
accompanied by compulsive coughing, spitting, blowing, or barking sounds. There
may also be echolalia, consisting of the repetition of words or short phrases immediately after the patient has heard them. Table 8.27 shows the frequency of
initial symptoms recorded in patients from 2 recent studies. In addition, some
patients are prone to compulsive self-mutilation, with biting of the oral cavity and
extremities and head banging, while others may express inappropriate aggressive
sexual or ritualistic behavior.

Diagnosis

The diagnosis of Gilles de la Tourette syndrome is clinical and requires careful
observation over a period of time. In 1977 Golden called attention to 5 major
difficulties in diagnosing the Tourette syndrome in childhood.

1. *Confusion with transient tics of childhood.* Initially, all patients manifest a
single movement, and although a diagnosis cannot be made at this point, the child
in whom the onset of blinking of both eyes is rather acute should be observed
closely. Progression to other tics with a changing pattern would then raise the
level of diagnostic suspicion.

2. *Failure to elicit a history of inarticulate sounds.* A child often will not manifest such sounds during an examination, and the physician must rely on a directed
history in order to uncover this symptom.

3. *Misinterpretation of coughing, throat clearing, and sniffing.* These symptoms,
in the absence of other medical findings that indicate disease of the respiratory
tract, do not call for medical therapy. When they occur in a child with tics, however, the suspicion of Tourette syndrome becomes quite strong.

4. *Reluctance to make the diagnosis in the absence of coprolalia and/or
echolalia.* Coprolalia occurred in approximately 50 percent of a series of 34 patients
and in Tourette's own cases; echolalia occurred even less frequently. These
symptoms may be present only transiently and can disappear spontaneously.

5. *Psychiatric referral without strong evidence for a personality or behavioral
disorder.* In many patients referral to a psychiatrist is made only on the basis of
the presence of tics, and such children are otherwise happy, stable, and well
adjusted. In others there are interpersonal or family problems that make this referral appropriate. The physician should continue to follow the motor symptoms in
children suspected of having the disorder.

Table 8.27. Tourette syndrome: Initial symptoms

Study	No. of cases	Motor tics		Sound(s)		Multiple	
		No.	%	No.	%	No.	%
Shapiro (1975)	145	63	43	11	8	71	49
Eldridge (1977)	21	11	52	6	29	4	19

Source: R. Eldridge et al., 1977, *Neurology* 27:115. Reprinted by permission of Raven Press,
New York.

Laboratory studies presently are not helpful in the diagnosis of Tourette syndrome.

Basic defect

The basic defect in Tourette syndrome is not known. Major investigative studies have been directed toward 2 areas. It was originally thought that these patients have an abnormality in the peripheral metabolism of dopamine beta-hydroxylase or norepinephrine. However, recent studies have not supported this contention, despite the fact that some patients show improvement of symptoms while taking the drug haloperidol (a substance known to block the postsynaptic receptor for dopamine).

The second area of investigation is concerned with a possible alteration in purine metabolism. In 1977 Van Woert and co-workers noted a decreased stability of the enzyme hypoxanthine-guanine phosphoribosyltransferase (HGPRTase) in several patients and in the parents of 1 affected child. Furthermore, upon isoelectric focusing of this enzyme they observed an abnormal pattern in their patients. Other investigators have not been able to document the instability of HGPRTase and its abnormal pattern upon isoelectric focusing in these patients.

From a histopathological viewpoint, no consistent change has been noted in the central nervous system or other tissues in the few cases that have been studied at autopsy.

Although in 1974 Merskey reported a patient with Tourette syndrome having a XYY karyotype, no chromosomal abnormality is known to be associated with this disorder.

Genetics

In 1945 Mahler and co-workers were among the first to suggest that Ashkenazi Jews are especially prone to this disorder. Several reports published since then (mainly from the New York City area) stress the high frequency of this condition among Jews. The overall average of Jews among these patients is 50 percent. Of 53 families from Toronto, Minneapolis, and Washington, D.C., 15 percent were of Ashkenazi Jewish ancestry.

Eldridge and co-workers looked for geographical clustering of the origins of 49 Jewish grandparents in 13 families but noted no special pattern (Figure 8.9). It would be worthwhile to have more data of this kind before drawing conclusions on the question of clustering.

In 1973 Abuzzahab and Anderson reviewed the geographical distribution of 485 cases of Tourette syndrome and found that most were from the U.S., France, Germany, and the United Kingdom. Their report did not mention Jewish ethnic origin. Scattered reports have also come from other countries in Europe and from Israel and Japan. Tourette syndrome seems to be rare among black Americans.

The genetic factors in Tourette syndrome are not well understood, although familial aggregation has long been recognized. Furthermore, inaccuracy in diagnosis has made the evaluation of family studies difficult. In support of a genetic etiology concordance has been observed in 3 of 4 pairs of monozygotic twins. Autosomal dominant, recessive, X-linked recessive, and multifactorial inheritance have all been postulated for this syndrome. Several cases of an affected father and son exclude X-linked transmission. Vertical transmission has been observed in many families, but penetrance is markedly reduced, and this raises doubts as to the possibility of autosomal dominant inheritance. On the basis of their family studies, Eldridge and co-workers favor autosomal recessive inheritance. Their explanation of the preponderance of affected males is that symptoms are more likely to remit in females. Consanguinity has not been noted among any of the Jewish families with this disorder.

The precise mode of inheritance of Tourette syndrome and its frequency among Ashkenazi Jews await clarification. Genetic heterogeneity may play a role in this syndrome.

Prognosis and treatment

Until recently no effective treatment of Tourette syndrome was known and the prognosis was poor in most cases. Many patients have had to be institutionalized

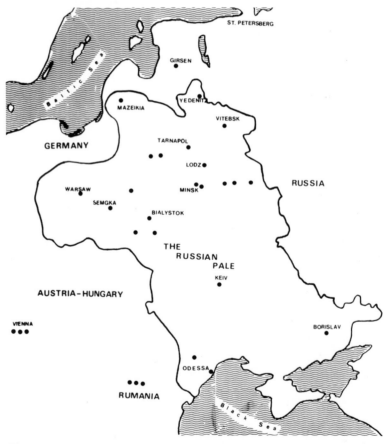

Figure 8.9. European origins of 49 Jewish grandparents in 13 families. No geographical clustering is noted. Courtesy of R. Eldridge, Bethesda, Maryland.

Table 8.28. Tourette syndrome: Response of patients to haloperidol

Study	Total no. of patients	Improved[a]		No change or discontinued		Worse or with serious side effects	
		No.	%	No.	%	No.	%
Moldofsky (1974)	15	6	40.0	5	33.3	4	26.6
Shapiro (1975)	65	57	87.7	8	12.3		—[b]
Eldridge (1977)	20	11	55.0	2	10.0	7	35.0

Source: R. Eldridge et al., 1977, *Neurology* 27:115. Reprinted by permission of Raven Press, New York.

Note: More than half the patients were on other medication as well.

[a] Fifty percent decrease in symptoms.

[b] Included in "discontinued."

or live as recluses. Recently, however, the tranquilizer haloperidol, a butyrophenone derivative, has been reported to be effective in several cases (Table 8.28). Moreover, pimozide, which has a more specific antidopaminagic activity than haloperidol, has been used in this disorder and seems to effectively reduce the number of tics in patients. Pimozide causes fewer side effects than haloperidol. Sedatives, antidepressants, central nervous system stimulants, anticonvulsants, and antiparkinsonian drugs have rarely provided any immediate or sustained therapeutic benefit.

Various neurosurgical procedures have been tried in the treatment of Tourette syndrome, but the results generally have not greatly improved the patient's condition.

Some physicians believe that the above treatments do not alter the eventual outcome of the disease. Some patients are troubled by symptoms all their lives, while others have a spontaneous remission.

References

Abuzzahab, F. S., and Anderson, F. O. 1973. Gilles de la Tourette's syndrome. *Minn. Med.* 56:492.

———. 1974. Gilles de la Tourette's syndrome: Cross-cultural analysis and treatment outcomes. *Clin. Neurol. Neurosurg.* 1:66.

Eldridge, R.; Sweet, R.; Lake, C. R.; Ziegler, M.; and Shapiro, A. K. 1977. Gilles de la Tourette syndrome: Clinical, genetic, psychological, and biochemical aspects in 21 selected families. *Neurology* 27:115.

Eldridge, R.; Wasserman, E. R.; Nee, L.; and Koerber, T. 1979. Gilles de la Tourette syndrome. In *Genetic diseases in Ashkenazi Jews*, ed. R. M. Goodman and A. G. Motulsky. New York: Raven Press, forthcoming.

Fernando, S. J. M. 1967. Gilles de la Tourette's syndrome: A report on four cases and a review of published case reports. *Br. J. Psychiatry* 113:607.

Friel, P. B. 1973. Familial incidence of Gilles de la Tourette's disease, with observations on aetiology and treatment. *Br. J. Psychiatry* 122:655.

Gilles de la Tourette, G. 1885. Étude sur une affection nerveuse caractérisée par l'incoordination motrice accompagnée d'écholalie et de coprolalie. *Arch. Neurol.* 9:158.

Golden, G. S. 1977. The effect of central nervous system stimulants on Tourette syndrome. *Ann. Neurol.* 2(1):69.

————. 1977. Tourette syndrome: The pediatric perspective. *Am. J. Dis. Child.* 131:531.

Itard, J. M. G. 1825. Mémoire sur quelques fonctions involontaires des appareils de la locomotion, de la préhension, et de la voix. *Arch. Gén. Méd.* 8:385.

Mahler, M. S.; Luke, J. A.; and Daltroff, W. 1945. Clinical and follow-up study of the tic syndrome in children. *Am. J. Orthopsychiatry* 15:631.

Merskey, H. 1974. A case of multiple tics with vocalization (partial syndrome of Gilles de la Tourette) and XYY karyotype. *Br. J. Psychiatry* 125:593.

Moldofsky, H.; Tullis, C.; and Lamon, R. 1974. Multiple tic syndrome (Gilles de la Tourette's syndrome): Clinical, biological, and psychological variables and their influence with haloperidol. *J. Nerv. Ment. Dis.* 15:282.

Rose, M. S., and Moldofsky, H. 1977. Comparison of pimozide with haloperidol in Gilles de la Tourette syndrome. *Lancet* 1:103.

Sanders, D. G. 1973. Familial occurrence of Gilles de la Tourette syndrome. *Arch. Gen. Psychiatry* 28:326.

Shapiro, A. K.; Shapiro, E.; and Wayne, H. L. 1973. The symptomatology and diagnosis of Gilles de la Tourette's syndrome. *J. Am. Acad. Child Psychiatry* 12:702.

————. 1973. Treatment of Gilles de la Tourette's syndrome with haloperidol: Review of 34 cases. *Arch. Gen. Psychiatry* 28:92.

Shapiro, A. K.; Shapiro, E.; Wayne, H. L.; and Clarlsen, J. 1972. The psychopathology of Gilles de la Tourette's syndrome. *Am. J. Psychiatry* 129:427.

Van Woert, M. H.; Yip, L. C.; and Balis, M. E. 1977. Purine phosphoribosyltransferase in Gilles de la Tourette syndrome. *N. Engl. J. Med.* 296:210.

MULTIPLE SCLEROSIS

Multiple sclerosis (MS) is one of the most common chronic neurological diseases in man. The term *multiple sclerosis* was coined 80 years ago by neuropathologists but it gives no inkling that the myelin sheath bears the brunt of the disease. The term was used to describe the disease's end-stage lesions, which are characterized by scarring or sclerosis resulting from glial overgrowth in the areas involved.

Classical features of the disorder include visual impairment, nystagmus, dysarthria, intention tremor, ataxia, impairment of perception of position and vibratory senses, bladder dysfunction, paraplegia, and alteration in emotional responses.

At present no absolutely reliable or completely pathognomonic laboratory examination exists for this disease. The determination of cerebrospinal fluid IgG (absolute value elevated in 74 percent of the cases) by electroimmunodiffusion, coupled with the family history and clinical findings, appears to be the most valuable diagnostic aid. For a detailed discussion of the clinical, therapeutic, and pathological features of this disease the reader is referred to any standard textbook of neurology.

In the early 1960s Alter and co-workers began to publish their findings from a survey of the Israeli Jewish population conducted from 1955 through 1959. Given the fact that the prevalence of MS decreases from a high rate in temperate latitudes to low rates in latitudes near the equator, Israel, with immigrants from over 100 countries (including regions of high and low prevalence of MS), presented an ideal testing ground for further assessment of this geographical factor. Alter's group found 282 patients with MS, 208 of whom were of European origin (Ashkenazim) and 61 of whom were of Afro-Asian origin (Sephardim and

Oriental Jews); this number also included 25 native Israelis. The prevalence of MS was more than 6 times higher among the Ashkenazim than among the Sephardim and Oriental Jews (Table 8.29).

The overall prevalence of MS in Israel was 15/100,000 population. Table 8.30 shows the prevalence in each national group in which cases of MS were identified. Among immigrants from countries in northern and central Europe the prevalence was high (30–51/100,000 population), while among those from southern Europe it was lower (9–18/100,000) and among those from North Africa lower still (6/100,000). The prevalence of MS among native Israelis was 4/100,000 population. Among immigrants from Yemen the rate was 3/100,000, the lowest rate among immigrant groups.

Since the rates for the countries reported in this study were derived from immigrant populations, it was important to determine whether or not the immigrants were representative of their countries of origin insofar as the prevalence of this disease is concerned. Indeed, the high prevalence observed among immigrants from northern European countries is very similar to rates reported from these countries. Unfortunately, there are few data from the African and Asian countries with which to compare the prevalence observed among immigrants from these areas. In U.S. communities at latitudes similar to those of these African and Asian countries (30°N–35°N), the prevalence of MS is low (6–18/100,000), similar to that found among Asian and African immigrants in Israel.

Despite the difference in prevalence, the clinical features of MS were remarkably similar in the European and Afro-Asian groups. No significant differences could be discerned in presenting symptoms, course of illness, exacerbation rate, and disability. The apparent earlier age of onset of MS among Afro-Asians was attributed to the fact that the mean age of Afro-Asians in the general Israeli population is lower than that of the Europeans. Duration of residence in the European environment ("exposure") did not influence the age of onset or subsequent disability.

Table 8.29. Multiple sclerosis: Age-specific prevalence among Israelis by area of origin, 1960

	Area of origin					
	Europe (Ashkenazim)			Afro-Asia (Sephardim and Oriental Jews)		
Age group (yr)	No. of patients	No. in general pop.	Rate/ 100,000 pop.	No. of patients	No. in general pop.	Rate/ 100,000 pop.
<20	0	71,641	—	8	708,603	1.1
20–29	15	69,805	21.5	23	194,806	11.8
30–39	43	134,480	32.0	10	120,344	8.3
40–49	68	158,636	42.9	11	70,641	15.6
50–59	64	130,910	58.9	8	55,025	14.5
60–69	13	64,938	20.0	—	28,533	—
70–79	3	34,171	8.8	1	16,308	6.1
Unknown	2	—	—	0	—	—
Total no. and average rate	208	664,581	31.3	61	1,194,260	5.1

Source: M. Alter et al., 1964, *J. Neurol. Neurosurg. Psychiatry* 27:522.

Table 8.30. Multiple sclerosis: Prevalence among national groups in Israel, 1958

Area and country of origin	Size of national group	Mean latitude (°N)	Accepted cases			Prevalence/ 100,000 pop. based on probable and possible cases
			Probable	Possible	Total	
Central Europe						
Germany-Austria	53,000	50	20	7	27	51
Hungary	31,000	47	7	7	14	45
Northeastern Europe						
Czechoslovakia	30,000	50	11	2	13	43
Romania	149,000	46	25	21	46	31
Russo-Poland	310,000	52	68	26	94	30
Northwestern Europe and South America						
France	⎫	47	3	—		
Holland	⎬ 20,000	52	1	—	6	30
England	⎪	54	—	1		
Argentina	⎭	35[a]	—	1		
Southeast Europe						
Greece	11,000	40	1	1	2	18
Yugoslavia	9,000	44	—	1	1	11
Bulgaria	43,000	43	4	—	4	9
Italy	—	41	1	—	1	—
Eastern Mediterranean						
Turkey	41,000	40	2	1	3	7
Iraq	130,000	34	4	5	9	7
Iran	31,000	33	—	2	2	7
Lebanon	—	34	2	1	3	—
Syria	—	35	2	—	2	—
North Africa						
Egypt	⎫		2	1		
Morocco	⎪ 226,000	31	3	—	14	6
Tunisia	⎬		2	1		
Libya	⎪		2	2		
Algeria	⎭		1	—		
Far East (China)	—	—	1	—	1	—
Israel	588,000	32	22	3	25	4
Arabian peninsula (Yemen, Aden)	63,000	14	1	1	2	3
Unknown	—	—	8	5	13	—
Total no. and average rate	1,735,000		193	89	282	15

Source: M. Alter et al., 1962, *Arch. Neurol.* 7:253. Copyright 1962, American Medical Association.

[a] °S.

What is known about the genetic factors involved in MS? Reports that certain HLA determinants are more common in MS than in controls has created much interest, since MS has been considered by many to have an immune basis. Several studies have shown that HLA-A3 and HLA-B7 loci are increased in MS and that the Dw2 locus is particularly common compared to the non-MS population. In 1977 Brautbar and co-workers showed that HLA-A3 and HLA-B7 were actually less common in Jews with MS than in matched controls, while Bw 40 loci were increased. This study and studies of Japanese MS patients refute the concept that HLA-A3 and HLA-B7 are universal markers of MS susceptibility.

The familial occurrence of MS is increasing. McAlpine concluded that the risk for a first-degree relative of a patient with MS is at least 15 times that for a member of the general population. However, the concordance rate in monozygotic twins is so low that it is difficult to conclude that genetic factors are of great importance in this disease.

In the survey conducted by Alter's group in Israel, genetic factors were investigated among the patients interviewed. No familial aggregation of MS was found. The rate of consanguinity among the parents of patients was found to be 2–3 times higher than that reported for the general population. Consanguineous marriages were noted in 3 percent of the immigrants from Europe and in 14 percent of those from Afro-Asian countries. However, among European immigrants with MS, 10 percent reported that their parents were related, while among parents of Afro-Asian patients the rate of consanguinity was 22 percent. Although Alter and co-workers suggest that this may indicate recessive transmission, there is very little in the literature to support this hypothesis. In actuality the rates quoted are not much higher than the rates estimated for that period (1955–1959), with the exception of the 10 percent consanguinity noted among the parents of affected European immigrants.

It has been suggested that the increased familial incidence of MS reflects common exposure to a similar environmental factor. One such factor could be a viral agent; in fact, antibody to measles has been shown to be higher in MS patients than in controls. Thus it has been postulated that MS may be a delayed host response to childhood infections.

In conclusion, the occurrence of MS in Jews, as in other ethnic groups, seems to correlate with the latitude of the country of origin of the various Jewish communities. Jews (mainly Ashkenazim) who have resided in a temperate climate have a far greater chance of contracting MS than those living in tropical or subtropical regions. In contrast to studies of other populations, no correlation was found between age at onset of the disease and latitude of country of origin. As expected, Ashkenazi Jews born in Israel showed a low prevalence of MS because of the latitude of their country of birth.

References

Alter, M. 1976. Is multiple sclerosis an age-dependent host response to measles? *Lancet* 1:456.
Alter, M., and Cendrowski, W. 1976. Multiple sclerosis and childhood infections. *Neurology* 26:201.
Alter, M.; Halpern, L.; Kurland, L. T.; Bornstein, B.; Leibowitz, U.; and Siberstein, J. 1962. Multiple sclerosis in Israel: Prevalence among immigrants and native inhabitants. *Arch. Neurol.* 7:253.
Alter, M.; Leibowitz, U.; and Halpern, L. 1964. Clinical studies of multiple sclerosis in Israel. 2: A comparison between European and Afro-Asian patients. *J. Neurol. Neurosurg. Psychiatry* 27:522.
Bornstein, M. B. 1973. The immunopathology of demyelinative disorders examined in organotypic cultures of mammalian central nerve tissues. In *Progress in neuropathology*, ed. G. H. M. Zimmerman, 2: 69–90. New York: Grune and Stratton.
Brain, L., and Walton, J. N. 1969. *Brain's diseases of the nervous system*, 7th ed., pp. 494–507. London: Oxford University Press.
Brautbar, C.; Cohen, I.; Kahana, E.; Alter, M.; Jørgensen, F.; and Lamm, L. 1977. Histocompatibility determinants in Israeli Jewish patients with multiple sclerosis. *Tissue Antigens* 10:291.

Leibowitz, U.; Halpern, L.; and Alter, M. 1967. Clinical studies of multiple sclerosis in Israel. 5: Progressive spinal syndromes and multiple sclerosis. *Neurology* 17:988.

Leibowitz, U.; Kahana, E.; and Alter, M. 1969. Multiple sclerosis in immigrant and native populations of Israel. *Lancet* 2:1323.

Merritt, H. A. 1973. *A textbook of neurology*, 5th ed. pp. 684–705. Philadelphia: Lea and Febiger.

Saito, S.; Naito, S.; Kawanami, S.; and Kuroiwa, Y. 1976. *Neurology* 26 (suppl.) : 49.

Tabira, T.; Webster, H. de F.; and Wray, S. H. 1976. Multiple sclerosis CSF produces myelin lesions in tadpole optic nerves. *N. Engl. J. Med.* 295:644.

NEOPLASTIC DISEASES

The interplay between environment and heredity is a crucial factor in the pathogenesis of a number of neoplastic diseases. Epidemiologists have long been trying to evaluate the role of each in the various forms of neoplasia. Through the years a number of clinical impressions (some well founded, others not) have come into being with regard to the incidence of certain neoplastic diseases among Jews. For the most part these impressions have pertained to the Ashkenazi Jewish community, for little was known about neoplastic disorders in the other Jewish ethnic groups. One such impression is that carcinoma of the cervix is rare among Jewish women and that carcinoma of the penis is infrequent among Jewish men.

The low incidence of these lesions has often been attributed to various Jewish religious customs and practices, but is that assumption correct? Other questions that need to be answered are: What is the incidence of neoplasia in the Sephardi and Oriental Jewish communities? How do the rates of specific neoplastic disorders in Israel (among the Jewish population) compare with those in other parts of the world (among the non-Jewish population)? The amount of data available is voluminous. In an attempt to present the reader with an intelligible frame of reference, I have turned primarily to the studies of Modan and co-workers in Israel and will discuss the subject from two vantage points: (1) the similarities and differences between the incidence of selected cancers among the Jewish population in Israel and among the white and black populations of the United States; and (2) comments on the relatively high-risk cancer sites among the various Jewish ethnic groups in Israel.

When Modan compared the incidence of various neoplasias in Israeli Jews of European (Ashkenazi), Asian (Oriental), and North African (Sephardi) origin with those observed in the white and black populations of the U.S. he noted a number of similarities: (1) there was a relatively higher incidence of most cancers in European-born Israelis and white Americans; (2) the pattern of occurrence of cancer of the corpus uteri, ovary, and breast was similar in Israel and the U.S., in contrast with that of uterine cervix cancer; (3) the ratio of incidence between European- and non-European-born Israelis and between U.S. whites and blacks was highest for cancer of the colon and rectum, intermediate for gastric cancer, and lowest for esophageal cancer, suggesting the operation of different etiological agents at each site; (4) the incidence of cancer of the thyroid was similar in the main ethnic groups in Israel and in black and white Americans; (5) there was a smaller spread in the sex ratio for cancer of the colon and rectum among non-European-born Israelis and black Americans; (6) both populations showed minimal interethnic differences in childhood for all tumor categories combined; (7) with time, the incidence of cancer among immigrants changed and tended to approach that in the native population. This last finding was most evident for gastric cancer, but Israeli data on leukemia and melanoma also provide supportive evidence.

The similarity in interethnic patterns for 4 cancer sites (brain, breast, colon and rectum, and thyroid) is shown in Figures 8.10–8.13. Modan attributes this striking parallelism in the patterns seen in white and black groups in the U.S. with the patterns seen in European-, Asian-, and North African-born Jews living in Israel to interethnic differences in socioeconomic status. Since the Israeli groups do not share a common genetic background with the American ethnic subgroups, such a postulate supports previous observations on the role of environmental factors in carcinogenesis.

Table 8.31 lists the relatively high-risk cancer sites in foreign-born Israeli Jews by major ethnic origin and sex. A few comments about some of these neoplastic disorders follow.

Nasopharyngeal cancer

Nasopharyngeal cancer is a relatively rare disease with a distinct population distribution. Various studies have demonstrated a high incidence among Chinese in diverse geographical locations. Other clusters have been reported in Southeast Asia, East Africa (Kenya) and North Africa (mainly Tunisia).

In 1978 Turgman and co-workers reported a nationwide study of this cancer

Table 8.31. Relatively high-risk cancer sites in foreign-born Israeli Jews by major ethnic origin and sex

High-risk cancer sites in European- and American-born Israeli Jews		High-risk cancer sites in Asian- and African-born Israeli Jews	
Males	Females	Males	Females
Lip	Lip	Nasopharynx	Nasopharynx
Salivary gland	Tongue	Liver	Mouth
Stomach	Salivary gland		Larynx
Small intestine	Stomach		Cervix
Colon	Colon		
Rectum	Rectum		
Pancreas	Gallbladder		
Breast	Pancreas		
Testis	Lung		
Kidney	Breast		
Melanoma	Corpus uteri		
Brain	Ovary		
Leukemia	Kidney		
	Melanoma		
	Eye		
	Brain		

Source: B. Modan et al., 1975, *Cancer Res.* 35:3503.

Note: Data are based on studies referred to in the text and data of the Israel Central Cancer Registry. Site has been considered high risk if age-adjusted rate was at least 50 percent higher than unadjusted rate (world population used for standardization).

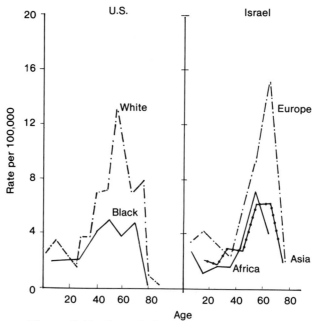

Figure 8.10. Interethnic comparison of mean annual incidence of malignant brain neoplasms in Israel and the United States. From B. Modan, 1974, *Israel J. Med. Sci.* 10:1112.

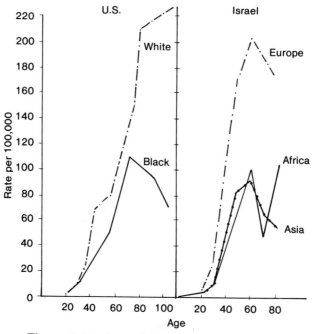

Figure 8.11. Interethnic comparison of mean annual incidence of breast cancer in Israel and the United States. From B. Modan, 1974, *Israel J. Med. Sci.* 10:1112.

in Israel during a nine year period (1960–1968). They found 150 cases, or a mean annual incidence of 1.0/100,000 in males and 0.4/100,000 in females. A significantly higher incidence was observed in North African–born residents (3.0/100,000 in males and 1.1/100,000 in females). The chances of survival were relatively better in females with lymphoepithelioma and in cases without neurological complications. Turgman and co-workers concluded that their findings support a possible environmental cause, although a genetic etiology cannot be ruled

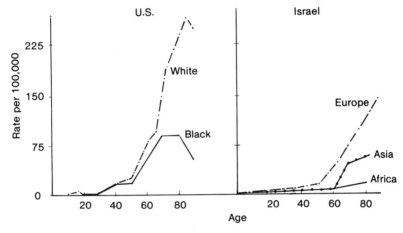

Figure 8.12. Interethnic comparison of mean annual incidence of cancer of the colon and rectum in Israel and the United States. From B. Modan, 1974, *Israel J. Med. Sci.* 10:1112.

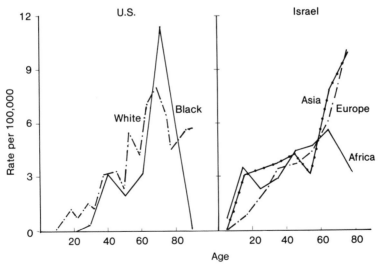

Figure 8.13. Interethnic comparison of mean annual incidence of cancer of the thyroid in Israel and the United States. From B. Modan, 1974, *Israel J. Med. Sci.* 10:1112.

out. Viral agents such as the Epstein-Barr virus have been postulated as a possible etiological factor. In 1971 Nevo and co-workers' report on this disease in dizygotic twins of Jewish Moroccan ancestry suggested that heredity may play a role.

Esophageal cancer

Between 1960 and 1966 the mean annual incidence of esophageal cancer in Israel was 2.3/100,000, with a male:female ratio of 1.6:1. The incidence was highest among the Asian-born segment of the population below 60 years of age. The majority of these patients originated from Iran and Turkey and to a lesser extent from Yemen. The most frequent localization of this cancer was the middle third of the esophagus, followed by the lower third. More than two-thirds of the patients were considered unsuitable for surgery. The overall rate of survival for 5 years was 5.8 percent.

Stomach cancer

Between 1961 and 1963 cancer of the stomach was diagnosed in 1,172 Jewish and 33 Arab patients in Israel, yielding an incidence rate of 23.4/1,000 in males and 15.0/1,000 in females. The incidence was significantly high in residents of European extraction, with a Europe:Africa age-adjusted ratio of 1.3:1 and a Europe:Asia ratio of 1.8:1. In all population groups the incidence of this cancer was significantly higher in new immigrants than in veteran immigrants. A higher proportion of "definite" cases (diagnosed on a histopathological basis), relative to "probable" cases (diagnosed clinically), was observed in males than in females, in younger than in older age groups, and in immigrants coming from Europe than in those coming from Asia and Africa.

Cancer of the colon and rectum

Between 1961 and 1965 the mean annual incidence of cancer of the colon and rectum in Israel was 15.4/100,000 (14.8/100,000 among males and 16.0/100,000 among females). The specific incidence for cancer of the colon was 9.0/100,000 and for cancer of the rectum 6.2/100,000. (In the remaining 0.2/100,000 the exact anatomical location was unclear.) The incidence of both cancer of the colon and cancer of the rectum was significantly higher among European-born patients than among those born in Asia and Africa. The European:Oriental ratio was considerably higher for these sites than for most other cancer sites. The incidence among Israeli-born patients was intermediate—close to the European-born group among males and to the non-European-born among females. This difference stemmed in part from a relatively higher incidence among Asian- and African-born females than among the respective male groups. The incidence of these cancers appeared to be higher in the urban, as compared to the rural, population.

Cancer of the cervix and endometrium

Between 1961 and 1965 the mean annual incidences of cervical and endometrial cancer were 4.7/100,000 and 6.5/100,000. Contrasting patterns of these disease entities were noted. Cervical cancer appeared most frequently in the younger age groups and was most prevalent among North African–born and married women, while the risk for endometrial cancer was higher in the older age groups among European-born and single women. A parallelism between the differential ethnic and marital incidence of endometrial and breast cancer was observed. These patterns emphasize a correlation with socioeconomic status and fertility, and point toward environmental etiological factors. Future elimination of interethnic differences in Israel would probably lead to a decrease in the incidence of cervical cancer and an increased incidence of endometrial cancer.

Additional comments on cervical cancer are warranted because this disease has traditionally been thought to have a low rate of occurrence among all Jewish women due to the circumcision of Jewish males. On the basis of the following observations this causal relationship is now considered to be a myth: (1) carcinoma of the cervix is common in other circumcized populations, such as the Turks, Iranians, and Israeli Arabs; (2) case control studies have not proved the existence of such a relationship; (3) the validity of information on circumcision obtained in case control studies is far from accurate; and (4) early reports were based on findings among Ashkenazi women from the United States and the United Kingdom, whereas the disease is known to be relatively common in Moroccan-born Jews.

Despite the high frequency of cervical cancer in Jewish women of Moroccan ancestry, the incidence of this disease is still low in the majority of Jewish women. Why? Current evidence suggests that this form of neoplasia is due to a sexually transmitted agent—probably a herpes 2 virus. Thus, it is conceivable that this virus has been rare in most Jewish communities. With changes in sexual attitudes, coupled with migration and intermarriage both in Israel and in the Diaspora, one would expect enhanced propagation of the virus, resulting in an increased incidence of this disease among Jewish women from various communities. This increased incidence is already being seen among Israeli-born women. At the same time, these changes have led to a decreased incidence in African-born Jewish women.

Brain cancer

Between 1960 and 1964 the mean annual incidence of brain tumors among Jews in Israel was 4.4/100,000 for malignant tumors, with a male:female ratio of 1.4:1, and 2.4/100,000 for benign tumors, with a male:female ratio of 0.6:1. The incidence among the Arab segment of the population was considerably lower, probably due to underdiagnosis. The incidence of malignant tumors was significantly higher among European- and Israeli-born residents than among both the Asian- and African-born. Similar differences were noted with regard to benign tumors, but these were of only borderline significance. Glioblastoma multiform constituted 40 percent of all malignant tumors, increasing from 11 percent in children to 58 percent in older patients. Medulloblastoma and astrocytoma were the dominant tumors in children. Meningioma constituted 72 percent of all benign tumors and close to 24 percent of all tumors combined.

Leukemia

In 1961 Modan's group reported a survey of 718 leukemia deaths registered during the years 1950–1958 and of a series of 150 leukemia patients observed consecutively in one hospital.

The mortality rate for leukemia rose during this period from 3.9/100,000 to 6.1/100,000. An increase occurred in all age groups and in different ethnic groups. The increase was most marked in immigrants from Afro-Asian countries below the age of 15. A causal link between this increase and exposure to X-ray is suggested.

The hospital series suggests a possible causal relationship between certain drugs and cases of leukemia.

To sum up: (1) European-born (Ashkenazi) Jews share a similar incidence of certain forms of neoplasia with the white population of the U.S., while Asian- and North African–born (Oriental and Sephardi) Jews share a similar incidence of certain forms of neoplasia with the black population of the U.S. (2) Distinct incidences and predispositions for various types of neoplasia characterize the different Jewish ethnic groups. (3) Findings from various epidemiological studies among the Jewish population of Israel stress environmental factors more than genetic considerations as causative agents in neoplasia.

References.

Aurelian, L.; Strandberg, J. D.; Melendez, L. V.; et al. 1971. Herpes virus 2 isolated from cervical tumor cells grown in tissue culture. *Science* 174:704.

Cohen, A., and Modan, B. 1968. Some epidemiologic aspects of neoplastic diseases in Israeli immigrant population. III: Brain tumors. *Cancer* 22:1323.

Davies, A. M.; Modan, B.; Djaldetti, M.; and de Vries, A. 1961. Epidemiological observations on leukemia in Israel. *Arch. Intern. Med.* 108:86.

Lilienfeld, A. M., and Graham, S. 1958. Validity of determining circumcision status by questionnaire as related to epidemiological studies of cancer of the cervix. *J. Natl. Cancer Inst.* 21:713.

Modan, B. 1974. Role of ethnic background in cancer development. *Israel J. Med. Sci.* 10:1112.

Modan, B.; Barell, V.; Lubin, F.; and Modan, M. 1975. Dietary factors and cancer in Israel. *Cancer Res.* 35:3503.

Modan, B.; Barell, V.; Lubin, F.; Modan, M.; Greenberg, R. A., and Graham, S. 1975. Low fiber intake as an etiological factor in cancer of the colon. *J. Natl. Cancer Inst.* 55:15.

Modan, B.; Eisenstein, Z.; and Virag, I. 1969. Thyroid cancer in Israel. *Br. J. Cancer* 23:488.

Modan, B.; Shani, M.; Goldman, B.; and Modan, M. 1969. Nodal and extranodal malignant lymphoma in Israel. *Br. J. Haematol.* 16:53.

Modan, B.; Sharon, Z.; Shani, M.; and Sheba, C. 1970. Some epidemiological aspects of cervical and endometrial carcinoma. *Pathol. Microbiol.* 35:192.

Movshovitz, M., and Modan, B. 1973. Role of sun exposure in the etiology of malignant melanoma: Epidemiologic inference. *J. Natl. Cancer Inst.* 51:777.

Nevo, S.; Meyer, W.; and Altman, M. 1971. Carcinoma of nasopharynx in twins. *Cancer* 28:807.

Pridan, H., and Lilienfeld, A. M. 1971. Carcinoma of the cervix in Jewish women in Israel, 1960–67. *Israel J. Med. Sci.* 7:1465.

Shani, M., and Modan, B. 1975. Esophageal cancer in Israel. *Am. J. Dig. Dis.* 20:951.

Shani, M.; Modan, B.; Steinitz, R.; and Modan, M. 1966. The incidence of breast cancer in Jewish females in Israel. *Harefuah* 71:337.

Steinitz, R. 1974. *Israel Cancer Registry*. Jerusalem: Ministry of Health.

Tulchinsky, D., and Modan, B. 1967. Epidemiological aspects of cancer of the stomach in Israel. *Cancer* 20:1311.

Turgman, J.: Modan, B.; Rappaport, Y.; and Shanon, E. 1978. Nasopharyngeal cancer in a total population: Selected clinical and epidemiological aspects. *Br. J. Cancer,* in press.

POLYCYTHEMIA VERA

In 1892 Vaquez published the first description of persistent polycythemia in which it was distinguished from the relative and transient forms of the disease. Case reports by Saundby and Russell in 1902 and Osler in 1903 established this disorder as a specific entity. In 1904 Türk pointed out the presence of leukocytosis and immaturely formed red and white cells, which indicated hyperplastic blood formation, and in 1906 Hutchinson and Miller described the associated megakaryo-cytic proliferation. The clinical picture was completed in 1910 with the recognition of thrombocytosis by Le Sourd and Pagniez. Thus, polycythemia vera came to be defined as a chronic disease of unknown etiology characterized by an absolute erythrocytosis, leukocytosis, thrombocytosis, and splenomegaly.

Owing to the infrequent occurrence of polycythemia vera (less than 1,000 new cases per year in the United States), few epidemiological investigations have been conducted. Most reports have been based on selected series of patients from hematology clinics and hospitals and are characterized by all the inherent problems and biases that such studies encompass.

Polycythemia vera is essentially a disease of the middle and later years. The peak age of onset is between 50 and 60 years in most large reported series, but the distribution ranges from adolescence to old age. Childhood cases are rare. Males are affected slightly more frequently than females, with the mean ratio of males to females in 26 large published series being 1.5:1.

The incidence of polycythemia vera in different ethnic and racial groups has been and still is a debatable issue. Nevertheless, it has generally been accepted that this disease occurs frequently in Ashkenazi Jews and rarely in blacks. As mentioned earlier, this picture has frequently been derived from personal experience, the bias of selected hospital or clinical populations, and selected practices of certain physicians.

In 1934/35 Reznikoff and co-workers examined the ethnic background of polycythemia vera patients in 6 hospital clinics in New York City. They found that 47.8 percent of the patients were Jews born in Eastern Europe, whereas the overall frequency of admission of East European Jews to these hospitals was approximately 9 percent. However, the clinic populations from which these patients were drawn were not necessarily representative of the total hospital populations, which supplied the "control" frequencies. Furthermore, in at least 3 of the 6 hospitals the ethnic background of admitted patients was only estimated.

In 1958 Damon and Holub compared the proportion of Jewish patients in their study group to that of patients who had received blood transfusions during a 6-month period at the same institution. Thirty-three percent of the polycythemia vera patients were Jewish, as compared to 16.1 percent of the transfusion group.

358   GENETIC DISORDERS AMONG THE JEWISH PEOPLE

When only white patients were analyzed, the percentage of Jews among the polycythemia patients was 34.2, while among the "controls" it was 19.7. The selection
of such a control group left much to be desired, and information regarding religion
provided by hospital records was not always complete or even present.

In 1965, in a well-designed study involving the Baltimore community, Modan
found that the percentage of Jewish patients with polycythemia vera was significantly
in excess of their relative proportion in the city—about fourfold compared to
Protestants and sixfold compared to Catholics. (The population of Baltimore at
that time was approximately 55 percent Protestant, 33 percent Catholic, and 8
percent Jewish.) Although these findings tended to support the observation that
Ashkenazi Jews are prone to develop polycythemia vera, Modan added two qualifying remarks regarding his observations. First, the number of patients he saw was
small; second, Jews tend to seek medical care more than non-Jews do.

Modan found the incidence of polycythemia vera in Israel to be significantly
higher among European-born immigrants than among Jews born in Asian and
North African countries. He also noted that the incidence among European-born
Israeli Jews was in the same range of magnitude as that among Baltimore Jews, the
vast majority of whom were of European ancestry (Table 8.32).

In contrast to these findings, in 1937 Blake, a Harvard Medical School student
who based his Ph.D. thesis on a 20-year survey of the records of the Peter Bent
Brigham Hospital in Boston, did not note a higher proportion of Jews with this
disease. Likewise, in his 1955 monograph on 303 cases of polycythemia vera
Lawrence found no preponderance of the disease in any particular ethnic or religious
group.

Modan's Baltimore-based study revealed an average annual incidence of 4.9/
million population. Affected males slightly outnumbered females by a ratio of
1.2:1. The mean age for newly discovered cases was 60.3 years. The lowest rates
were observed among the blacks of the city (see Table 8.32). Whereas blacks

Table 8.32. Polycythemia vera: Annual age-specific rates per million Baltimore City
residents and Israeli Jews originating from Europe, Asia, and Africa

	Baltimore City					
	Whites				Total	
	Jews		Non-Jews			
Age (yr)	No.	Rate	No.	Rate	No.	Rate
<10	—	—	—	—	—	—
10–19	—	—	—	—	—	—
20–29	—	—	—	—	—	—
30–39	—	—	—	—	—	—
40–49	1	9.5	2	2.4	3	3.2
50–59	6	66.8	8	11.3	14	17.5
60–69	2	30.3	10	19.2	12	20.4
70+	2	46.1	10	29.2	12	31.1
Total no. and average rate	11	14.2	30	4.9	41	6.1
Age-adjusted rates		10.6		3.6		4.5

Sources: B. Modan, 1965, *Blood* 26:657; B. Modan et al., 1971, *Blood* 37:172. Reprinted by
permission of Grune & Stratton, Inc.

comprise 35 percent of the population of Baltimore, only 8 percent of the affected study population were blacks. Modan suggested that less concern for medical care and a lower "normal" red blood cell level may contribute to bias in ascertainment. It is possible that this disease is not as rare among blacks as was once thought.

In Israel, Modan found that the average annual incidence of polycythemia vera was 6.7/million population—higher than that in Baltimore. The male:female ratio was 1.1:1 and the peak age at onset for both sexes was 60–69 (Table 8.32).

Very few familial cases of this disorder have been well documented. In fact, many of the cases reported have not been polycythemia vera. In reviewing the literature in light of the question of the familial nature of polycythemia vera, Modan accepted that diagnosis in only 3 families, and in these only sibs were affected (2 sibs in 2 families and 3 sibs in another).

Other investigators have tried to show an association between polycythemia vera and specific blood groups but without success.

Much has been written on the chromosomal changes that result from polycythemia vera. The problem in interpreting these data is that most studies have been done on patients who have been treated with P^{32} or various myelosuppressive drugs. Thus it has been impossible to determine whether chromosomal abnormalities observed are related to the disease itself or to the cytotoxic therapy. Some investigators have reported normal chromosomal studies in patients who had not received prior myelosuppressive therapy; others have noted in untreated patients chromosomal changes similar to those found in patients previously treated with P^{32}. Whether one speaks of a Philadelphia chromosome or alterations in the C, F, or G groups in polycythemia vera, it is not possible at this time to state that this disease is characterized by a specific chromosomal aberration.

In conclusion, available evidence indicates that polycythemia vera is more common in the Ashkenazi Jewish community than in other ethnic groups, but additional epidemiological studies are needed to better document this observation.

| Baltimore City | | | | Israel | | | | | |
| Nonwhites | | Total pop. | | Europeans | | Asians & Africans | | Total pop. | |
No.	Rate	No.	Rate	No.	Rate	No.	Rate	No.	Rate
—	—	—	—	—	—	—	—	—	—
—	—	—	—	—	—	—	—	—	—
—	—	—	—	1	1.2	—	—	1	0.3
1	2.2	1	0.7	8	5.4	1	0.9	9	3.0
—	—	3	2.3	27	14.4	3	3.8	31	11.0
—	—	14	13.5	38	22.9	8	13.5	46	19.5
3	23.4	15	20.9	40	45.3	6	16.7	48	37.0
1	14.9	13	28.6	17	36.6	3	14.7	20	28.6
—	—	—	—	—	—	—	—	—	—
5	1.8	46	4.9	131	16.2	21	3.2	155	6.7
	2.0		4.0		8.5		3.3		6.8

Genetic studies on this disorder provide little data to support the concept that hereditary factors play a primary etiological role in polycythemia vera. On the other hand, there is no adequate explanation—genetic or environmental—for the fact that Ashkenazi Jews are more prone to this disease than other ethnic groups.

References

Blake, D. 1937. Unpublished student thesis, Harvard University Medical School.

Chievitz, E., and Thiede, T. 1962. Complications and causes of death in polycythemia vera. *Acta Med. Scand.* 172:513.

Damon, A., and Holub, D. A. 1958. Host factors in polycythemia vera. *Ann. Intern. Med.* 49:43.

Erf, L. A. 1956. Radioactive phosphorous in the treatment of primary polycythemia (vera). *Prog. Hematol.* 1:153.

Erkman, B.; Hazlett, B.; Crookston, J. H.; and Conen, P. E. 1967. Hypodiploid chromosome pattern in acute leukemia following polycythemia vera. *Cancer* 20:1318.

Hutchinson, R., and Miller, C. H. 1906. A case of splenomegalic polycythemia, with report of post-mortem examinations. *Lancet* 1:744.

Kay, H. E.; Lawler, S. D.; and Millard, R. E. 1966. The chromosome in polycythemia vera. *Br. J. Haematol.* 12:507.

Kemp, N. H.; Stafford, J. L.; and Tanner, R. K. 1961. Cytogenetic studies in polycythaemia vera. In *Proc. 8th Cong. Eur. Soc. Hematol.*, 1:92. Basel: Karger.

Kiossoglou, K. A.; Mitus, W. J.; and Dameshek, W. 1966. Cytogenetic studies in the chronic myeloproliferative syndrome. *Blood* 28:241.

Lawrence, J. H. 1955. *Polycythemia: physiology, diagnosis, and treatment based on 303 cases.* Modern Medical Monographs. New York: Grune and Stratton.

Lawrence, J. H., and Goetsch, A. T. 1950. Familial occurrence of polycythemia and leukemia. *Calif. Med.* 73:361.

Le Sourd, L., and Pagniez, P. 1910. Les plaquettes sanguines dans certaines polyglobulies. *C. R. Soc. Biol.* 68:746.

Levin, W. C.; Houston, E. W.; and Ritzmann, S. E. 1967. Polycythemia vera with Ph[1] chromosomes in two brothers. *Blood* 30:503.

MacDiarmid, W. D. 1965. Chromosomal changes following treatment of polycythaemia with radioactive phosphorus. *Quart. J. Med.* 34: 133.

Meytes, D.; Akstein, E.; and Modan, B. 1977. Cytogenetic findings in polycythemia vera: A review and reevaluation. *Israel J. Med. Sci.* 13:1226.

Millard, R. E.; Lawler, S. D.; Kay, H. E.; and Cameron, C. B. 1968. Further observations on patients with a chromosomal abnormality associated with polycythemia vera. *Br. J. Haematol.* 14:363.

Modan, B. 1965. An epidemiological study of polycythemia vera. *Blood* 26:657.

———. 1971. *The polycythemic disorders.* Springfield, Ill.: Charles C Thomas.

Modan, B.; Kallner, H.; Zemer, D.; and Yoran, C. 1971. A note on the increased risk of polycythemia in Jews. *Blood* 37:172.

Modan, B.; Padeh, B.; Kallner, H.; Akstein, E.; Meytes, D.; Cyerniak, P.; Ramot, B.; Pinkhas, J.; and Modan, M. 1970. Chromosomal aberrations in polycythemia vera. *Blood* 35:28.

Osler, W. 1903. Chronic cyanosis with polycythemia and enlarged spleen: A new clinical entity. *Am. J. Med. Sci.* 126:187.

Reznikoff, P.; Foot, N. C.; and Bethea, J. M. 1935. Etiologic and pathologic factors in polycythemia vera. *Am. J. Med. Sci.* 189:753.

Reznikoff, P.; Foot, N. C.; Bethea, J. M.; and Dubois, E. F. 1934. Racial and geographic origin of patients suffering from polycythemia vera and pathological findings in blood vessels of bone marrow. *Trans. Assoc. Am. Physicians* 49:273.

Türk, W. 1904. Beiträge zur kenntnis des symptomenbildes Polyzythämie mit Milztumor und Zyanose. *Wien Klin. Wochenschr.* 17:153.

Vaquez, H. 1892. Sur une forme spéciale de cyanose s'accompanant d'hyperglobulie excessive et persitente. *C. R. Soc. Biol.* 4:384.

Wintrobe, M. M.; Lee, G. R.; Boggs, D. R.; Bithell, T. C.; Athens, T. C.; and Foerster, J. 1974. *Clinical hematology*, 7th ed., pp. 968–1008. Philadelphia: Lea and Febiger.

REGIONAL ENTERITIS
(CROHN DISEASE)

In 1932 Crohn and co-workers first defined the clinical and pathological features of a disorder they called "regional ileitis." In subsequent reports involvement of the duodenum, stomach, esophagus, and any region of the small bowel and colon was noted and the disease became known as regional enteritis.

The disease is best defined as a chronic, inflammatory, granulomatous condition of the small bowel. Although the terminal ileum is most often involved, the disease may affect any part of the gastrointestinal tract from the esophagus to the anus. The spread of regional enteritis is usually segmental, with diseased regions of the bowel separated by apparently healthy segments. Inflammation extends through all layers of the gut wall and involves mesentery and regional lymph nodes. The disease is characterized by a wide variety of clinical manifestations and a prolonged, complicated, and indolent course, with unpredictable exacerbations and remissions.

For details concerning the pathology, diagnosis, clinical course, and treatment of regional enteritis the reader is referred to any standard textbook on gastroenterology or medicine.

Regional enteritis occurs throughout the world, but for the most part, meaningful comparisons of incidence and prevalence among various populations are not available. However, reports from urban centers in England, Scotland, Norway, and the United States indicate that among the industrialized white population 1 or 2 persons per 100,000 develop the disease annually. In Oxford, England, a 10-year study based on a population of 250,000 revealed an annual incidence of 0.8/ 100,000 and a prevalence of 9/100,000. Rates based on first hospitalizations are shown in Table 8.33.

Table 8.33. Regional Enteritis: Average annual first hospitalization rate per 100,000 population

Population	Rate
White	
England (Oxford area)	0.95
Baltimore	1.35
Norway	0.25
Scotland	1.30
Nonwhite	
Baltimore	0.04

Source: A. I. Mendeloff et al., 1966, *Gastroenterology* 51:748. © 1966 The Williams & Wilkins Co., Baltimore.

Regional enteritis is slightly more common in males than in females. It has been reported in newborns as well as in octogenarians, but symptoms usually develop when the patient is in his twenties.

Most investigators agree that whites develop the disease 2–5 times more often than nonwhites (see Table 8.33). However, the validity of this difference is difficult to determine because the number of nonwhites studied has been small and diagnostic facilities have not always been comparable.

In contrast to possible discrepancies in the incidence of this disease in whites and blacks, careful surveys done in the United States have consistently shown that regional enteritis is more common in Jews than in non-Jews. Table 8.34 shows the rates for Jews and non-Jews obtained from a study done in the Baltimore area and reported in 1967 by Monk and co-workers. For males the ratio of Jews to non-Jews is approximately 6:1; for females it is about 3:1. Similarly, in 1973 Acheson reported a fourfold greater frequency of regional enteritis among Jewish dischargees from Veterans Administration hospitals than among non-Jewish dischargees.

The investigators in the Baltimore study were well aware of the possibilities of diagnostic bias and of differential rates of hospitalization for Jews and non-Jews as a possible explanation for these differences. After further analysis of such factors, they concluded that even if one allows for a greater possibility of Jews (Ashkenazi) in Baltimore being hospitalized for this disease, it did not seem reasonable that differences in demand or receipt of medical care could explain the differences in rates between Jews and non-Jews.

Evidence from other studies also suggests that neither diagnostic bias nor frequency of hospitalization can wholly account for ethnic differences in the incidence and prevalence of either regional enteritis or ulcerative colitis. In the study from Oxford, England, where all persons with ulcerative colitis and regional enteritis were included, whether hospitalized or not, the incidence of these diseases was higher among Jews than among non-Jews.

The etiology of regional enteritis is not known. Various efforts have been made to ascertain a possible genetic component of the disease. Some have argued that the high frequency of this disease and ulcerative colitis among Jews is evidence

Table 8.34. Regional enteritis: Number and annual rate of total
and first hospitalizations by sex and religion (white patients only)

| Patients | Total hospitalizations | | | | First hospitalizations (definite regional enteritis) | |
| | Definite regional enteritis | | Possible regional enteritis | | | |
	No.	Rate	No.	Rate	No.	Rate
Males						
Jews (a)	19	19.65	4	4.14	7	7.24
Non-Jews (b)	33	3.21	20	1.95	21	2.04
Ratio (a:b)		6.12		2.12		3.55
Females						
Jews (a)	9	8.42	4	3.74	0	
Non-Jews (b)	34	3.03	23	2.05	15	1.34
Ratio (a:b)		2.78		1.82		0

Source: M. Monk et al., 1967, *Gastroenterology* 53:198. © 1967 The Williams & Wilkins Co., Baltimore.

Note: Annual rates per 100,000 population are based on the 1960 Baltimore area census.

of a genetic etiology. Familial aggregation has long been recognized in patients with regional enteritis. Several reports indicate that 3–11 percent of such patients have a family history of regional enteritis or ulcerative colitis. Table 8.35 shows the work of Almy and Sherlock on the familial occurrence of these two diseases either individually or together. Four cases of concordance in monozygotic twins have been recorded. Although this number is small, the chance occurrence of concordance for regional enteritis in monozygotic twins is 1 in over 6 billion persons. The information shown in Table 8.35 suggests that genetic factors may be operating, but it does not eliminate the possibility of latent environmental influences.

It has been pointed out by various observers that the incidence of regional enteritis is increasing in large urban populations of the Western world, but it is not clear whether this rising incidence is real or merely reflects an increased awareness of the disease. Similarly, it is not clear whether this disorder is really more frequent in industrialized Western countries or simply is not recognized in the less-developed nations of the world.

In conclusion, it appears that Ashkenazi Jews are more prone to regional enteritis than are non-Jewish populations. The reason for this selective ethnic distribution is not known. A detailed epidemiological study of this disease remains to be done in Israel. Such an investigation would be of immense importance, not only in comparing the incidence of the disease in the Ashkenazi community of Israel and the Diaspora, but also in determining the rate of occurrence of regional enteritis among non-Ashkenazi Jews.

References

Acheson, E. D. 1960. The distribution of ulcerative colitis and regional enteritis in United States veterans with particular reference to the Jewish religion. *Gut* 1:291.

————. 1965. Epidemiology of ulcerative colitis and regional enteritis. In *Recent advances in gastroenterology*, ed. J. Badenoch and B. N. Brooke. London: J. and A. Churchill.

Almy, T., and Sherlock, P. 1966. Genetic aspects of ulcerative colitis and regional enteritis. *Gastroenterology* 51:757.

Brown, P. W.; Bargen, J. A.; and Weber, H. M. 1934. Chronic inflammatory lesions of small intestine (regional enteritis). *Am. J. Dig. Dis. Nutrit.* 1:426.

Table 8.35. Familial ulcerative colitis (UC) and regional enteritis (RE)

Relationship	No. of families affected		
	UC	RE	UC and RE
Parent and one child[a]	39	14	3
Parent and multiple children	1	2	2
Two sibs	43	19	3
Three or more sibs	5	5	3
Monozygotic twins	3	4	0
Dizygotic twins	1	2	0
Collateral relatives	13	10	6
Husband and wife	2	0	0

Source: T. P. Almy and P. Sherlock, 1966, *Gastroenterology* 51:757. © 1966 The Williams & Wilkins Co., Baltimore.

[a] Two instances of father and son; 21 instances of mother and son; 8 instances of mother and daughter; 8 instances of father and daughter.

Crohn, B. B. 1969 Regional enteritis. In *Gastroenterologic medicine*, ed. M. Paulson, pp. 855–65. Philadelphia: Lea and Febiger.

Crohn, B. B.; Ginzburg, L.; and Oppenheimer, G. D. 1932. Regional ileitis: A clinical and pathological entity. *JAMA* 99:1323.

Crohn, B. B., and Janowitz, H. D. 1954. Reflections on regional ileitis, twenty years later. *JAMA* 156:1221.

Evans, J. G., and Acheson, E. D. 1965. An epidemiological study of ulcerative colitis and regional enteritis in the Oxford area. *Gut* 6:311.

Freysz, H.; Haemmerli, A.; and Kartagener, M. 1958. Ileitis regionalis, bei einem weiblichen Zwillingspaar [regional ileitis in female twins]. *Gastroenterologia* 89:75.

Gjone, E.; Orning, O. M.; and Myren, J. 1966. Crohn's disease in Norway, 1956–1963. *Gut* 7:372.

Kirsner, J. B., and Spencer, J. A. 1963. Family occurrences of ulcerative colitis, regional enteritis, and ileocolitis. *Ann. Intern. Med.* 59:133.

Kyle, J., and Blair, D. W. 1965. Epidemiology of regional enteritis in North-east Scotland. *Br. J. Surg.* 52:215.

Lockhart-Mummery, H., and Morson, B. 1960. Crohn's disease (regional enteritis) of the large intestine and its distinction from ulcerative colitis. *Gut* 1:87.

Mendeloff, A. I.; Monk, M.; Siegel, C. I.; and Lilienfeld, A. 1966. Some epidemiological features of ulcerative colitis and regional enteritis: A preliminary report. *Gastroenterology* 51:748.

Monk, M.; Mendeloff, A. I.; Siegel, C. I.; and Lilienfeld, A. 1967. An epidemiological study of ulcerative colitis and regional enteritis among adults in Baltimore. I: Hospital incidence and prevalence, 1960 to 1963. *Gastroenterology* 53:198.

————. Monk, M.; Mendeloff, A.; Siegel, C.; and Lilienfeld, A. 1969. An epidemiological study of ulcerative colitis and regional enteritis among adults in Baltimore. II: Social and demographic factors. *Gastroenterology* 56:847.

Niederle, B., and Sebek, V. 1960. Terminal ileitis in monozygotic twins. *Cas. Lek. Cesk.* 99:1038.

Sherlock, P.; Bell, B. M.; Steinberg, H.; and Almy, T. P. 1963. Familial occurrence of regional enteritis and ulcerative colitis. *Gastroenterology* 45:413.

Singer, H. C.; Anderson, J. G. D.; Frischer, H.; and Kirsner, J. B. 1971. Familial aspects of inflammatory bowel disease. *Gastroenterology* 61:423.

Steigman, F., and Shapiro, F. 1961. Familial regional enteritis. *Gastroenterology* 40:215.

TAKAYASU ARTERITIS

Historical note

Although this form of arteritis was probably recognized in the 19th century, it was not until the 20th century that a report by Japanese ophthalmologist Migito Takayasu stimulated interest in the condition. Over the years this form of arteritis has become known as a distinct clinical entity but has acquired a number of names, such as Takayasu disease, pulseless disease, and aortitis syndrome. Its ethnic distribution originally centered in the countries of the Far East, but later it was observed among the blacks of South Africa, the Spanish population of Central and South America, and, to a lesser extent, among the whites of the United States and northern Europe. In 1974 Deutsch and co-workers reported the unique distribution of this disease among the various ethnic communities of Israel.

Clinical features

The onset of Takayasu arteritis has been reported in patients 11 and 64 years of age. Most patients are female and the onset of symptoms usually occurs between the ages of 20 and 40 years. During the acute stage some patients complain of fever or night sweats. The main symptom is ischemia involving primarily the brain, eyes, face, and upper extremities. Specific manifestations of the ischemia include the following: vertigo, syncope, convulsions, aphasia, headache, transient episodes of cerebral ischemia, hemiparesis, bouts of blindness, amblyopia, photophobia, muscular atrophy of the face, ulcerated nose and palate, claudication of muscles of mastication, and a variety of symptoms indicating vascular insufficiency of the upper extremities.

Physical findings are variable but they all reflect obstructive changes in arterial blood flow with concomitant changes in venous return.

Diagnosis

Diagnosis of Takayasu arteritis should be suspected in any individual who presents with the above symptoms and has decreased or absent arterial pulses in the neck or upper extremities.

Leukocytosis and an elevated sedimentation rate are common.

Because the disorder may be detected from the deformation and irregularities of the aorta seen in plain film chest roentgenograms, patients with characteristic presenting symptoms should receive careful roentgenological attention. Diagnosis is confirmed, however, on the basis of angiographic studies, which should include the entire aorta and proximal peripheral arteries.

Basic defect

The basic defect in Takayasu arteritis is not known, but most investigators believe it is an autoimmune disease.

Histologically, the lesions are characterized by arteritis of all layers of the involved vessels, with giant cell infiltration and obliteration of the lumen.

Genetics

In contrast to Buerger disease in Jews, which affects mainly the Ashkenazim, Takayasu arteritis in Jews is seen almost exclusively in the Oriental and Sephardi communities. In the 22 patients reported from Israel by Deutsch and co-workers, 9 were Arabs or Bedouins and 13 were Jewish—8 Oriental and 5 Sephardi (Table 8.36). The ratio of females to males in this study group was 1.2:1, which is quite different from the 8:1 ratio usually noted for this disease. The average age of onset in these patients was 29.9 years. Family histories did not reveal other similarly affected members, but family studies were not done.

Variations in the vessels and types of lesions involved in this disorder appear to reflect the geographical origins of patients. For example, in Europe, Japan, and the United States, vascular stenoses or occulsions are common and aneurysms are rare, while in India, Thailand, and Africa, aneurysms are a prominent feature of

Table 8.36. Takayasu arteritis: Age, sex, and ethnic distribution of 22 Israeli patients

Ethnic origin	Age (yr)	Sex	Ethnic origin	Age (yr)	Sex
Oriental Jews			Sephardi Jews		
India	18	F	Bulgaria	42	F
India	22	F	Ethiopia	26	M
India	12	F	Greece	45	M
India	22	M	Tunisia	21	F
Iran	30	F	Turkey	38	F
Iraq	36	F	Bedouins	40	M
Syria	26	F		40	M
Yemen	24	M		23	F
Arabs	40	M		27	F
	24	F		40	M
	36	M			
	27	M			

Source: V. Deutsch et al., 1974, *Am. J. Roentgenol. Rad. Therapy Nucl. Med.* 122:13.

the disease. In the Israeli group studied by Deutsch and co-workers, all 4 Jewish patients from India had aneurysms of the thoracic aorta, while only 3 other patients had similar aneurysms. Occlusion or stenosis of the abdominal aorta was a predominant feature in 3 of 5 Bedouins from the Sinai Peninsula and in 3 of 4 Arabs from Gaza, a finding which suggests that ethnic origin may be a factor influencing the pattern of regional involvement. Reports of distal aortic involvement are common only in Africa, but it is likely that an African influence is to be found among the Israeli Arabs and particularly the Sinai Bedouins. As confirmed in genetic studies, the proximity of Africa and the Sinai Peninsula has led to the introduction of many African genes in the Sinai Bedouins.

Although very little has been written about genetic factors in Takayasu arteritis, it would seem that this disease, with its distinct geographical distribution and possible autoimmune factor, is an ideal one to evaluate genetically using a variety of markers, including the HLA-antigens.

Prognosis and treatment

The natural history of Takayasu arteritis has not been fully elucidated, but it is thought that the disorder progresses at an unpredictable rate. Patients usually die of cerebral ischemia or heart disease.

Long-term anticoagulant treatment has been recommended in an effort to prevent arterial thrombosis. Surgical treatment involving endarterectomy, local resection, and vessel grafts may be indicated in certain cases.

Proper therapy may impede the progression of the vascular lesions but will not reverse the changes already present.

References

Deutsch, V.; Wexler, L.; and Deutsch, H. 1974. Takayasu's arteritis: An angiographic study with remarks on ethnic distribution in Israel. *Am. J. Roentgenol. Rad. Therapy Nucl. Med.* 122:13.

Hirsch, M. S.; Aikat, B. K.; and Basu, A. K. 1964. Takayasu's arteritis: Report of five cases with immunological studies. *Bull. Johns Hopkins Hospital* 115:29.

Judge, D. R.; Currier, D. R.; Gracie, A. W.; and Figley, M. M. 1963. Takayasu's arteritis and aortic arch syndrome. *Am. J. Med.* 32:397.

Kinare, S. G. 1968. Etiopathological aspects of non-specific aortitis. In *Cardiology: Current topics and progress,* ed. H. Eliakim and H. N. Neufeld, pp. 322–25. New York: Academic Press.

Kozuka, T.; Nosaki, T.; Soto, K.; and Ihara, K. 1968. Arteritis syndrome with special reference to pulmonary vascular changes. *Acta Radiol. [Diagn.]* 7:25.

Kozuka, T.; Nosaki, T.; Soto, K.; and Tachiri, H. Aneurysm associated with aortitis syndrome. *Acta Radiol [Diagn.]* 7:314.

Lande, A., and Gross, A. 1972. Total aortography in diagnosis of Takayasu's arteritis. *Am. J. Roentgenol. Rad. Therapy Nucl. Med.* 116:165.

Poloheimo, J. A. 1967. Obstructive arteritis of Takayasu's type: Clinical, roentgenological, and laboratory studies on 36 patients. *Acta Med. Scand.* [Suppl.] 4:1.

Ueda, H. 1968. Etiology and clinical manifestations of "aortitis disease." In *Cardiology: Current topics and progress,* ed. H. Eliakim and H. N. Neufeld, pp. 320–21. New York: Academic Press.

Vinijchaikul, K. 1968. Pathological spectrum of sclerosing aortitis. In *Cardiology: Current topics and progress,* ed. H. Eliakim and N. H. Neufeld, pp. 326–28.

ULCERATIVE COLITIS

In 1875 Wilks and Moxon first used the term *ulcerative colitis* and clearly distinguished between this disease and other forms of colitis caused by bacilli or parasites. Over the years, however, pathologists have noted a number of similarities between ulcerative colitis and regional enteritis. Some resected specimens have shown features of both diseases, and in several cases the findings have been completely compatible with either diagnosis. Some investigators believe that these disorders share a common cause and differ only in tissue reaction to some unknown, harmful agent. Nevertheless, ulcerative colitis can be defined as an inflammatory disease of unknown cause which affects mainly the mucosa of the rectum and left colon, but in many instances the entire organ. A chronic disease with remissions and exacerbations, ulcerative colitis is characterized by rectal bleeding and diarrhea and occurs principally in youth and early middle age. The disease may produce serious local and systemic complications. Therapy is nonspecific and life expectancy is reduced.

As in the case of regional enteritis, this discussion will center on certain epidemiological and genetic features of the disease.

It has long been considered that ulcerative colitis is more common in Ashkenazi Jews than in other ethnic groups. In 1950 Sloan and co-workers found that 9.4 percent of their 2,000 ulcerative colitis patients were Jewish. In the same year Paulley compared the proportion of Jewish patients with ulcerative colitis in 2 London hospitals with the proportion of Jews among all patients discharged. He found twice as many Jews among the ulcerative colitis patients as among the dischargees. In 1944 Acheson and Nefzger reported U.S. Army records of 525 cases of ulcerative colitis and controls matched for date of birth, race, and rank. They found that Jewish males were affected more than twice as frequently as non-Jewish males, regardless of size and place of birth or residence within the United States. An excess risk was found among white officers, and although a large number of the officers were Jewish, the matching procedure controlled for this factor. White officers were affected almost twice as frequently as white enlisted men, but there was no significant difference between the rates for white and black enlisted men.

In 1960 Acheson's report on 2,320 male veterans discharged from 174 hospitals of the Veterans Administration throughout the United States showed that the proportion of Jews among patients discharged for ulcerative colitis, regional enteritis, or mixed forms of the disease was 4 times greater than the proportion of Jews in samples of all general medical and surgical patients. When the cases of ulcerative colitis and regional enteritis were analyzed by region of birth, there was a higher porportion of Jews among them than in the control group in every region except one. The single exception (patients with regional enteritis born in the West) may be attributed to the small numbers involved.

Studies in Oxford, England, and Baltimore, Maryland, support the impression of a higher incidence of ulcerative colitis among Jews than among non-Jews. Table 8.37 lists the annual rates of hospitalization for ulcerative colitis according to sex and religion as observed in the Baltimore study. From this table it is possible to conclude that both the number and rate of hospitalizations for ulcerative colitis are higher among Jews than among non-Jews—especially the rate of hospitalizations for ulcerative colitis among Jewish women.

The Baltimore group found that the rate of hospitalization for ulcerative colitis in Baltimore fell within the general range of figures obtained for other countries (Table 8.28). The rate of first hospitalizations in New Zealand was only slightly higher than that in Baltimore; in Norway the rate was less than half the Baltimore rate. In Oxford, England, where the rate was based on records from physicians and outpatient clinics as well as from hospitals, the incidence was somewhat higher than in either Baltimore or New Zealand. It is possible that the inclusion of non-hospitalized cases may account for the higher rate in England. As in their study of regional enteritis, the Baltimore investigators concluded that it was unlikely that diagnostic bias and differential likelihood of hospitalization could account for the difference in rates between Jews and non-Jews.

Table 8.37. Ulcerative colitis: Number and annual rate of total and first hospitalizations per 100,000 population by sex and religion (white patients only)

	Total hospitalizations				First hospitalizations (definite ulcerative colitis)	
	Definite ulcerative colitis		Possible ulcerative colitis			
Patients	No.	Rate	No.	Rate	No.	Rate
Males						
Jews (a)	23	23.78	9	9.31	9	9.31
Non-Jews (b)	59	5.74	40	3.89	35	3.40
Ratio (a:b)		4.14		2.39		2.74
Females						
Jews (a)	34	31.82	4	3.74	18	16.85
Non-Jews (b)	77	6.87	53	4.73	46	4.10
Ratio (a:b)		4.63		0.79		4.11

Source: M. Monk et al., 1967, *Gastroenterology* 53:198. © 1967 The Williams & Wilkins Co., Baltimore.

Note: Annual rates per 100,000 population are based on the 1960 Baltimore area census.

Table 8.38. Ulcerative colitis: Average annual incidence and first hospitalizations per 100,000 population by sex (selected countries and years)

Country	Males	Females	Total pop.
		Average annual incidence	
Oxford, England, 1951–1960	1.0	1.3	1.15
		Average annual first hospitalizations	
Norway			
1946–1955	1.1	1.3	1.20
1956–1960	2.0	2.1	2.05
New Zealand			
1954–1958	—	—	5–6
United States (Baltimore)			
1960–1963 (whites only,			
20 yr and older)	3.9	5.2	4.6

Source: M. Monk et al., 1967, *Gastroenterology* 53:198. © 1967 The Williams & Wilkins Co., Baltimore.

The 1960 study by Birnbaum and co-workers supports the concept that, among Jews, mainly the Ashkenazim are prone to develop this disease. Eighty percent of the hospitalized Jewish patients studied were of Ashkenazi descent, while the remaining 20 percent were of Oriental or Sephardi origin (Table 8.39). On the basis of this hospital population Birnbaum and co-workers concluded that ulcerative colitis was more than 3 times as prevalent among Jewish patients of Ashkenazi background as among Jews of Oriental or Sephardi origin.

In 1974 Gilat and co-workers reported an overall annual incidence of ulcerative colitis of about 3.7/100,000 population for the period 1961–1970 in the Tel Aviv area. Earlier data from Baltimore had shown a markedly higher incidence of

Table 8.39. Ulcerative colitis: Number of patients hospitalized in Israel, 1952–1956, by country of birth

Country of birth	No. of patients	%
Asia & Africa		
Iraq	2	
Persia	3	
Turkey	2	
Yemen and Aden	2	
Libya	2	
Total	11	20
Europe & America		
Russia	4	
Poland	17	
Lithuania	2	
Romania	7	
Bulgaria	4	
Greece	1	
Germany	4	
Austria	1	
Czechoslovakia	2	
Hungary	1	
Total	43	80
Total born abroad	54	100
Israel	8	
Country of birth not stated	14	

Source: D. Birnbaum et al., 1960, *Arch. Intern. Med.* 105:843. Copyright 1960, American Medical Association.

ulcerative colitis in American Jews (Ashkenazim) than in Israelis, and this led Gilat and co-workers to analyze whether or not the incidence of ulcerative colitis differed among Israeli Jews born in Asia, Africa, Europe, America, and Israel. They found that the prevalence rates for Israelis born in Africa and Asia were 18.5/ 100,000 and 18.9/100,000, respectively. These rates were lower than the rate of 25.8/100,000 noted for persons born in Israel and considerably lower than the rate of 37.3/100,000 observed for those persons born in Europe and America who later migrated to Israel. These differences in rates may reflect differences in concern for medical care. In addition, because these rates indicate prevalence rather than incidence or first hospitalization, some of the differences among the groups may reflect differences in duration of the disease. If ulcerative colitis tended to be more protracted in the Ashkenazim than in the non-Ashkenazim, the prevalence rate among the Ashkenazim would be higher. This would be true even if the incidence, which is the measure of actual risk, were the same in all groups. Thus the observations of Gilat and co-workers must be carefully scrutinized.

Many theories have been proposed to explain the etiology of ulcerative colitis, and the most common have involved infectious, psychosomatic, immunologic, and genetic mechanisms. Currently much attention is being directed toward cell-mediated immune responses in this disease. Lymphocytes from patients with ulcerative colitis are cytotoxic for colonic epithelial cells in tissue culture.

There is a vast amount of literature on the psychosomatic aspects of this disease, but most of it is anecdotal or deals with studies lacking controls. The personality of the ulcerative colitis patient has been variously described as obsessive-compulsive and immature, or passive, anxious to avoid conflict, and above the norm in intelligence. In an effort to explain the high incidence of the disease among Jews, some have expressed the view that these patients are guided by maternal dominance and possessiveness. However, recent studies have challenged this view. In a well-designed epidemiological study in Baltimore in 1962, Monk and co-workers surveyed patients with ulcerative colitis, normal control subjects, and control patients with irritable colons in an effort to identify psychosocial factors unique to patients with ulcerative colitis. They could not find any precipitating stresses in the ulcerative colitis patients versus the control population, and in general the social and occupational background of the patients resembled that of the normal population. In a study by Feldman and co-workers published in 1967 extensive psychiatric evaluation of 34 patients with ulcerative colitis did not reveal a higher incidence of psychiatric aberration than was observed in a control population similarly examined. Although psychological factors may influence the course of various diseases, it is doubtful that they play a major causative role in ulcerative colitis.

There is some evidence for a genetic hypothesis, but the data are far from confirmatory. The finding that the incidence of ulcerative colitis is higher among Ashkenazi Jews among than non-Jews and lower among blacks than among whites suggests that genetic factors may be operating. Furthermore, it is known that the disease occurs with much greater frequency (10–15 percent) in families of patients with ulcerative colitis than in families of control patients without the disease. Several affected members of the same family have been reported and the disorder has been observed in monozygotic twins (see Table 8.35). In addition, ulcerative colitis has a high rate of association with ankylosing spondylitis, a disease with a known genetic component, and a low frequency in Rh− individuals. Multifactorial inheritance has been postulated by some, but more data are needed to clarify the role of heredity in this disorder. Continued research efforts in the direction of genetics and immunology seem warranted for this disorder and regional enteritis.

References

Acheson, E. D. 1960. An association between ulcerative colitis, regional enteritis, and ankylosing spondylitis. *Quart. J. Med.* 29:489.

————. 1960. The distribution of ulcerative colitis and regional enteritis in United States veterans, with particular reference to the Jewish religion. *Gut* 1: 291.

————. Acheson, E. D. 1965. Epidemiology of ulcerative colitis and regional enteritis. *Recent advances in gastroenterology*, ed. J. Badenoch and B. N. Brooke. London: J. and A. Churchill.

Acheson, E. D., and Nefzger, M. D. 1963. Ulcerative colitis in the United States army in 1944. Epidemiology: comparisons between patients and controls. *Gastroenterology* 44:7.

Almy, T., and Sherlock, P. 1966. Genetic aspects of ulcerative colitis and regional enteritis. *Gastroenterology* 51:757.

Birnbaum, D.; Groen, J. J.; and Kallner, G. 1960. Ulcerative colitis among the ethnic groups in Israel. *Arch. Intern. Med.* 105:843.

Bonnevie, O.; Riis, P.; and Anthonisen, P. 1968. An epidemiological study of ulcerative colitis in Copenhagen County. *Scand. J. Gastroenterol.* 3:432.

Boyd, W. C.; Heisler, M.; and Orowan, E. 1961. Correlation between ulcerative colitis and Rh blood groups. *Nature* 190:1123.

Engle, G. L. 1955. Studies of ulcerative colitis. III: The nature of the psychological processes. *Am. J. Med.* 19:231.

Evans, J. G., and Acheson, E. D. 1965. An epidemiological study of ulcerative colitis and regional enteritis in the Oxford area. *Gut* 6: 311.

Feldman, F.; Cantor, D.; Soll, S.; and Bachrach, W. 1967. Psychiatric study of a consecutive series of 34 patients with ulcerative colitis. *Br. Med. J.* 2:14.

Gilat, T.; Ribak, J.; Benaroya, Y.; Zemishlany, Z.; and Weissman, I. 1974. Ulcerative colitis in the Jewish population of Tel-Aviv Jafo. I: Epidemiology. *Gastroenterology* 66:335.

Gjone, E., and Myren, J. 1964. Colitis ulcerative i Norge. *Nord. Med.* 71:143.

Kirsner, J. B., and Spencer, J. A. 1963. Familial occurrences of ulcerative colitis, regional enteritis, and ileocolitis. *Ann. Intern. Med.* 59:133.

Maur, M.; Toranzo, J. C.; and Marcelo, F. A. 1964. ABO and Rh blood groups in colonic disease. *Semana Med.* (Buenos Aires) 124:634.

Mendeloff, A. I.; Monk, M.; Siegel, C. I.; and Lilienfeld, A. 1970. Illness experience and life stresses in patients with irritable colon and with ulcerative colitis. *N. Engl. J. Med.* 282:14.

Monk, M.; Mendeloff, A. I.; Siegel, C. I.; and Lilienfeld, A. 1967. An epidemiological study of ulcerative colitis and regional enteritis among adults in Baltimore. I: Hospital incidence and prevalence, 1960–1963. *Gastroenterology* 53:198.

————. An epidemiological study of ulcerative colitis and regional enteritis among adults in Baltimore. II: Social and demographic features. *Gastroenterology* 56:847.

————. 1970. An epidemiological study of ulcerative colitis and regional enteritis among adults in Baltimore. III: Psychological and possible stress-precipitating factors. *J. Chronic Dis.* 22:565.

Nefzger, M. D., and Acheson, E. D. 1963. Ulcerative colitis in the United States Army in 1944: Follow-up. *Gut* 4:183.

Paulley, J. W. 1950. Ulcerative colitis: A study of 173 cases. *Gastroenterology* 16:566.

Sedlack, R. E.; Nobrega, F. T.; Kurland, L. T.; et al. 1972. Inflammatory colon disease in Rochester, Minnesota, 1935–1964. *Gastroenterology* 62:935.

Sherlock, P.; Bell, B. M.; Steinberg, H.; and Almy, T. P. 1963. Familial occurrence of regional enteritis and ulcerative colitis. *Gastroenterology* 45:413.

Sloan, W. P., Jr.; Bargen, J. A.; and Gage, R. P. 1950. Symposium on diseases of colon: Life histories of patients with chronic ulcerative colitis; review of 2000 cases. *Gastroenterology* 16:25.

Thayer, W. R., and Bove, J. R. 1965. Blood groups and ulcerative colitis. *Gastroenterology* 48:326.

Ustvedt, H. J. 1958. Ulcerative colitis in Norway. In *Recent studies in Epidemiology*, ed. J. Pemberton and H., Willard. Oxford: Blackwell Scientific Publications.

Wigley, R. D., and Maclaurin, B. P. 1962. A study of ulcerative colitis in New Zealand, showing a low incidence in Maoris. *Br. Med. J.* 2:228.

Wilks, S., and Moxon, W. 1875. *Lectures on pathological anatomy*, 2nd ed., p. 672. London: J. and A. Churchill.

9

Nonpathological genetic traits and variants

A NUMBER of nonpathological conditions common to certain Jewish communities, along with a few isolated defects, are discussed in this chapter. It is essential that physicians properly inform their patients of the benign nature of these disorders, for occasionally, through misinformation, a patient may be treated for a more serious condition.

BENIGN FAMILIAL HEMATURIA

Historical note

In 1962 Livaditis and Ericsson called attention to persistent or recurrent hematuria in otherwise healthy children. In 1965 Ayoub and Vernier noted the familial occurrence of this disorder and in 1966 McConville and co-workers documented the autosomal dominant transmission of this form of benign hematuria. In 1979 Eisenstein and co-workers reported the unusually high occurrence of this entity among Jewish children from non-Ashkenazi communities in Israel.

Clinical features

The onset of this painless form of hematuria may occur any time from early childhood through adulthood. It is not associated with renal disease, deafness, or ocular anomalies. The hematuria is usually microscopic in nature and may be persistent or recurrent.

Diagnosis

The diagnosis of benign familial hematuria is usually one of exclusion unless the physician is aware of the trait in other family members. A thorough renal evaluation is necessary, however, even in patients with a history of benign familial hematuria.

373

Table 9.1. Benign hematuria: Clinical information on 23 Israeli families

Patients	No. of males	No. of females	Age at time of investigation (yr)	Age at time of detection (yr)	Length of follow-up (yr)
Probands	8	15	9:6–18:6	1:6–13:0	3:0–8:6
Affected family members	33	46			

Source: B. Eisenstein et al., 1979, Benign familial hematuria among Israeli children *J. Med. Genet.*, in press.

Eisenstein and co-workers have studied 23 families with this disorder. Table 9.1 shows the age, sex, age at time of detection, and duration of the hematuria in the cases they studied. Hematuria was discovered in some relatives of probands only as a result of investigating the proband. In several instances its presence had been known for a period of years. In most cases the hematuria was asymptomatic, although 13 patients complained of occasional abdominal pain and 9 of rare dysuria. These complaints probably were not related to the hematuria. In only 5 cases had the hematuria ever been macroscopic, and in 1 case, persistently so for 4 years. Microscopic hematuria was found to be constant in 36 individuals and intermittent in 38. Proteinuria was absent or minimal (less than 200 mg/24 hr). In 12 of the 23 probands, hematuria was first detected during or shortly after an upper respiratory tract infection.

Physical examination did not contribute to the diagnosis. Blood pressure was normal in all cases. Numerous renal tests and audiometric studies failed to reveal any pathology.

Basic defect

The basic defect in this disorder is not known, but electron microscopic studies in some cases have shown focal thinning of the glomerular basement membrane and especially of the lamina densa (see Figure 9.1).

Genetics

Figure 9.2 shows the abbreviated pedigrees of the 23 Jewish families studied by Eisenstein and co-workers. In 3 families 3 generations were affected, in 16 families 2 generations were affected, and in 4 families only 1 generation was affected, although in this last group each family had 2 affected children. Consanguinity was present in 5 families, 3 of which originated from Iraq and 2 of which came from Morocco and Afghanistan. However, the presence of consanguinity in these families is considered to be an incidental finding. Of the 83 affected individuals, 48 were females and 35 were males. In several families male-to-male transmission was noted. These observations suggest that the most likely mode of transmission is autosomal dominant with decreased penetrance and variable expressivity. Previous family studies tend to confirm the autosomal dominant inheritance of this condition.

Of the 23 affected families, 18 (78 percent) were of non-Ashkenazi Jewish (Asian or African) descent, while 5 families (22 percent) were of Ashkenazi

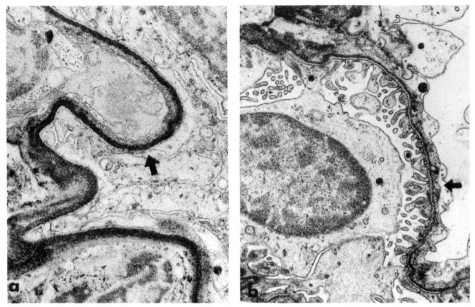

Figure 9.1. (a) Electron micrograph of normal renal glomeruli from a 10-year-old child. (b) Electron micrograph of renal glomeruli from a 9-year-old child with benign familial hematuria. Note the marked thinning of the lamina densa in (b) compared to the normal glomeruli in (a) (arrows). Courtesy of H. Stark, Israel.

origin. Of the non-Ashkenazi families, 8 (35 percent) were of Jewish Iraqi origin. Due to the lack of adequate statistical data it is not possible to state definitely whether or not this disorder occurs more frequently in the non-Ashkenazi Jewish community, although there is a trend in that direction. Additional genetic studies are needed to better clarify the frequency and ethnic distribution of the trait among the various Jewish communities of Israel.

Prognosis and treatment

The prognosis in this disorder is excellent, for it is not considered to be pathological. No treatment is indicated.

References

Arneil, G. C.; Lam, C. N.; McDonald, A. M.; and McDonald, M. 1969. Recurrent haematuria in 17 children. *Br. Med. J.* 2:235.

Ayoub, E. M., and Vernier, R. L. 1965. Benign recurrent hematuria. *Am. J. Dis. Child.* 109:217.

Eisenstein, B.; Stark, H.; and Goodman, R. 1979. Benign familial hematuria among Israeli children. *J. Med. Genet.*, in press.

Glasgow, E. F.; Monerief, M. W.; and White, R. H. R. 1970. Symptomless haematuria in childhood. *Br. Med. J.* 2:687.

Livaditis, A., and Ericsson, N. O. 1962. Essential hematuria in children: Prognostic aspects. *Acta Paediatr.* 51:630.

Rogers, P. W.; Kurtzman, N. A.; Bunn, S. M., Jr.; and White, M. G. 1973. Familial benign essential hematuria. *Arch. Intern. Med.* 131:257.

COLOR BLINDNESS

In 1926, in her classic monograph on the genetics of color blindness, Bell ascribed to Plato the first suggestion, derived possibly from Heraclitus, that individual colors do not necessarily appear the same to all people. In 1688 Boyle described at least one person who was color-blind. Descriptions by Huddart of a family of X-linked color defectives in 1777 and by Scott of a similar family in 1778 were later mentioned in several publications, but serious interest in defective color vision did not develop until 16 years later, when Dalton, a famous chemist, reported on this condition. Dalton and 2 of his brothers were affected, and in 1794 he reported "extraordinary facts relating to the vision of colors." These early observers were well acquainted with the finding that this defect occurs mainly in men, and in

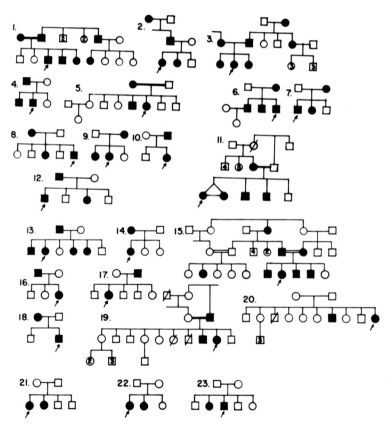

Figure 9.2. Abbreviated family pedigrees of 23 probands with benign familial hematuria. Courtesy of H. Stark, Israel.

1861 Sedgwick recognized the essentials of what is now called X-linked recessive inheritance in relation to this visual abnormality. In 1876 Horner showed that color blindness is transmitted in the same way as Nasse had shown hemophilia to be inherited. He was also able to explain the apparent contradiction of direct transmission from father to son, for in his family, where this occurred, the mother was a carrier.

Much research into the pathophysiology, genetics, and world-wide distribution of color blindness has been done since these early descriptive studies, but many questions remain unanswered. Adam has been the key investigator of this defect among the various Jewish ethnic groups in Israel, and he has personally examined cases in a number of populations throughout the world. Table 9.2 shows the frequency and distribution of color blindness in various world populations. These data are based on tests with the anomaloscope, which provides a more refined and accurate assessment of the problem than do other techniques. As seen in Table 9.2, Ashkenazi Jews have one of the highest rates of overall "red-green blindness" in the world (9.1), while the rate for Yemenite Jews is among the lowest (3.8) and the rest of non-Ashkenazi Jewish groups show an average of 6.1.

One of the current controversies among investigators of color blindness centers on the reason for the high rates of red-green blindness among European and a few Asian populations. The contention of one group is that these high rates characterize old civilizations and reflect relaxed selection. Adam has cogently challenged this theory on a number of grounds and points out possible advantages of color blindness for primitive man which may have counteracted natural selection. Furthermore, he states that any discussion of selection and relaxation should be based on data that differentiate between mild and severe defects. Such data are obtainable only

Table 9.2. Frequency of dichromatic and trichromatic red-green deficiencies
in human populations

Population	No. of males examined	Dichro-macies	Trichro-macies	Overall red-green blindness
Jews				
Ashkenazi	778	2.6	6.5	9.1
Other, non-Ashkenazi[a]	635	2.0	4.1	6.1
Yemenite	1,128	1.8	2.0	3.8
Asians				
Japanese	6,586	2.1	2.9	5.0
New Guinena Highlanders[a]	1,135	3.3	1.6	4.9
Papuans[a]	3,685	2.4	2.2	4.6
Southern Chinese	669	2.8	2.9	5.7
Thais	1,658	3.5	2.1	5.6
Europeans				
Various populations	50,264	2.1	5.3	7.4
Other				
Israeli Arabs (2 villages)	1,684	2.4	6.1	8.5
Israeli and Sinai Bedouins[a]	826	1.8	1.6	3.4
Mexican aboriginal Indians[a]	367	1.6	—	1.6
Mexican mestizos and mixed-bloods[a]	795	3.8	1.9	5.7
Chilean Aymara Indians[a]	140	2.9	3.5	6.4

Source: A. Adam, 1969, *Soc. Biol.* 16:197.

[a] Comprising several samples of isolates, sometimes with a wide range of frequencies.

through the use of the anomalscope and thus are lacking for the majority of non-European populations. In addition, most surveys based on pseudoisochromatic plates probably underestimate the rates of trichromatic defects.

In conclusion, available data do not explain why color blindness is most prevalent among European and some Asian populations, or why it is high among Ashkenazi Jews and low among Yemenite Jews.

References

Adam, A. 1969. A further query on color blindness and natural selection. *Soc. Biol.* 16:197.

Adam, A.; Doron, D.; and Modan, B. 1967. Frequencies of protan and deutan alleles in some Israel communities and a note on the selection-relaxation hypothesis. *Am. J. Phys. Anthropol.* 26:287.

Bell, J. 1926. *Colour blindness: Treasure of human inheritance,* vol. 2, pt. 2, pp 125–268. Cambridge: At the University Press.

Kalmus, H. 1965. *Diagnosis and genetics of defective colour vision.* New York: Pergamon Press.

Neel, J. V., and Post, R. H. 1963. Transitory "positive" selection for color blindness? *Eugen. Quart.* 10:33.

Pickford, R. W. 1963. Natural selection and colour blindness. *Eugen. Rev.* 55:97.

Post, R. H. 1965. Notes on relaxed selection in man. *Anthropol. Anz.* 29:186.

Sorsby, A. 1970. *Ophthalmic Genetics,* 2nd ed. New York: Appleton-Century-Crofts.

ESSENTIAL PENTOSURIA

Historical note

Pentosuria was first described in 1892 by Salkowski and Jastrowitz. In 1906 Janeway reported this entity in 2 brothers and stressed the innocuousness of the condition. In 1908 Garrod included this condition among his list of "inborn errors of metabolism" and noted its familial occurrence primarily in Jewish families.

From 1933 to 1955 Enklewitz and Lasker clarified the nature of urinary sugar and accurately described the clinical and genetic features of pentosuria. Various investigators have contributed to our current understanding of the biochemical defect in this disorder, but the foundation for these studies was the work of Touster and associates during the period 1955–1957.

Clinical features

No clinical features or disturbed functions have been demonstrated to result from pentosuria. Unfortunately, some patients have been mistakenly diagnosed and treated for diabetes mellitus, occasionally with severe consequences.

Diagnosis

Pentosuria should be suspected in individuals (particularly those of Ashkenazi Jewish origin) who have none of the symptoms of diabetes mellitus but in whose urine a small quantity of reducing substance is consistently found. The diagnosis can be confirmed by various procedures ranging from the reduction of Benedict's reagent at low temperature, use of paper chromatography, or actual demonstration of the enzymatic defect in the erythrocytes of patients. Chromatography is the most convenient and unequivocal diagnostic method.

The types and causes of pentosuria are listed in Table 9.3.

Basic defect

This metabolic disorder is a manifestation of the defect in the glucuronic acid oxidation pathway which is caused by reduced activity of the NADP-linked xylitol dehydrogenase, the enzyme that catalyzes the conversion of L-xylulose to xylitol.

Genetics

Pentosuria is found predominantly in Ashkenazi Jewish families of Polish-Russian extraction, although a few cases have been reported in non-Jewish Lebanese families.

In one study the rate of consanguinity in marriages that produced pentosuric off-spring was 12.6 percent. Family studies confirm the autosomal recessive transmission of this trait. The incidence in American Jews is estimated to be 1:2,000–1:2,500 births, while in Israel it has been calculated to be 1:5,000 births. The gene frequency among Ashkenazi Jews is approximately 0.02. Heterozygotes can be detected by demonstrating either an intermediate level of erythrocyte activity of the enzyme xylitol dehydrogenase or increased serum or urinary levels of L-xylulose, or both, in a glucuronolactone-loading test.

Prognosis and treatment

Pentosuria is totally benign and no treatment, other than properly informing those who are affected, is indicated.

Table 9.3. Pentosuria: Types and causes

Diagnosis	Urine pentose	Amount of pentose excreted (g/24 hr)	Contributing factor
Normal	L-xylulose	Up to 0.060	
	D-ribose	Up to 0.015	
	D-ribulose	Traces	
"Ribosuria"	D-ribose	Up to 0.030	Muscular dystrophy
Alimentary pentosuria	L-arabinose	Less than 0.100	Excessive fruit intake
	L-xylose	Less than 0.100	Excessive fruit intake
Essential pentosuria	L-xylulose	1.0–4.0	Metabolic error

Source: H. H. Hiatt, 1972, Pentosuria, in *The metabolic basis of inherited disease*, ed. J. B. Stanbury, J. B. Wyngaarden, and D. S. Fredrickson, 3rd ed. (New York: McGraw-Hill), p. 119.

References

Hiatt, H. H. 1972. Pentosuria. In *The metabolic basis of inherited disease*, ed. J. B. Stanbury, J. B. Wyngaarden, and D. S. Fredrickson, 3rd ed., pp. 119–30. New York: McGraw-Hill.

Hollman, S., and Touster, O. 1957. The L-xylulose-xylitol enzyme and other polyol dehydrogenases of guinea pig liver mitochondria. *J. Biol. Chem.* 225:87.

Khachadurian, A. K. 1962. Essential pentosuria. *Am. J. Hum. Genet.* 14:249.

Lasker, M.; Enklewitz, M.; and Lasker, G. W. 1936. The inheritance of L-xyloketosuria (essential pentosuria). *Hum. Biol.* 8:243.

Mizrachi, O., and Ser, I. 1963. Essential pentosuria. In *Genetics of migrant and isolate populations*, ed. E. Goldschmidt, p. 300. Baltimore: Williams and Wilkins.

Politzer, W. M., and Fleischmann, H. 1962. L-xylulosuria in a Lebanese family. *Am. J. Hum. Genet.* 14:256.

Roberts, P. D. 1960. The inheritance of essential pentosuria. *Br. Med. J.* 1:1478.

Salkowski, E., and Jastrowitz, M. 1892. Ueber eine bisher nicht beobachtete Zuckerart im Harn. *Abl. Med. Wiss.* 30:337.

Touster, O.; Reynolds, V. H.; and Hutcheson, R. M. 1956. The reduction of L-xylulose to xylitol by guinea pig liver mitochondria. *J. Biol. Chem.* 221:697.

Wang, Y. M., and Van Eys, J. 1970. The enzymatic defect in essential pentosuria. *N. Engl. J. Med.* 282:892.

FAMILIAL HYPERGLYCINURIA

Historical note

In 1973 Greene and co-workers reported a new genetic variant of familial hyperglycinuria in an Ashkenazi Jewish father and his 2 sons.

Clinical features

The proband, a 22-year-old male college student (III-1), was discovered to have hyperglycinuria at the age of 17 years, when he was a volunteer at the Clinical Center, National Institutes of Health. His past medical history was unremarkable except for a lifelong impaired sense of smell, and his physical examination was normal except for the anosmia.

The proband's 20-year-old brother (III-2) was first evaluated in 1966, at which time his medical history and physical examination were unremarkable. His sense of smell was normal.

The father, a 57-year-old man (II-2), had had several episodes of flank pain compatible with renal colic but had never passed stones or had hematuria. His past history indicated a somewhat reduced sense of smell.

A 58-year-old paternal aunt (II-3) had passed 2 renal stones, neither of which was analyzed. Her 2 sons (III-1 and III-4) were asymptomatic, and the past history of all 3 indicated normal olfaction.

Diagnosis

In the above cases hyperglycinuria was demonstrated by measuring the 24-hour rate of urinary glycine excretion by high voltage electrophoresis and confirming it by column chromatography. The results are shown in Table 9.4. No other amino

Table 9.4. Familial hyperglycinuria: Rate of
urinary glycine excretion per 24 hours

Subject	Mg of glycine excreted/24 hr	Mg of glycine excreted/g creatinine/24 hr
III-1	1,003	463
III-2	1,140	581
II-2	414	207
II-1	105	104
II-3	151	151
III-3	120	53
III-4	218	142

Source: M. L. Greene et al., 1973, *Am. J. Med.* 54:265.
Note: The normal range is 50–300 mg/24 hours.

acids were abnormally excreted; detailed studies of case III-2 showed that the patient's urinary proline excretion rate was 0–10 mg/24 hours, while the rate of excretion of urinary hydroxyproline was 0–5 mg/24 hours. Plasma glycine concentrations were normal in father and sons. The rate of urinary glycine excretion after oral or intravenous loading increased in both sons. Intravenous proline infusion in the younger son (III-2) showed a normal maximal transport rate (Tm) for proline, but, consistent with a "Km" mutation affecting proline binding, there was a marked splay in the renal tubular titration curve for proline reabsorption. Glycine reabsorption was not further depressed by proline infusion. Intestinal glycine absorption and amino acid content of sweat were normal.

Basic defect

The basic defect in familial hyperglycinuria is not known. Greene and co-workers postulate that the transport defect in the above family is limited to the kidney and affects the renal transport system for glycine, proline, and hydroxyproline. They further propose that this mutation be designated, iminoglycinuria type II (see "Familial iminoglycinuria" and "Glycinuria associated with nephrolithiasis").

Genetics

The mode of transmission of this disorder is not entirely clear (Figure 9.3), for investigators lack the information needed to determine whether the sons are homozygous for a previously undescribed type of mutation or are doubly heterozygous for two different mutations affecting the renal transport of glycine and the imino acids. To date, this defect has been described only in the above family, but it is possible that this genetic abnormality is the same as the one described by de Vries and co-workers in Israel in 1957 (see "Glycinuria associated with nephrolithiasis").

Prognosis and treatment

From the information presented it would seem that this inborn error of metabolism is a benign disorder. The renal colic in 1 family member and the anosmia in 2 others may be chance happenings and may not be associated with the metabolic defect.

Reference

Greene, M. L.; Lietman, P. S.; Rosenberg, L. E.; and Seegmiller, J. E. 1973. Familial hyperglycinuria: New defect in renal tubular transport of glycine and imino acids. *Am. J. Med.* 54:265.

FAMILIAL IMINOGLYCINURIA

In 1958 Joseph and co-workers first described familial iminoglycinuria and attributed it to a defect in renal tubular transport. Much has been learned about this disorder since its original description, but a reproducible clinical picture has not emerged from the study of patients with this metabolic defect. Patients have ranged from 1 to 42 years of age. Some have been mentally retarded, but because they were detected in urinary screening programs in retarded children, it is thought that the association between retardation and iminoglycinuria is only fortuitous. Congenital nerve deafness has been noted in 2 boys, but, again, they were detected because of this disability; other cases with deafness have not been recorded. One child with familial iminoglycinuria also had congenital achromatopsia with severe amblyopia.

Individuals with this inborn error of metabolism should be considered healthy. However, because they are well, detection of the disorder depends on screening programs or amino acid studies or other reasons. Homozygotes can be detected without difficulty by using paper chromatographic or electrophoretic studies of urinary amino acid levels (increased presence of the imino acids, proline, and hydroxyproline plus glycine). Determination of plasma proline and hydroxyproline concentrations is necessary to exclude hyperprolinemia and hydroxyprolinemia, which can produce the same aminoaciduria, but for different reasons.

The basic defect in this autosomal recessive inborn error of metabolism is not known. What is known is that glycine and the imino acids are transported in the renal tubules and the intestines by a genetically controlled system with selective

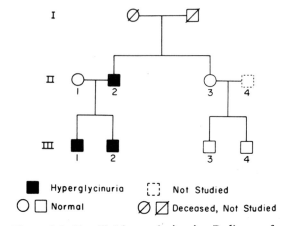

Figure 9.3. Familial hyperglycinuria: Pedigree of the affected family. From M. L. Greene et al., 1973, *Am. J. Med.* 54:265.

affinity for these substances. Furthermore, this shared system is not the only transport mechanism for glycine or the imino acids in the kidney and gut.

As of 1976, familial iminoglycinuria had been reported in approximately 25 unrelated families, several of which have more than a single affected member. Although these families represent different ethnic backgrounds, 3 unrelated families are of Ashkenazi Jewish origin. This seemingly high proportion has suggested to some investigators that the disorder may be more frequent in Ashkenazi Jews than other ethnic groups. However, more information is needed before this impression can be confirmed.

In a screening survey in the United States, Levy found that the frequency of iminoglycinuria was 1:20,000, which approximates that of cystinuria. Genetic heterogeneity in iminoglycinuria is suggested by the fact that some apparent homozygotes show a defect in intestinal absorption of L-proline, whereas others do not, and some obligate heterozygotes show hyperglycinuria upon glycine loading and some do not (see Table 9.5).

In conclusion, this benign inborn error of metabolism requires no treatment. On the basis of presently available information, it should not be considered more common in Ashkenazi Jews than in other populations. (See "Glycinuria with or without oxalate urolithiasis.")

References

Joseph, R.; Ribinerre, M.; Job, J. C.; and Girault, M. 1958. Maladie familiale associante des convulsions à début trés précoce, une hyperalbuminorachie et une hyperaminoacidurie. *Arch. Franç. Pediatr.* 15:374.

Procopis, P. G., and Turner, B. 1971. Iminoaciduria: A benign renal tubular defect. *J. Pediatr.* 79:419.

Rosenberg, L. E.; Durant, J. L.; and Elsas, L. J., II. 1968. Familial iminoglycinuria: An inborn error of renal tubular transport. *N. Engl. J. Med.* 278:1407.

Scriver, C. R. 1972. Familial iminoglycinuria. In *The metabolic basis of disease*, ed. J. B. Stanbury, J. B. Wyngaarden, and D. S. Frederickson 3rd ed., pp. 1520–35. New York: McGraw-Hill.

Scriver, C. R., and Rosenberg, L. E. 1973. *Amino acid metabolism and its disorders*, pp. 178–86. Philadelphia: W. B. Saunders.

Statter, M.; Ben Zvi, A.; Shina, A.; Schein, R.; and Russell, A. 1976. Familial iminoglycinuria with normal intestinal absorption of glycine and imino acids in association with profound mental retardation: A possible "cerebral phenotype." *Helv. Paediatr. Acta* 31:173.

Table 9.5. Familial iminoglycinuria: Indications of genetic heterogeneity

Type	Urinary glycine and imino acids in homozygotes	Intestinal absorption of L-proline in homozygotes	Urinary glycine in heterozygotes
I	Increased	Impaired	Normal
II	Increased	Normal	Normal
III	Increased	Normal	Increased

Source: C. R. Scriver and L. F. Rosenberg, 1973, *Amino acid metabolism and its disorders* (Philadelphia: W. B. Saunders), p. 184.

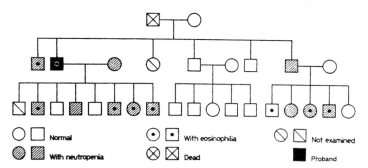

Figure 9.4. Pedigree of a representative Jewish Yemenite family with neutropenia and eosinophilia.

Tancredi, F.; Guazzi, G.; and Auricchio, S. 1970. Renal iminoglycinuria without intestinal malabsorption of glycine and imino acids. *J. Pediatr.* 76:386.

Whelan, D. J., and Scriver, C. R. 1968. Cystathioninuria and renal iminoglycinuria in a pedigree: A perspective on counselling. *N. Engl. J. Med.* 278:924.

FAMILIAL NEUTROPENIA

Familial neutropenia was first reported in 1941 by Gäensslen, who described it as an asymptomatic trait transmitted in an autosomal dominant manner. In 1958 de Vries and co-workers observed the first case of this condition in Israel in a Jewish family originating from Libya. In 1961 Djaldetti and his group collected data on 11 Jewish Yemenite families with familial neutropenia. In 1968 Feinaro and Alkan reviewed the medical records of 780 Jewish patients of Yemenite origin and found 16 cases of unequivocal neutropenia. In a study of 104 relatives of these 16 patients, 80 were found to have persistent neutropenia. An average of 1,533 neutrophils/mm^3 was found among this neutropenic group, with a range of 380–2,840/mm^3. This neutropenia remained constant in 5 patients when they developed intercurrent infections. Neither a shift to the left nor any morphologic changes were observed in the white blood cells of these patients.

Thirty-three (42 percent) of the 80 neutropenics had an absolute eosinophilia (more than 250/mm^3), with a range of 350–850/mm^3, while only 3 of 40 controls were found to have an eosinophilia of 320/mm^3. The red blood cells and thrombocytes of these patients were normal, as were all aspects of clotting.

Family studies confirmed the autosomal dominant transmission of both the neutropenia and the concomitant eosinophilia in some cases (Figure 9.4). No causative factor was found that would explain the eosinophilia.

Neutropenia is considered to be a benign disorder and is not known to be associated with any other malformation or disease. Although approximately 2 percent of the 800 Yemenite Jews screened for neutropenia in Feinaro and Alkan's study showed a persistent neutropenia, additional genetic studies are needed to better assess the frequency of this trait among the Yemenite Jewish community of Israel. Further investigative studies are also needed to clarify the possible relationship between neutropenia and eosinophilia in this disorder, in cyclic neutropenia, and in an entity referred to as lethal congenital neutropenia with eosinophilia.

References

Andrews, J. P.; McClellan, J. T.; and Scott, C. H. 1960. Lethal congenital neutropenia with eosinophilia occurring in two siblings. *Ann. J. Med* 29:358.

Cutting, H. O., and Lang, J. E. 1964. Familial benign chronic neutropenia. *Ann. Intern. Med.* 61:876.

De Vries, A.; Peketh, L.; and Joshua, H. 1958. Leukemia and agranulocytosis in a member of a family with hereditary leukopenia. *Acta Med. Orient.* 17:26.

Djaldetti, M.; Joshua, H.; and Kalderon, M. 1961. Familial leukopenia in Yemenite Jews. *Bull. Res. Coun. Israel* 9:24.

Feinaro, M., and Alkan, W. J. 1968. Familial neutropenia in Jews of Yemenite origin. *Proc. 9th Int. Cong. Life Ass. Med.*, p. 172. Basel: Karger.

Gäensslen, M. 1941. Konstitutionelle familiäre Leukopenie (Neutropenie). *Klin. Wochenschr.* 37:922.

Morley, A. A.; Carew, J. P.; and Baikie, A. G. 1967. Familial cyclical neutropenia. *Br. J. Haematol.* 13:719.

HAIRY EARS

In 1960 Dronamraju's report on coarse hairs on the pinna of the ear supported the earlier hypothesis that this trait is Y-linked. In 1963 Slatis and Apelbaum, reporting on hairy ears in just under 900 men from various Israeli populations, concluded that the potential for hair on the pinna of the ear is present in about a quarter of Israeli Jews (Table 9.6). According to their studies, the age of onset of this trait is variable and late. The earliest age of onset on record is 20 years, but penetrance does not appear to be complete until very late in life. Slatis and Apelbaum also concluded that this trait is determined by a gene on the Y chromosome.

However, controversy exists as to whether this trait is Y-linked, autosomal, or perhaps both. In 1970 Rao proposed that hairy ears result from the interaction of 2 loci, 1 on the homologous segments of the X and Y chromosomes and 1 on the nonhomologous segment of the Y chromosome.

Table 9.6. Frequency of hairy pinna among Jewish Israeli men according to community of origin and age

Age group (yr)	Ashkenazim		Iraqi-Iranians		North Africans		Yemenites		Others		All men			% with HP
	N	HP	N	HP	N	HP	N	HP	N	HP	N	HP	Total	
18–29	226	3	47	0	27	0	7	1	62	0	369	4	373	0.011
30–39	30	1	23	2	12	0	4	2	12	0	81	5	86	0.058
40–49	36	4	12	2	5	1	2	0	5	4	60	11	71	0.155
50–59	68	6	16	2	9	3	1	1	5	2	99	14	113	0.124
60–69	57	12	23	10	7	2	7	0	5	5	99	29	128	0.227
70–99	43	13	13	9	7	1	5	1	4	1	72	25	97	0.258

Source: H. M. Slatis and A. Apelbaum, 1963, *Am. J. Hum. Genet.* 15:74–85. Copyright, 1963, Grune & Stratton, Inc., for the American Society of Human Genetics. Reprinted by permission of The University of Chicago Press.

Note: N = normal; HP = hairy pinna.

Among Ashkenazi men the gene for hairy ears seems to occur most often as an allele that causes hair to grow at the top of the ear. Among Iraqi-Iranian Jewish men the most common allele seems to cause hair to grow at the side of the ear (Figure 9.5). Among Indians there may be a hairy pinna allele that causes an early onset of the trait. Among all men of European ancestry (Jewish and non-Jewish) the frequency of the trait is much higher than previously suspected. The reason for this is that among affected Europeans the hair about the ears is less likely to be obvious: (1) in men with brown, blond, or red hair, the hairs on the pinna may be unpigmented; (2) the site of these hairs is less often the side of the ear, which is the most easily observed position; (3) age of onset of hairy ears is later in Europeans, which reduces the frequency of affected men at a given gene frequency; and (4) this hair is probably cut.

Observations have also been made on hair on other parts of the body, including the tragus of the ear, head, surface of the nose, and chest. Some interrelationships have been found but are not striking. Some are due to separate correlations with age. After correction for the age effect a correlation remains between hair on the pinna and hair on the tragus, but growth at these two sites appears to be controlled by basically independent events.

References

Dronamraju, K. R. 1960. Hypertrichosis of the pinna of the human ear: Y-linked pedigrees. *J. Genet.* 57:230.

Rao, D. C. 1970. A contribution to the genetics of hypertrichosis of the ear rims. *Hum. Hered.* 20:486.

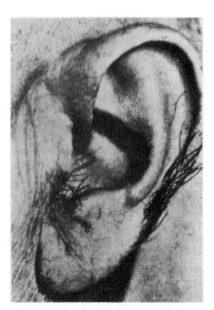

Figure 9.5. Hairy ear. Note the coarse hairs on the side of the pinna and around the tragus.

———. 1972. Hypertrichosis of the ear rims: Two remarks on the two-gene hypothesis. *Acta Genet. Med. Gemellol.* 21:216.

Slatis, H. M., and Apelbaum, A. 1963. Hairy pinna of the ear in Israeli populations. *Am. J. Hum. Genet.* 15:74.

HEREDITARY DEFICIENCY OF PEROXIDASE AND PHOSPHOLIPIDS IN EOSINOPHILIC GRANULOCYTES
(PRESENTEY ANOMALY)

Various genetic anomalies involving leukocytes have been reported in the literature. One of the more recent ones was first described by Presentey in 1968 and pertains to the eosinophilic granulocytes. This anomaly is characterized by a deficiency of peroxidase and phospholipids in the eosinophilic granules and occasionally by hypersegmentation of the nucleus with hypogranulation (see Figures 9.6 and 9.7). No illness is known to be associated with this finding. The biochemical defect that causes this morphologic variant is not known, but it is transmitted by an autosomal recessive gene.

When this genetic anomaly was first reported it was thought to occur primarily among the North African and Asian Jewish communities, with an especially high frequency among Yemenite Jews. More recent studies show that this morphologic trait is also common among Israeli Arabs, and a few cases have been found in the Ashkenazi Jewish community and in non-Jewish European populations. Table 9.7 lists the frequencies among the various Israeli Jewish and Arab communities.

References

Joshua, H.; Spitzer, A.; and Presentey, B. 1970. The incidence of peroxidase and phospholipid deficiency in eosinophilic granulocytes among various Jewish groups in Israel. *Am. J. Hum. Genet.* 22:574.

Joshua, H.; Zucker, A.; and Presentey, B. 1976. Peroxidase and phospholipid deficiency

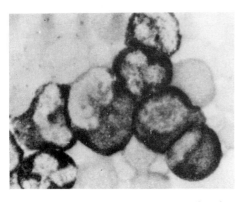

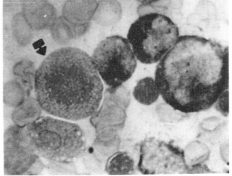

Figure 9.6. Normal bone marrow showing staining for phospholipids with Sudan Black using Lison's method. Courtesy of B. Presentey, Israel.

Figure 9.7. Negative reaction of an eosinophil myelocyte (arrow) to Sudan Black stain.

Table 9.7. Frequency of Presentey anomaly in various ethnic groups in Israel

Ethnic group	No. of individuals	Frequency of affected individuals	Frequency of carriers	Gene frequency
Jews				
Yemenites	1,166	1:116	1:6.9	0.092
North Africans	1,096	1:365	1:9.6	0.052
Iraqis, Persians	799	1:799	1:14.3	0.035
Arabs	1,182	1:591	1:12.2	0.041

Source: H. Joshua et al., 1976, *Israel J. Med. Sci.* 12:71.

in eosinophilic granulocytes among Arabs of the Nazareth district. *Israel J. Med. Sci.* 12:71.

Presentey, B. Z. 1968. A new anomaly of eosinophilic granulocytes. *Tech. Bull. Reg. Med. Technol.* 38:887.

———. 1969. Cytochemical characterization of eosinophils with respect to a newly discovered anomaly. *Am. J. Clin. Pathol.* 51:451, 1969.

———. 1970. Partial and severe peroxidase and phospholipid deficiency in eosinophils: Cytochemical and genetic considerations. *Acta Haematol.* 44:345.

LACK OF PERMANENT UPPER CANINES AND LACK OF WISDOM TEETH

In 1936 Grüneberg reported an Ashkenazi Jewish family with 2 independent genetically determined anomalies of the teeth. The husband lacked permanent upper canines, his wife lacked wisdom teeth, and various combinations of these defects were present in their offspring.

Grüneberg rightly pointed out that the absence of these teeth causes no more than a cosmetic disturbance and went on to state that the biological importance of lack of permanent upper canines must be viewed in terms of the species in which it is noted. If, for example, the same anomaly were observed in the lion, it would be considered a very serious handicap and would probably be classified as a sublethal trait.

In view of the troubles so often encountered at the eruption of wisdom teeth, the lack of 2 or more such teeth in the mother and in 4 of her 5 children may be regarded as a favorable trait, having possibly a slight positive selective value.

Lack of permanent upper canines and lack of wisdom teeth are transmitted as autosomal dominant traits. The combination of the 2 anomalies in the same family is rare (no other cases reported to date), but there is little reason to consider these genetic abnormalities as being limited to Ashkenazi Jews. Independently the 2 findings are not rare.

References

Dolamore, W. H. 1925. Absent canines. *Br. Dent. J.* 46:5.
Gorlin, R. J., and Goldman, H. M. 1970. *Thoma's oral pathology*, 6th ed., 1:148–54. St. Louis: C. V. Mosby.
Grüneberg, H. 1936. Two independent inherited tooth anomalies in one family. *J. Hered.* 27:225.

LACTOSE INTOLERANCE

Historical note

In 1881 Traube described his own lactose intolerance and expressed his great personal satisfaction with the laxative effect of 9–15 g taken in milk every morning. In 1911 Finkelstein recognized that some infants with diarrhea tolerated carbohydrates poorly. However, lactose intolerance in infants as it is known today was first described by Durand in 1958. The first reports on lactose intolerance appeared in 1963 with confirmation of lactase deficiency and the demonstration that the activity of other disaccharidases was normal. In 1966 Bayless and Rosensweig called attention to the racial and ethnic features of this defect. In 1968 and 1970 two reports showed the relatively high frequency of this disorder among most of the Jewish ethnic groups of Israel.

Clinical features

The clinical features of lactose intolerance (LI) vary markedly and the first symptoms usually appear in the late teens. Many people with LI are asymptomatic, while others who ingest milk complain of mild diarrhea with or without cramps and borborygmi upon ingestion of threshold quantities of milk or lactose. Stools after the intake of such quantities are watery, may have a sour odor, and are frothy in appearance.

The quantity of milk required to produce symptoms of LI varies considerably and is not related to the absolute level of lactase activity in the mucosa. Thus, some patients with LI tolerate normal or large amounts of milk, while others are sensitive to small quantities.

Steatorrhea occurs only where there is a clear predisposition, as in rapid intestinal transit due to hyperthyroidism. In general, steatorrhea is not considered to be a clinical feature of LI in adults.

Diagnosis

Oral lactose tolerance tests with analyses of blood sugar at various time intervals have been advocated as highly reliable in ascertaining LI, but 30 percent of patients with normal lactase activity by assay of intestinal biopsy show flat responses when venous blood is analyzed. Use of capillary blood eliminates these falsely flat tests but apparently produces a falsely normal increase in blood sugar in 40 percent of lactose intolerant patients. It has been suggested that administering the capillary lactose tolerance test after ingestion of 1 gram of sugar per kilogram body weight yields few false positive or negative results.

Table 9.8 shows the frequency of symptoms that occur with lactose tolerance tests in lactose intolerant patients and in hospital patients with normal lactase activity.

Littman points out the pitfalls in mucosal assay by emphasizing that only a single area of the small intestine is sampled and some mucosal lesions have a patchy distribution. Thus, a single specimen may overestimate or underestimate the capacity of the small intestine to digest and absorb disaccharides.

Table 9.8. Frequency of symptoms occurring with
lactose tolerance tests in 104 Israeli patients

Symptom	% with normal lactase activity	% with deficient lactase activity
Cramps	9.9	45.4
Diarrhea	7.0	36.4
Distention	4.2	18.2
One or more of the above symptoms	15.5	66.7
None of the above symptoms	84.5	33.3

Source: A. Littman et al., 1968, *Israel J. Med. Sci.* 4:110.

Final confirmation of a diagnosis of LI is the dramatic response usually noted when the sugar is completely eliminated from the diet.

Basic defect

The basic defect in LI is a deficiency of intestinal lactase activity. Most mammals other than man have abundant intestinal lactase at birth which wanes within days to months with weaning. It has been suggested that the loss of lactase occurs with maturation and is probably the normal condition for man.

Genetics

Table 9.9 shows the distribution of LI in various populations of the world. Gilat and co-workers found that approximately two-thirds of the Jewish population in Israel is lactase deficient. Table 9.10 shows a breakdown of this deficiency among the Jewish ethnic groups based on results of lactose tolerance tests. This table also points out the important clinical finding that most lactose intolerant patients are not aware of milk intolerance. Thus, the condition tends to be relatively benign and asymptomatic among the Jews of Israel.

The frequency of this defect among Israeli Jews is not homogenous and the differences among some groups were found to be significant. Geographical location, socioeconomic conditions, and milk-drinking habits proved to be of no importance in this study. This correlates well with other studies, for the major determinant is the ethnic origin of the population being studied.

The frequency of lactase deficiency in healthy adults from several racial groups (Table 9.9) suggests that this enzyme deficiency is genetically transmitted. Good evidence indicates autosomal recessive inheritance, but some investigators support autosomal dominant transmission of this trait.

Two theories have been offered to explain the great difference in frequency of LI between African and Asian populations (high incidence) and Europeans and their descendants (low incidence). One theory proposes that conditions of genetic selection may have led some groups to have persistently high levels of intestinal lactase and others not. A low incidence of tolerance would develop over time in a group that had an abundant milk supply, that had alternate food stuffs inadequate in amount and quality, and that consumed milk in lactose-rich forms. Since such

Table 9.9. Lactase deficiency in various world populations

Population and country studied	Ethnic group	No. of subjects studied	% of subjects lactase deficient
Europeans			
England	English	67	22
	Greek Cypriots	17	88
Switzerland	Swiss	17	6
U.S.	Caucasians	447	11 (2–19)
Australia	Caucasians	12	16
Blacks			
U.S.	Blacks	107	74 (70–77)
Uganda	Bantu	52	90
	Other tribes	63	9–44
Far Easterners			
U.S.	Chinese, Japanese, Koreans	11	100
	Chinese, Filipinos	20	95
Australia	Chinese, Indian	20	85
Others			
Australia	Aborigines	44	80–90
Colombia	Antioqueños	29	38
	Mestizos	16	25
U.S.	American Indians	3	67
Israel	Jews	354	68 (44–85)

Source: T. Gilat et al., 1970, *Am. J. Dig. Dis.* 15:895.

selection could not have occurred among groups that did not use milk, areas of nonmilking in the modern world are the first to be delimited. The origins and diffusion of dairying are then sketched to determine the length of time that milk has been consumed in various regions (Figure 9.8), and thus the present-day high and low incidences of intolerance in various Old World groups are explained. The groups within traditional nonmilking areas show high incidences of intolerance. American blacks, whose ancestors came from nonmilking regions, also have high

Table 9.10. Results of lactose tolerance tests among Israeli Jews

Ethnic group	No. of subjects studied	Glucose rise < 20		Glucose rise > 20		% with glucose rise < 20
		No. with symptoms (lactose intolerant)	No. without symptoms	No. with symptoms	No. without symptoms (lactose tolerant)	
Yemenites	36	15	1	—	20	44.4
Sephardim						
North African	32	17	3	—	12	62.5
Others	36	24	2	2	8	72.2
Ashkenazim	53[a]	32	10	3	8	79.2
Iraqis	38	31	1	1	5	84.2
Orientals (others)	20	13	4	—	3	85.0
Total and average	215	132	21	6	56	71.1

Source: T. Gilat et al., 1970, *Am. J. Dig. Dis.* 15:895.

[a] Two Ashkenazim, in whom symptoms were not adequately recorded, are not included in this table.

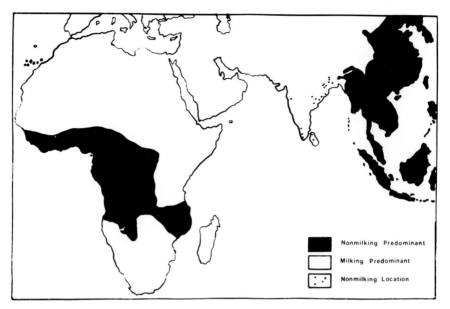

Figure 9.8. Traditional areas of milking and nonmilking. From F. J. Simoons, 1970, *Am. J. Dig. Dis.* 15:695.

incidences of intolerance. Moreover, within the milking areas of Africa and Europe, the known group differences in tolerance are in accord with this postulate.

A different view suggests that the advantage conveyed by the adult LI gene(s) lies in an improvement of calcium absorption by lactose tolerant individuals; this, in turn, prevents rickets and osteomalacia in an environment where the nutritional supply of vitamin D is low and its production in the skin is insufficient because of low ultraviolet irradiation.

Each postulate seems plausible, but how does one explain the puzzling high frequency among most of the Jewish ethnic groups? Perhaps the latter theory is reasonable, since Jews originated from an area with much sunshine and thus did not need to maintain a high level of lactose tolerance. The similar frequency of this trait in most of the Jewish communities (lower among Yemenite Jews) has been cited by some geneticists to support the theory of the common ancient Mideastern ancestry of the Jewish people.

Prognosis and treatment

The prognosis in the adult form of LI is excellent as long as individuals with symptoms refrain from ingesting lactose.

References

Bayless, T. M., and Rosensweig, N. S. 1966. A racial difference in incidence of lactase deficiency. *JAMA* 197:968.

Bayless, T. M., et al. 1975. Lactose and milk tolerance: Clinical implications. *N. Engl. J. Med.* 292:1156.

Charney, M., and McCracken, R. D. 1971. Intestinal lactase deficiency in adult non-human primates: Implications for selection pressures in man. *Soc. Biol.* 18:416.

Durand, P. 1958. Lattosuria idiopatica in una paziente con diarrea cronica et acidosi. *Minerva Pediatr.* 10:706.

Flatz, G., and Rotthauwe, H. W. 1973. Lactose nutrition and natural selection. *Lancet* 2:76.

Gilat, T.; Kuhn, R.; Gelman, E.; and Mizrahy, O. 1970. Lactase deficiency in Jewish communities in Israel. *Am. J. Dig. Dis.* 15:895.

Kretchmer, N. 1972. Lactose and lactase. *Scientific American*, no. 4, p. 70.

Littman, A. 1976. *Disaccharidase deficiencies in gastroenterology*, ed. H. L. Bockus, 3rd ed., 2: 334–60. Philadelphia: W. B. Saunders.

Rozen, P., and Shafrir, E. 1968. Behavior of serum free fatty acids and glucose during lactose tolerance tests. *Israel J. Med. Sci.* 4:100.

Sahi, T. 1974. The inheritance of selective adult-type lactose malabsorption. *Scand. J. Gastroenterol.* 9 (suppl. 30): 1.

Simoons, F. J. 1970. Primary adult lactose intolerance and the milking habit: A problem in biologic and cultural interrelations. II. A culture historical hypothesis. *Am. J. Dig. Dis.* 15:695.

Traube, M. 1881. Ueber den Milchzucker als Medicament. *Dtsch. Med. Wochenschr.* 7:113.

LEFT-HANDEDNESS

The frequency of left-handedness in man ranges from 1 percent to 30 percent. This great variability is influenced by such factors as age, sex, and method of ascertainment. It would appear from reports in the literature that the frequency of left-handedness also varies among ethnic groups. However, it is often impossible to compare these frequencies because studies are designed so differently and the definitions of phenotypes are far from uniform.

In 1972 Goodman and Adam conducted a survey of the frequency of left-handedness among the various Jewish ethnic groups in Israel. The survey was carried out in 8 secondary schools in the Tel Aviv area and involved 3,463 students between the ages of 14 and 18 years. The schools were selected on the basis of parental representation of the major Jewish ethnic communities in Israel: Ashkenazi, Iraqi, North African (in this sample, mainly Moroccan and Libyan), Yemenite (including Aden), and Sephardi (mainly the Balkan countries and Turkey). Each student filled out a detailed questionnaire containing family questions and queries concerning the use of the hands. On the basis of the numerous combinations of replies, 5 "phenotypes" were defined: (1) *left-handed*, a person who has never switched to the right and performs all tasks with the left hand; (2) *predominantly left-handed*, a person who writes with the left hand, but does one or more tasks with the right or both hands, or a person who writes and may perform more tasks with the right hand, but was born left-handed and later changed; (3) *ambidextrous*, a person who writes and does other tasks with both hands equally well (frequently having been left-handed in the past); (4) *predominantly right-handed*, a person who writes with the right hand, but does one or more other tasks with the left or both hands (without ever having been left-handed); (5) *right-handed*, a person who performs all tasks with the right hand and has never been left-handed.

Table 9.11. Distribution of handedness among 3,463 Jewish teen-agers in Israel
by sex and community

Sex and community	Phenotypes[a]						
	L	pL	Amb.	pR	R	Total	% L + pL
Males							
Ashkenazi	42	56	7	75	417	597	16.4
Iraqi	20	12	4	43	187	266	12.0
North African	6	7	—	22	86	121	10.8
Yemenite	5	4	1	27	104	141	6.4
Sephardi	15	13	3	16	97	144	19.4
Mixed, other	13	11	4	25	134	187	12.8
Total and average	101	103	19	208	1,025	1,456	14.0
Females							
Ashkenazi	50	39	7	76	652	824	10.8
Iraqi	28	15	1	51	283	378	11.4
North African	11	3	2	29	165	210	6.7
Yemenite	3	7	1	28	148	187	5.3
Sephardi	6	15	—	18	140	179	11.7
Mixed, other	20	17	1	12	179	229	16.2
Total and average	118	96	12	214	1,567	2,007	10.4

[a] L = left-handed; pL = predominantly left-handed; Amb. = ambidextrous; pR = predominantly right-handed; R = right-handed.

The distribution of the 5 phenotypes among the population samples is shown in Table 9.11. Males and females are listed separately. In each section of the table an additional row ("Mixed, other") comprises students whose 4 grandparents were not from identical communities or belonged to small or unknown communities.

The combined percentages of left and predominantly left-handedness appear in the last column and are used in the following analyses. Note that overall there is a significantly higher rate of left-handedness among males (14 percent) than among females (10.4 percent), with $\chi^2 = 8.88$ and $p < .01$.

Except for the mixed group, the rate of left-handedness is higher among males in each of the communities, but this is statistically significant only for the largest subsample, "Ashkenazi."

A marked heterogeneity is evident among the communities, the highest frequencies being more than double those of the lowest. Again, excluding the mixed group, the ranking of communities by rate of left-handedness is similar (though not identical) for males and females, with the Sephardim having the highest frequencies and the Yemenites the lowest.

A comparison of the frequencies of left and predominantly left-handedness to all others proves that the heterogeneity among the communities is statistically significant ($p < .01$) for males ($\chi^2 = 15.35$) and females ($\chi^2 = 16.76$).

One hundred and seven students (3.1 percent of the whole sample) stated that they had been left-handed in childhood but had switched to the right. In most cases the change had been initiated by their parents.

The rate of consanguinity was lower among parents of the left-handed than among parents of the others, but the difference was not statistically significant.

Despite the fact that it is extremely difficult to compare the frequencies of handedness in this study with those from other surveys, some comments can be made regarding the findings. With regard to the sex distribution of handedness, the observations from the above study agree with most previous ones, that more males than females are left-handed, but the usually stated male:female ratio of 2:1 was not found among the individual Jewish communities in Israel.

Although much variability exists in the rates of handedness reported among various populations, Lord Brain stated in 1965 that "it is safe to say that between 5 and 10 percent of the population of Great Britain and the U.S.A. are left-handed." If this statement is valid, the overall rate of left-handedness among Jews in Israel—14.0 percent in males and 10.4 percent in females—is higher than that found among non-Jews in England and the U.S. Again, the even higher frequency of left-handedness among the individual Jewish ethnic groups (exceptions being the Yemenite and North African communities) suggests differing frequencies in different ethnic groups. At the same time, within the overall Jewish population of both males and females, one finds a wide range in the rate of left-handedness.

It is important to note that the Israeli students who were surveyed all attended schools for normal children. Thus, the higher frequency of left-handedness in children with speech disorders or certain forms of mental retardation was not a factor in the frequency found in this survey. There were no known monozygotic twins in the survey, which also would increase the frequency of left-handedness.

Many theories have been proposed to explain the etiology of handedness. From questions asked in the above survey pertaining to handedness in other family members, it would seem that genetic factors are operating. They are probably multifactorial in nature, so it is unlikely that handedness is determined by simple Mendelian inheritance.

Before firm comparative conclusions can be drawn regarding the frequency of left-handedness in Jews versus non-Jews, similar studies must be done in other populations.

References

Annett, M. 1964. A model of the inheritance of handedness and cerebral dominance. *Nature* 204:59.
———. 1973. Handedness in families. *Ann. Genet.* 37:93.
Bakan, P. 1971. Handedness and birth order. *Nature* 229:195.
Brain, W. R. 1965. *Speech Disorders: Aphasia, apraxia, and agnosia*, 2nd ed. pp. 23–31. London: Butterworths.
Coren, S., and Porac, C. 1977. Fifty centuries of right-handedness: The historic record. *Science* 198:631.
Goodman, R. M. and Adam, A. 1972. Handedness among teenagers in Israel. Unpublished data.
Hecaen, H., and de Ajuriaguerra, J. 1964. *Left-handedness: Manual superiority and cerebral dominance*. New York: Grune and Stratton.
Huheey, J. E. 1977. Concerning the origin of handedness in humans. *Behav. Genet.* 7:29.
Levy, J. 1976. A review of evidence for a genetic component in the determination of handedness. *Behav. Genet.* 6:429.
Levy, J., and Nagylaki, T. 1972. A model for the genetics of handedness. *Genetics* 72:117.

Rife, D. C. 1940. Handedness with special reference to twins. *Genetics* 25:178.

Sutton, P. R. N. 1963. Handedness and facial asymmetry: Lateral position of the nose in two racial groups. *Nature* 198:909.

OVOID PUPILS

In 1937 White and Fulton described a very rare pupillary defect in female monozygotic twins and their Ashkenazi Jewish mother. An extensive search of the literature has failed to show other cases of this defect.

Clinically, all affected members were well and the genetic abnormality of the pupils did not interfere with visual acuity. Upon physical examination the pupils were found to be extremely large and irregular. They responded to light and accommodation only in the superior temporal quadrant and (very slightly) in the inferior nasal quadrant (Figure 9.9). Peripheral visual fields and visual acuity were normal as were the ophthalmoscopic examinations. The findings in the twins were identical except that one twin (C.L.), under the strain of strong illumination, showed a more marked constriction of the right pupil.

The characteristic pupillary features of this abnormality are: (a) dilation, (b) irregularity, and (c) reaction to constricting stimuli only in the superior temporal quadrant and to a lesser extent in the inferior nasal quadrant. Slit-lamp examination did not reveal definite evidence of coloboma in either the iris or the choroid. There was a small retinal nevus in the right eye of C.L., a finding often noted in the presence of colobomata.

The basic defect in ovid pupils is not known. It has been suggested that the deformity represents an inherent deficiency in the sphincter iridis muscle.

The pedigree shown in Figure 9.10 is compatible with autosomal dominant transmission with possibly reduced penetrance. The fact that only females are affected makes it plausible that this is an X-linked dominant or even a sex-influenced trait.

Since ovoid pupils is not associated with a pathological state, the prognosis is excellent and no treatment is indicated.

Reference

White, B. V., Jr., and Fulton, M. N. 1937. A rare pupillary defect inherited by identical twins. *J. Hered.* 28:177.

PERSISTENT MILD HYPERPHENYLALANINEMIA

Approximately one-quarter of all patients with hyperphenylalaninemia have a "mild" or "benign" type of hyperphenylalaninemia without phenylketonuria (PKU). In the beginning this metabolic defect was recognized in North Americans of Mediterranean background, and thus this association fostered the eponym "Mediterranean hyperphenylalaninemia." The term has now been abandoned because the trait is known to occur widely among Anglo-Saxons (particularly Scots), Central Europeans, Arabs, and Jews (including Ashkenazim, among whom classical PKU is very rare) (see section on PKU, p. 179).

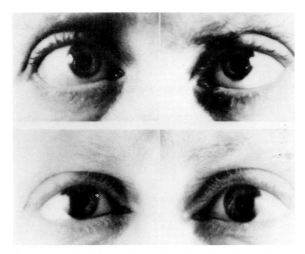

Figure 9.9. Ovoid pupils. In bright light the pupils can contract only in certain regions and thus take on an ovoid shape.

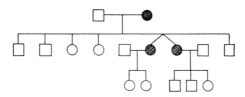

Figure 9.10. Ovoid pupils: Family pedigree showing the mother and her affected twin daughters.

Table 9.12 shows the ethnic distribution of the persistent mild hyperphenylalaninemia observed in Israel from 1964 to 1972. Fifty-seven percent of all sibships were of Sephardi or Oriental Jewish origin—the majority of these being from North Africa—while almost 20 percent of the total number of sibships were Ashkenazi. Another interesting finding was that only 3 marriages were consanguineous, which is well within the normal consanguinity rate for these ethnic groups.

A total of 62 cases in 48 families revealed multiple cases in some families. All parents had normal phenylalanine levels, which supports the concept of autosomal recessive transmission of this trait. The different ethnic distribution and consanguinity rates for this disorder and PKU led Cohen and co-workers to conclude that PKU and hyperphenylalaninemia are genetically different metabolic defects possibly caused by an allele of the PKU gene. This concept has also been proposed by others.

From a clinical and laboratory viewpoint, the postnatal rise in plasma phenylalanine is usually slower in persistent mild hyperphenylalaninemia than in classical PKU, and the plateau reached is below 1 mM, even when the dietary intake of phenylalanine is unrestricted. Phenylpyruvate and its derivatives are not formed in significant amounts. Normal development of cognitive functions in affected children

Table 9.12. Cases of persistent mild
hyperphenylalaninemia in Israel

Ethnic group	No. of sibships	Consanguinity	No. of cases
Jews from:			
North Africa	13	2	23
Iran	3		4
Yemen	4		4
Syria	1		1
Iraq	3		3
Mixed	4		4
Ashkenazim	10		12
Israeli Arabs	8	1	9
Unknown	2	–	2
Total	48	3	62

Source: B. E. Cohen et al., 1973, *Israel J. Med. Sci.*
9:1393.
Note: The IQ of only 2 individuals was less than 80.

in the absence of treatment is the most important clinical feature of this form of hyperphenylaninemia.

Phenylalanine-loading tests show that the rate of clearance of phenylalanine from plasma is slower than normal in the probands, yet faster than that in homozygotes with classical PKU. Another distinguishing feature is that the level of plasma tyrosine rises in the hyperphenylalaninemic patient after a phenylalanine load, but it does not in the PKU patient.

The enzymatic mechanism of hyperphenylalaninemia has been examined by several investigators. In each case a significant level of residual phenylalanine hydroxylation activity was found in the biopsied liver material. This residual activity, which was about 10–20 percent of normal, could be increased at least threefold by the addition of synthetic cofactor (dimethyltetrahydropterin) to the incubation mixture. It has been speculated that the substrate (phenylalanine) could inhibit a mutant form of the enzyme in the presence of the natural coenzyme *in vivo* and that this inhibition could perhaps be alleviated by the therapeutic use of synthetic cofactor.

In conclusion, this form of hyperphenylalaninimia should be considered a non-pathological trait. No therapeutic measures are indicated.

References

Cohen, B. E.; Szeinberg, A.; Pollak, S.; Peled, I.; Likverman, S.; and Crispin, M. 1973. The hyperphenylalaninemias in Israel. *Israel J. Med. Sci.* 9:1393.

Levy, H. C.; Shih, V. E.; Karolkewicz, V.; Frerich, W. A.; Carr, J. R.; Cass, V.; Kennedy, J. L., Jr.; and McCrady, R. A. 1971. Persistent mild hyperphenylalaninemia in the untreated state: A prospective study. *N. Engl. J. Med.* 285:424.

Scriver, C. R. 1967. Diagnosis and treatment: Interpreting the positive screening test in the newborn infant. *Pediatrics* 39:764.

Scriver, C. R., and Rosenberg, L. E. 1973. *Amino Acid Metabolism and Its Disorders*, pp. 390–37. Philadelphia: W. B. Saunders.

Woolf, L. I.; Goodwin, B. C.; Cranston, W. I.; Wade, D. N.; Woolf, F.; Hudson, F. P.;

and McBean, M. S. 1968. A third allele at the phenylalalanine-hydroxylase locus in mild phenylketanuria (hyperphenylalaninemia). *Lancet* 1:114.

STUB THUMBS

Brachydactyly of the terminal phalanx of the thumb (stub thumbs) has been observed in various ethnic groups. In 1963 the late Dr. Chaim Sheba called to my attention the common occurrence of this malformation among Jews in Israel (Figure 9.11). Soon thereafter, a genetic survey of this trait was undertaken to determine its frequency among the various ethnic groups in Israel.

Table 9.13 shows the prevalence of this trait among various populations in Israel and Table 9.14 gives the distribution of this trait in the families of 61 probands. No significant difference in the prevalence of this genetic malformation was observed among the various Jewish communities. Approximately 1.6 percent of the Jewish population and 3 percent of the Israeli Arab population were affected, half of them bilaterally. Males and females were affected equally. Autosomal dominant inheritance was confirmed and penetrance was approximately 40 percent.

The frequency of stub thumbs among non-Jews is extremely low. In 1957 Stecher noted frequencies of 0.41 percent and 0.1 percent, respectively, in U.S. white and black populations. The higher frequency found among Israeli Arabs may be due to bias in ascertainment. It would be of interest to know whether the frequency is comparable in Arab populations of other countries.

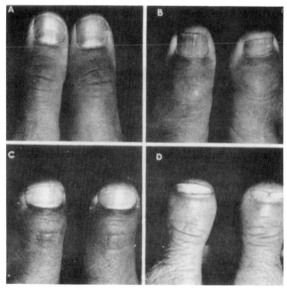

Figure 9.11. (A) Normal thumbs. (B) Only right thumb affected. (C) Bilaterally affected thumbs. (D) Severely affected thumbs. Note the extremely short, wide nails and the flaring of the distal ends of the abnormal thumbs.

Table 9.13. Prevalence of stub thumbs in Israeli communities (random samples)

Community	Sex	No. examined	People with affected thumbs				%	± standard error
			Right	Left	Both	Total		
Jews								
Ashkenazim (Central and Eastern Europe)	M	584	5	1	2	8	1.66	0.44
	F	261	—	3	3	6		
Sephardim								
Southern Europe	M	182	—	2	1	3	1.89	0.94
	F	30	—	—	1	1		
North Africa	M	254	—	—	2	2	0.99	0.57
	F	48	—	—	1	1		
Orientals, Iraqis, and Iranians	M	250	1	2	1	4	1.80	0.80
	F	28	—	—	1	1		
Yemenites	M	179	1	1	1	3	1.41	0.81
	F	34	—	—	—	—		
Total no. and average rate	M and F	1,850	7	9	13	29	1.57	0.29
Arabs (Israeli)	M	496	1	5	6	12		
	F	391	4	2	9	15		
Total no. and average rate	M and F	887	5	7	15	27	3.05	0.58

Source: R. M. Goodman et al., 1965, *J. Med. Genet.* 2:116.

Table 9.14. Distribution of stub thumbs in families of 61 Israeli probands

No. of thumbs affected	No. of probands	Parents				Sibs				Offspring			
		No. affected	No. not affected	Unknown	Total	No. affected	No. not affected	Unknown	Total	No. affected	No. not affected	Unknown	Total
Both	32	14	40	10	64	15	62	29	106	3	18	4	25
One	29	11	33	14	58	9	33	17	59	1	11	4	16
Total	61	25	73	24	122	24	95	46	165	4	29	8	41

Source: R. M. Goodman et al., 1965, *J. Med. Genet.* 2:116.

Unilaterally and bilaterally affected individuals were observed in the same family in the Israeli study, but when 2 or more members of a family were affected unilaterally, the defect always occurred on the same hand (Figure 9.12).

A significant increase in the frequency of whorls was noted on affected thumbs. Among the anomalies that appeared in association with stub thumbs, the most common was a short fourth toe.

Radiographic studies have shown that the deformity in this trait is confined to the distal phalanx of the thumb. Breitenbecher compared radiographs of the distal phalanx of the affected thumb with those of the normal thumb and found the distal phalanx in the affected thumb to be half the length of that in the normal thumb. Stecher observed that the distal phalanx of the affected thumb is about two-thirds the usual length. Goodman and co-workers have shown that there can be considerable variation in the expression of this trait (Figure 9.11). Roentgenographic studies show that this abnormality results from a partial fusion or premature closing involving the epiphysis of the distal phalanx of the thumb.

Stub thumbs is an insignificant genetic malformation and no treatment is indicated.

References

Breitenbecher, J. K. 1923. Hereditary shortness of thumbs. *J. Hered.* 14:15.

Goodman, R. M.; Adam, A.; and Sheba, C. 1965. A genetic study of stub thumbs among various ethnic groups in Israel. *J. Med. Genet.* 2:116.

Stecher, R. M. 1957. The physical characteristics and heredity of short thumbs. *Acta Genet. (Basel)* 7:217.

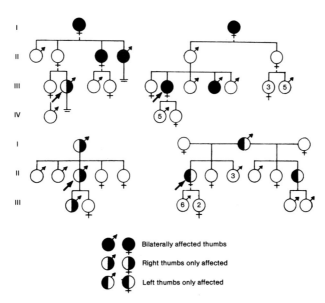

Figure 9.12. Pedigrees of families with stub thumbs. Figures inside symbols indicate number of subjects.

TYROSINOSIS

Historical note

In 1927 Medes and co-workers reported an unusual reducing substance in the urine of an Ashkenazi Jewish man with myasthenia gravis. Five years later Medes isolated and identified the reducing compound as p-hydroxyphenylpyruvic acid, the alpha-keto acid of tyrosine, and termed the condition *tyrosinosis*. In 1934 Blatherwick searched for additional cases among more than 20,000 persons who showed a weakly positive response to the test for glucose in the urine but failed to uncover any new ones. At present, the only case of this particular inborn error of metabolism on record is the patient reported by Medes.

Clinical features

The 49-year-old Russian Jewish man reported by Medes had myasthenia gravis, which is not at all related to tyrosinosis. Other than findings related to myasthenia gravis, no abnormal features were present. Tyrosinosis, like pentosuria, iminoglycinuria, and familial hyperglycinuria, is a benign metabolic condition and is not known to be associated with any disease state.

Diagnosis

Medes and co-workers identified the unusual reducing substance in the patient's urine as p-hydroxyphenylpyruvic acid and noted that the level of the other tyrosine metabolites increased proportionately to increased intake of dietary phenylalanine and tyrosine.

La Du and Gjessing have suggested that, on the basis of the metabolites excreted in the urine of the patient, and in order to emphasize the excretion of p-hydroxyphenylpyruvic acid, a more appropriate term for this condition would be *tyrosyluria*. This inborn error of metabolism could then be referred to as *essential* or *idiopathic tyrosyluria*, to distinguish it from other conditions in which tyrosyluria is a secondary finding.

Basic defect

The basic defect in tyrosinosis is not known. In 1932, on the basis of the tyrosine metabolites found in the urine, Medes proposed that the defect results from the lack of p-hydroxyphenylpyruvic acid oxidase activity. In a scholarly review of Medes's excellent and detailed study, La Du and Gjessing suggested that her findings are compatible with a deficiency of tyrosine aminotransferase activity. Technological limitations at the time of her study prevented Medes from demonstrating hypertyrosinemia, which theoretically should have been present if her patient had a deficiency of the above enzyme.

Scriver and Rosenberg have commented that the block in tyrosine metabolism in Medes's patient was relatively greater at high levels of tyrosine intake than at low levels. Furthermore, they point out that no p-hydroxyphenyllactic acid was formed at any time, which suggests that most of the urinary p-hydroxyphenylpyruvic acid was formed in the kidney (presumably by deamination) and immediately excreted into the urine. Their findings suggest a tissue-specific enzyme deficiency—in this instance perhaps a deficiency of renal tyrosine aminotransferase—but we shall remain in the dark concerning the basic defect in this disorder until another patient is diagnosed.

Genetics

Autosomal recessive inheritance is the most likely mode of transmission of this trait.

Prognosis and treatment

Tyrosinosis does not appear to be associated with any disease state and thus no treatment is indicated. The fact that only one patient with this disorder has been recognized should serve as a note of caution in our search for a better understanding of this condition.

References

Blatherwick, N. R. 1934. Tyrosinosis: A search for additional cases. *JAMA* 103:1933.

La Du, B., and Gjessing, L. R. 1972. Tyrosinosis and tyrosinemin. In *The metabolic basis of inherited disease,* ed. J. B. Stanbury, J. B. Wyngaarden, and D. S. Fredrickson, 3rd ed., pp. 296–307. New York: McGraw-Hill.

Medes, G. 1932. A new error of tyrosine metabolism: Tyrosinosis, the intermediary metabolism of tyrosine and phenylalanine. *Biochem. J.* 26:917.

Medes, G.; Berglund, H.; and Lohmann, A. 1927. An unknown reducing urinary substance in myasthenia gravis. *Proc. Soc. Exp. Biol. Med.* 25:210.

Scriver, C. R., and Rosenberg, L. E. 1973. *Amino acid metabolism and its disorders,* p. 345. Philadelphia: W. B. Saunders.

10

Misconceptions

THE PURPOSE of this chapter is to clarify the status of a number of disorders, not all of which have a definite genetic etiology, but which nevertheless have been thought to afflict mainly Ashkenazi Jews. These misconceptions have arisen for a number of reasons, such as lack of adequate control studies, biases in ascertaining data, and the promulgation of medical misinformation. Well-designed studies are still needed to determine conclusively whether or not some Jewish communities actually have a high rate of occurrence of certain disorders. Whenever possible, an effort has been made to trace the origins of these misconceptions.

ACROMEGALY

In 1920 Davidoff, a physician working at the Peter Bent Brigham Hospital in Boston, reported 100 cases of acromegaly and noted that 21 percent of the patients with this disorder were Jewish (most probably Ashkenazim). He pointed out that this proportion was far in excess of the number of Jews living in America at that time. (According to the 1920 census, the total population was 105,710,614; the number of Jews was 3,600,350.) What Davidoff failed to realize was that a large number of Jews were living in the Boston area, and that he, a prominent Jewish endocrinologist, had undoubtedly attracted Jews who were ill with endocrine problems. In his paper Davidoff went on to mention that in 1903 both Lorand and Sternberg had published reports on the incidence of acromegaly in Europe and they too had thought this disorder was common among Jews. Davidoff speculated that perhaps "the more highly strung nervous make-up so frequently observed in members of this race is associated with some instability in the endocrine mechanism."

In 1928 Sir Humphry Rolleston touched on the subject of acromegaly among Jews. He mentioned that L. P. Mark in his "Apologia of an Acromegalic" had raised the question of a special predisposition of Jews to this pituitary disease on the admittedly slender evidence that 4 of 12 patients were Jewish. Rolleston postulated that because the rate of diabetes mellitus is high among Jews, and because there is an association between diabetes and acromegaly, perhaps this was additional evidence that acromegaly is common to Jews. Prudently, however, Sir Humphry continued with an interesting statement: "Some physicians in a position to know have told me that they do not know of any evidence of a higher incidence of acromegaly among Jews than in other nations, and have warned me that any assumption that the *frustes* forms of the condition are common in Jews should be entertained with caution, because more or less prognathism and thick negroid lips are frequent among Jews, especially when compared with Anglo-Saxons."

At present there is no evidence to suggest that Jews are exceptionally prone to acromegaly. As a matter of fact, acromegaly is not characteristic of any ethnic group.

The majority of cases of acromegaly are sporadic, although some families have been reported in which many members were said to be affected. A word of caution is necessary regarding these familial cases. Only in a very few cases has the lesion been anatomically confirmed, and in none have high HGH levels been documented by radioimmunoassay. Furthermore, certain genetic disorders may mimic acromegaly clinically. In some instances such patients have been reported to have familial acromegaly, but when evaluated more carefully have been found to have one of the genetic syndromes presenting similar features.

In conclusion, acromegaly, like other disorders in this chapter, has suffered from severe biases in reporting.

References

Davidoff, L. M. 1926. Studies in acromegaly. III: The anamnesis and symptomatology in one hundred cases. *Endocrinology* 10:461.
Lorand, A. 1903. *Die Ehtstehung der Zuckerkrankheit*, p. 1063. Berlin: Verlag von A. Hirschwald.
Rimoin, D. L., and Schimke, R. N. 1971. *Genetic disorders of the endocrine glands,* pp. 53–54. St. Louis: C. V. Mosby.
Rolleston, H. 1928. Some diseases in the Jewish race. *Bull. Johns Hopkins Hospital* 43:117.
Steinberg, M. 1903. *Acromegaly.* Eng. transl. London: New Synderham Society.

CYSTIC FIBROSIS
(MUCOVISCIDOSIS)

Among peoples of northern European extraction cystic fibrosis (CF) is the most frequent lethal Mendelian disease of childhood. Its symptomatology is well known to most pediatricians and consists of alteration of the exocrine function of the pancreas (malabsorption), the intestinal glands (meconium ileus), the biliary tree (biliary cirrhosis), the bronchial glands (chronic bronchopulmonary infections with emphysema), the sweat glands (high sweat electrolyte with depletion in a hot environment), and infertility in males and females due to obstructive degenerative changes in the male transport ducts and altered cervical mucus in the female.

The occurrence of CF is worldwide, yet there are some racial groups in which it is rarely seen or has never been reported. For example, CF is rare in the black American population and certain Mediterranean populations and has not been reported in black Africans or among Mongolians. Steinberg and Brown have estimated the phenotype frequency among the white population of the United States to be about 1:3,700, a value only about one-fourth that of previous estimates. The gene frequency is approximately 0.016 and about 3 percent of the white population

Table 10.1. Cystic fibrosis: Ethnic origin of cases
and families in Israel, 1954–1975

Ethnic origin	No. of cases	No. of families
Ashkenazi	71	55
Sephardi	37	30
Ashkenazi-Sephardi	5	4
Ashkenazi-Oriental	1	1
Yemenite	2	1
Unknown (Jewish)	6	5
Arab	15	13
Total	137	109

Source: D. Katznelson, Israel.

are heterozygotes. In a study from Connecticut, Honeyman and Siker arrived at higher estimates—1:489 (maximal) and 1:1,863 (minimal). Among the white populations of Europe the phenotypic frequency ranges from 1:2,000 to 1:4,000 live births.

Prior to 1955 CF was rarely diagnosed in Israel. In 1963 Levin surveyed the number of diagnosed cases and reported on 38. He estimated the phenotypic frequency among the Israeli Ashkenazi community to be about 1:5,000 live births, which suggests that the frequency of the disease is lower in the Ashkenazi community than in other white populations of the world. He also found that the number of cases among the Sephardi Jewish community was only two-thirds of the total. For several years thereafter it was generally assumed that CF was rare among the Ashkenazim and seldom occurred among the other Jewish ethnic groups.

In 1978 Katznelson reported the results of a survey of the Israeli population from 1954 to 1975 in which he found 137 cases in 109 families. All cases fit the classical description of the disease spectrum and no differences were noted among Israel's various ethnic groups. Table 10.1 shows the distribution of these cases by ethnic origin. The absence of cases in families originating from Iraq and Iran is conspicuous, and in only 2 cases (1 family) are the parents from Yemen.

Consanguinity among CF families is rare, as substantiated by the results from a recent survey in Israel (see Table 10.2) in which 50 of the 109 families surveyed were personally interviewed by the investigators. There were no instances of consanguinity among the Ashkenazi families, and the few that occurred among the

Table 10.2. Ethnic distribution and degree of consanguinity in
Israeli cystic fibrosis cases, 1954–1975

Ethnic group	No. of families interviewed	No. of consanguineous marriages	Degree of consanguinity
Ashkenazi	34	0	—
Sephardi	11	1	Second cousins
Intercommunity (Ashkenazi-Sephardi)	3	0	—
Oriental	1	1	First cousins
Arab	1	1	First cousins

Source: D. Katznelson, Israel.

other groups merely reflect the overall increase in consanguinity that is known to be occurring in these communities (see Chapter 12).

Although no attempt was made in this survey to calculate the gene frequency of CF in the various communities, it is thought that the frequency among Ashkenazi Jews is similar to that among other white populations of the world. The earlier impression of a lower frequency of CF in the Ashkenazi Jewish community of Israel probably reflects the lack of awareness and poor diagnostic techniques that existed during that period.

A comprehensive study of CF among the various Jewish communities in Israel remains to be done. However, some evidence suggests that this disease is very rare among the Oriental Jews and uncommon among the Sephardi Jewish communities. Both of these populations are of darker skin pigmentation than Ashkenazi Jews, and such an observation is in keeping with the overall concept that this autosomal recessive disorder affects primarily the white populations of the world.

The basic defect in CF is not known, but it is hoped that in the very near future we shall better understand and thus better treat this disorder.

References

Honeyman, M. S., and Siker, E. 1965. Cystic fibrosis of the pancreas: An estimate of the incidence. *Am. J. Hum. Genet.* 17:461.

Hösli, P., and Vogt, E. 1977. Cystic fibrosis, a multiple leakage of intracellular digestive tract enzymes into the extracellular space: Prospects for neonatal and prenatal diagnosis and for carrier detection. *Hum. Hered.* 27:185.

Katznelson, D., and Ben-Yishay, M. 1978. Cystic fibrosis in Israel: Clinical and genetic aspects. *Israel J. Med. Sci.* 14:204.

Levin, S. 1963. Fibrocystic disease of the pancreas. In *Genetics of migrant and isolate populations*, ed. E. Goldschmidt, p. 294. Baltimore: Williams and Wilkins.

Lobeck, C. C. 1972. Cystic fibrosis. In *The metabolic basis of inherited disease*, ed. J. B. Stanbury, J. B. Wyngaarden, and D. S. Fredrickson, 3rd ed., p. 1605. New York: McGraw-Hill.

Schaap, T.; Hodes, M. E.; and Cohen, M. M. 1978. Cystic fibrosis: Problems and Prospects. *Israel J. Med. Sci.* 14:201.

Steinberg, A. G., and Brown, D. C. 1960. On the incidence of cystic fibrosis of the pancreas. *Am. J. Hum. Genet.* 12:416.

CREUTZFELDT-JAKOB DISEASE

Creutzfeldt-Jakob disease (CJD) is a rapidly progressive, fatal "degenerative" disease of the central nervous system which is generally thought to be one of the unconventional slow virus diseases of man. There are many familial reports of this disorder in the literature, and in several instances passage of the disease from affected individuals to certain primates has been accomplished. Despite this, no slow virus has been isolated.

In the late 1960s it was suggested that Libyan Jewish immigrants living in Israel might be unusually predisposed to CJD. Prior to that time no ethnic focus of the disease had been recognized. In 1974 Kahana and co-workers reported the results of a survey of CJD cases in Israel. Their study produced 29 patients, 16 of whom were histopathologically confirmed as definite CJD cases, 7 as probable cases, and 6 as possible cases. Table 10.3 shows the incidence of CJD among the various Jewish ethnic groups in Israel. The average annual age-adjusted incidence of CJD varied in the narrow range of 0.4–1.9 per million population for all ethnic groups except the Jewish immigrants from Libya. In this group it was 31.3 per million population, or at least 16–78-fold higher. Even after age adjustment to another standard population (United States, 1970) and after exclusion of possible cases of CJD, an extraordinary Libyan focus was still apparent.

A comparison of the clinical characteristics of CJD in the Libyan ethnic group and in other Jewish groups as a whole showed an average age at onset of 56 years for both groups and a male:female ratio of 1.2:1 and 3.0:1, respectively ($p > .05$). The average duration of the illness was 4.4 months for Libyans and 11.0 months for others ($p < .05$). The general clinical manifestations of the disease were similar in both groups. The percentage of histopathologically confirmed cases was almost identical in the Libyan and other ethnic groups. All of the Libyan cases, but only 63 percent of the others, were classified as definite or probable CJD, which suggests that criteria for diagnosis of the Libyans were, if anything, more stringent. There were no familial cases of CJD in this Israeli series, but we now know of a father and son of Jewish Libyan ancestry with the disease.

In their search for the source of this slow virus, investigators have noted that kuru, which is pathologically similar to CJD, can be acquired from deceased victims of the disease through cannibalism during burial rituals. Indeed, kuru declined in frequency when cannibalism was prohibited. Scrapie, a disease of sheep that is also like CJD, is transmitted orally through the ingestion of the scrapie agent from fields where the animals graze. It has been suggested that CJD may be transmitted to man through ingestion of infected sheep's eyeballs or brains, which are considered to be a gastronomic delicacy among various North African Arabs and also among Libyan Jews. Not only is there evidence in the literature to document this finding, but in the recently discovered Libyan Jewish family with an affected father and son, both gave a history of frequently eating sheep's brains.

Table 10.3. Creutzfeldt-Jakob disease among Jewish ethnic groups in Israel

Place of birth	No. of patients	Pop. at risk	Average annual incidence/ million pop. (1963–1972) age-adjusted to pop. of	
			Israel, 1968	U.S., 1970[a]
Libya[b]	13 (13)	30,792	31.3 (31.3)	33.0
Iraq	3 (2)	117,587	1.9 (1.3)	2.5
Western & Central Europe	4 (3)	199,300	1.0 (0.6)	1.1
Israel	2 (1)	1,020,411	1.0 (0.5)	1.0
Morocco, Algeria, Tunisia	2 (1)	275,432	0.8 (0.3)	0.9
Eastern Europe	5 (3)	509,317	0.4 (0.2)	0.5
Total	29 (23)			

Source: E. Kahana et al., 1974, *Science* 183:90. Copyright 1974 by the American Association for the Advancement of Science.

Note: Numbers in parentheses exclude "possible" CJD cases.

[a] Based on total CJD cases.

[b] Three additional cases are known among Libyan Jews, 1 of which involves a father and son.

In a recent epidemiological study of CJD in England and Wales, Matthews found evidence for geographical clustering and possible contact between cases but no definite source of natural transmission. The eating of swine's brains was ruled out. However, 2 patients had come in contact with ferrets, which may prove to be of interest since mink encephalopathy is caused by a slow virus that is transmissible to the white ferret.

Epidemiological studies in Israel and various North African countries would help to clarify the natural mode of transmission of this disease and to explain its length of incubation. Even at this early stage of investigation, it would seem wise for populations to abandon such "delicacies" as sheep's eyeballs and brains.

References

Alter, M. 1974. Creutzfeldt-Jakob disease: Hypothesis for high incidence in Libyan Jews in Israel. *Science* 186:848.

Alter, M.; Frank, Y.; Doyne, H.; and Webster, D. D. 1975. Creutzfeldt-Jakob disease after eating ovine brains? *N. Engl. J. Med.* 292:927.

Brownell, B.; Campbell, M. J.; Greenham, L. W.; and Peacock, D. B. 1975. Experimental transmission of Creutzfeldt-Jakob disease. *Lancet* 2:186.

Duffy, P.; Wolf, J.; Collins, G.; de Voe, A. G.; Streeten, B.; and Cowen, D. 1974. Possible person-to-person transmission of Creutzfeldt-Jakob disease. *N. Engl. J. Med.* 290:692.

Gajdusek, D. C., and Gibbs, C. J., Jr. 1976. Survival of Creutzfeldt-Jakob disease virus in formol-fixed brain tissue. *N. Engl. J. Med.* 294:553.

Gibbs, C. J., Jr.; Gajdusek, D. C.; Asher, D. M.; Alpers, M. P.; Beck, E.; Daniel, P. M.; and Matthews, W. B. 1968. Creutzfeldt-Jakob disease (spongiform encephalopathy): Transmission to the chimpanzee. *Science* 161:388.

Herzberg, L.; Herzberg, B. N.; Gibbs, C. J., Jr.; Sullivan, W.; Amyx, H.; and Gajdusek, D. C. 1974. Creutzfeldt-Jakob disease: Hypothesis for high incidence in Libyan Jews in Israel. *Science* 186:848.

Kahana, E.; Alter, M.; Braham, J.; and Sofer, D. 1974. Creutzfeldt-Jakob disease: Focus among Libyan Jews in Israel. *Science* 183:90.

Matthews, W. B. 1975. Epidemiology of Creutzfeldt-Jakob disease in England and Wales. *J. Neurol. Neurosurg. Psychiatry* 38:210.

Roos, R.; Gajdusek, D. C.; and Gibbs, C. J., Jr. 1973. The clinical characteristics of transmissible Creutzfeldt-Jakob disease. *Brain* 96:1.

Zlotnik, I.; Grant, D. P.; Dayan, A. D.; and Earl, C. J. 1974. Transmission of Creutzfeldt-Jakob disease from man to squirrel monkey. *Lancet* 2:435.

HEMORRHOIDS

Hemorrhoids are probably the most common of all anal diseases. Their pathogenesis is not entirely clear, but there is little evidence of a genetic etiology. Despite this fact, hemorrhoids have long been thought to be very common among Jews.

The earliest reference to hemorrhoids can be found in the Bible (Deut. 28:27) in the Hebrew *opoilim*, meaning "swellings." This term has caused a great deal of confusion among the exegesists of the Scriptures. In some old manuscripts the term *t'choirim* appears instead of *opoilim*. The former term is used in the Targum (Aramaic translation of the Bible) and is derived from *t'chor*, which means "to strain at stool"; hence *t'choirim* is taken to refer to hemorrhoids. In the Psalms (78:66) one finds that "the Lord afflicted his oppressors with *ochoir*." Rashi explains that the term *ochoir*, which literally means "the posteriors," represents *tochoir*, or hemorrhoids. In the Midrash (Midr. Sam. 10) the term *tochoir* refers to "one who sits straining himself like a sufferer from hemorrhoids."

According to Friedenwald, who has researched this disorder extensively, in 1305 Bernard de Gordon wrote a Latin text entitled *Lilium Medicinae* which was translated into Hebrew in 1387 by Jekuthiel ben Solomon of Narbonne. In this text, the prevalence of hemorrhoids among Jews is described as follows:

> It is to be noted that the Jews suffer greatly from hemorrhoids for three reasons: first because they are generally sedentary and therefore the excessive melancholy humors collect; secondly, because they are usually in fear and anxiety and therefore the melancholy blood becomes increased, besides (according to Hippocrates) fear and faint-heartedness, should they last a long time, produce the melancholy humor; and thirdly, it is the divine vengeance against them (as written in Psalms 78:66), and "he smote his enemies in the *hinderparts*, he put them to a perpetual reproach."

Jekuthiel ben Solomon is said to have translated the first and second reasons, but when he reached the third, he stated with indignation, "sheker shekosaf veamaminim skeker"—i.e., "what is written is a lie and they, who believe it, lie."

In 1777 Elcan Isaac Wolf, a Jewish physician of Mannheim, wrote a small book entitled *Von den Krankheiten der Juden* in which he addressed himself to the "misery and poverty of his brethren . . . because their diseases are so intimately related to their sad fate." He pictured frightful poverty, unsanitary homes, improperly prepared and insufficient food, uncleanliness, daily anxiety to earn a livelihood, continual sorrow, and the resulting lean bodies, living corpses, sallow complexions, excessive nervous irritability, and frequency of hypochondriasis, melancholia, and hemorrhoids. He warned his people against excessive indulgence in coffee and tea because of their depressing injurious effects and the danger of hemorrhoids.

Hemorrhoids have been a part of Jewish folklore for such a long time that the subject has found its way into such Yiddish proverbs as "A jüdische jrüische is a gildene uder" ("A Jew's inheritance is a golden vein [i.e., hemorrhoids]") and "Wus jarsch'enen jüden? Zurojss ün meriden!" ("What is the Jew's inheritance? Sore troubles and hemorrhoids!").

It is doubtful that hemorrhoids should continue to be thought of as an occupational disease among Jews. Although the Jews' troubles may not have decreased, certainly their sedentary ways are not markedly different from other Western populations. The common occurrence of the condition among most peoples would seem to preclude singling out any one ethnic group. However, those who believe that Jews have a special predisposition to hemorrhoids should note that the present Israeli Jewish community, with its varying ethnic groups, would be an ideal setting in which to gain information on the precise frequency and distribution of this disorder. It is thought that the Ashkenazi Jewish community shares this affliction equally with non-Ashkenazi Jews and with non-Jews in general, but only a well-designed study will provide the answer.

References

Brim, C. J. 1936. *Medicine in the Bible*, p. 22. New York: Froben Press.

Friedenwald, H. 1944. *The Jews and medicine: Essays*, 2: 523–28. Baltimore: The Johns Hopkins Press.

HEREDITARY HEMORRHAGIC TELANGIECTASIA
(RENDU-OSLER-WEBER DISEASE)

In 1919 Libman and Ottenberg described what they thought was a new clinical form of hereditary hemoptysis in 7 members of 3 generations of a Russian Jewish family living in New York City. Their presentation of this so-called new genetic entity was published in a book dedicated to Sir William Osler on his seventieth birthday.

The original pedigree of this family is shown in Figure 10.1. All affected members presented with hemoptysis during or after the age of puberty. Of the 7 affected individuals, only 3 were examined by Libman and Ottenberg. One of these patients also had a history of intermittent hematuria. Although the skin lesions that are characteristic of this disorder were not noted in these 3 patients, the nature of their bouts of hemoptysis, combined with occasional hematuria in 1 individual and with a similar clinical history in 4 other family members spanning 3 generations, certainly speaks for the diagnosis of hereditary hemorrhagic telangiectasia (HHT). After carefully reading the report of Libman and Ottenberg, I find there is little question that the correct diagnosis is indeed HHT.

In his article "Some diseases in the Jewish race" Sir Humphry Rolleston mentioned the 1919 report of Libman and Ottenberg but did not draw any conclusions as to its possible significance. In discussing the ethnic distribution of HHT with some of my medical colleagues, I have found that some believe that HHT may be more common among Ashkenazi Jews. In 1950 Garland and Anning reviewed the literature and found that the disease had been reported in 264 different families. Many details were available on 112 of these families, but ethnic origins were not

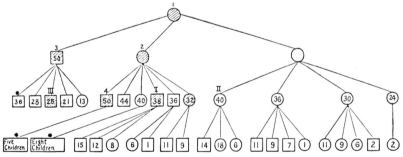

Circles = Females; Squares = Males; * = in Europe; no Details Obtainable. Shading Indicates Bleeders. The Numbers Inscribed in Squares or Circles Represent the Present Age of Each Individual. The Numbers above Squares or Circles Refer to Numerals in the Text; the Roman Numerals (I, II, III) Indicate Individuals Actually Examined by Us, the Arabic Figures (1, 2, 3) Bleeders That Were Not Available for Examination.

Figure 10.1. Hereditary hemorrhagic telangiectasia: Family pedigree prepared by Libman and Ottenberg in 1919. Note the details recorded by the authors.

stated. To this list of 112 families Garland and Anning added 19 families of their own, 2 of which were of Jewish descent. In their discussion they made the following statement: "Hereditary hemorrhagic telangiectasia has been observed in families of most of the European races and in a number of Jewish families. In our series the two Jewish families in a total of 19 families from this district may be compared with the Jewish 2.77% of all who attended the out-patient department of this hospital in 1948. The defect would appear to be relatively more common among Jews than Gentiles, and is probably more common in most communities than is generally realized."

It is possible that the influx of Jews into England after World War II introduced a bias into the cases reported by Garland and Anning, for other reviews do not mention an unusually high frequency of this disease among Jews.

HHT is an autosomal dominant disorder transmitted with equal frequency by males and females and its ethnic distribution is known to be world-wide. Whether or not this condition is more frequent in Jews than in non-Jews cannot be determined from presently available data. Since this disorder is relatively common, few cases are reported today. It is conceivable that a well-designed genetic and epidemiological study would not show an increased frequency of HHT among Jews. In Israel, HHT has not been observed to be unduly common in any of the Jewish ethnic groups.

References

Garland, H. G., and Anning, S. T. 1950. Hereditary haemorrhagic telangiectasia: A genetic and bibliographical study. *Br. J. Dermat. Syph.* 62:289.

Hodgson, C. H.; Burchell, H. B.; Good, C. A.; and Clagett, O. T. 1959. Hereditary hemorrhagic telangiectasia and pulmonary arteriovenous fistula: Survey of a large family. *N. Engl. J. Med.* 261:625.

Libman, E., and Ottenberg, R. 1919. Hereditary hemoptysis. In *Contributions to medical and biological research dedicated to Sir William Osler,* pp. 632–39. New York: Paul B. Hoeber.

Rolleston, H. 1928. Some diseases in the Jewish race. *Bull. Johns Hopkins Hospital* 43:117.

INGUINAL HERNIA

In 1963, as mentioned in the Preface to this text, the late Dr. Chaim Sheba introduced me to the subject of genetic diseases among the Jewish people. During ward rounds he frequently discussed disease processes and their occurrence in the various Jewish ethnic groups. On one occasion I recall his mentioning that he thought inguinal hernia was very common among Ashkenazi Jews. It is important to know that his clinical impression gained a foothold while Dr. Sheba was studying medicine in Vienna prior to World War II. By oral transmission it found its way into the medical genetics literature, and in Dr. Victor McKusick's catalog *Mendelian Inheritance in Man* (4th edition) it is listed under "Ashkenazi Jews" in a table entitled "The Ethnicity of Disease: Disorders in which the Genetics is Complex or Genetic Factors are not Proved."

In an attempt to document this clinical impression, I have searched the medical literature, but nowhere have I found a statement suggesting that the occurrence of inguinal hernia is high in Jews. However, the story does not end here. In conversation with some of my surgical colleagues in Israel, and in particular with Prof. Mark Moses of the Chaim Sheba Medical Center, I heard an interesting story concerning inguinal hernia in young Jewish males. Prof. Moses received his medical education and surgical training in Warsaw, Poland, prior to World War II. There he learned that young Jewish males at the turn of the century and even much earlier had not been keen on spending many years in the service of the Russian army. Since the army took only men in excellent health, an inguinal hernia or signs of its repair was sufficient grounds for deferment of service. Therefore, many of these young men had sought surgical intervention for a nonexistent hernia or had produced a hernia to be repaired. Thus, Dr. Sheba's clinical impression, stemming from his early medical training in Europe, has some credence, but it is doubtful that it is related to a genetic predisposition of Ashkenazi Jews to inguinal hernia.

However, it would be a mistake to completely dismiss a possible genetic component from the etiology of some cases of inguinal hernia. In a brief review article in 1949 Weimer cited several cases as evidence of the genetic transmission of this defect. He himself reported a family in which 1 male in 4 successive generations had bilateral inguinal hernia. In 1974 Edwards and Simpson and co-workers also described families with familial inguinal hernia. Moreover, the rate of occurrence of inguinal hernia is high among those who suffer from certain heritable disorders of connective tissue—e.g. Marfan syndrome.

In conclusion, it seems plausible to assume that certain families (without a known heritable disorder of connective tissue) are genetically predisposed to inguinal hernia. Since more males than females are commonly affected with this type of hernia, the mode of transmission may be variable, such as sex-influenced autosomal dominant or Y-linked. There is little evidence, however, that the frequency of this defect is unusually high among Jews. Nevertheless, there may be differences in the frequency of the condition among various populations of the world, but at present such data are not available.

References

Edwards, R. H. 1974. Familial hernia. *Birth Defects* 16:329.
McKusick, V. A. 1975. *Mendelian inheritance in man*, 4th ed., p. liv. Baltimore: The Johns Hopkins University Press.
Simpson, J. L.; Morillo-Cucci, G.; and German, J. 1974. Familial inguinal hernia affecting females. *Birth Defects* 16:332.
Weimer, B. R. 1949. Congenital inheritance of inguinal hernia. *J. Hered.* 40:219.

KALLMANN SYNDROME
(HYPOGONADOTROPIC HYPOGONADISM WITH HYPOSMIA;
DYSPLASIA OLFACTOGENITALIS OF DE MORSIER)

Historical note

In 1918 Glaser described a Russian Jewish family in which 3 generations were affected with anosmia or hyposmia. He also noted that this family had other abnormalities, such as "much stammering, early and complete loss of the incisors, frequent hernia, a thumb nearly twice the normal width, excessive sex interest and very considerable mental powers." In 1944 Kallmann and co-workers described in 9 men from 2 Russian Jewish families a familial syndrome of eunuchoidism and anosmia. In 1954 de Morsier coined the term *olfactogenital dysplasia* and used it to describe any combination of unilateral or bilateral, partial or complete, absence of olfactory bulbs associated with gonadal abnormalities, with or without other CNS and/or somatic malformations, in individuals of both sexes who were at times also known to have had anosmia.

Clinical features

Today the term *Kallmann syndrome* is applied primarily to males with hyposmia or anosmia and eunuchoidism. The eunuchoid features usually manifested are obese body habitus, arm span equal to or greater than height, high-pitched voice, lack of secondary sex characteristics, small or infantile penis, cryptorchidism or very small testes, hypoplastic scrotum, no palpable prostate, gynecomastia, and female escutcheon. Other findings include hypotelorism, borderline normal intelligence or mild mental retardation, various skeletal anomalies, and unilateral renal aplasia with ipsilateral absence of the testis.

Heterozygous females may show manifestations of anosmia, hypogonadism, and internal genital malformation.

Diagnosis

Diagnosis of Kallmann syndrome is made by demonstrating hyposmia in an individual with secondary hypogonadism. Anosmia must be inquired about in all cases of hypogonadism because patients rarely volunteer this information. The hypogonadism is characterized by a chromatin negative buccal smear, a normal karyotype, decreased plasma and urinary concentrations of LH and FSH, and decreased plasma testosterone concentration.

Testicular biopsies have shown a decreased number of germ cells and a spermatogenic state at the primary spermatocyte stage. Leydig cells are not histologically identifiable.

Basic defect

The basic defect in this disorder is not known. The hypogonadism has been found to be secondary to a deficiency of the pituitary gonadotropins, while the anosmia has been shown to be secondary to agenesis of the olfactory lobes of the brain. Hypoplasia of the hypothalamus and the mammillary bodies has been observed in several autopsied cases; thus it has been postulated that the hypogonadism may be secondary to a deficiency of gonadotropin-releasing factors caused by a developmental anomaly of the hypothalamus. In 1974 extensive endocrine studies by Antaki and co-workers showed the complete integrity of the adenohypophysis and led them to conclude that "the hypogonadotropic hypogonadism is of hypothalamic origin."

Genetics

The mode of transmission in Kallmann syndrome is still unclear, although the majority of well-documented cases strongly suggests X-linked recessive or male-limited autosomal dominant inheritance. However, evidence is mounting in support of genetic heterogeneity in Kallmann syndrome.

The early report of anosmia in an Ashkenazi Jewish family by Glaser in 1918, followed by the description of this disorder by Kallmann and co-workers in 1944 in 9 men from 2 unrelated Russian Jewish families, led some investigators to conclude that Kallmann syndrome occurs more frequently in the Ashkenazi Jewish community than among non-Jews. As late as 1970 Krikler mentioned this possibility. Yet a search of the current literature does not support this contention. The disease has been reported in a number of ethnic groups, but no special predisposition has been noted.

Prognosis and treatment

Kallmann syndrome is not a life-threatening disorder, but the lower intelligence of some affected individuals may be a limiting factor in terms of their work potential. Full secondary sexual development can be restored in males by means of testosterone therapy. The usefulness of HCG has been questioned, but it should be tried if fertility is desired. Combined gonadotropin therapy has been used successfully to induce ovulation in affected females.

The presence of an associated unilateral renal aplasia in some affected individuals warrants proper care and treatment of all renal diseases in such patients.

References

Antaki, A.; Somma, M.; Wyman, H.; and Van Campenhout, J. 1974. Hypothalamic-pituitary function in the olfacto-genital syndrome. *J. Clin. Endocrinol. Metab.* 38:1083.

De Morsier, G. 1954. Études sur les dysraphies cranioencéphaliques. 1. Agénésie lobes olfactifs (téléncephaloschizis latéral) et des commissures calleuse et anterieure (téléncephaloschizis médian): La dysplasie olfactogénitale. *Schweiz. Arch. Neurol. Neurochir. Psychiatr.* 74:309.

Glaser, O. 1918. Hereditary deficiencies in the sense of smell. *Science* 48:647.

Kallmann, F. J.; Schoenfeld, W. A.; and Barrera, S. E. 1944. The genetic aspects of primary eunuchoidism. *Am. J. Ment. Defic.* 48:203.

Krikler, D. M. 1970. Diseases of Jews. *Postgrad. Med. J.* 46:687.

Rimoin, D. L., and Schimke, R. N. 1971. *Genetic disorders of the endocrine glands*, pp. 26–28. St. Louis: C. V. Mosby.

Wegenke, J. D.; Uehling, D. T.; Wear, J. B., Jr.; Gordon, E. S.; Bargman, J. G.; Deacon, J. S. R.; Hermann, J. P. R.; and Opitz, J. M. 1975. Familial Kallmann syndrome with unilateral renal aplasia. *Clin. Genet.* 7:368.

KAPOSI SARCOMA

Historical note

Kaposi sarcoma is named after the Hungarian Jewish physician Kaposi, whose name was originally Moricz Kohn. Changing a Jewish family name to a specifically non-Jewish one was not an uncommon practice among Jews in the early 18th century. Names that told the place of origin of a person were favored. The name Kaposi indicated that Kohn came from Kaposvár, or the burg of Kapos. In centuries past, noblemen whose ancestors actually founded a community or built a castle on the hilltop of the city carried the name of this community, but with an adjectival *y* and not an *i* at the end of the name. Kaposi could not have changed his name to Kaposy with a *y*, because this would have indicated nobility, which he could not claim, but to change it to Kaposi with an *i* was a simple matter requiring only the filling out of an application and 24 cents for the official stamps.

Since Kaposi's description of this disease in 1872, many have considered this disorder to be rare and virtually confined to Ashkenazi Jews and to peoples of the Mediterranean region.

In 1961 an international symposium on Kaposi sarcoma was held in Uganda, and since that conference there has been an upsurge of interest in and research on this disease.

Clinical features

Kaposi sarcoma tends to occur in men between the ages of 50 and 70 years. The early lesions first appear most frequently on the arches of the feet, forearms, hands, legs, and soles as reddish, bluish-black, or violaceous macules and patches that spread and coalesce to form large plaques or nodules. These nodules have a firm, rubbery consistency and appear as dusky violaceous angiomas. Onset may be accompanied by a brauny edema of the affected parts. Later the macules and nodules may appear on the face, ears, trunk, and in the mouth, especially on the soft palate.

Internally, the gastrointestinal tract is most frequently affected, followed by involvement of the lungs, heart, liver, adrenal glands, and the lymph nodes of the abdomen.

Diagnosis

Diagnosis can easily be made clinically. There is considerable variation in histopathology, depending on the stage of the disease. Early lesions show chronic inflammation or are granulomatous in nature, with new and dilated lymph and blood vessels, edema, hemorrhages, blood pigment, and dense perivascular infiltrations of lymphocytes, plasma, and mast cells. The endothelial cells of the capillaries are large and protrude into the lumen like buds. The individual lesions are made up of capillaries and a fibrosarcoma-like tissue in varying proportions, and often the capillaries show a marked tendency to anastomose. At this stage the lesion looks like a hemangioma or angiosarcoma. In the later stages there is wild connective-tissue proliferation, which may be difficult to distinguish from sarcoma.

Occasionally, the peripheral blood shows monocytosis and, less frequently, eosinophilia.

Basic defect

The basic defect in Kaposi sarcoma is not known. Some investigators think the tumor arises from the vascular periepithelial cells and that it is composed mostly of 2 types of cells—proliferating endothelial cells and proliferating perithelial cells. Others consider this to be a disease of reticuloendothelial tissue derivation.

Genetics

There is little evidence that Kaposi sarcoma is genetically determined, but 5 unrelated families, most with 2 affected generations, have been reported with this disease (Figure 10.2). Only 1 of the 5 families was of Ashkenazi Jewish origin. If these few familial examples are not caused by some common environmental factor, the pattern of transmission suggests autosomal dominance with incomplete penetrance. However, proof of a genetically transmitted form is still lacking, and it is perhaps significant that no cases involving identical twins have been reported.

It is known that this disease occurs world-wide, but predominantly in Europe and Africa. In 1931 Dörffel reviewed the literature and noted that 31.4 percent of the cases were Italians, 14 percent were Russians, and 12.6 percent were Jews. He commented that of the 50 cases reported by de Amicis, not a single one was a Jew, and he concluded that the distribution of the disease is geographical rather than racial.

In 1950 McCarthy and Pace reported 36 patients with this disorder and noted that 30 (83 percent) were Jews and Italians by origin. In 1959 Cox and Helwig reported 50 cases from the Armed Forces Institute of Pathology in Washington, D.C.; among these none was known to be Jewish and 8 were of Italian descent.

Upon careful examination of the literature, it becomes apparent that little can be said about the true frequency of occurrence of Kaposi sarcoma in the Ashkenazi Jewish community. So much bias has crept into past reports that only a well-designed epidemiological study will determine the frequency of this disease among Jews. In Israel, where the Ashkenazi community makes up about 48 percent of the total Jewish population, the disease is rare.

In Africa, Kaposi sarcoma appears to be prevalent only south of the Sahara. It

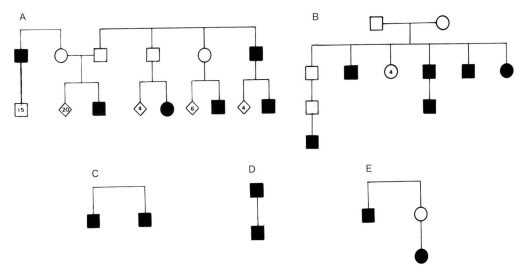

Figure 10.2. Pedigrees of families with Kaposi sarcoma collected from the literature.

is more common among children in tropical Africa. In the temperate zones of Africa and elsewhere, adults in their fifties are most frequently affected. Males generally outnumber females 10 to 1, but in South Africa, white women outnumber white men, and in Durban, whites outnumber blacks.

Prognosis and treatment

The course of Kaposi sarcoma is extremely variable. Death may occur within a few years, or the disease may last for years, with death ensuing from other causes.

It is known that Kaposi sarcoma may occur in conjunction with a variety of other diseases, such as malignant lymphomas, Hodgkin disease, mycosis fungoides, lymphosarcoma, sarcoidosis, leukemia, and other forms of carcinoma.

Treatment consists of external radiation or the use of various chemotherapeutic agents, such as antimetabolites, antibiotics, alkylating agents, and other antitumor drugs. Although the lesions may regress in response to a variety of therapeutic measures for a period of several months, in no instance has complete tumor involution been observed.

References

Bluefarb, S. M. 1957. *Kaposi's sarcoma: Multiple idopathic hemorrhagic sarcoma*, p. 171. Springfield, Ill.: Charles C Thomas.
Cook, J. 1962. The treatment of Kaposi's sarcoma with nitrogen mustard. *Acta Un. Int. Cancr.* 18:494.
Cox, F. H., and Helwig, E. B. 1959. Kaposi's sarcoma. *Cancer* 12:289.
Domonkos, A. N. 1971. *Andrews' diseases of the skin*, pp. 712–16. Philadelphia: W. B. Saunders.
Dörffel, J. 1932. Histogenesis of multiple idopathic hemorrhagic sarcoma of Kaposi. *Arch. Dermatol.* 26:108.
Gordon, J. A. 1967. Kaposi's sarcoma: A review of 136 Rhodesian African cases. *Postgrad. Med. J.* 43:513.
Kaposi, M. 1872. Indiopathisches multiples Pigmentsarkom der Haut. *Arch. Dermatol. Syph.* 4:265.
McCarthy, W. D., and Pack, G. T. 1950. Malignant blood vessel tumors: A report of 56 cases of angiosarcoma and Kaposi's sarcoma. *Surg. Gynecol. Obstet.* 91:465.
Oettlé, A. G. 1962. Geographical and racial differences in the frequency of Kaposi's sarcoma as evidence of environmental or genetic causes. *Acta Un. Int. Cancr.* 18:330.
Rothman, S. 1962. Some remarks on Moricz Kaposi and on the history of Kaposi's sarcoma. *Acta Un. Int. Cancr.* 18:322.
———. 1962. Remarks on sex, age, and racial distribution of Kaposi's sarcoma and on possible pathogenetic factors. *Acta Un. Int. Cancr.* 18:326.
———. 1962. Some clinical aspects of Kaposi's sarcoma in the European and North American population. *Acta Un. Int. Cancr.* 18:364.

LEGG-CALVÉ-PERTHES DISEASE
(PERTHES DISEASE)

Historical note

Osteochondritis deformans coxae juvenilis was first described in 1909 by Legg and in 1910 by Calvé and Perthes. Today the disorder is called Legg-Calvé-Perthes disease, or simply Perthes disease.

There is some evidence that a genetic component may be operating in this disease. In 1963 Wamoscher and Farhi reported the occurrence of this disorder in 8 members of an Ashkenazi Jewish family spanning 3 generations. In 1970, writing on diseases of Jews, Krikler mentioned that this condition may occur more frequently in the Ashkenazi Jewish community than in the other Jewish ethnic groups, but this point needs clarification.

Clinical features and diagnosis

In sporadic cases males tend to be affected more than females, but in familial cases the sex distribution is equal. Symptoms occur between the ages of 3 and 10 years. In sporadic cases involvement is usually unilateral, whereas in familial cases bilateral expression is not uncommon. Three stages are usually described, each lasting from about 9 months to a year. The first stage is marked by aseptic necrosis, and the patient usually presents with symptoms of pain and restricted movement of the hip joint—a limp may be present. Roentgenographically, there may be no change during the first weeks, after which a relative opacity of the epiphysis becomes evident. The second stage consists of revascularization, during which the epiphysis becomes mottled and fragmented. In the third stage reossification occurs and serial roentgenograms demonstrate gradual re-formation of the head of the femur.

Basic defect

The basic defect in Legg-Calvé-Perthes disease is not known. Vulnerability to injury of the blood vessels supplying the head and neck of the femur is a commonly accepted theory. A fracture, strain, or twist could shut off the blood supply to these vessels. Some consider that toxic thrombolus is involved. Others have postulated that the defect consists of a congenital abnormality in the vascular supply of the femoral head and neck.

Genetics

Table 10.4 presents a rather thorough review of the familial report of this disorder. The number of affected families cannot be ignored. Whether the mode of transmission for one form of this disease is autosomal dominant with variable expressivity, or multifactorial as suggested by Gray and co-workers, cannot be resolved at this time.

There is no evidence at present to support the concept that this disorder has an unusually high rate of occurrence in the Ashkenazi Jewish community. Wamoscher and Farhi's 1963 report of this disease in 8 members of a Jewish family spanning 3 generations lends weight to a possible genetic etiology, but it does not infer any ethnic predisposition. In 1974 Axer discussed the treatment of this condition in 208 patients, but because his report dealt primarily with treatment, very little genetic information was obtained. He did state, however, that he did not find any unusual distribution of this disease among the various Jewish ethnic groups in Israel. As most studies have noted, in sporadic (nonfamilial) cases there is a preponderance of affected males. Axer observed that in his group male children predominated 4:1. In familial cases the ratio of males to females tends to be closer to 1:1.

Table 10.4. Reports of familial Legg-Calvé-Perthes disease

Authors	Year	Country	Ethnic background	Family members affected
Perthes	1910	Germany	?	Several members
Eden	1912	Germany	?	Father and son
Brandes	1920	Germany	?	Several members
Calvé	1921	France	?	Brother and sister
Müller	1922	Germany	?	Father and daughter
Brill	1927	Germany	?	Several members in 6 generations
Kaiser	1928	Germany	?	Members in 4 generations
Hagen	1939	U.S.	Italian	2 brothers
Lindemann	1941	Germany	?	Dizygotic and monozygotic twins in unrelated families
Stephens and Kerby	1946	U.S.	Welsh	28 affected members in 5 generations
McComas	1946	Australia	?	4 members in 2 generations
Hamsa and Campbell	1953	U.S.	?	3 brothers
Giannestras	1954	U.S.	?	Monozygotic twins
Goff	1954	U.S.	?	20% of cases reported had family history of the disease
Ruckerbauer	1958	Canada	?	Monozygotic twins
Wansbrough et al.	1959	Canada	?	12 of 129 cases had known affected relatives. 7 patients had unexamined relatives with a limp or hip trouble of unknown cause
Dunn	1960	U.S.	?	Monozygotic twins
Inglis	1960	U.S.	?	Monozygotic twins
Wamoscher and Farhi	1963	Israel	Ashkenazi Jewish	8 members in 3 generations
Gray, Lowry, and Renwick	1972	Canada	?	37 of 267 patients, or 14% with a positive family history
McKusick	1975	U.S.	?	Father and son

In 1976 Harper and co-workers did a population study on the occurrence of Perthes disease in South Wales over a 25-year period. The risk to sibs was less than 1 percent, and the risk to offspring of an affected parent was about 3 percent.

Prognosis and treatment

The principle of treatment is avoidance of weight bearing, for the head of the femur tends to flatten and become mushroom-shaped, causing incongruity between the head and the acetabulum, with degenerative changes later in life. The main prognostic factors as far as the eventual shape of the head of the femur is concerned are the age of the child at the time of onset, the amount of involvement shown radiographically, and whether dislocation of the hip or some other predisposing condition has been present in the past. In recent years surgical intervention has been advocated by some in order to maintain the spherical shape of the femoral head, but the merits of this approach have not been proved.

References

Axer, A. 1974. Perthes disease in Israel. *Harefuah* 86:239.

Brandes, M. 1920. Nachuntersuchungen und weitere Beobachtungen zum Krankheitsbilde der Osteochondritis deformans juvenilis coxae. *Dtsch. Z. Chir.* 155:216.

Brill, W. 1927. Beitrag zur Ätiologic der Perthesschen Erkrankung des Hüftgelenkes und der Köhlerschen Metatarsalerkrankung. *Arch. Orthop. Unfall-Chir.* 24:64.

Calvé, J. 1921. Coxa plana. *Presse Méd.* 29:383.

Dunn, A. W. 1960. Coxa plana in man. *J. Bone Joint Surg.* 42A:178.

Eden, R. 1912. Über Osteoarthritis deformans coxae juvenilis. *Dtsch. Z. Chir.* 117:148.

Giannestras, N. 1954. Legg-Perthes disease in twins. *J. Bone Joint Surg.* 36A:149.

Goff, C. W. 1954. *Legg-Calvé-Perthes syndrome and related osteochondroses of youth.* Springfield Ill.: Charles C Thomas.

Gray, I. M.; Lowry, R. B.; and Renwick, D. H. G. 1972. Incidence and genetics of Legg-Perthes disease (Osteochondritis deformans) in British Columbia: Evidence of polygenic determination. *J. Med. Genet.* 9:197.

Hagen, W. H. 1939. Coxaplana: Report of two bilateral cases in brothers. *J. Bone Joint Surg.* 21:1028.

Hamsa, W. R., and Campbell, L. S. 1953. Osteochondritis deformans coxae juvenilis. *Am. J. Dis. Child.* 86:54.

Harper, P. S.; Brotherton, J.; and Cochlin, D. 1976. Genetic risks in Perthes disease. *Clin. Genet.* 10:178.

Inglis, A. 1960. Genetic implications in coxa plana. *J. Bone Joint Surg.* 42A:711.

Kaiser, H. 1928. Über familiäres Auftreten von Osteochondritis deformans coxae (Perthes). *Wien. Arch. Inn. Med.* 16:61.

Legg, A. T. 1910. An obscure affection of the hip-joint. *Boston Med. Surg. J.* 162:202.

Lindenmann, K. 1941. Daserbliche Vorkommen der angeborenen Coxa Vara. *Z. Orthop.* 72:326.

McComas, E. 1946. Perthes' disease and its occurrence as a familial condition. *Med. J. Aust.* 2:584.

McKusick, V. A. 1975. *Mendelian inheritance in man,* 4th ed., p. 199. Baltimore: The Johns Hopkins University Press.

McNutt, W. 1962. Inherited vascular pattern of the femoral head and neck or a predisposing factor to Legg-Calvé-Perthes disease. *Tex. Rep. Biol. Med.* 20:525.

Müller, W. 1922. Beobachtungen zur Frage des Verlaufes, der Endausgänge sowie des familiären Auftretens der Osteochondritis deformans coxae juvenilis. *Arch. Orthop. Unfall-Chir.* 20:327.

Perthes, G. C. 1910. Über Arthritis deformans juvenilis. *Dtsch. Z. Chir.* 107:111.

Ruckerbauer, G. M. 1958. Genetical factors in Legg-Calvé-Perthes disease. M. A. thesis, University of Toronto.

Stephens, F. E., and Kerby, J. P. 1946. Hereditary Legg-Calvé-Perthes Disease. *J. Hered.* 37:153.

Wamoscher, Z., and Farhi, A. 1963. Hereditary Legg-Calvé-Perthes disease. *Am. J. Dis. Child.* 106:97.

Wansbrough, R. M.; Carrie, A. W.; Walker, N. F.; and Ruckerbauer, G. M. 1959. Coxa plana: Its genetic aspects and results of treatment with the long Taylor walking caliper. *J. Bone Joint Surg.* 41A:135.

MENTAL ILLNESS

Perhaps more has been written on mental illness in Jews than on any other disorder discussed in this chapter. The older medical literature abounds with reports implying that the rate of occurrence of a variety of mental illnesses is high among Jews (see section on mental retardation). Explanations for this allegedly high rate of affliction have been many and varied through the years. For example, some have claimed that mental illness has been passed from such Biblical personalities as King Saul; others have maintained that it is due to the frequent consanguineous marriages among Jews; some have emphasized the fact that Jews have been urban dwellers—i.e., living in stressful surroundings—for such a long period; others have postulated that mental illness is inherent in the nature of the Jew or have laid the blame on the great difficulties Jews have encountered throughout history. Although much has been written on the subject, it is extremely difficult to determine whether or not mental illnesses are indeed more frequent among Jews than among non-Jews. In discussing this question with a number of psychiatrists and leaders in the mental health field, I have found that most agree that the necessary data are lacking to make a decision concerning the frequency of certain forms of mental illness in Jews.

Partial exceptions can be found in the data obtained from two studies. The first is that of Malzberg, who collected an enormous amount of information on the incidence of mental diseases among Jews and non-Jews admitted to all hospitals, public and private, in New York State from 1939 to 1961. The second is the report of Gershon and Liebowitz, who analyzed the data (sociocultural and demographic) on all persons hospitalized at a psychiatric facility in Jerusalem between 1969 and 1972. Because these studies differ considerably in methodology and in the composition of the Jewish communities evaluated, they will be discussed separately; however, when possible, comparisons will be made between the two.

Although the work of Malzberg does not cover the entire spectrum of mental illness, it does represent a major segment. The biases in Malzberg's data are obvious to those trained in epidemiology, but because he has seriously tried to deal with the question of the frequency of certain mental illnesses in Jews, some attention must be given to his work. In 1973 he reported on 5,514 Jewish and 34,707 white non-Jewish first admissions (a total of 40,221) to all mental hospitals, public and private, in New York State from April 1959 to March 1961.

Table 10.5 summarizes his main findings, and the statements below reflect the conclusions he reached.

General paresis. Jews were differentiated from non-Jews with respect to the incidence of general paresis in that the average annual rate of first admissions for

Table 10.5. Mental illness: Jewish and white non-Jewish first admissions to all mental

| Mental disorder | Jews | | | | |
| | | | Total | | Average annual rate/ 100,000 pop. |
	Males	Females	No.	%	
General paresis	—	—	—	—	—
Alcoholic	17	2	19	0.3	0.4
With cerebral arteriosclerosis	381	521	902	16.4	18.2
Senile	178	277	455	8.3	9.2
Involutional	238	571	809	14.7	16.4
Manic-depressive	95	183	278	5.0	5.6
Schizophrenia	813	916	1,729	31.4	34.9
Psychoneuroses	246	467	713	12.9	14.4
Other	329	280	609	11.0	12.4
Total no. and rate	2,297	3,217	5,514	100.0	111.5

Source: B. Malzberg, 1973, *Acta Psychiatr. Scand.* 49:479. © 1973 Munksgaard International

Jews was zero, whereas the rate for non-Jews, although very low, was still 0.2 per
100,000.

Alcoholic psychoses. The incidence of alcoholic psychoses was significantly lower
for Jews than for non-Jews. The average annual rate was 0.4/100,000 among Jews,
compared to 8.2/100,000 among non-Jews. After standardizing for age, Malzberg
obtained a rate of 0.7 for Jews and 13.0 for non-Jews.

Psychoses with cerebral arteriosclerosis. The average annual rates per 100,000
population were 18.2 for Jews and 26.8 for non-Jews, indicating a lower incidence
of this disorder among Jews than among non-Jews of New York State.

Senile psychoses. The incidence of disorders in this category was lower among
Jews than among non-Jews. The average annual rates per 100,000 population were
9.2 for Jews and 12.5 for non-Jews.

Involutional psychoses. The incidence of such disorders was higher among Jews
than among non-Jews. The average annual rates per 100,000 population were 16.4
for Jews and 10.8 for non-Jews. When standardized, the rates became 34.4 for
Jews and 22.5 for non-Jews.

Manic-depressive psychoses. The incidence of this condition was higher among
Jews than among non-Jews. The average annual rates per 100,000 population were
5.6 for Jews and 3.2 for non-Jews. The standardized rates were 7.9 for Jews and
4.3 for non-Jews.

Schizophrenia. The incidence of this disease was higher among Jews than among
non-Jews. The average annual rates per 100,000 population were 34.9 for Jews
and 38.7 for non-Jews. When standardized, the rates became 50.8 for Jews and
44.4 for non-Jews.

hospitals in New York State, 1960–1961, classified according to mental disorders

Non-Jews					
		Total		Average annual rate/ 100,000 pop.	
Males	Females	No.	%		Mental disorder
39	6	45	0.1	0.2	General paresis
1,630	464	2,094	6.0	8.2	Alcoholic
3,298	3,583	6,881	19.8	26.8	With cerebral arteriosclerosis
1,266	1,941	3,207	9.2	12.5	Senile
812	1,964	2,776	8.0	10.8	Involutional
268	540	808	2.3	3.2	Manic-depressive
4,136	4,490	8,626	24.9	38.7	Schizophrenia
1,676	2,644	4,320	12.5	16.9	Psychoneuroses
3,987	1,963	5,950	17.1	18.1	Other
17,112	17,595	34,707	100.0	135.4	Total no. and rate

Publishers Ltd., Copenhagen, Denmark.

Psychoneuroses. The incidence of these disorders was lower among Jews than among non-Jews. The average annual rates per 100,000 population were 14.4 for Jews and 16.9 for non-Jews. The standardized rates were 20.7 for Jews and 23.0 for non-Jews.

Malzberg stated that these findings agreed with those in similar studies done by him under the same conditions in New York State during the periods 1939–1941 and 1949–1951. Furthermore, he stressed that his more recent observations were also in agreement with findings from a similarly designed Canadian study. It has been thought that the close Jewish family unit and the nonexcessive use of alcohol by Jews (see page 301) could explain the low rates of general paresis and alcoholic psychoses found by Malzberg, but the high or low rates noted for the other disorders are not explained as readily, nor is there a consensus as to the validity of these findings.

In 1975 Gershon and Liebowitz reported their findings on 833 Jewish residents of Jerusalem admitted to psychiatric hospitals for the first time during the period 1969–1972. The average annual incidence of psychiatric illness was 1.90/1,000 for the population aged 15 years or older. Table 10.6 lists the average annual incidence by diagnostic subdivision. A lower incidence of first hospitalizations was observed among Oriental and Sephardi Jews than among the Ashkenazim (see Tables 10.7 and 10.8). At that time the non-Ashkenazi community comprised 34 percent of the Jerusalem population aged 15 or older but accounted for only 25 percent of the city's psychiatric patients ($p < 0.001$).

Comparison of the incidence of psychiatric hospitalization of Ashkenazi Jews in Jerusalem with that of Jews from New York State (almost all were Ashkenazim in Malzberg's studies) reveals a slightly higher incidence in the Jerusalem population: 1.9/1,000 for the Jerusalem Ashkenazim versus 1.1/1,000 for Jews in New York State. Moreover, Malzberg noted that the incidence for white non-Jews was 1.35/1,000. When a correction for age was introduced, the psychiatric hospitalization rates became about the same in the Jerusalem and in New York State studies.

As seen in Table 10.9, the lifetime prevalence of psychiatric hospitalization was approximately 10.4 percent for both Jerusalem and New York State Jews. It should be noted that the rate of hospitalization was slightly lower for Jews than for white

Table 10.6. Mental illness: Average annual rate of hospitalization according to diagnosis, Jerusalem study

Diagnosis	No. of cases	%	Rate[a]
Affective disorders	155	19	0.354
Functional psychoses	280	34	0.640
Organic retarded	122	15	0.278
Neuroses (personality disorders)	133	13	0.258
Behavioral disorders	99	12	0.226
Attempted suicide	29	3	0.068
Observation	35	4	0.078
Total no. and average rate	833	100	1.902

Source: E. Gershon and J. L. Liebowitz, 1975, *J. Psychiatr. Res.* 12:37. Reprinted by permission of Pergamon Press, Ltd.

[a] Based on estimated population figures for January 1, 1971, expressed as new cases per 1,000 population aged 15 years or over.

Table 10.7. Mental illness: Average annual first hospitalization rates
according to birthplace, Jerusalem study

Diagnosis	No. of cases	Rates[a]		
		Israel	Asia and Africa	Europe and America
Affective disorders	154	0.24	0.22	0.63
Functional psychoses	276	0.77	0.45	0.69
Organic retarded	120	0.29	0.21	0.32
Neuroses (personality disorders)	113	0.36	0.21	0.20
Behavioral disorders	98	0.34	0.15	0.19
Attempted suicide	28	0.07	0.07	0.05
Observation	34	0.16	0.04	0.02
Total no. and average rate	823[b]	2.22	1.37	2.19
Total no. of patients	823	338	203	282
Population over age of 14 yr	145,777	50,580	49,161	45,092

Source: E. Gershon and J. L. Liebowitz, 1975, *J. Psychiatr. Res.* 12:37. Reprinted by permission of Pergamon Press, Ltd.

Note: $\chi^2 = 32.16$; D.F. $= 2$; $p < 0.001$.

[a] Rates per 1,000 population aged 15 years or over according to estimated population on January 1, 1961.

[b] Data not available for 10 patients.

non-Jews. However, Jews seem to have a higher lifetime prevalence of hospitalization for the affective disorders included in the data of Malzberg, which suggests a higher prevalence of affective illness among Jews than among non-Jews in New York. In the Jerusalem study the lifetime prevalence of hospitalization for affective disorders was 2.4 percent. Gershon and Liebowitz point out that no comparable figure can be computed for Jews in New York because diagnostic categories in the 2 studies differ.

Gershon and Liebowitz concluded that the diagnosis of affective disorders in the Jerusalem study was associated with status—higher social class, Ashkenazi ethnicity, birth abroad, older age, sex, and marital status. A multivariate analysis indicated

Table 10.8. Mental illness: Ethnic distribution of diagnoses, Jerusalem study

Diagnosis	No. of cases	Ashkenazim (%)	Sephardim[a] (%)
Affective disorders	154	68	32
Functional psychoses	271	57	43
Organic retarded	118	53	47
Neuroses (personality disorders)	111	42	58
Behavioral disorders	96	35	65
Attempted suicide	27	41	59
Observation	37	27	73
Total no. and average rate	811[b]	52	48

Source: E. Gershon and J. L. Liebowitz, 1975, *J. Psychiatr. Res.* 12:37. Reprinted by permission of Pergamon Press, Ltd.

[a] *Sephardim* here refers to both Oriental and Sephardi Jews.

[b] Data were not available for an additional 22 patients.

Table 10.9. Mental illness: Lifetime prevalence of affective disorders and psychiatric hospitalization after the age of 15, Jerusalem and New York State studies

Study		Rates[a]	
		Psychiatric hospitalization	Affective disorders
Jerusalem, 1969–1972[b]			
Jewish population		0.1044	0.0240
Western born (Europe or the Americas)		0.1340	0.0350
Eastern born (Asia or Africa)		0.0797	0.0148
Native Israeli		0.1141	0.0194
New York State, 1960–1961[c]		Manic-depressive	Involutional psychosis
Jews	0.1034	0.0047	0.0152
Non-Jews (whites)	0.1082	0.0026	0.0096

Source: E. Gershon and J. L. Liebowitz, 1975, *J. Psychiatr. Res.* 12:37.

[a] For the Jerusalem study, rates are based on population figures for January 1, 1971, expressed as new cases per 1,000 population aged 15 or over; for the New York State study, rates are annual averages per 100,000 population.

[b] Incomplete data for 22 of 833 patients.

[c] Malzberg's data.

that the sociocultural factors were relatively less important than the demographic ones in determining diagnosis.

When it comes to discussing the genetics of mental disorders, one soon realizes that very little is known about such a role in most of them. Much has been written about genetic factors in schizophrenia, but the key investigators are far from agreement on a monogenic versus a polygenic cause. Some even argue that specific pathogenic genes are not involved.

Much remains to be learned about the basic mechanism(s) of most forms of mental illness and about the distribution and frequency of mental illnesses among the various Jewish ethnic groups. Thus, what once seemed certain in the minds of many—that the rate of mental illness among Jews is extremely high—can no longer be accepted as a truism. As our knowledge of the biochemistry of these disorders increases, it will be possible to design better epidemiological and genetic studies to answer some of the questions raised in this discussion.

References

Davies, A. M., and Kaplan-Dinur, A. 1961. Suicide in Israel: An epidemiological study. *Int. J. Soc. Psychiatry* 8:32.

Ebstein, W. 1902. *Die Medizin im Alten Testament.* Stuttgart: n.p.

Fishberg, M. 1911. *The Jews: A study of race and environment.* New York: Charles Scribner's.

Gershon, E., and Liebowitz, J. L. 1975. Sociocultural and demographic correlates of affective disorders in Jerusalem. *J. Psychiatr. Res.* 12:37.

Gregory, I. 1960. Genetic factors in schizophrenia. *Am. J. Psychiatry* 116:961.

Grewel, F. 1967. Psychiatric differences in Ashkenazim and Sephardim. *Neurol. Neurochir. Psychiatr. Pol.* 70:339.

Malzberg, B. 1960. *Mental disease among Jews in New York State.* New York: Intercontinental Medical Book Corp.

————. 1962. The distribution of mental disease according to religious affiliation in New York State, 1949–1956. *Ment. Hygiene* 4:510.

————. 1963. *Mental disease among Jews in Canada.* Albany, N.Y.: Research Foundation for Mental Hygiene.

————. 1963. *The mental health of Jews in New York State, 1949–1951.* Albany, N.Y.: Research Foundation for Mental Hygiene.

————. 1966. *Ethnic variations in mental disease in New York State, 1949–1951.* Albany, N.Y.: Research Foundation for Mental Hygiene.

————. 1971. *Studies of mental illness among Jews.* Albany, N.Y.: Research Foundation for Mental Hygiene.

————. 1973. Mental disease among Jews in New York State, 1960–1961. *Acta Psychiatr.* Scand. 49:479.

Miller, H. 1967. Depression. *Br. Med. J.* 1:257.

Myerson, A. 1920. The "nervousness" of the Jew. *Ment. Hygiene* 4:65.

Rosenthal, D., and Ketty S. 1968. *The transmission of schizophrenia.* New York: Pergamon Press.

White, W. A.; Davis, T. K.; and Frantz, A. M., ed. 1931. *Manic-depressive psychosis.* Baltimore: Williams and Wilkins.

MENTAL RETARDATION

The older literature on mental retardation (mainly European from the mid- and late 19th and early 20th centuries) is filled with claims of a high rate of mental retardation among Jews. Table 10.10, a sample of this literature, compares the number of Christians and Jews admitted to Prussian mental asylums from 1882 to 1900.

During the years of heavy Jewish immigration to the United States and England several published studies purported to show the high frequency of mental deficiency among the new immigrants. In 1928 Sir Humphry Rolleston said of the Jews: "This race [is] remarkable for the contrasts it presents of high culture and intellectual ability, wealth and luxury, on the one hand, with, on the other hand, an incidence of mental defectives said to be higher than [that] in any other civilized race."

Evaluating the older literature on mental retardation is difficult, whether the data involve Jews or other ethnic groups. Past criteria for diagnosis are inadequate by today's standards, test settings were frequently biased, and most studies were

Table 10.10. Number of Christian and Jewish idiots (severely retarded patients) per 1,000,000 population admitted to mental asylums in Prussia, 1882–1900

Years	No. of Christians/ 1,000,000 pop.	No. of Jews/ 1,000,000 pop.
1882–1885	25.9	95.5
1886–1890	28.6	88.1
1891–1895	53.4	122.7
1896–1900	62.1	140.2

Source: M. Fishberg, 1911, *The Jews: A study of race and environment* (New York: Charles Scribner's), p. 333.

poorly designed and lacked control groups. Considering these facts, should all such literature be ignored, or could there be some element of truth in these reports inferring a high frequency of mental deficiency among Ashkenazi Jews? In attempting to answer this complex question, the following points should be taken into account: (1) several genetic disorders in which mental deficiency is a key feature are known to affect the Ashkenazi community (see Chapter 5); (2) there is a correlation between the rate of consanguinity among normal parents and offspring who suffer from mental retardation of unknown etiology. If one assumes that those disorders associated with mental retardation occurred frequently in the Ashkenazi community some 100 years ago but were not diagnosed, and that the rate of consanguinity in this group was higher (which it must have been) than it is at present, it is conceivable that mental retardation was a common event in Jewish communities of the past (see also the discussion of marriage patterns in Chapter 13). However, to say that mental retardation occurred predominantly in Jews in the proportions recorded in the older literature would be more exaggeration than fact.

Because most studies today approach mental retardation from an etiological viewpoint (genetic [chromosomal or biochemical] or environmental) rather than from the perspective of ethnic distribution, there are few data with which to examine the supposition that the frequency of mental retardation is high among Jews.

Costeff and co-workers have investigated the influence of parental consanguinity on mentally retarded Jewish children. In 1972 they reported their findings on the rate of parental consanguinity in 972 cases of mental retardation from 904 families. Table 10.11 shows the extent of parental consanguinity in the various types of mental retardation. A significantly higher rate of first-cousin marriages was observed in the following groups: (1) familial retardates, severe (34 percent); (2) idiopathic retardates, mild (19.5 percent); and (3) idiopathic retardates, severe (15.5 percent).

In view of the higher rate of parental consanguinity among the more severe cases of familial retardation, all familial retardates were analyzed in more detail

Table 10.11. Number of Jewish Israeli families with familial retardation by major diagnostic category, degree of retardation, and parental consanguinity

Degree of retardation	Diagnostic category	First cousins	Loosely related	Un-related	Total	
Mild	Obviously nonfamilial	3	1	15	19	$\chi^2 = 2.94$
	Obviously familial	11	10	70	91	D.F. = 1
	Pathology of uncertain etiology	0	1	6	7	$0.1 > p > 0.05$
	Idiopathic[a]	36	16	133	185	
	Total	50	28	224	302	
Severe	Obviously nonfamilial	9	12	86	107	$\chi^2 = 40.0$
	Obviously familial[a]	40	7	72	119	D.F. = 6
	Pathology of uncertain etiology	3	1	16	20	$p < 0.001$
	Idiopathic[a]	52	24	265	341	
	Total	104	44	439	587	

Source: H. Costeff et al., 1972, *Acta Paediatr. Scand.* 61:452.
Note: Dotted lines indicate division of table for χ^2 calculation.
[a] Group with significantly high rate of parental consanguinity.

Table 10.12. Number of Jewish Israeli families with familial retardation by diagnostic category, degree of retardation, and parental consanguinity

Degree of retardation	Diagnostic category	First cousins	Loosely related	Unrelated	Total	
Mild	Heredofamilial diseases	1	0	6	7	$\chi^2 = 1.97$
	Unlabeled syndromes	3	0	2	5	D.F. $= 1$
	Nonsyndromic, parents normal	5	6	34	45	$p > 0.1$
	Nonsyndromic, parent(s) apparently retarded	2	4	28	34	
	Total	11	10	70	91	
Severe	Heredofamilial diseases	10	0	4	14	$\chi^2 = 14.6$
	Unlabeled syndromes	3	1	6	10	D.F. $= 3$
	Nonsyndromic, parents normal	21	5	28	54	$p < 0.001$
	Nonsyndromic, parent(s) apparently retarded	6	1	34	41	
	Total	40	7	72	119	
Mixed	Heredofamilial diseases	1	0	0	1	
	Unlabeled syndromes	2	0	0	2	
	Nonsyndromic, parents normal	2	0	7	9	
	Nonsyndromic, parent(s) apparently retarded	0	1	2	2	
	Total	5	1	9	15	

Source: H. Costeff et al., 1972, *Acta Paediatr. Scand.* 61:452.
Note: Dotted lines indicate division of table for χ^2 calculation.

by Costeff's group. Each type of retardation was classified as one of the following: heredofamilial disease of known cause (e.g., phenylketonuria); retardation as part of an unclassified or unlabeled familial syndrome; retardation without syndromic findings in sibs only; retardation without syndromic findings proved in at least one sib and suspected in at least one parent.

Table 10.12 details the consanguinity trends among the familial retardates. It shows that the rate of parental consanguinity in families with apparently retarded parents or mildly retarded parents is not significantly higher than the approximately 10 percent rate of first-cousin marriages found among nonfamilial retardates. All other categories of severe familial retardation and of familial retardation of mixed degree (mild and severe in the same family) show greatly increased parental consanguinity.

Since the Israeli Jewish population consists of a number of ethnic groups with different rates of inbreeding, Costeff's group compared the consanguinity trends noted in Tables 10.11 and 10.12 with those occurring in the major ethnic groups. Tables 10.13 and 10.14 show a significant link between parental consanguinity and both severe familial cases and, with the exception of the Yemenites, severe idiopathic cases when these cases are compared either to a control group of nonfamilial retardates or to the prevailing rates of consanguineous marriages in these same ethnic groups. With the exception of the Ashkenazi Jews, who do not show a higher rate of parental consanguinity, the same trend prevails among parents with mild idiopathic mental retardation.

This study shows that among the various Jewish ethnic groups in Israel there

Table 10.13. Parental consanguinity by ethnic group and diagnostic classification: Severe idiopathic cases

Ethnic group	Familial non-syndromic (I.Q. < 50)		Idiopathic (I.Q. < 50)		Obviously non-familial (all degrees)		Prop. of consanguineous marriages in pop. at large
	Consanguineous	Unrelated	Consanguineous	Unrelated	Consanguineous	Unrelated	
Ashkenazi Jews (European)	2	3	6	93	0	36	1.52
Iraqi Jews	9	7	14	31	4	15	22.8
Yemenite Jews	2	5	6	37	2	12	12.2
Moroccan Jews	3	2	5	16	1	6	9.0
Persian Jews	2	1	10	10	0	5	26.0
Total observed	18	18	41	187	7	74	
Total expected (based on data of Goldschmidt et al.)[a]	5.8	30.2	24.1	203.9	8.5	72.5	
χ^2	30.3		13.3		0.30		
p	0.001		0.001		n.s.		

Source: H. Costeff et al., 1972, *Acta Paediatr. Scand.* 61:452.

Note: Consanguineous = first cousins and uncle-niece pairs; lesser degrees of consanguinity have been omitted from all calculations.

[a] Data are taken from the population survey of Goldschmidt et al.

is a strikingly high consanguinity rate among parents who are normal but have 2 or more severely retarded children. A moderately high rate of parental consanguinity was also observed in patients whose retardation was of unknown etiology and who had no retarded sibs. It should be mentioned that similar surveys from other countries have shown the same correlation. This feature of parental consanguinity has not been significant in parents who themselves appeared retarded, nor has it been found among families with 2 or more mildly retarded children.

Autosomal recessive inheritance appears to play a primary role in severe familial retardation of children of normal parents and a significant one in all degrees of isolated idiopathic retardation.

In conclusion, the question of the overall frequency of mental retardation among Jews remains unanswered. However, it is apparent that Jewish ethnic groups (mainly non-Ashkenazi) in which the rate of consanguinity is high (see Chapter 12) will have a greater proportion of children with familial idiopathic retardation than will groups with lower rates of consanguinity.

References

Åkesson, H. O. 1961. *Epidemiology and genetics of mental deficiency: Swedish population.* Uppsala: Almqvist and Wiksell.

Costeff, H. 1977. Consanguinity analysis in heterogeneous populations. *Am. J. Hum. Genet.* 29:329.

Costeff, H.; Cohen, B. E.; and Weller, L. 1972. Parental consanguinity among Israeli mental retardates. *Acta Paediatr. Scand.* 61:452.

Costeff, H.; Cohen, B. E.; Weller, L.; and Rahman, D. 1977. Consanguinity analysis in Israeli mental retardates. *Am. J. Hum. Genet.* 29:339.

Dewey, W. J.; Barrai, I.; Morton, N. F.; and Mi, M. P. 1965. Recessive genes in severe mental defect. *Am. J. Hum. Genet.* 17:237.

Drillien, C. M.; Jameson, S.; and Wilkinson, E. M. 1966. Studies in mental handicap. Part 1: Prevalence and distribution by clinical type and severity of defect. *Arch. Dis. Child.* 41:528.

Fishberg, M. 1911. *The Jews: A study of race and environment.* New York: Charles Scribner's.

Goddard, H. H. 1912. Feeble-mindedness and immigration. *Training School Bulletin* 9(6):1.

———. 1928. Mental tests and the immigrant. *J. Delinq.* 2:243.

Goldschmidt, F.; Ronen, A.; and Ronen, I. 1960. Changing marriage systems in the Jewish communities of Israel. *Ann. Hum. Genet.* 24:191.

Rolleston, H. 1928. Some diseases in the Jewish race. *Bull. Johns Hopkins Hospital* 43:117.

MYOPIA

Many of the early studies on myopia among Jews were done in London between 1925 and 1929. In 1925 Pearson and Moul, two eugenicists, began publishing a fascinating series of articles dealing with the question of whether or not Jews (Ashkenazi Jews) were fit for immigration to Great Britain. Visual acuity was one of many things these investigators evaluated. In the introduction to their study they stated the following: "The purport of this memoir is to discuss whether it is desirable in an already crowded country like Great Britain to permit indiscriminate immigration, or, if the conclusion be that it is not, on what grounds discrimination should be based." They readily mentioned that they had nothing against Jews, but merely wanted to know if Polish and Russian Jews were fit for English society. "In the case of Russian and Polish Jews," they wrote, "there has been more or less continuous oppression, nay, a veritable selection going on for a much longer period. Such a treatment does not necessarily leave the best elements of a race surviving."

With regard to visual acuity, they found a high rate of myopia among Jewish children of Polish-Russian extraction, but concluded that poor environmental conditions did not contribute to this defective vision: "Our final conclusion here must be that poor environment is not a source of defective vision in these Jewish boys and the inference is that it will not be found to be so either in the case of Gentile children."

In 1928 Sourasky (who later changed his name to Sorsby), a Jewish ophthalmologist working in London, also investigated the frequency of myopia in both Jewish and non-Jewish boys and girls from London. There were a number of interesting sidelights to his study: (1) it was carried out under the auspices of the Jewish Health Organization of Great Britain; (2) his main publications on the subject of myopia in Jewish and non-Jewish children do not refer to the work of Pearson and Moul, which was done during the same period and in the same city; and (3) it seems that he was selected to do this study in order to counteract any ill effects on Jewish immigration brought about by the studies of Pearson and Moul.

Being Jewish, Sourasky wrote a different kind of introduction in his article on myopia among the Jewish population in the East End of London:

It will not be out of place to say a few words about social conditions among Jews in the East End. As immigration into this country has practically ceased since 1914, the children attending the elementary schools are almost all born in this country, though in the vast majority of cases their parents are of Polish or Russian origin.

The children are brought up in very much the same way as the non-Jewish child population, except in the cases of the boys, who in addition to attending the ordinary elementary day school also attend classes for the study of Hebrew for two and a half to three hours every evening (except Friday and usually also Saturday, when there is no attendance, and Sunday, when attendance is in the morning).

Those acquainted with the Hebrew alphabet know how tiring its letters are on account of the alternate thick and thin strokes, and the little difference (such as a slightly longer thin stroke) that exists between one letter and another. Difficult as these conditions are they are made still more difficult by the fact that the books in use are almost all badly printed, poor type on poor paper; and as the schools are supported by voluntary contributions they experience the usual financial embarrassment associated with such institutions, so that in most schools only one book is provided for the use of two pupils. All this together with improper use or the total absence of desks, must throw a strain on the eyes, such as the non-Jewish boys can hardly experience.

What were Sorsby's findings? Table 10.14 shows the proportions of good and defective vision among Jewish and non-Jewish boys in the East End of London. At the end of his investigations Sorsby drew the following conclusions:

(1) The incidence of visual defects among Jewish boys in the East End is over 40 percent—double that of the non-Jewish boys.

(2) This heavy incidence of defect among Jewish boys is stationary all through their school life; it is practically no heavier at the age of 14 than it is at 7.

(3) The incidence of the defects is, therefore, not increased with school life, and apparently not produced by the excessive amount of close work done by Jewish boys.

(4) Comparative analysis of the refractive errors seen among the defectives of the Jewish and non-Jewish children reveals but little difference in the distribution of errors apart from a rather higher incidence of myopia and of low hypermetropia among the Jewish children.

(5) There is but little difference in the percentage of myopes in the early years of school life (5–9 years) in the two groups. The greater incidence of myopia among Jewish children becomes marked in the later years (10–14 years).

(6) It is argued that the greater increase in myopia in the later years among Jewish children is not the result of excessive close work, but of the greater incidence of low hypermetropia among the young Jewish children.

(7) When the analyses are carried further to bring out any distinction in the

Table 10.14. Myopia: Good and defective vision among Jewish and non-Jewish boys in London's East End, 1928

Subjects	Total no.	Age (yr)	Vision of 6/9 and 6/6 (%)	Vision of 6/12 and 6/18 (%)	Vision less than 6/18 (%)
Jewish boys	1,649	6–14	56.8	22.1	21.1
Non-Jewish boys	600	8–14	78.3	15.0	6.7

Source: A. Sourasky 1928, *Br. J. Ophthalmol.* 12:197.

increase of the number of myopes among Jewish boys as compared with girls, it is found that the increase is decidedly greater among the boys (who do much more close work).

(8) However, the same is seen to be true of the non-Jewish boys (who do not do an excessive amount of close work) as compared with the non-Jewish girls.

(9) It is therefore suggested that there is a sex-determined factor which controls the growth of the eye.

(10) The excessive incidence of myopia among Jewish boys is explained by the racial factor of the great prevalence of low hypermetropia and the sex-determined (and nonracial) factor which allows for a greater or longer development of the length of the eye.

Duke-Elder has noted that a similar ratio of myopia among Jews and Gentiles was found in Germany by Weiss in 1885 and by Kirchner in 1889, while Gallus, in 1922, noted an unusually high occurrence of myopia among Jews. In 1914 Tenner evaluated 4,800 school children in the New York City area and stated the following: "As to nationality, myopia is prevalent in Germany, and it is interesting to note that the proportionate amount of myopia was greatest among the children of German stock, viz., thirty-five percent. The Russians, being mainly Jews, came next with 34.5 percent. The children of American parents showed almost as great a proportion of myopia, 30 percent, the Irish, 27 percent, and the Italians, a comparatively low porportion 23.8 percent." Since Tenner recorded only the place of birth of the parents of these myopic children, I suspect that the rate of myopia was highest in the Jewish children in his study.

High frequencies of myopia are not restricted to Jews, however. Well-documented studies show that the occurrence of this condition is also high among the Japanese, Chinese, and West Europeans.

In none of the previously mentioned studies was any attempt made to evaluate the presence of myopia in the families of affected children. However, there are many well-documented studies on the familial occurrence of myopia. Mild to moderate myopia has been shown to be transmitted as an autosomal dominant trait in many families, while pronounced myopia is usually inherited as an autosomal recessive trait. Nevertheless, autosomal dominant inheritance of pronounced myopia has been reported in some families. Some investigators think that myopia is multifactorial in etiology, while Karlsson has recently claimed that most cases of myopia are due to autosomal recessive inheritance. It seems apparent from reviewing the literature that there is much heterogeneity in myopia, and proper genetic studies are needed to distinguish the various types.

On the basis of available data, it would be wrong to conclude that myopia occurs most frequently among Jews. However, it can be said that myopia is common in Jews and apparently favors the Ashkenazi community. How common it is and its exact frequency and distribution among the various Jewish ethnic groups are questions that remain to be answered.

It seems appropriate to end this historical account of myopia with a hopeful clinical note written by an ophthalmologist.

Poor distant vision is the main symptom of this defect. Curiously, in its milder form it may in many cases appear to be an advantage. Accustomed to defective vision from the time he began to look upon the world intelligently, the myope frequently fails to recognize his limitations. Especially when his close attention is required largely for near work, as so often happens under civilized conditions of life, he accepts a blurring of distant objects as normal and neglects it. In the middle of life, when his accommodation fails, he has the advantage that he does not require glasses for reading; and in old age, as his contracting pupil cuts down his diffusion circles, and as the senile changes in his lens bring on a relative hypermetropia, he is in the happy position that at 80 he is the envy of his hypermetropic contemporaries and the pride of his bespectacled presbyopic children.

References

Duke-Elder, S., ed. 1970. *System of ophthalmology*, vol. 5: *Ophthalmic optics and re-fraction*, pp. 238–39, 268–74. St. Louis: C. V. Mosby.

Francois, J. 1967. *Heredity in ophthalmology*, pp. 194–201. St. Louis: C. V. Mosby.

Karlsson, J. L. 1974. Concordance rates for myopia in twins. *Clin. Genet.* 6:142.

———1975. Evidence for recessive inheritance of myopia. *Clin. Genet.* 7:197.

Pearson, K., and Moul, M. 1925–1926. The problem of alien immigration into Great Britain, illustrated by an examination of Russian and Polish children: Part 1. *Ann. Eugen.* 1:5.

———. 1927. The problem of alien immigration into Great Britain, illustrated by an examination of Russian and Polish children: Part II. *Ann. Eugen.* 2:111.

———. 1928. The problem of alien immigration into Great Britain, illustrated by an examination of Russian and Polish children: Part III. *Ann. Eugen.* 3:1.

Sorsby, A. 1934. The pre-myopic state: Its bearing on the incidence of myopia. *Trans. Ophthalmol. Soc. U.K.* 54:459.

Sourasky, A. 1928. Race, sex, and environment in the development of myopia. *Brit. J. Ophthalmol.* 12:197.

Tenner, A. S. 1915. Refraction in school children: 4,800 refractions tabulated according to age, sex, and nationality. *N.Y. Med. J.* 102:611.

Waardenburg, P. J. 1963. *Genetics and opthalmology*, vol. 2, p. 1232. Springfield, Ill.: Charles C Thomas.

OBESITY

In the older medical literature pertaining to diseases in Jews, many sources either suggest or declare that obesity is common in Jews. Since most of the reports are from the European literature (mainly German), one can assume that such statements refer to Ashkenazi Jews. In 1928 Sir Humphry Rolleston wrote the following on obesity among Jews: "The subject of obesity, which is so common in Jews, is of interest in connection not only with the high incidence of diabetes in Jews, but also with other evidence of their special liability to disorders of fat metabolism, as shown by the comparative frequency of Gaucher's splenomegaly and Niemann's disease in Hebrews." Perhaps Rolleston would be even more convinced today of the predisposition of Ashkenazi Jews to obesity if he knew that other lipid disorders, such as abetalipoproteinemia, mucolipidosis type IV, Tay-Sachs disease, and possibly spongy degeneration of the central nervous system, also are common to the Ashkenazi Jewish community. However, there is probably no connection whatsoever between the above disorders and obesity. Furthermore, diabetes mellitus has not been proven to be exceptionally frequent in Jews (see page 334).

Table 10.15. Familial aggregation in obesity

Investigator	Year	Place	Observations
Gurney	1936	U.S.	9% of children obese when both parents normal
Rony	1940	U.S.	250 obese patients—69% with 1 or both parents obese
Bauer	1945	Vienna	1,000 obese patients—73% with 1 or both parents obese
Angel	1949	U.S.	Series of obese children—80% with 1 or both parents obese One parent obese—50% of offspring obese Both parents obese—66% of offspring obese

The early statements on obesity in Jews were almost always personal accounts, for the concept of control studies did not exist at that time. The question of obesity in Jews—Ashkenazi or non-Ashkenazi— remains unanswered, for proper epidemiological studies are lacking to evaluate this matter.

Most authorities in the field recognize that the tendency to obesity can be inherited, regardless of whether the direct cause is metabolic, psychological, or something else. It is commonly observed that obese individuals often come from obese families (see Table 10.15). However, because of the problem of assortative matings (e.g., obese individuals marry obese and thin marry thin) and because family groups share common eating habits, the genetic significance of such studies is difficult to interpret. Although studies of twins have been criticized for similar reasons, they do suggest that identical twins are more closely related in weight than are fraternal twins or sibs taken at the same age. For example, Newman and co-workers found a much closer correlation of weight in monozygotic twins than in dizygotic twins or sibs. The mean pair difference in the weight of the sibs was 10.4 pounds, compared with 10.0 pounds for the dizygotic twins and 4.1 pounds for the monozygotic twins.

The role of heredity in familial obesity is probably multifactorial. The weights of sibs of obese index cases are unimodally distributed, with a higher modal weight than the control population, as one would expect with multifactorial inheritance. It is conceivable that the number and size of adipose tissue cells are genetically determined, but much remains to be learned about the precise role of heredity in obesity.

References

Angel, J. L. 1949. Constitution in female obesity. *Am. J. Phys. Anthropol.* 7:433.

Bauer, J. 1945. *Constitution and disease.* New York: Grune and Stratton.

Goldstein, J. L., and Motulsky, A. 1974. Genetics and endocrinology. In *Textbook of endocrinology,* ed. R. H. Williams, p. 1025. Philadelphia: W. B. Saunders.

Gurney, R. 1936. Hereditary factor in obesity. *Arch. Intern. Med.* 57:557.

Krinkler, D. M. 1970. Diseases of Jews. *Postgrad. Med. J.* 46:687.

McCracken, B. H. 1962. Etiological aspects of obesity. *Am. J. Med. Sci.* 243:153.

Newman, H. H.; Freeman, R. N.; and Holzinger, J. J. 1937. Twins: A study of heredity and environment. Chicago: The University of Chicago Press.

Rimoin, D. L., and Schimke, R. N. 1971. *Genetic disorders of the endocrine glands,* pp. 151–66. St. Louis: C. V. Mosby.

Rolleston, H. 1928. Some diseases in the Jewish race. *Bull. Johns Hopkins Hospital* 43:117.

Rony, H. R. 1940. *Obesity and leaness.* Philadelphia: Lea and Febiger.

PEMPHIGUS VULGARIS

Historical note

According to Lever, the first case in the medical literature to which the diagnosis pemphigus vulgaris might possibly be applied is that described by Koenig in 1681. In 1777 Macbride reported cases definitely identifiable as pemphigus vulgaris and referred to the condition as *morbus vesicularis*. In 1791 Wichmann described the disease lucidly and was the first to use the term *pemphigus.*

In the 1940s, medical surveys from metropolitan centers of the eastern United States began reporting that pemphigus vulgaris was common among Ashkenazi Jews. This observation soon became entombed in textbooks of dermatology and thus was perpetuated. In 1964, however, Ziprkowski and Schewach-Millet's report on the disease did not confirm an unusually high frequency in the Ashkenazi Jewish community and furthermore showed that one-third of the cases in Israel are found among non-Ashkenazi Jews.

Clinical features

Pemphigus vulgaris occurs with equal frequency in men and women and usually presents itself during the fifth and sixth decades of life. It is characterized by bullae on apparently normal skin and mucous membranes. The fluid in the bullae is clear at first, but later may become hemorrhagic or seropurulent. These bullae arise momentarily and are tense, but soon become flaccid and rupture to form erosions with raw surfaces that ooze and bleed easily. The large denuded areas then become partially covered with crusts and spread extensively by confluence. The healed lesions are usually hyperpigmented but show little or no scarring.

The lesions usually appear first in the mouth and later in the groin. Other sites frequently affected are the scalp, face, neck, axillae, and genitals. Involvement of the paronychial areas may come first, with the oral lesions. In the beginning the bullae are usually sparse and seem inconsequential, but extensive generalized lesions may develop within a few weeks or may be limited to one or more sites for several months.

Diagnosis

Clinical findings in conjunction with a skin biopsy usually make for an easy diagnosis. Characteristic histopathological findings are acantholysis, intraepidermal cleft and blister formation, and acantholytic cells (Tzanck cells) lining the bulla as well as lying free in the bulla cavity.

Many of the acantholytic cells are detached or loosely attached to neighboring cells, or lie in clusters within the bulla. These cells are separate and show no intercellular bridges; the large nuclei are surrounded by a lightly staining halo in the cytoplasm and then a darkly staining cytoplasm at the periphery of the cell.

The histological finding of suprabasal intraepidermal bullae with acantholysis is characteristic of pemphigus and usually differentiates it from other similar diseases.

Table 10.16. Pemphigus vulgaris: Familial cases resulting in death

Author	Year	Familial occurrence
Feldman	1936	2 brothers
Greenbaum	1940	Father and son; 2 sisters
Ferrari	1947	Twin brother and sister
Granirer	1948	Sister and 2 brothers
Miller and Frank	1949	Sister and 2 brothers
Velentej	1960	Mother and daughter

Basic defect

The basic defect in pemphigus vulgaris is not known. The presence of inter-cellular antiepithelial antibodies in the serum of patients with all forms of pemphigus suggests that this is an autoimmune disease.

Genetics

Although there have been scattered reports (Table 10.16) of familial cases of pemphigus vulgaris, there is little evidence that this is a genetically determined disorder.

Pemphigus vulgaris has been reported in many populations throughout the world, but certain groups, such as Ashkenazi Jews, Italians, Greeks, Arabs, and East Indians, have been reported to have a greater predisposition for the disease.

Table 10.17 lists the number of cases reported in Ashkenazi Jews from various large cities of the world. One cannot completely ignore the figures in Table 10.17, but it is important to realize the degree of bias in such reporting. The fact that these cities are known to have large Ashkenazi Jewish populations, that Jews tend to seek medical care more than other ethnic groups, that many of the physicians reporting their experience with this disease were Jews themselves and thus attracted Jewish patients—all are cogent factors in introducing bias.

Although Ziprkowski and Schewach-Millet's 1964 report was concerned mainly with the treatment of this disease, it also showed that Jews other than those of Ashkenazi origin are predisposed to pemphigus. In their review of 48 cases reported

Table 10.17. Pemphigus vulgaris: Cases observed in Ashkenazi Jews from various cities of the world

Author	City	Time period	Total no. of patients	No. of Jewish patients	Jewish %
Gellis and Glass	N.Y.C. Belevue Hosp.	1911–1941	170	84	49
Tappeiner	Vienna—Allgemeine Krankenhaus	1920–1937	227	66	29
Eller and Kest	N.Y.C. Hosp.	1941	77	56	73
Gombes and Canizares	N.Y.C. Bellevue Hosp.	1941–1950	82	59	72
Costello, Jaimovich, and Dannenberg	N.Y.C. Bellevue Hosp.	1951–1955	52	30	58
Sheklakov	Moscow	1961	162	65	40
Lever	Boston	1971	65	39	60

438   GENETIC DISORDERS AMONG THE JEWISH PEOPLE

from 1949 to 1963, 33 were Ashkenazi, 13 were Sephardi, and 2 were of Yemenite origin. Dermatologists in Israel have stated that they are not aware of an exceptionally high number of Jewish patients with this disease.

These scattered bits of information and impressions should be better documented and a well-designed epidemiological study should be undertaken to place in proper perspective the ethnic distribution of this disease not only among Jews but in other groups as well. Genetic and family studies also may be worthwhile since some consider pemphigus vulgaris to be an autoimmune disease.

Prognosis and treatment

The prognosis in pemphigus was a guarded one before the use of corticosteroids, for nearly all patients died. In some instances the disease progressed rapidly and death occurred within a few weeks. Usually several months and occasionally even a few years passed before the patient succumbed to the disease. Only rarely did a patient survive.

Lever has commented that in his experience this disease usually progresses more rapidly in Jewish patients than in other patients.

Skin lesions may be sprayed with corticosteroids or 2 percent procaine hydrochloride. Corticosteroids are always given systemically and the dosage depends on the extent of the lesions and the patient's response to therapy. Supportive therapy involving antibiotics, fluids, electrolytes, anabolic agents, etc., is indicated, depending upon the patient's condition. Various immunosuppressive drugs, such as methotrexate and cytoxan, also are being used. With the proper course of treatment there is much hope for pemphigus patients, and many eventually become free of the lesions and lead normal lives.

References

Combes, F. C., and Canizares, O. 1950. Pemphigus vulgaris: A clinopathological study of 100 cases. *Arch. Dermatol. Syph.* 62:786.

Costello, M. J.; Jaimovich, L.; and Dannenberg, M. 1957. Treatment of pemphigus with corticosteroids. *JAMA* 165:1249.

Eller, J. J., and Kest, L. H. 1941. Pemphigus: Report of seventy-seven cases. *Arch. Dermatol. Syph.* 44:337.

Feldman, S. 1936. Pemphigus in brothers. *Arch. Dermatol. Syph.* 33:730.

Ferrari, A. V. 1947. Sopra tre casi di pemfigo volgare in una famiglia (pemfigo familiare). *Ann. Ital. Dermatol. Sif.* 2:271.

Gellis, S., and Glass, F. A. 1941. Pemphigus: Survey of 170 patients admitted to Bellevue Hospital between 1911 and 1941. *Arch. Dermatol. Syph.* 44:321.

Granirer, L. W. 1948. Three cases of pemphigus in the same family: Report of one case. *Conn. Med. J.* 12:623.

Greenbaum, S. S. 1940. Cases of familial and of conjungal pemphigus vulgaris. *Arch. Dermatol. Syph.* 41:1073.

Lever, W. F. 1971. Pemphigus. In *Dermatology in general medicine*, ed. T. B. Fitzpatrick, K. A. Arndt, W. H. Clark, A. Z. Eisen, E. J. Van Scott, and J. H. Vaughan, pp. 644–59. New York: McGraw-Hill.

Lever, W. F., and Talbott, J. H. 1942. Pemphigus: A historical study. *Arch. Dermatol. Syph.* 46:800.

Macbride, D. 1777. *A Methodical Introduction to the Theory and Practice of the Art of Medicine*, 2nd ed. 1:239 and 2:493. Dublin: W. Watson.

Miller, O. B., and Frank, L. J. 1949. Familial pemphigus vulgaris. *Arch. Dermatol. Syph.* 59:484.

Sheklakov, N. D. 1962. Pemphigus, Moscow, 1961. *Excerpta Medica*: Dermatol. *Venerol.* 16:309.

Tappeiner, S. 1954. Pemphigus and Rasse. *Z. Haut. Geschlkr.* 16:360.

Velentej, N. N. 1960. Pemphigus vulgaris in mother and daughter. *Vestn. Dermatol. Venerol.* 34:72.

Wichmann, J. E. 1791. *Beytrag zu Kenntnis des Pemphigus. Erfurt*s G. A. Keyser.

Ziprkowski, L., and Schewach-Millet, M. 1964. A long-term study of pemphigus. *Proc. Tel-Hashomer Hosp.* 3:46.

WILSON DISEASE

This inborn error of metabolism was first described by Wilson in 1912. Although he was aware of the familial nature of the disorder, he did not think that it was a genetically determined disease. It was Hall in 1921 who first presented evidence of the recessive nature of the disease.

Clinically, Wilson disease occurs predominantly in young adults and is associated with cirrhosis of the liver and degeneration of the basal ganglia of the brain. Pathological lesions give rise to the characteristic symptomatology. Tremor and rigidity of the extremities, coupled with a fixed expression of the face, are the usual neurological symptoms. Jaundice and signs of hepatic decompensation are rather uncommon but may dominate the clinical picture. Occasionally, evidence of neurological disease is entirely absent. A golden-brown ring at the limbus of the cornea (Kayser-Fleischer ring) is pathognomonic of the disease. For a detailed account of the clinical and therapeutic features of this disease the reader is referred to any standard textbook of medicine.

With regard to the occurrence of Wilson disease among Jews, Bearn published a genetic analysis of 32 patients from 30 New York City families in 1960. Because his study was done in the city with the largest Jewish population in the world—at that time approximately 3 million—it is not surprising that 14 of his 32 patients, or 43.75 percent (representing 13 families), were Ashkenazi Jews originating from the border areas of Russia and Poland. Eight patients, or 25 percent (representing 7 families), were Italians originating from Sicily and the southernmost tip of Italy. Thus, both main groups came from geographically circumscribed areas. Although the groups differed somewhat in the manifestations of the disease, the differences were not significant statistically.

Bearn's study tended to influence various medical writers, who accepted his observations, biased as they were, and thereby aided in promulgating the theory that the frequency of Wilson disease was high among Ashkenazi Jews.

Today we know that this disorder is world-wide in distribution and affects various ethnic groups. It is particularly common in populations with a high inbreeding coefficient. As noted in Chapter 12, the inbreeding coefficient for the Ashkenazi Jewish community today is not high. Three or four generations ago it was undoubtedly higher, but at that time Wilson disease was not recognized.

In 1977 Passwell and co-workers reported the results of a survey of Wilson

Table 10.18. Wilson disease: Ethnic distribution of 50 cases in Israel

Origin of families	No. of families	No. of patients		
		Definite	Probable	Total
Jews				
Ashkenazi	9	9	3	12
Moroccan	2	3	—	3
Iraqi	2	3	—	3
Yemenite	4	7	1	8
Iranian	6	7	1	8
Turkish	1	1	—	1
Non-Jews				
Arabs[a]	5	6	3	9
Druze[b]	3	4	2	6
Total	32	40	10	50

Source: J. Passwell et al., 1977, *Israel J. Med. Sci.* 13:15.

[a] Includes one family from Nablus.

[b] Includes 2 families from the Golan Heights.

disease among the various populations of Israel. Forty definite and 10 probable cases of the disorder were identified in 32 families, only 2 of whom were related. The disease was distributed among all major Israeli ethnic groups, with a relatively high prevalence among Arab and Druze patients (Table 10.18). A striking finding was the very early onset of the disease in this group. Onset of the disease by the age of 10 was found in all but 1 of the 14 Arab patients, whereas among Jews only 9 of 31 patients presented with symptoms at such an early age. The probability that this age distribution in the ethnic groups is due to chance alone is extremely small ($\chi^2 = 13.3; p_1 < .001$). In most of the non-Jewish patients the onset of cirrhosis was early and the disease often followed a rapidly fatal course. Frequently, early signs of neurological involvement also were present. The types, age at onset, and course of the disease in the Jewish communities were not unusual.

In their genetic analysis of 20 of the families they surveyed, Passwell and co-workers noted a high rate of consanguineous marriages in the Arab and non-Ashkenazi Jewish communities (see Table 10.19). This is in keeping with the high rates of consanguinity known to exist in these populations.

Although these investigators were not able to obtain adequate information on all known cases of Wilson disease in Israel, they postulated that the frequency of the gene among the large Jewish communities probably is not markedly different from the reported rate of about 1:200 in an American population, or an incidence of about 1 affected child per 40,000 live births. However, the rate among the

Table 10.19. Wilson disease: Details of familial genetic analysis

Ethnic groups	No. of sibships		No. of offspring		
	Total	Consanguineous	Affected	Nonaffected	Total
Ashkenazi Jews	5	1	7	8	15
Non-Ashkenazi Jews	8	7	16	38	54
Arabs & Druzes	7	7	14	32	46
Total	20	15	37	78	115

Source: J. Passwell et al. 1977, *Israel J. Med. Sci.* 13:15.

Jewish communities formerly of Yemen and Iran and in the Israeli Arab population appears to be considerably higher.

Most series report a higher incidence in males. When all patients in the Israeli study were considered, the sex ratio was equal. However, differences were noted in the Arab and non-Ashkenazi populations. A recent finding is the unexplained tendency of families to have affected cases of one sex and unaffected sibs of the other. This trend was not significant in the Israeli cases, nor were there clinical differences with regard to type of disease or age at onset between the sexes within any of the population groups. The number of patients in this series was too small to merit any significant conclusion regarding the predisposition of either sex to this disorder, but such a liability may operate as a modifying factor in the disease.

Genetic heterogeneity is now a well-recognized feature of Wilson disease. It is evident that the disease is not confined to Ashkenazi Jews, and the relatively large number of Arab and Oriental Jewish patients suggests that Wilson disease may be widely distributed in the Middle East.

Further genetic studies on Wilson disease in Israel and other parts of the Middle East should yield a better understanding of the distribution and frequency of this disease. Greater appreciation of the genetic variants can be achieved only after the basic defect has been identified.

References

Arina, M., and Sano, I. 1968. Genetic studies of Wilson's disease in Japan. *Birth Defects* 4:54.

Bearn, A. G. 1960. A genetical analysis of thirty families with Wilson's disease (hepatolenticular degeneration). *Ann. Hum. Genet.* 24:33.

―――. 1972. Wilson's disease. In *The metabolic basis of inherited disease*, ed. J. B. Stanbury, J. B. Wyngaarden, and D. S. Fredrickson, 3rd ed., pp. 1033–50. New York: McGraw-Hill.

Cox, D. W.; Fraser, F. C.; and Sass-Kortsak, A. 1972. A genetic study of Wilson's disease: Evidence for heterogeneity. *Am. J. Hum. Genet.* 24:646.

Hall, H. C. 1921. *La dégénerescence hépato-lenticulaire: Maladie de Wilson— Pseudosclérose.* Paris: Masson.

Passwell, J.; Adam, A.; Garfinkel, D.; Streiffler, M.; and Cohen, B. E. 1977. The heterogeneity of Wilson's disease in Israel. *Israel J. Med. Sci.* 13:15.

Strickland, G. T.; Frommer, D.; Leu, M. L.; Pollard, R.; Sherlock, S.; and Cumings, J. N. 1973. Wilson's disease in the United Kingdom and Taiwan. I: General characteristics of 142 cases and prognosis. II: A genetic analysis of 88 cases. *Quart. J. Med.* 42:619.

Strickland, G. T., and Leu, M. L. 1975. Wilson's disease: Clinical and laboratory manifestations in 40 patients. *Medicine* 54:113.

Wilson, S. A. K. 1912. Progressive lenticular degeneration: A familial nervous disease associated with cirrhosis of the liver. *Brain* 34:295.

WOLMAN DISEASE

Historical note

In 1956 Abramov, Schorr, and Wolman described a Jewish Iranian infant from consanguineous parents who presented with abdominal distention, hepatosplenomegaly, and massive calcification of the adrenals. The child died at 2 months of age. In 1961 Wolman and co-workers reported 2 more affected sibs from the same family. Although it was originally thought that this disorder is more common among Jews than among non-Jews, it is now known that Wolman disease occurs in various ethnic groups throughout the world. In 1969 Patrick and Lake demonstrated a deficiency of an acid lipase which apparently leads to the progressive accumulation of triglycerides and cholesterol esters in the lysosomes of tissues of affected individuals.

Clinical features

With few exceptions the course of Wolman disease is remarkably similar in all cases, and death usually occurs in the first few months of life. The disorder manifests itself in the first weeks of life with persistent and forceful vomiting associated with severe abdominal distention. Diarrhea with watery stools also may be present. Jaundice and a persistent low-grade fever have been noted in a few cases. Hepatosplenomegaly is a constant finding and may be present as early as the fourth day of life. The abdominal distention is greater than that produced by the hepatosplenomegaly alone. By the sixth week of life anemia is present and it becomes more severe as the disease progresses.

Characteristic clinical findings related to the central nervous system are uncommon in this disorder, but neurological development is not normal. Although affected infants appear alert up to the age of 6 weeks, by 9 weeks there is usually a marked reduction in their activity. It is not certain whether this change is due to a neurological deficit or the severely debilitated state of the infant. In rare cases a Babinski sign, exaggerated tendon reflexes, ankle clonus, and opisthotonus have been observed.

Diagnosis

Wolman disease should be suspected in any infant who fails to thrive, has hepatosplenomegaly with a markedly distended abdomen, and upon roentgenographic examination of the abdomen shows calcification and enlargement of the adrenal glands. Figure 10.3 shows the histopathological changes in the adrenal gland.

Vacuolization of peripheral lymphocytes is usually observed and the vacuoles are both intracytoplasmic and intranuclear. Lipid-laden histiocytes have been found in bone marrow aspirates by the sixth week of life, and as the disease progresses similar cells are noted in the peripheral blood. Plasma lipids are usually normal, although 1 patient has had hyperlipidemia and another hypolipoproteinemia.

A definitive diagnosis is obtained by means of a liver biopsy. Acid lipase activities should be evaluated if possible, and cholesterol, cholesteryl ester, triglyceride, and phospholipid concentrations should be determined.

Other laboratory studies may show evidence of malabsorption, with a significant impairment in fat absorption. Such alterations in the small intestine, due to flattening of the villi with infiltration of the lamina propria by foam cells, can be noted in Figure 10.4. ACTH-stimulation tests have shown depressed adrenal responsiveness.

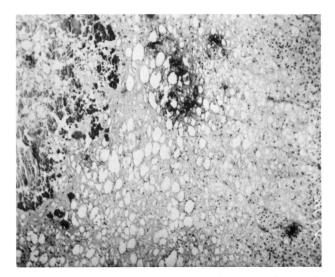

Figure 10.3. Wolman disease: Histopathological changes in the adrenal gland. On the right, note the remnants of preserved cortical tissue, followed by a zone of progressively accumulating lipids with eventual loss of nuclei, followed by areas of necrosis with calcification. Courtesy of M. Wolman, Israel.

Basic defect

The basic defect in Wolman disease has not been elucidated, but it is thought to involve some alteration in lipid metabolism which permits the accumulation of both cholesteryl esters and triglycerides in many organs. The tissue concentrations of diglycerides, monoglycerides, and free fatty acids also are elevated. These lipids seem to collect in progressively increasing quantities. It is not known whether one lipid accumulates first and the others secondarily.

Recent studies have demonstrated a total deficiency of acid lipase activity directed toward the hydrolysis of triglycerides and cholesteryl esters in the liver and spleen.

Prenatal diagnosis of this disorder is now possible. Upon culturing, a deficiency in acid lipase activity can be detected in fibroblasts obtained by aminocentesis.

Genetics

Because this inborn error of lipid metabolism was first reported in a Jewish family of Iranian origin (Figure 10.5) the initial impression was that this was another genetic disease common to Jews. However, reports of other cases from non-Jewish ethnic groups (Japanese, English, Irish, Greek, Dutch, and German-Irish-English) soon made it clear that the gene for this disorder did not reside solely within the Jewish community. Although one other case has been reported in a Jewish Iraqi family, there is no evidence that the frequency of Wolman disease is higher in the Oriental Jewish community than in any other.

Males and females seem to be affected equally, and this, in combination with

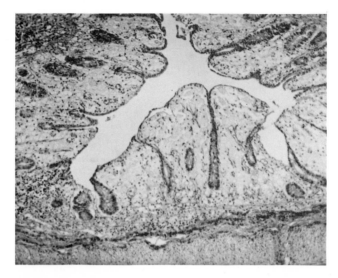

Figure 10.4. Wolman disease: Histopathological changes in the small intestine. Note the flattening of the villi due to infiltration of the lamina propria by foam cells. Courtesy of M. Wolman, Israel.

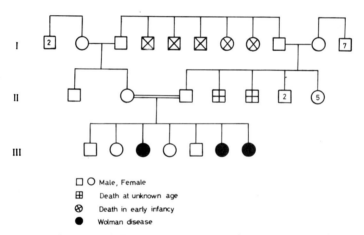

□ O Male, Female
⊞   Death at unknown age
⊗   Death in early infancy
●   Wolman disease

Figure 10.5. Wolman disease: Pedigree of the family reported by Wolman and co-workers. From M. Wolman et al., 1961, *Pediatrics* 28:742. Copyright American Academy of Pediatrics 1961.

unaffected parents, occurrence of the disease in sibs, and parental consanguinity in a few cases, supports an autosomal recessive mode of transmission.

This disorder may exhibit genetic heterogeneity, for the disease has been reported in an 8-year-old child who is apparently living and well and has only hepatomegaly. The authors in this case have shown that their patient has the same enzyme deficiency and have suggested that the general term *acid lipase deficiency* be applied to the whole group, with Wolman disease being reserved for the acute infantile form.

Prognosis and treatment

Most infants with Wolman disease die by the age of 5 months. One child has survived to the age of 14 months, and the 8-year-old child mentioned above most probably has a different form of the disorder. Therapy consists of symptomatic care.

References

Abramov, A.; Schorr, S.; and Wolman, M. 1956. Generalized xanthomatosis with calcified adrenals. *J. Dis. Child.* 91:282.

Lake, B. D., and Patrick, A. D. 1970. Wolman's disease: Deficiency of 600-resistant acid esterase activity with storage of lipids in lysosomes. *J. Pediatr.* 76:262.

Patrick, A. D., and Lake B. D. 1969. Deficiency of an acid lipase in Wolman's disease. *Nature* 222:1067.

Sloan, H. R., and Fredrickson, D. S. 1972. Rare familial diseases with neutral lipid storage. In *The metabolic basis of inherited disease*, ed. J. B. Stanbury, J. B. Wyngaarden, and D. S. Fredrickson, 3rd ed., pp. 808–17. New York: McGraw-Hill.

Wolman, M.; Sterk, V. V.; Gatt, S.; and Frenkel, M. 1961. Primary familial xanthomatosis with involvement and calcification of the adrenals: Report of two more cases in siblings of previously described infant. *Pediatrics* 28:742. 1961.

Young, E. P., and Patrick, A. D. 1970. Deficiency of acid esterase activity in Wolman's disease. *Arch. Dis. Child.* 45:664.

11

Prevention and treatment

DURING THE PAST DECADE significant advances have been made in the prevention of some genetic diseases. Unfortunately, in the area of treatment no major breakthroughs have been achieved, and thus most genetic disorders are treated at the symptomatic level. This does not mean that efforts are not being directed toward treatment; on the contrary, much research is taking place in this sphere, and it is hoped that in the near future certain inborn errors of metabolism will become properly treatable. Various approaches to prevention and treatment are discussed in this chapter, as are the ethical issues they raise.

UNDERSTANDING PATIENTS WITH GENETIC DISEASES

Most patients with genetic diseases live with their malady from birth to death. Both they and their families know the afflictions and the psychological problems created by their disorder. The special problems of each genetic disease, combined with the unique personality of each individual, produce a situation the dimensions of which are unknown to those who have been blessed with good health.

Genetic diseases give rise to emotions that are deep and complex. How do such individuals feel when they realize that their disease is caused by the fact that their parents are closely related; that as Jews they are at a higher risk than non-Jews for a number of genetic disorders; or that their mother is the carrier of an X-linked recessive disease that will threaten half her sons with early death?

Patients with genetic diseases have special problems and therefore must be dealt with differently than most medical patients. Unfortunately, many physicians are not fully cognizant of the psychological stresses produced by genetic diseases. Only by deepening our understanding of these problems will it be possible to provide better care for these patients and their families.

GENETIC COUNSELING

In the chapters of this text that deal with diseases no mention is made of genetic counseling, but in all cases it is an integral part of treatment.

Counseling may be done by one individual or by a group of qualified people. There are pros and cons to each approach. Personal attention and intimacy may be lacking in the group approach, but on the other hand, the group approach may provide a variety of views and a broader range of experience. In large genetic units the group approach tends to be favored, but exceptions must be made for patients who insist on the privacy of a one-to-one relationship.

Genetic counseling must be done by capable people. What are the qualifications for a genetic counselor? Knowledge of the basic fundamentals of genetics does not imply knowledge of genetic diseases or vice versa. Erudition in one area and not in the other could easily result in the transmission of incorrect information. Yet proficiency in both of these spheres is not enough. The genetic counselor must be understanding, flexible in thought, and must not let personal feelings interfere with the patient's decision making. On the other hand, some very qualified people argue that the genetic counselor should be directive and should not hesitate to express opinions, for in the opinion of these people the counselor can best assess the situation and decide on the proper course of action. Certain aspects of genetic counseling are by nature controversial, and because of this counselors will be guided by different attitudes. Each counselor must individualize each case and present the patient with information and advice accordingly.

The role of the genetic counselor is not only to state the risk factors involved but also to relate to the overall health and care of the affected patient and family. Admittedly, for some this is much too broad an undertaking. Reasons for expanding the role of the genetic counselor are many, but they center on the fact that patients often require varied forms of therapy and are shuttled from one specialist to another without anyone's knowing the interrelationships and dimensions of the patient's disease or how he relates to the disease. Patients and their families are often confronted with complex problems that can be seen in proper perspective only by someone knowledgeable in the area of genetic diseases. Ideally, that person will also be capable of counseling and guiding the patient and his family in the direction of better health and care.

Genetic counseling should be thought of as an open-ended process, the length of which is determined by the nature of the disease and the needs of the patient and his family. It should not be considered a one-visit consultation.

In their zeal to practice modern-day medicine, physicians and other health-care professionals are often eager to refer patients to the genetic counselor. However, as in all referrals, the patient should be properly prepared. He should know why the referral is being made and what can be achieved by it. Patients are often referred without knowing why. Such a situation may prove embarrassing for the patient and the counselor, resulting in communication problems. For example, before referring a patient to a specialist for prenatal diagnosis, the physician should know what diseases can be diagnosed prenatally. If such information is not at hand, he should not create false hopes that a given disease can be diagnosed *in utero*. The physician who sends patients to the genetic counselor should be familiar with the laws regarding abortion. One cannot overemphasize the psychological trauma that can be caused patients by inaccurate statements or false hopes based on lack of information. When in doubt about how to prepare or refer a patient for genetic counseling, the referrer should communicate with the genetic counselor beforehand.

PRENATAL DIAGNOSIS

The development of intrauterine diagnostic techniques has greatly enhanced the value and precision of genetic counseling. These techniques include amniocentesis, ultrasound, roentgenographic studies, and fetoscopy—the most useful technique at present being amniocentesis. In addition to the various chromosomal abnormalities that can be detected using amniocentesis, a number of metabolic disorders also can be diagnosed. Table 11.1 lists the diagnosable metabolic diseases commonly found in Jews. The basis for making a prenatal diagnosis of a genetic disease involving an inborn error of metabolism has been the recognition of the biochemical defect in a given disorder. However, in certain lysosomal storage diseases, such as mucolipidosis type IV (see page 92), the basic defect is not known; only by utilizing ultrastructural findings from electron micrographs of cultured fibroblasts is it possible to make this diagnosis *in utero*.

Cytogenetic abnormalities are known to exist in Bloom syndrome (see page 73) and ataxia-telangiectasia (see page 124) and with further studies it may be possible to use such observations as an aid in diagnosing these disorders *in utero*.

The diagnostic contributions of amniocentesis are well recognized, but the procedure raises several crucial questions. First and foremost is the matter of diagnostic indications for performing amniocentesis. Table 11.2 lists some of the more common diagnostic indications for amniocentesis in genetic diseases. The qualifying term *certain* is used to indicate that although some genetic diseases may be diagnosable *in utero* by amniocentesis and other means, such a procedure is not always indicated. In general, amniocentesis is not performed if the parents are opposed to interrupting the pregnancy if the findings are abnormal or if the physician feels that the procedure is not indicated.

The term abnormal conjures up many questions. Are there not degrees of abnormality? Who is to determine the dividing line? Should the decision be solely in the hands of the parents, with the physician merely obeying their wishes? Does the physician have the right to refrain from aborting a fetus with a "minor defect" that can easily be repaired. Once the decision to interrupt the pregnancy has been agreed upon by the parents and the physician, must the diagnosis be confirmed

Table 11.1. Metabolic disorders diagnosable *in utero*
and commonly found in Jews

Disorder	Jewish ethnic group
Tay-Sachs disease	Ashkenazi
Niemann-Pick disease	Ashkenazi
Gaucher disease (chronic adult noncerebral form)	Ashkenazi
Ichthyosis vulgaris (X-linked)	Oriental
Mucolipidosis IV	Ashkenazi
Glycogen storage disease type III	Sephardi

Table 11.2. Amniocentesis: Indications and order of frequency for use in prenatal
diagnosis of genetic disorders

Indication	Frequency[a]
A previously affected infant with a *certain* diagnosable inherited disease	C
A previous child with Down syndrome	C
Mother over 35 years of age	C
Mother proved or thought to be a carrier of *certain* X-linked recessive disorders	MC
Parents who have not had children and are known to be carriers of *certain* diagnosable metabolic inherited diseases	MC
Balanced translocation in one parent	R
A previous child with *certain* nondisjunction chromosomal syndromes	R
Exposure in one parent (or both) to a heavy dose of a mutagenic or teratogenic agent prior to or early in pregnancy	R
History of multiple offspring dying from similar multiple malformations that may or may not suggest a specific diagnosis	R
History of multiple abortions	R

[a] R = rare; MC = moderately common; C = common.

on the aborted fetus? What is the time limit for aborting a fetus? What risks do the mother and fetus face during amniocentesis? Should parents be told the sex of the fetus once a given test is normal? In conditions other than X-linked diseases, do parents have the right to demand an interruption of the pregnancy solely on the basis of the sex of the fetus? These questions are real, as genetic counselors will attest.

Although only a few of the many questions concerning prenatal diagnosis have been raised, physicians directly associated with these procedures must take a stand on such issues. Much thought has been and is still being given to the ethical aspects of amniocentesis. Because many questions remain unresolved, there is continued need for dialogue among the public, religious authorities, and health professionals.

By their nature ultrasound and fetoscopy have definite limitations as diagnostic tools. At the present time fetoscopy is used in women at high risk of having a fetus with a malformation that is easily recognizable upon visual examination. Fetoscopy is also being used to obtain fetal blood and skin biopsy samples in order to diagnose a variety of genetic disorders. Leprechaunism, Meckel syndrome, and acrocephalopolysyndactyly type IV, discussed in this text, could be diagnosed *in utero* using fetoscopy.

Ultrasound is a benign procedure that is gaining in diagnostic stature. It can be used (1) directly to outline skeletal and soft-tissue defects; (2) indirectly to show the abnormal growth patterns characteristic of infants with certain disorders; and (3) indirectly to localize the placenta and fetus prior to amniocentesis. More specifically, neural tube defects such as anencephaly, hydrocephaly, microcephaly, and major defects of the spine may be detected *in utero* by means of ultrasound. The diagnosis of soft-tissue defects involving the fetal kidneys, heart and heart valves, genitalia, and other organ systems will improve as techniques for better resolution are developed. Ultrasound, in conjunction with cytogenetic studies, may be useful in evaluating fetal size in Bloom syndrome (infants with this disorder are characteristically small at birth). The combination of amniocentesis, which measures alpha-fetoprotein levels in amniotic fluid, and ultrasound is proving to be a valuable means of diagnosing various neural tube defects. This combination would also seem useful in the prenatal diagnosis of Meckel syndrome.

In addition to these ongoing procedures, entirely new methods await discovery—methods that will undoubtedly raise further moral questions.

GENETIC SCREENING

A vital stimulus in creating awareness of genetic diseases among Jews has been the screening for Tay-Sachs disease (TSD) carried out in various Jewish communities throughout the world. This screening has raised many important social and ethical issues. For example, is the cost of such a program warranted in view of the small number of affected infants born? In terms of dollars, it is estimated that the intensive care of an affected child over its brief life span of 3–4 years would cost approximately $35,000. Since about 50 cases of TSD occur every year in the United States, the annual cost amounts to $1,750,000. Research advances now permit the identification of carriers, intrauterine diagnosis, and elective abortion of affected fetuses. The research developments that led to these advances in preventive medicine cost less than a single year's expenditures for the care of affected children. Aside from economic savings, families can be spared the tragedy of watching their affected child slowly die from this disease. On the surface, the reasons are cogent enough to screen all childbearing Ashkenazi Jews for the presence of this gene. Yet, convincing as the argument may seem, there is another side to the story. What are the psychological implications of being told one is the carrier of a presently fatal genetic disease? Who should be screened and what is the best method of informing people that they are carriers? In an initial voluntary screening survey in Israel, Ashkenazi couples were screened prior to marriage. Some couples who were told that both were TSD carriers canceled their marriages. It has also been learned that labeling an individual a carrier of a lethal disease may produce serious psychological problems for some. In their study of persons who had been screened for TSD, Childs and co-workers found that the feelings of some heterozygotes could be allayed by genetic counseling but that others evidenced residual unease. They suggested that such anxiety would be less prominent and more easily reduced if screening were done under conditions of ordinary primary medical care rather than outside the conventional system. Furthermore, their studies showed the need for physicians to learn the relationship of genetics to preventive medicine and the need for the public to know more about the biology of man.

Although most medical geneticists acknowledge the value of genetic screening, many issues must be resolved before such programs can provide the best in preventive health care. Important questions, such as the most appropriate age for testing and the circumstances under which it should be done, still need to be clarified.

Screening for phenylketonuria, which among Jews affects primarily those of Yemenite origin, can easily be done at birth. Such a survey has been under way in Israel for a number of years. Screening for glucose-6-phosphate dehydrogenase deficiency also can be done at birth. In Israeli Oriental and Sephardi Jewish communities at risk for this disorder, such surveys have been going on for some time. Since the latter disorder can easily be diagnosed and treated properly, concern for early recognition is not as great as in more life-threatening conditions.

As the number of genetic diseases amenable to screening increases, so will detection of genetic disorders common to Jews. As Childs and co-workers noted in their study of TSD screening, there is a real need for medical geneticists to educate not only the segment of the public that is being screened but also the physicians involved. Without proper knowledge on the part of both, it will be difficult to deal with the many social, ethical, educational, and legal questions that such a procedure raises. Some of these questions are unique and are not commonly considered in ordinary office practice. They include the legal rights of the fetus and whether new statutes are needed to protect the unborn child; confidentiality and the dissemination of information about an individual's genetic constitution; and new ethical issues in the physician-patient relationship, particularly the ways in which physicians use or misuse techniques and knowledge.

As new screening tests become available it will be necessary to demonstrate their benefits in well-designed and controlled studies before they are widely employed and integrated into public health programs or routine office procedure. Moreover, every effort must be made to educate the public and medical professionals that screening will *not* make it possible for everyone to have "normal" babies. The true purpose of genetic screening is to increase options so that individuals can make informed, educated choices.

SPECIFIC THERAPEUTIC MEASURES

A number of therapeutic approaches to the treatment of genetic diseases are currently being used or are under investigation. Each of these methods is discussed briefly below and when possible is illustrated with one or more of the disorders mentioned earlier in this text.

Substrate limitation

Substrate limitation is a well-established method that alters the body's abnormal biochemistry, usually by dietary manipulation. In phenylketonuria (see page 179), mental retardation can be prevented by early phenylalanine restriction. Low-phenylalanine diets have been used successfully in treating this disorder for the past 15 years.

Replacement of product

Clinical symptoms in genetic disorders resulting from a deficiency of a product rather than from toxic precursors can be alleviated by means of replacement. Products farther along the metabolic pathway can still be manufactured and feedback inhibition can occur in those pathways where it is a regulatory phenomenon.

Among the diseases common to Jews, the coagulation disorders PTA deficiency (see page 106), combined factor V and factor VIII deficiency (see page 227), and Glanzmann thrombasthenia (see page 160) are being treated by replacement of the missing product through the administration of fresh plasma, fresh whole blood, platelets, or cryoprecipitate as indicated by the specific disorder.

In pituitary dwarfism II (Laron type, see page 184) the administration of human growth hormone can give added height to these patients, although they are all pre-destined to be dwarfed.

In selective vitamin B_{12} malabsorption, found mainly in the Tunisian Jewish community (see page 196), patients respond to replacement therapy involving the administration of parenteral B_{12}.

In type III glycogen storage disease (see page 170) the metabolic problem is that glucose cannot be liberated from glycogen in the usual manner. By doing a portacaval shunt in these patients, it is possible to provide them with greater quantities of glucose. The glucose absorbed from the intestinal tract is diverted from its usual storage depot in the liver, thus causing hepatic glycogen to be formed at a diminished rate. Furthermore, this procedure provides glucose-rich blood to the brain, heart, and other tissues, allowing carbohydrate rather than lipid to be used as the primary source of energy. Portacaval shunts are potentially hazardous, however, and should be done only after careful evaluation.

Toxicity limitation

In genetic disorders in which the substrate produces symptoms, toxicity limitation is aimed at converting the substrate to a less toxic agent or at limiting its toxicity by various physical or chemical means. Treatment of Wilson disease (see page 439) is a case in point. Since copper is the incriminating agent in Wilson disease, chelation of free copper is achieved through the oral administration of D-penicillamine, which allows for the excretion of excess copper in the urine. BAL, another chelating agent, also has been used in treating this disease, but D-penicillamine is the drug of choice.

Avoidance of drugs

In certain genetic disorders symptoms are not manifested unless the affected individual comes in contact with specific stressful stimuli. Drug-sensitivity states of genetic origin are a prime example.

G6PD deficiency (see page 163), so common among Kurdish Jews and Jews from other Oriental communities, may not become apparent until affected individuals ingest fava beans or take a variety of drugs that affect the oxidative reactions of the pentose-phosphate pathway. Avoidance of such oxidants will prevent hemolytic crises in many variants of G6PD deficiency.

Cofactor or coenzyme therapy

Some enzymes are known to have an absolute requirement for certain cofactors, usually vitamins. Mutations producing diminished affinity of the enzyme for its cofactor or altered cofactor appearance tend to limit formation of "active" catalysts. By increasing the concentration of the cofactor it is possible in some cases to increase the amount of "active" enzyme formed. When such cofactors are vitamins, oral or parenteral supplements permit normalization of metabolism in certain genetic disorders. These disorders are termed vitamin-dependency states and can be illustrated by the use of vitamin B_{12} in one form of methylmalonic aciduria and vitamin B_6 in various pyridoxine-dependent states, including one form of homocystinuria.

Correction of enzyme defect

Induction of "deficient" mutant enzymes in the patient and actual administration of exogenous "normal" enzyme are two methods used to correct enzyme defects.

Patients with Crigler-Najjar syndrome who have minimal but measurable levels of enzyme seem to respond to the administration of phenobarbitol. Phenobarbitol somehow increases the complexity of smooth endoplasmic reticulum, thereby inducing the production of microsomal enzymes. At present such induction therapy is not applicable to any of the genetic diseases involving Jews.

Experimentation is under way to bring about enzyme induction by means of viruses. Viruses may serve as a vehicle for the transport of specific nucleic acids into the protein-deficient cells of a patient. The problems posed by such means of therapy are numerous, and many questions must be answered before this can become an accepted mode of therapy (see the section in this chapter on gene therapy).

Enzyme replacement

Enzyme replacement has been tried *in vitro* and *in vivo* in cases of certain inborn errors of metabolism and shows promise in a few disorders such as Fabry disease and Gaucher disease (see page 86). The findings in patients with the adult form of Gaucher disease are encouraging because enzyme replacement may be required relatively infrequently and the enzyme itself may not be a potent immunogenic substance. On the other hand, enzyme replacement in Tay-Sachs disease (intravenously and intrathecally) has not proved to be an adequate form of therapy.

Much more work is needed to determine the long-range effects of enzyme replacement in hereditary diseases. In particular, attention must be devoted to the following problems: (1) therapy must be continuous or repeated at frequent intervals; (2) the enzyme must be delivered to an exact target tissue, cell, or cell organelle; (3) a method must be found to deliver the enzyme across the blood-brain barrier without producing serious toxicity; and (4) the enzyme may be recognized by the body as a foreign protein and thus would serve as an antigenic stimulus.

Insoluble or encapsulated enzyme preparations may provide a means of supplying therapeutic enzymes in a more stable and less immunogenic form.

Organ transplantation

Genetic disorders in which a single organ system is involved (excluding the central nervous system) lend themselves to consideration for organ homograft transplantation. This approach has produced relief of symptoms and biochemical changes in several instances. In patients with childhood cystinosis (see page 133) and other genetic disorders of the kidney, renal transplantation has shown encouraging results in some cases. For those suffering from various immune deficiencies the only effective mode of therapy may be bone marrow transplantation.

At present, organ transplantation should be considered only when the organ to be replaced is the major organ impaired in a disease associated with severe morbidity and mortality. Although a number of genetic disorders lend themselves to this approach, too many questions remain unanswered to advocate widespread use of this method.

Gene therapy

To view gene therapy from the proper perspective it is necessary to realize that medical science is a long way from applying such a method to the treatment of human genetic diseases. Although it is now possible to isolate and even manufacture the messenger RNA for a gene, its safe introduction into the nucleus of a specialized cell, followed by normal function, remains exceedingly problematic. Most experts agree that gene therapy of somatic cells will occur in the distant future, while gene therapy of gonadal tissue and ultimate genetic cure may never be achieved.

Gene therapy by means of viral transduction raises serious ethical questions due to the possibility of such untoward consequences as neoplasia. The few genetic diseases that are conceptually amenable to gene therapy are very rare. The more common genetic diseases tend to be multifactorial and would not respond to gene therapy unless a major manipulatable gene were found. In conclusion, it is apparent that prenatal diagnosis and abortion of defective fetuses will play a greater role in the control of genetic disorders than will gene therapy.

A NOTE ON JEWISH VIEWS ON ETHICAL ISSUES IN MEDICAL GENETICS

The question could well be asked, How does Judaism speak to the ethical issues raised by genetic diseases common to the Jewish people? From the outset it must be understood that there is no one Jewish point of view with regard to such matters. Within the framework of Orthodox Judaism, which is governed by the *Halacha* (Jewish Law based on Biblical and rabbinical law), one can find varying opinions on such questions. For example, on the issue of abortion some Orthodox authorities interpret the Law strictly and rule that an abortion can be performed only when the mother's life is endangered. However, other Orthodox leaders agree that if one can show conclusively that the fetus is destined to be severely deformed and/or mentally retarded, it is permissible for the mother to have an abortion, providing it is done prior to the 21st week of embryogenesis. Jews who identify with the non-Orthodox sphere of Judaism, be it Conservative or Reform, tend to interpret the Law more freely, and on the issue of abortion often make their decision on the basis of personal choice.

Thus, Jewish views on ethical issues of a medical nature range from Orthodox religious doctrine to personal preference. Since it is beyond the scope of this text to present an in-depth discussion of the varying Jewish approaches to these ethical questions, appropriate references are provided for those interested.

REFERENCES

Ethical considerations

Baumiller, R. C. 1974. Ethical issues in genetics. *Birth Defects* 10, no. 10: 297.

Blumberg, B. D.; Golbus, M. S.; and Hanson, K. H. 1975. The psychological sequelae of abortion performed for a genetic indication. *Am. J. Obstet. Gynecol.* 122:799.

Burnet, M. 1971. *Genes, dreams, and realities.* Aylesbury, Great Britain: Medical and Technical Publishing Co.

Carr, E. F., and Oppé, T. E. 1971. The birth of an abnormal child: Telling the parents. *Lancet* 2: 1075.

Fletcher, J. 1975. Moral and ethical problems of prenatal diagnosis. *Clin. Genet.* 8:251.

Friedenwald, H. 1917. The ethics of the practice of medicine from the Jewish point of view. *Bull. Johns Hopkins Hospital* 28:256.

Gordis, R. 1978. Abortion: Major wrong or basic right. *Midstream* 24:44.

Ingle, D. J. 1967. Ethics of genetic intervention. *Med. Opin. Rev.* 3:54.

Jakobovits, I. 1959. *Jewish medical ethics.* New York: Bloch.

Lederberg, J. 1967. A geneticist looks at contraception and abortion: The changing mores of biomedical research. Ann. Intern. Med. 67, suppl. 7: 25.

Medawar, P. 1967. The genetical impact of medicine: The changing mores of biomedical research. *Ann. Intern. Med.* 67, suppl. 7: 28.

Milunsky, A., and Annas, G. J., ed. 1976. *Genetics and the law.* New York: Plenum.

Muller, H. F. 1959. The guidance of human evolution. *Perspect. Biol. Med.* 3:1.

Tendler, M. D., ed. 1975. *Medical ethics: A compendium of Jewish moral, ethical, and religious principles in medical practice.* New York: Federation of Jewish Philanthropies of New York.

Torrey, E. F., ed. 1968. *Ethical issues in medicine.* Boston: Little, Brown.

Genetic counseling

Carter, C. O. 1970. Prospects in genetic counseling. In *Modern trends in human genetics,* ed. A. E. H. Emery, pp. 339–49. London: Butterworths.

———. Current status of genetic counseling and its assessment. In *Birth defects,* ed. A. G. Motulsky and W. Lenz, pp. 277–80. Amsterdam: Excerpta Medica.

Emery, A. E. H.; Watt, M. S.; and Clack, E. R. 1973. Social effects of genetic counseling. *Br. Med. J.* 1:724.

Epstein, C. J. 1973. Who should do genetic counseling, and under what circumstances? *Birth Defects* 9, no. 4: 39.

Fraser, F. C. 1974. Genetic counseling. *Am. J. Hum. Genet.* 26:636.

Goodman, R. M., and Gorlin, R. J. 1977. *An atlas of the face in genetic disorders,* 2nd ed. St. Louis: C. V. Mosby.

Hecht, F., and Holmes, L. B. 1972. What we don't know about genetic counseling. *N. Engl. J. Med.* 287:464.

Leonard, C. O.; Chas, G. A.; and Childs, B. 1972. Genetic counseling: A consumer's view. *N. Engl. J. Med.* 287:433.

Murphy, E. A. 1975. Analytical aspects of genetic counseling. In *Modern trends in human genetics,* ed. A. E. H. Emery, 2nd ed., pp. 372–403. London: Butterworths.

Stevenson, A. C.; Davison, B. C. C.; and Oakes, M. W. 1970. *Genetic counseling.* London: Heinemann Medical Books.

Wilson, M. G. 1975. *Genetic counseling: Current problems in pediatrics,* pp. 1–51. Chicago: Year Book Medical Publishers.

Prenatal diagnosis and screening

Adinolfi, A.; Adinolfi, M.; and Lessof, M. H. 1975. Alpha-fetoprotein during development and in disease. *J. Med. Genet.* 12:138.

Atkins, L.; Milunsky, A.; and Shahood, J. M. 1974. Prenatal diagnosis: Detailed chromosomal analysis in 500 cases. *Clin. Genet.* 6:317.

Benzie, R. J., and Doran, T. A. 1975. The "fetoscope": A new clinical tool for prenatal genetic diagnosis. *Am. J. Obstet. Gynecol.* 121:460.

Bergsma, D., ed. 1971. Intrauterine diagnosis. *Birth Defects* 8, no. 5: 1.

Brock, D. J. H.; Scrimgeour, J. B.; and Nelson, M. M. 1975. Amniotic fluid alphafetoprotein measurements in the early prenatal diagnosis of central nervous system disorders. *Clin. Genet.* 7:163.

Burton, B. K.; Gerbie, A. B.; and Nadler, H. L. 1974. Present status of intra-uterine diagnosis of genetic defects. *Am. J. Obstet. Gynecol.* 118:718.

Campbell, S. 1974. The antenatal detection of fetal abnormality by ultrasonic diagnosis. In *Birth defects*, ed. A. G. Motulsky and W. Lenz, pp. 240–47. Amsterdam: Excerpta Medica.

Chaube, S., and Swinyard, C. A. 1975. The present status of prenatal detection of neural tube defects. *Am. J. Obstet. Gynecol.* 121:429.

Childs, B. 1975. *Genetic screening: Programs, principles, and research.* Washington, D.C.: National Academy of Sciences.

Childs, B.; Gordis, L.; Kaback, M. M.; and Kazazian, H. H., Jr. 1977. Tay-Sachs screening: Motives for participation and knowledge of genetics and probability. *Am. J. Hum. Genet.* 28:537.

———. 1977. Tay-Sachs screening: Social and psychological impact. *Am. J. Hum. Genet.* 28:550.

Emery, A. E. H. 1972. The prevention of genetic disease in the population. *Int. J. Environ. Stud.* 3:37.

———. 1974. Antenatal diagnosis: Limitations and future prospects. *Birth Defects* 10, no. 10: 289.

———, ed. 1973. *Antenatal diagnosis of genetic disease.* Edinburgh: Churchill Livingstone.

Golbus, M. S.; Conte, F. A.; Schneider, E. L.; and Epstein, C. J. 1974. Intra-uterine diagnosis of genetic defects: Results, problems, and follow-up of one hundred cases in a prenatal genetic detection center. *Am. J. Obstet. Gynecol.* 118:897.

Hösli, P. 1974. Microtechniques for rapid prenatal diagnosis in early pregnancy. In *Birth defects*, ed. A. G. Motulsky and W. Lenz, p. 226. Amsterdam: Excerpta Medica.

Kaback, M. M.; Zeiger, R. S.; Reynolds, L. W.; and Sonneborn, M. 1974. Tay-Sachs disease: A model for the control of recessive genetic disorders. In *Birth defects*, ed. A. G. Motulsky and W. Lenz, pp. 248–62. Amsterdam: Excerpta Medica.

Littlefield, J. W.; Milunsky, A.; and Atkins, L. 1974. An overview of prenatal genetic diagnosis. In *Birth defects, ed.* A. G. Motulsky and W. Lenz, pp. 221–25. Amsterdam: Excerpta Medica.

Milunsky, A. 1973. *The prenatal diagnosis of hereditary disorders.* Springfield, Ill.: Charles C Thomas.

Milunsky, A., and Alpert, E. 1974. The value of alpha-fetoprotein in the prenatal diagnosis of neural tube defects. *J. Pediatr.* 84:884.

Niermeijer, M. F.; Sachs, M.; Jahodova, C.; Tichelaar-Kleeper, C.; Kleijer, W. J.; and Galjaard, H. 1976. Prenatal diagnosis of genetic disorders. *J. Med. Genet.* 13:182.

Robinson, A.; Bowes, W.; Droegemueller, W.; Puck, M.; Goodman, S.; Shikes, R.; and Greenshur, A. 1973. Intrauterine diagnosis: Potential complications. *Am. J. Obstet. Gynecol.* 116:937.

Scrimgeour, J. B. 1974. Fetoscopy. In *Birth defects*, ed. A. G. Motulsky and W. Lenz, pp. 234–39. Amsterdam: Excerpta Medica.

Scriver, C. R.; Laberge, C.; and Clow, C. L. 1977. Genetic screening and allied services: Structure, process, and objective. In *Medico-social management of inherited metabolic disease*, ed. D. N. Raine, p. 21. Lancaster: MTP Press.

Treatment

Brady, R. O.; Pentchev, P. G.; and Gal, A. E. 1975. Investigations in enzyme replacement therapy in lipid storage diseases. *Fed. Proc.* 34:1310.

Brady, R. O.; Pentchev, P. G.; Gal, A. E.; Hibbert, S. R.; and Dekaban, A. S. 1974. Replacement therapy for inherited enzyme deficiency: Use of purified glucocerebrosidase in Gaucher's disease. *N. Engl. J. Med.* 291:989.

Evans, P. R. 1975. Hereditary disease and its control. *Br. Med. J.* 3:141.

Mertens, T. R. 1975. *Human genetics: Readings on the implications of genetic engineering*. New York: John Wiley.

Nadler, H. L., and Booth, C. W. 1975. Treatment of genetic disease. In *Modern trends in human genetics*, ed. A. E. H. Emery, 2nd ed., pp. 449–82. London: Butterworths.

Smith, C. 1970. Ascertaining those at risk in the prevention and treatment of genetic disease. In *Modern trends in human genetics*, ed. A. E. H. Emery, pp. 350–69. London: Butterworths.

Stanbury, J. B.; Wyngaarden, J. B.; and Fredrickson, D. S. 1972. Inherited variation and metabolic abnormality. In *The metabolic basis of inherited disease*, ed. J. B. Stanbury, J. B. Wyngaarden, and D. W. Fredrickson, 3rd ed., pp. 3–28. New York: McGraw-Hill.

Stevenson, R. E., and Howell, R. R. 1972. Some medical and social aspects of the treatment for genetic-metabolic diseases. *Ann. Am. Acad. Polit. Soc. Sci.* 339:30.

12

The reasons?

THE REASONS why some genetic disorders are common among specific Jewish groups are found in the history and culture of the Jewish people, as well as in their genetic makeup. Some aspects of these contributing factors are understood, but many intricacies cannot be adequately explained at present. Certain answers are missing because we lack genetic information about non-Jewish population centers where Jews formerly resided. The absence of other answers reflects the primitive state of our understanding of the complex interrelationships between environment and heredity. This chapter deals with the genetic mechanisms that are known to influence the distribution and frequency of hereditary disorders in Jews owing to certain features of Jewish history and culture previously discussed.

THE AUTOSOMAL RECESSIVE NATURE OF THE DISEASES

The genetic disorders that characteristically afflict Jews (or any other ethnic group for that matter) are usually transmitted in an autosomal recessive manner. Autosomal dominant disorders are severely selected against, since most carriers of these genes manifest clinical symptoms. X-linked recessive diseases also are not generally characteristic of any large ethnic group, for affected males are selected against, while female heterozygotes are usually normal. However, in autosomal recessive diseases, selective pressures are much less effective because most of the genes are carried by asymptomatic heterozygotes. Severe dominant diseases are the result of new mutations, whereas severe recessive conditions are maintained in the carrier state. For these reasons the gene frequencies of autosomal recessive diseases are higher among various ethnic groups than those of disorders inherited in other ways.

MECHANISMS AFFECTING FREQUENCY

High mutation rates

Theoretically, a high mutation rate among Jews could account for the elevated frequencies of the various autosomal recessive diseases from which they suffer. Meals calculated that for lethals the necessary rate of mutation would have to be equal to the frequency of the trait in the population. Thus, the mutation rate for Tay-Sachs disease would be approximately 1:6,000 gametes/generation among Ashkenazi Jews and 1:500,000 among other populations. Meals went on to point out that there is no precedent for such a vast difference in mutation rate (eighty-fold) in either human or animal genetic studies. Furthermore, it is known that natural selection eliminates persons afflicted with deleterious mutations, thus preventing the accumulation of mutants beyond a certain incidence in the population. Therefore, mutation alone does not explain the high frequencies of genetic diseases among Jews.

Hybridization and gene flow

It is conceivable that migration and occasional outbreeding with local non-Jews could account for certain genetic disorders in Jews, if these conditions occurred with any appreciable frequency in the surrounding non-Jewish populations. However, there is little evidence that the characteristic genetic disorders found among the various Jewish ethnic groups are also present among the non-Jewish populations of Eastern Europe, the Middle East, or North Africa. It is difficult to prove or disprove that these diseases previously existed in non-Jewish communities. The disorders could have disappeared from non-Jewish populations owing to differences between their environment and that of the Jews. Possible environmental differences include such factors as dietary habits and urban versus rural life.

In general, migration has been considered a factor in explaining differences in gene frequency, and some disease distribution could be accounted for by gene flow from one population to another, but unfortunately historical documentation of such a mechanism is not available. As Motulsky mentioned, these events occurred in prehistoric times or during periods when history was not recorded. Therefore, most geneticists do not invoke this mechanism to explain differences in gene frequency and distribution of genetic disorders among Jews.

Genetic drift and founder effect

Genetic drift can be defined as a random fluctuation in gene frequency from one generation to the next which is based on the finite size of the effective breeding population. Thus, two generations of a population may have different frequencies for the same gene, even though these frequencies were originally identical. Essentially the influence of drift on gene frequency is inversely proportional to the size of the population. For example, the chance predominance of one genotype over another within a population will be greater, the smaller the population.

Founder effect is a special feature of drift in which some genes carried by the founders of a new community will by chance differ in frequency from those in the original, or parent, population.

Genetic drift has been shown to strongly influence the frequencies of nonlethal genes in neighboring but genetically isolated communities. The mechanism of drift could explain the variations in gene frequency in such conditions as essential pentosuria, PTA deficiency, and Gaucher disease, for these disorders do not clearly reduce the fertility of affected individuals.

Using computer simulations, Livingstone has shown that even lethal recessive genes can attain high frequencies in a population through the founder effect. For example, in a founding population of 80 individuals, one of whom was a carrier of a lethal autosomal recessive disease (i.e., the frequency of the gene in the founding population is 0.00625), the frequency in 5 percent of the randomly generated populations after 5 generations was greater than 0.04. Starting with fewer founders and calculating for more generations, the changes in gene frequency are even more dramatic. Rao and Morton have shown that chance alone can explain the high frequency of Tay-Sachs disease among Ashkenazi Jews, but they acknowledge the fact that similar disorders (Niemann-Pick disease, Gaucher disease, etc.) provide an argument against drift.

Just how relevant are genetic drift and founder effect in accounting for genetic diseases among Jews? Chase and McKusick, and more recently Fraikor, favor this mechanism as an explanation for the high frequency of Tay-Sachs disease and some of the other disorders that affect predominantly Ashkenazi Jews. They contend that the relatively high frequencies of these genetic diseases can be accounted for by founder effect and/or drift operating in a manner comparable to that which McKusick and co-workers demonstrated in the separate Amish demes. Their reasoning is that the Jewish populations that previously resided in Eastern Europe were established by small numbers of Jews migrating eastward into Poland and Lithuania during the 13th and 14th centuries, and that this pattern of migration (small bands of people) is not unlike the formation of the Amish demes.

As noted in Chapter 1, these early Jewish settlements in Poland and Lithuania were composed of many small groups that often consisted of no more than a handful of families. These groups were relatively isolated genetically, not only from their gentile neighbors but also from other Jewish communities. Thus, the historical background of Ashkenazi Jewry, with its numerous small founding groups and relative genetic isolation, fits well with the features of genetic drift and founder effect and accounts for the establishment of the now characteristic Ashkenazi Jewish diseases. As these founding groups grew in size, became mobile, and were subjected to diluting forces, the frequency of these genes was diluted, although never to the low frequencies observed in the surrounding non-Jewish populations. The latter point is of interest not only to geneticists but also to Jewish historians, for it reflects in some measure the degree of cohesiveness of Ashkenazi Jewry.

The importance of genetic drift in the various Ashkenazi diseases can be seen in the information obtained on the ancestral origins of patients with these disorders. Moreover, Meals and others showed that for many of these diseases there is a geographical aggregation of origins, a finding which supports the role of founder effect in these disorders (see Figure 12.1).

Aspects of genetic drift and founder effect are also discussed in this chapter under the heading "Reasons for genetic disorders among the Oriental and Sephardi Jewish communities."

Heterozygous advantage

Heterozygous advantage is an important causative factor in the persistence of many genes, but unfortunately very little is known about the mechanisms involved. It is thought that if a carrier of the gene for an autosomal recessive disorder has selective advantage over a homozygous normal individual, the gene frequency of that disorder will increase to a balance point, even though the disorder itself is lethal. By definition, selective advantage is an increase in the number of offspring who attain fertility and thus produce proportionately more carriers. The examples usually given as evidence for balanced polymorphism are the malaria-dependent traits of glucose-6-phosphate dehydrogenase deficiency (see page 163), sickling, and thalassemia. Motulsky has pointed out, however, that direct mortality data are available only for the sickle cell trait, and these show that among sickle cell trait carriers, death from falciparum malaria is negligible. Malarial parasites are fewer in number in G6PD-deficient red cells (GdA—) or in those with G6PD variant A+ than in carriers of normal G6PD. These data suggest that mortality may be lower in carriers of such variants.

In evaluating other selective forces that may influence the gene frequencies of various diseases among Jews, Motulsky mentioned urbanization, endemic diseases, intelligence, and nutritional causes.

Regarding *urbanization*, large populations of Jews have lived in cities longer than most other ethnic groups. The crucial selective environment would be pre-

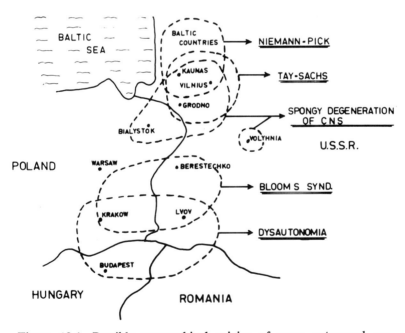

Figure 12.1. Possible geographical origins of some autosomal recessive diseases observed among Ashkenazi Jews. From R. A. Meals, 1971, *J. Chronic. Dis.* 23:547. Reprinted by permission of Pergamon Press, Ltd.

industrial towns. Crowd diseases appear to be more prevalent among city dwellers than among hunters, gatherers, and pastoralists.

Endemic diseases have accounted for the deaths of children for many generations. Thus, tuberculosis and malaria are better selective agents than are epidemics of plague. Genes that protect against endemic diseases have considerable selective advantages.

Selection for *intelligence* also has been invoked as a factor affecting gene frequency. It has been stated that the scholar or rabbi in East European Jewish communities married the most desirable girl (see page 472) and had more children than did other men. If true, this would have resulted in selection for the type of rational intelligence valued by present-day Western societies.

With regard to *nutritional factors*, Neel has suggested that genetic factors which predispose an individual to diabetes and atherosclerosis may give survival advantages under famine conditions by more readily mobilizing carbohydrate or fat reserves.

Various investigators have utilized certain of these selective factors in an effort to explain the high frequency of some diseases among Ashkenazi Jews. For example, Myrianthopoulos and Aronson have postulated that the heterozygous carrier of the Tay-Sachs disease gene has increased resistance (selective advantage of the heterozygote) to tuberculosis. According to their data, this protective advantage led to increased fertility, thus increasing the gene frequency of this disease among Ashkenazi Jews emigrating primarily from the northern Baltic countries.

Myrianthopoulos and Aronson's study also showed that a selective advantage of about 1.25 percent for the heterozygote over the homozygote would be sufficient to maintain the TSD gene at equilibrium, despite its mass elimination by homozygosity.

In terms of fertility, Myrianthopoulos and Aronson studied the grandparents rather than the parents of TSD patients because the grandparents' reproductive performance was not modified by the occurrence of offspring with a lethal defect. Fertility estimates were based on a comparison of the number of surviving offspring of a control group. The study group consisted of 1,244 sibs within 388 sibships. The control group (matched for country of birth, age, number of children, and current geographical distribution) consisted of 2,848 sibs within 812 sibships. The results showed that the fertility of grandparents of TSD patients was slightly higher than the fertility of the controls. This difference was greatest in the number of offspring born in Eastern Europe and surviving to the age of 21—a finding which conforms to the theory that a selective advantage acts in the East European environment. The differences in fertility were small, however, and not statistically significant. Meals has rightly pointed out that the results obtained would be statistically significant only if the differences in fertility were large, or if the number of individuals in the sample were greatly increased. Neither criterion can be met because the hypothesis requires a small (1.25 percent) advantage only for the heterozygote in order to account for the observed differences. Furthermore, TSD is a relatively rare disorder, which means that accurate and complete fertility data on the grandparents of affected individuals are difficult to obtain. In conclusion, the evidence for heterozygote advantage in TSD is suggestive but far from decisive.

Eldridge has postulated that in the autosomal recessive form of torsion dystonia enhanced intelligence may be a factor in the selective advantage of the heterozygote (see page 100).

Eight of the 11 genetic disorders found predominantly among Ashkenazi Jews involve the central nervous system either primarily or secondarily. Gaucher, Tay-Sachs, and Niemann-Pick disease are all biochemically related sphingolipidoses. The basic alterations in familial dysautonomia, mucolipidosis type IV, abetalipo-proteinemia, primary torsion dystonia, and spongy degeneration of the brain remain unknown.

In discussions of selection versus founder effect and genetic drift, significance is given not only to the clustering of central nervous system involvement among Ashkenazi Jews, but even more to the fact that the three sphingolipidoses (Tay-Sachs, Gaucher, and Niemann-Pick disease) are closely related in their biochemical degradation of sphingolipids. For some the latter point supports the selection hypothesis. Suggesting that on the contrary this may be due to chance, McKusick points out that several forms of recessively inherited dwarfism among the Amish have been attributed to founder effect and genetic drift. However, at present there is no adequate explanation for the high frequency of the three sphingolipidoses or the clustering of certain neurological diseases among Ashkenazi Jews.

The controversy that has been raging between proponents of the importance of random genetic drift and those who cite heterozygous advantage to explain the high gene frequencies of certain genetic disorders among Jews has perhaps been quieted by the 1978 study of Chakravarti and Chakraborty. These investigators suggest that "heterozygote advantage together with random genetic drift should be considered as the most probable mechanism for the elevation of TSD gene frequency among the Ashkenazic Jews." Unfortunately, not even this compromising conclusion can be accepted as the final answer.

Consanguinity

Consanguinity refers to the mating of genetically related individuals, a process which increases homozygosity, with a resulting increase in rare recessive disorders. The frequency with which such matings occur in a given population depends in part on the population size and its social customs. Whereas the ancient Egyptians and the Incas favored marriages of brothers and sisters of the reigning dynasty, very close consanguineous matings are avoided in most present-day societies.

All states in the U.S. prohibit marriages between sibs and between parent and child. Most states also declare that marriages between a person and his parent's sibs—i.e., between niece and uncle, or nephew and aunt—are illegal. Marriages between first cousins are forbidden in more than one-third of the states, but in some states Jews are exempt from these laws because Judaism does sanction certain forms of consanguineous marriages. In other states even more distant degrees of consanguineous matings are prohibited. However, in most other countries no objection is raised against consanguineous marriages, with the exception of those between sibs and between parents and children.

Consanguineous marriages played an important role in the early history and development of the Jewish people, as witnessed by the fact that in the Patriarchal Period several marriages were consanguineous (see Figure 1.1, page 9). Even today, consanguinity is not uncommon in certain Oriental and Sephardi Jewish communities. In the past the rate of consanguineous marriages among all Jewish ethnic groups was much higher than it is today, for the following reasons: (1) Jewish communities were often small and geographically isolated from one another, so the choice of marriage partners was limited; (2) government and religious laws prohibited Jews from marrying non-Jews; (3) because of strong family, religious, and socioeconomic ties, Jews frequently chose to marry within families, and such marriages were often prearranged when the future partners were quite young; (4) according to Jewish Law, certain forms of consanguinity not only were sanctioned but were considered to be blessed.

The *Halacha* (Jewish Law) states that a man may marry: (a) his stepsister, his stepfather's wife (divorced or widowed), his niece, or his full- or half-brother's or half-sister's daughter-in-law; (b) his cousin, his stepson's wife (divorced or widowed), or his deceased wife's sister. A woman may marry: (a) her stepbrother or her stepmother's former husband; (b) her cousin or her deceased sister's husband, whether full- or half-sister; (c) her uncle.

The following quotations are from Jewish sources and reflect scholarly thought on some of the approved forms of consanguineous marriage within the Jewish community.

> One who married his sister's daughter—on him the Bible says: "They thou will call and G-d will answer" (Talmud, order Nashim, tractate Yevamot, 62b).

> It is a *mitzvah* [a good act] for a man to marry his sister's daughter or his brother's daughter (Shulkan Arukh, Even ha-Ezer, chapter 2).

In 1960 the late Professor Goldschmidt and her colleagues published their findings on the marriage patterns of 11,424 Jews from the major Jewish communities in Israel. Table 12.1 lists their observations with regard to consanguineous, exopatric, and intercommunity marriages. In 1972 Tsafrir and Halbrecht did a similar study on 1,625 Jews, and their findings are listed in Table 12.2. Table 12.3 compares the percentages of consanguinity involving first cousins or closer relatives in some of the Jewish ethnic groups from these two studies. The figures from the 1972 Israeli report must be questioned, for in some instances the numbers were quite small and the area in which the investigation was done may not be truly representative of all the communities. Nevertheless, it is possible to conclude that there has been a definite decrease in consanguineous matings in most of the Jewish ethnic groups.

Despite this decrease, consanguineous marriages still occur in the non-Ashkenazi communities, and it is this fact that accounts for most of the rare and isolated genetic syndromes discussed in Chapter 7. As the rate of consanguinity continues to decline among Jews of Oriental and Sephardi ancestry, the frequency of such rare genetic disorders also will be reduced. Consanguinity today plays essentially no role in most of the recessive disorders common to Ashkenazi Jews.

Ascertainment bias

Reported differences in gene frequencies among various ethnic groups do not always reflect real differences, but in fact may represent only measured differences.

Table 12.1. Rates of consanguineous, endopatric, exopatric, and intercommunity marriages among the various Jewish communities of Israel, 1960

Origin of parents	Total no.	Consanguineous partners — First cousins and closer relationships: 1st cousins (no.)	Uncle-niece (no.)	Total no.	%	±S.E.	More distant relationships: No.	%	Endopatric marriages of unrelated partners: No.	%	Exopatric marriages: No.	%	Inter-community marriages: No.	%
Total	11,424	596	56	652	—	—	454	—	5,558	—	2,190	—	2,570	—
Total Ashkenazim	4,734	64	2	66	1.4	—	50	—	2,078	—	2,190	—	350	—
Czechoslovakia	297	4	—	4	1.4	0.7	2	0.7	90	30.3	184	62.0	17	5.7
Germany, Austria	367	2	2	4	1.1	0.5	1	0.3	116	31.6	204	55.6	42	11.4
Hungary	249	7	—	7	2.8	1.0	3	1.2	102	41.0	121	48.6	16	6.4
Poland	1,794	29	—	29	1.6	0.3	23	1.3	1,050	58.5	569	31.7	123	6.9
Romania	908	18	—	18	2.0	0.5	10	1.1	530	58.4	303	33.4	47	5.2
U.S.S.R. (Ashkenazim)	373	1	—	1	0.3	0.3	3	0.8	114	30.6	223	59.8	32	8.6
Other Ashkenazim	746	3	—	3	0.4	0.2	8	1.1	76	10.2	586	78.4	73	9.8
Total non-Ashkenazim	6,690	532	54	586	8.8	—	404	—	3,480	—	—	—	2,220	—
Aden	119	9	4	13	10.9	2.9	8	6.7	44	37.0	—	—	54	45.4
Bulgaria	365	—	—	—	—	—	—	—	256	70.1	—	—	109	29.8
Egypt	427	17	1	18	4.2	1.0	12	2.8	246	57.4	—	—	151	35.4
Greece	187	6	—	6	3.2	1.3	9	4.8	82	43.8	—	—	90	48.1
Iraq	1,450	238	16	254	17.5	1.0	162	11.2	862	59.4	—	—	172	11.9
Libya	298	18	2	20	6.7	1.4	12	4.0	206	69.1	—	—	60	20.1
Morocco	504	26	10	36	7.1	1.1	18	3.6	366	72.6	—	—	84	16.7
Persia	427	68	7	75	17.6	1.8	37	8.7	214	50.1	—	—	101	23.6
Syria, Lebanon	406	15	2	17	4.2	1.0	16	3.9	200	49.3	—	—	173	42.6
Tunisia	149	16	2	18	12.1	2.7	2	1.3	92	61.8	—	—	37	24.8
Turkey	607	19	2	21	3.5	0.7	27	3.8	326	53.7	—	—	233	38.4
U.S.S.R.	160	20	1	21	13.1	2.7	6	3.8	54	33.7	—	—	79	49.4
Yemen	628	50	4	54	8.6	1.1	61	9.9	388	61.8	—	—	125	19.9
Others	963	30	3	33	3.4	0.6	34	3.5	144	15.0	—	—	752	78.2

Source: E. Goldschmidt et al, 1960, *Ann. Hum. Genet.* 24:191. Reprinted by permission of Cambridge University Press.

Table 12.2. Rates of consanguineous, endopatric, exopatric, and intercommunity marriages among the various Jewish communities of Israel, 1972

Country of origin	No.	First-cousin or closer relationship		More distantly related		Endopatric, unrelated		Exopatric		Intercommunity		% of total pop.
		No.	%	No.	%	No.	%	No.	%	No.	%	
Poland	485	4	0.8	3	0.6	223	46.0	184	37.9	71	14.6	39.0
Romania	240	—	—	3	1.3	117	48.7	94	39.2	26	10.8	19.3
Russia, Czechoslovakia[a]	316	—	—	5	1.6	57	18.0	211	66.8	43	13.6	25.2
Yugoslavia[b]	9	—	—	—	—	2	22.2	6	66.7	1	1.1	0.7
Germany[c]	96	—	—	1	1.0	12	12.5	72	75.0	11	11.5	7.7
Israel	69	—	—	—	—	3	4.3	56	81.2	10	14.5	5.5
Various	27	—	—	—	—	4	14.8	18	66.7	5	18.5	2.2
Yemen	690	34	4.9	70	10.1	511	74.1	58	8.4	17	2.5	36.0
Iraq[d]	550	60	10.9	54	9.8	302	54.9	91	16.5	43	7.8	28.6
Morocco[e]	236	14	5.9	12	5.1	139	58.9	48	20.3	23	9.7	12.3
Egypt[f]	138	6	4.3	14	10.0	43	31.1	54	39.1	21	15.2	7.2
Syria[g]	32	1	3.1	—	—	4	12.5	22	68.7	5	15.6	1.7
Turkey[h]	155	2	1.3	6	3.9	52	33.5	67	43.2	28	18.1	8.1
Israel	44	—	—	—	—	3	6.8	24	54.5	17	38.6	2.3
Various	38	1	2.6	—	—	2	5.3	21	55.3	14	36.8	1.9
India	33	—	—	—	—	22	66.7	6	18.2	5	15.1	1.7

Source: J. Tsafrir and I. Halbrecht, 1972, *Ann. Hum. Genet.* 35:343. Reprinted by permission of Cambridge University Press.
Note: Among "various" are included Jews from West European countries, the United States, South America, South Africa, Australia, England, etc.
[a] Plus Hungary and Lithuania.　[b] Plus Bulgaria.　[c] Plus Austria.　[d] Plus Iran and Afghanistan.　[e] Plus Algeria.　[f] Plus Libya and Tunisia.
[g] Plus Lebanon.　[h] Plus Bulgaria and Yugoslavia.

Table 12.3. Comparative rates of consanguinity
involving first cousins or closer relatives in some of the
Jewish ethnic groups in Israel, 1960 versus 1972

Country of origin	1960 (%)	1972 (%)
Ashkenazim		
Czechoslovakia	1.4	—
Germany	1.1	—
Poland	1.6	0.8
Romania	2.0	—
Russia	0.3	—
Non-Ashkenazim		
Egypt	4.2	4.3
Iraq	17.5	10.9
Morocco	7.1	5.9
Syria, Lebanon	4.2	3.1
Yemen	8.6	4.9

Source: E. Goldschmidt et al., 1960, *Ann. Hum. Genet.* 24:191; J. Tsafrir and I. Halbrecht, 1972, *Ann. Hum. Genet.* 35:343.

For example, if one ethnic group receives more frequent and better medical care than another, it is likely that a given disease will be diagnosed and reported more often among patients of the former group. Ascertainment bias also occurs if one investigates an unrepresentative sample population. In general, Jews tend to seek medical care more frequently than other ethnic groups. Moreover, many of the early reports on diseases in Jews came from the large Jewish population centers in Europe or the United States, mainly New York City. Ascertainment bias comes into play with regard to the conditions discussed in Chapter 10, but it is not considered to be a crucial factor in the observed differences in frequency of most of the other disorders discussed in this text.

Linkage to an advantageous gene

Another mechanism that has been postulated to explain ethnic variations in genetic disorders is linkage to an advantageous gene. Whenever a given allele increases in frequency because of selective advantage, a small chromosome segment in the region of the relevant locus also increases in frequency to some extent— passively, because of the linkage. The segment is carried along for a while with the advantageous allele. If such a chromosome segment happens to include a recessive allele, the frequency of the latter also increases. Evidence for such a mechanism among the various genetic diseases common to Jews has never been documented.

MULTIFACTORIAL DISEASES

Some of the diseases listed in Chapter 8 can be considered multifactorial disorders, as can certain forms of mental illness and mental retardation and some of the rare malformation syndromes listed in Chapter 7.

Differential population frequencies are known to exist for a number of these and other conditions, but our understanding of the interactions between heredity and environment that would explain these differences remains for the most part at a primitive level. Although various theories have been proposed to explain the high frequency of a certain type of neoplasia among Jews or why Jews are more prone to develop ulcerative colitis and regional enteritis than non-Jews, the true reasons remain unknown. Motulsky has suggested that our understanding of polygenic diseases will be advanced as we increase our knowledge of and search for genetic markers that are pathophysiologically related to a given disease. He points out, however, that random search for associations of genes to disease is usually fruitless.

COMMENTS ON REASONS FOR GENETIC DISORDERS IN THE ORIENTAL AND SEPHARDI JEWISH COMMUNITIES

Historically the communities making up Oriental and Sephardi Jewry (see Chapter 1) became much more fragmented than those of Ashkenazi Jewry and as such developed into more isolated and distinct ethnic subgroups. Ashkenazi Jewry has its subgroups with their characteristic diseases, but the lines of demarcation are not as sharp as those of the non-Ashkenazi communities. Thus, with a few exceptions (familial Mediterranean fever [FMF] primarily in Sephardi Jews; G6PD deficiency in Jews of Babylonian ancestry or in Oriental Jews), one does not observe a number of genetic diseases that are common to all of the major non-Ashkenazi groups. Rather the disorders tend to be characteristic of the various non-Ashkenazi subgroups (See Appendix 1).

Familial Mediterranean fever is found among all the Sephardi communities and also among the Oriental community of Iraqi Jews. It is also present among such non-Jewish populations as the Armenians, Turks, Syrians, and Egyptians. It has reached a very high frequency among Libyan Jews (1:600 individuals, compared to approximately 1:3,000–1:5,000 in other Sephardi communities [mainly North African] and only 1:80,000 among the Ashkenazim).

The fact that the FMF observed in Armenians seems to be clinically different from that observed in non-Ashkenazi Jews suggests that there may be at least two different allelic forms of the disease. The high frequency of FMF among Sephardi Jews and Armenians may be due to some common selective factor. Since amyloid is an immunologic complication of FMF, perhaps individuals who are heterozygous for the FMF gene are protected against some forms of infection. Genetic drift is a possibility, but the semilethality of the disease calls for a serious effort to identify other reasons for the presence of the genes in these populations.

Most geneticists agree that the high frequency of G6PD deficiency among Oriental Jews is due to the selective advantage of heterozygotes in malarial regions.

A number of autosomal recessive diseases have been found in relatively high frequencies among specific subgroups of Oriental and Sephardi Jewry. For example, Dubin-Johnson syndrome and selective hypoaldosteronism occur mainly in Jews of Iranian ancestry; phenylketonuria in Yemenite Jews; Glanzmann thrombasthenia in Iraqi Jews; selective vitamin B_{12} malabsorption with proteinuria in Tunisian Jews; and glycogen storage disease type III, congenital adrenal hyperplasia, and ataxia-telangiectasia among Moroccan Jews. The occurrence of these disorders could well be explained by the mechanisms of genetic drift and founder effect, but to employ such an explanation for all these disorders is not totally reasonable, for information is lacking concerning the frequency of most of these diseases among non-Jews of the same areas. In the case of Dubin-Johnson syndrome, there is evidence that this disease is rare among the non-Jewish population of Iran. Selection in favor of heterozygotes would further increase the frequency of some of these genes. Until more information is available, one can only postulate the reasons for the high frequency of certain genetic diseases among the various subgroups of Oriental and Sephardi Jewry.

REFERENCES

Adam, A. 1973. Genetic diseases among Jews. *Israel J. Med. Sci.* 9:1383.

Aronson, S. M.; Herzog, M. I.; Brunt, P. W.; McKusick, V. A.; and Myrianthopoulos, N. C. 1967. Inherited neurologic diseases of Ashkenazic Jewry: Demographic data suggesting non-random gene frequencies. *Trans. Am. Neurol. Assoc.* 92:117.

Bodmer, W. F., and Cavalli-Sforza, L. I. 1976. *Genetics, evolution, and man.* San Francisco: W. H. Freeman.

Cavalli-Sforza, L. I., and Bodmer, W. F. 1971. *The genetics of human populations.* San Francisco: W. H. Freeman.

Chakravarti, A., and Chakraborty, R. 1978. Elevated frequency of Tay-Sachs disease among Ashkenazic Jews unlikely by genetic drift alone. *Am. J. Hum. Genet.* 30:256.

Chase, G. A., McKusick, V. A. 1972. Founder effect in Tay-Sachs disease. *Am. J. Hum. Genet.* 24:339.

Cohen, T. 1971. Genetic markers in migrants to Israel. *Israel J. Med. Sci.* 7:1509.

Fraikor, A. 1977. Tay-Sachs disease: Genetic drift among the Ashkenazi Jews. *Soc. Biol.* 24:117.

Goldschmidt, E., and Cohen, T. 1964. Inter-ethnic mixture among the communities of Israel. *Cold Spring Harbor Symp. Quant. Biol.* 29:115.

Goldschmidt, E.; Ronen, A.; and Ronen, I. 1960. Changing marriage systems in the Jewish communities of Israel. *Ann. Hum. Genet.* 24:191.

Goodman, R. M. 1975. Genetic disorders among the Jewish people. In *Modern trends in human genetics,* ed. A. E. H. Emery, 2nd ed. London: Butterworths.

Knudson, A. G., Jr.: Founder effect in Tay-Sachs disease. *Am. J. Hum. Genet.* 25:108.

Knudson, A. G., and Kaplan, W. D. 1962. Genetics of the sphingolipidoses. In *Cerebral sphingolipidoses,* ed. S. M. Aronson and B. W. Volk, p. 395. New York: Academic Press.

Livingstone, F. B. 1969. The founder effect and deleterious genes. *Am. J. Phys. Anthropol.* 30:55.

McKusick, V. A. 1973. Ethnic distribution of disease in non-Jews. *Israel J. Med. Sci.* 9:1375.

———. 1979. The non-homogeneous distribution of recessive diseases. In *Genetic diseases among Ashkenazi Jews,* ed. R. M. Goodman and A. G. Motulsky. New York: Raven Press, forthcoming.

———, ed. 1978. *Medical genetic studies of the Amish: Selected papers.* Baltimore: The Johns Hopkins University Press.

Meals, R. A.: Paradoxical frequencies of recessive disorders in Ashkenazi Jews. *J. Chronic Dis.* 23:547.

Motulsky, A. G. 1973. Significance of genetic diseases for population studies. *Israel J. Med. Sci.* 9:1410.

Motulsky, A. G., and Gartler, S. M. 1959. Consanguinity and marriage. *Practitioner* 183:170.

Myrianthopoulos, N. C., and Aronson, S. M. 1966. Population dynamics of Tay-Sachs disease. I: Reproductive fitness and selection. *Am. J. Hum. Genet.* 18:313.

Myrianthopoulos, N. C.; Naylor, A. F.; and Aronson, S. M. 1972. Founder effect in Tay-Sachs disease unlikely. *Am. J. Hum. Genet.* 24:341.

Neel, J. V. 1969. Current concepts of the genetic basis of diabetes mellitus and the biological significance of the diabetic predisposition in diabetes. *Excerpta Medica, Int. Cong. Ser.*, no. 5, p. 68.

Ozdemir, A. I., and Sokmen, C. 1969. Familial Mediterranean fever among the Turkish people. *Am. J. Gastroenterol.* 51:311.

Rao, D. C., and Morton, N. E. 1973. Large deviations in the distribution of rare genes. *Am. J. Hum. Genet.* 25:594.

Schwabe, A. D., and Peter, R. S. 1974. Familial Mediterranean fever in Armenians: Analysis of 100 cases. *Medicine* 53:453.

Shaw, R. F., and Smith, A. P. 1969. Is Tay-Sachs disease increasing? *Nature* 224:1214.

Sheba, C. 1971. Jewish migration in its historical perspective. *Israel J. Med. Sci.* 7:1333.

Sohar, E.; Gafni, J.; Pras, M.; and Heller, H. 1967. Familial Mediterranean fever: A survey of 470 cases and review of literature. *Am. J. Med.* 43:227.

Tsafrir, J., and Halbrecht, I. 1972. Consanguinity and marriage systems in the Jewish communities in Israel. *Ann. Hum. Genet.* 35:343.

13

Present and future trends

THE MAIN FACTORS that will influence the prevalence of genetic
disorders among the Jewish people are medical and sociological in
nature. In this chapter some current and projected trends in both
areas are discussed.

MEDICAL CONSIDERATIONS

There is every reason to believe that medical science will continue to provide
man with greater family planning options, which in turn will increase his chances
of having healthier offspring. Genetic counseling, screening programs, and prenatal diagnostic methods will become more advanced, and more people will
utilize these services. Jews, and members of other populations at risk for genetic
disorders, will know much more about their genetic make-up prior to marriage,
and such information could well influence their choice of a marital partner. For
certain genetic diseases this information is already available (see Chapter 11).

Advances in the treatment of genetic diseases also will be made, but research
in this area is much more complex and probably will not keep pace with the strides
being made in the area of prevention.

Some geneticists are concerned that as medical science offers better treatment
and prevention of autosomal recessive diseases, there will be a tremendous build-up
of the carrier state, with a resulting increase in recessive disorders. Calculations
show, however, that it would take approximately 50 generations, or more than
1,000 years, for a doubling of treatable autosomal recessive disorders to occur—
a problem of concern, but one that does not require immediate attention.

Thus medical science, through various preventive means, will contribute greatly
to a reduction in the number of Jewish children born with certain of these debilitating diseases. It is also hoped that better means of treatment will become
available.

SOCIOLOGICAL CONSIDERATIONS

A number of sociological changes within the various Jewish communities of the world will contribute to the reduction in the number of children born with genetic disorders. The main sociological areas of concern here are Jewish marriage patterns and family size. However, because there is nothing permanent about present trends, predictions for the future must be considered of limited value.

Marriage customs

Before discussing present-day marriage patterns among Jews, it may be worth-while to consider some features of Jewish matrimonial customs of the past, for they shed light on factors that influence the occurrence of certain genetic disorders, and in a sense even affect current marital considerations.

Medieval Jews and Jews in Central Europe as late as the mid-19th century followed the rabbinical ordinances implicitly. Most Jewesses were married before they reached the age of 16, and their husbands usually were not much older. Oriental and Sephardi Jews tended to marry at an even earlier age than the Ashkenazim.

The selection of a mate was paramount and in most cases was done by the parents of the couple to be wed, often with the aid of a professional marriage broker. One of the main parental concerns was to match intellect and social status. The families most desirable for matrimonial alliances were classified by the rabbis in the following order: those of the scholar; the most prominent man in the community; the head of the community; the head of the congregation; the collector of charity; and the teacher of children. The children of an ignorant man were to be avoided.

The wealthy sought young men with attainments in learning, and when they could not find suitable young scholars of their own social and economic standing, they did not hesitate to take poor but learned young men for their daughters. The wealthy cared little for the physical appearance of the men they chose to be their sons-in-law. Their prime concern was intellectual attainment. Physical deformities usually did not interfere with the selection of prospective bridegrooms, provided the young men were scholars of promise or eminence. On the other hand, parents of the young men were quite concerned about the appearance of their prospective daughters-in-law, for it is in keeping with Jewish tradition that a man should endeavor to marry a pleasant looking, if not a beautiful, woman.

What can be said regarding the other side of the coin—the very poor, young men who did not have scholarly abilities, and young women who were not physically attractive? How were their matrimonial matters settled? In cases where young men or women were either too poor to venture into marriage or had some physical or mental infirmity that made it difficult to find a mate, organizations provided opportunities and funds to unite such individuals. Most physically and mentally handicapped individuals were encouraged to marry and procreate. Occasionally individuals were even forced into matrimony and parenthood. Public-spirited Jews, especially Jewesses, collected money to provide these unfortunates with trousseaus, cash dowries, and a variety of necessities for establishing a home. Undoubtedly, the mating of physically and mentally defective individuals contributed to a number of abnormal offspring.

Among certain segments of Orthodox Jewry, and even in less religious circles, "match-making" continues to play a prime role in matrimonial matters. This may be done by parents, friends, or a professional marriage broker. The criteria for matching couples have not changed dramatically, and in many places today dating services use computers to match couples according to levels of learning, interests, abilities, physical features, and economic status.

Intermarriage between the Jewish communities

When Jews from one ethnic group marry Jews from another, the chances of like heterozygous individuals mating is markedly reduced. This process of intermarriage between the Jewish communities is probably greatest in Israel. The population structure of Israel is such that approximately half the Jews are Ashkenazim while the other half are Sephardim and Oriental Jews. In no other country of the world is there such an equal division. The social and cultural differences between the various groups are gradually disappearing, and as a result Jews in Israel are marrying Jews from different ethnic backgrounds. The exact rate of intermarriages of this type is difficult to determine because adequate information is not recorded at the time a marriage license is obtained. Marriage license records note only the origins (Ashkenazi or non-Ashkenazi) of the partners' fathers (not of their mothers). If the father was born in Israel, no information is recorded. Table 13.1 thus reflects the trend (minimal, for the above reasons) between 1955 and 1974. The rate of intermarriage will most likely continue to increase among Israeli Jews, and for the immediate future will serve to lessen the occurrence of hereditary diseases that are characteristic of the various Jewish ethnic groups (see Appendixes 1 and 2). Because of the population make-up of Diaspora Jewry, it is doubtful that intermarriage between the Jewish communities there will be a significant factor in the dispersal of certain mutant genes.

Consanguinity

Consanguinity among the various Jewish ethnic groups was discussed in detail in Chapter 12. The point to be emphasized here is that the rate of closely consanguineous marriages is decreasing among the Oriental and Sephardi Jewish com-

Table 13.1. Rate of marriage of Ashkenazi Jews to non-Ashkenazi Jews
in Israel, 1955–1974

Year	%	Year	%	Year	%
1955	11.8	1965	13.8	1970	17.6
1960	14.5	1966	13.6	1971	18.5
1961	14.6	1967	15.5	1972	18.4
1962	14.9	1968	16.2	1973	18.6
1963	15.4	1969	17.5	1974	19.1
1964	15.1				

Source: *Statistical Abstract of Israel, 1976,* no. 27.

munities of Israel, and this trend will probably continue in the future. Consanguinity still exists among the Ashkenazim, but at such a low level that it can no longer be considered a major factor contributing to the frequency of most of the genetic diseases that are characteristic of this group.

Proselytism and Conversion

Proselytism (a process whereby Jews seek to convert non-Jews to Judaism) has varied in intensity from antiquity to the present. The act itself has often been the source of controversy, but from a genetic standpoint it serves to reduce the risk of parents having children with a genetic disorder common to one of the Jewish ethnic groups. Some Jewish leaders advocate that proselytism be actively pursued, but this has not been the case for the past 1,000 years of Jewish history. Although adequate information is lacking regarding the role of proselytism in increasing the size of the Jewish population, it can be stated with a high degree of certainty that the process currently has a minimal influence on the genetic make-up of the Jewish people.

Conversion (a process whereby non-Jews seek to convert to Judaism) to the Jewish religion in most instances takes place when a non-Jewish partner is about to marry a Jew or Jewess. In the majority of cases today the process involves a non-Jewish woman converting to Judaism. Information on the rate of conversion to Judaism is not easily obtained, but in 1954 reports from 785 U.S. congregational rabbis revealed that approximately 3,000 persons were being converted to Judaism annually. The number in the United States has been increasing yearly, but precise figures are not known.

From 1948 to 1968, 2,288 converts were accepted by the rabbinical courts of Israel. More recently the rabbinical authorities in Israel have taken a more lenient attitude toward conversion, but the annual rate of conversion remains small.

Some demographers in the United States point out that as the rate of intermarriage (mixed marriage) increases, there is a proportionate increase in the rate of conversion of the non-Jewish spouse to Judaism. Since there is a definite upward trend in intermarriage, one might predict a concomitant increase in the number of non-Jews converting to Judaism. The net result would be a subsequent decline in the occurrence (in the immediate future) of the genetic diseases common to Jews and, in America, of those disorders characteristically found among Ashkenazi Jews.

Intermarriage with assimilation

Intermarriage with assimilation, like proselytism, although a more active force, has long been a part of Jewish history, but present-day rates of intermarriage are difficult to obtain and are frequently misleading. Nevertheless, it is known that rates of intermarriage between Jews and non-Jews are quite high in the U.S.S.R. and in parts of the world where there are small local Jewish populations. The rates of intermarriage in these small communities range from 25 percent to 75 percent.

In the United States various surveys have been carried out in an effort to evaluate the rate of intermarriages involving Jews. The percentages noted vary tremendously depending upon where, when, and how the study was done. Such data include Rosenthal's overall rate of 42.2 percent for Iowa during the period 1953–1959, the

U.S. Bureau of the Census's 1957 rate of 7.2 percent, and Sanua's 1967 figure of 17 percent. A frequently quoted study is that of Massarik, who found that from 1966 to 1972 the percentage of intermarriages involving Jews in the United States was 31.7 percent. However, Massarik defines *intermarriage* as any marriage in which a Jew by birth marries a non-Jew, irrespective of whether or not that person converted to Judaism before the marriage. Thus, he includes in this category about 30 percent of the former non-Jews who had become Jewish converts, which, technically speaking, reduces the intermarriage rate to a little more than one-fifth of all marriages involving a Jew.

Some demographers feel that according to a strict definition of *intermarriage* (that between a Jew by birth and a non-Jew irrespective of conversion) the current rate in the United States is about 30 percent, of which 20 percent actually assimilate. These figures may not be totally accurate, but the process of intermarriage with assimilation is today considered to be a significant one in certain segments of the Jewish population. The future trend is difficult to project, but such processes will contribute to a reduction in the occurrence of genetic disorders in Jews. Although a few may conclude from this discussion that active proselytism and intermarriage with or without conversion are acceptable means of reducing the rate of certain genetic diseases among the Jewish people, fewer would endorse such an approach.

Family size

Small family size is the current trend among married couples in most developed countries of the world. Although religious and cultural ties have a strong influence, most Jews (with the exception of Orthodox Jews) are adhering to this pattern. Furthermore, evidence shows that Jewish families are frequently smaller than non-Jewish families from the same country or region.

In the United States the fertility rate has dropped from a peak of 3.76 children per woman in 1957 to a record low of 1.75 in 1976. Although it may rise in the next 30 years, most demographers feel it is highly improbable that in the foreseeable future Americans will again engage in the great procreational spree of the post–World War II years. Some nations have already reached their goal of zero population growth (the theoretical point at which deaths and births balance). It is predicted that this may be reached in the United States by the year 2025.

In 1977 the world-wide average reproduction rate was estimated to be 20–30 persons per 1,000, but the average annual reproduction rate for American Jews during the last 25 years has been only about 8 per 1,000.

The current average Jewish family size in the United States is estimated to be between 3.1 and 3.3. Although accurate figures are not available, it is conceivable that Jewish families in other parts of the Diaspora also are small.

In 1978 Sittner wrote a series of articles on Jewish family size in Israel. He stated that non-Ashkenazi Jewish women, who on the average had almost 6 offspring in 1955, had only 3.66 in 1976 (the last year for which precise figures are available). Ashkenazi Jewish women, on the other hand, have slightly increased their fertility rate from 2.63 offspring in 1955 to 2.96 in 1976. While there is a moderate trend among Ashkenazi Israelis to increase their family size, there is a significant proclivity among non-Ashkenazi Israelis to reduce their family size.

CONCLUSIONS

Current trends in marriage patterns and family size among the Jewish people strongly support a decline in the number of Jewish children destined to be afflicted with one of the genetic disorders common to Jews. If one adds to these sociological patterns present-day genetic counseling, prenatal diagnosis with selective abortion, and genetic screening programs, additional impetus is given to this decline. However, it would be wrong to expect this diminution in genetic diseases to occur with great rapidity. Furthermore, the entire question of hereditary diseases among Jews should not be thought of as a passing event. Unfortunately, the problem will remain. The task of medical science will be to reduce the prevalence of genetic disease so that families who know its tragedy or who come to learn its fate will be encouraged by the hope that, some day, others will not have to suffer as they have suffered.

REFERENCES

American Jewish Year Book. 1950–1977. Philadelphia: Jewish Publication Society of America.

Davis, M. 1968. Mixed marriages in Western Jewry: Historical background to the Jewish response. *Jewish J. Sociol.* 10:177.

Eichhorn, D. M. 1974. *Jewish intermarriages: Fact and fiction.* Satellite Beach, Fla.: Sattellite Books.

Genetic disorders: Prevention, treatment, and rehabilitation. 1972. WHO Tech. Rep. Ser., no. 497. Geneva: World Health Organization.

Goldschmidt, E., and Cohen, T. 1964. Inter-ethnic mixture among the communities of Israel. *Cold Spring Harbor Symp. Quant. Biol.* 29:115.

Gordon, A. I. 1959. *Jews in suburbia.* Boston: Beacon Press.

Patai, R., and Wing, J. P. 1975. *The myth of the Jewish race.* New York: Charles Scribner's.

Schereschewsky, B. Z. 1972. Mixed marriage. In *Encyclopaedia Judaica*, ed. C. Roth and G. Wigoder, 12:164–70. Jerusalem: Keter Publishing House.

Sidorsky, D., ed. 1973. *The future of the Jewish community in America.* Philadelphia: Jewish Publication Society of America.

Sittner, A. 1978. Large Sephardi family on the way. *Jerusalem Post*, March 7, p. 2.

Sklar, M., ed. 1958. *The Jews: Social patterns of an American group.* New York: The Free Press.

Genetic disorders classified according to ethnic group and community

Disorders by ethnic group and community	Mode of genetic transmission[a]	Special status[b]
ASHKENAZI		
Abetalipoproteinemia	AR	
Acute hemolytic anemia with familial ultrastructural abnormality of the red-cell membrane	AD	I
Aldolase A deficiency	AR	I
Bloom syndrome	AR	
Buerger disease	NG	
Color blindness	XR	NP
Coronary heart disease	M?	
Essential pentosuria	AR	
Familial dysautonomia	AR	
Familial hyperglycinuria	U	I
Familial iminoglycinuria	AR	F
Gaucher disease type I	AR	
Gilles de la Tourette syndrome	U	
Glycinuria associated with nephrolithiasis	AD?	I
Mucolipidosis type IV	AR	
Multiple sclerosis	NG	
Niemann-Pick disease (infantile type)	AR	
Oculopharyngeal muscular dystrophy	AR	I
Ovoid pupil	AD	I+NP
Polycythemia vera	M?	
Primary torsion dystonia	AR	
PTA (plasma thromboplastin antecedent) deficiency	AR	
Regional enteritis (Crohn disease)	M?	
Spongy degeneration of the central nervous system	AR	
Tay-Sachs disease	AR	I
Tyrosinosis	AR	
Ulcerative colitis	M?	
Upper limb–cardiovascular syndrome type I	C	I
Upper limb–cardiovascular syndrome type II	U	I
X-linked gout due to mutant feedback-resistant phosphoribosylpyrophosphate synthetase	XR	I
Werner syndrome	AR	F

Disorders by ethnic group and community	Mode of genetic transmission[a]	Special status[b]
ORIENTAL		
KURDISTAN		
Glucose-6-phosphate dehydrogenase deficiency	XR	
Thalassemia (alpha)	AR	
Thalassemia (beta)	AR	
INDIA		
Ichthyosis vulgaris (autosomal dominant type)	AD	
Takayasu arteritis	U	F
Thalassemia (alpha)	AR	
Thalassemia (beta)	AR	
IRAN		
Acrocephalopolysyndactyly type IV: A new syndrome	AR	I
Camptodactyly with fibrous tissue hyperplasia and skeletal dysplasia	AR	I
Combined factor V and factor VIII deficiency	AR	F
Cutis laxa: A new variant	AR	I
Dubin-Johnson syndrome	AR	
Glucose-6-phosphate dehydrogenase deficiency	XR	
Hairy ears	AD (Y-linked)	NP
Metachromatic leukodystrophy: A new variant	AR	I
Persistent mild hyperphenylalaninemia	AR	NP
Pituitary dwarfism II (Laron type)	AR	
Pseudocholinesterase deficiency	AR	
Selective hypoaldosteronism	AR	
Wrinkly skin syndrome	AR	I
IRAQ		
Benign familial hematuria	AD	NP
Blue sclerae and keratoconus	AR	I
Bronchial asthma	M?	
Cleidocranial dysplasia (autosomal recessive type)	AR	F
Combined factor V and factor VIII deficiency	AR	F
Congenital hepatic fibrosis and nephronophthisis	AR	I
Congenital ichthyosis with atrophy, mental retardation, dwarfism, and generalized aminoaciduria	AR	I
Familial infantile renal tubular acidosis with congenital nerve deafness	AR	I
Familial Mediterranean fever	AR	
Glucose-6-phosphate dehydrogenase deficiency	XR	
Glanzmann thrombasthenia	AR	
Glycoproteinuria, osteopetrosis, and dwarfism	AR?	I
Hairy ears	AD (Y-linked)	NP
Ichthyosis vulgaris (X-linked type)	XR	
Meckel syndrome	AR	
Pituitary dwarfism II (Laron type)	AR	
Pseudocholinesterase deficiency	AR	
Pyloric atresia	AR	F
Spondyloenchondrodysplasia	AR	I
X-linked recessive retinal dysplasia	XR	I
Wrinkly skin syndrome	AR	I
YEMEN		
Celiac disease	M?	
Cystic lung disease	M?	
Familial neutropenia	AD	
Familial syndrome of central nervous system and ocular malformations	AR	I
Hereditary deficiency of peroxidase and phospholipids in eosinophilic granulocytes	AR	NP
Meckel syndrome	AR	
Metachromatic leukodystrophy: Late infantile type among the Habbanites	AR	

Disorders by ethnic group and community	Mode of genetic transmission[a]	Special status[b]
Persistent mild hyperphenylalaninemia	AR	F+NP
Phenylketonuria	AR	
Pituitary dwarfism II	AR	
Hemoglobin Bart's (thalassemia syndrome)	AR	

SEPHARDI

EGYPT
Combined factor V and factor VIII deficiency	AR	F

LIBYA
Cystinuria	AR	
Familial Mediterranean fever	AR	

MOROCCO
Ataxia-telangiectasia	AR	
Deaf mutism with total albinism	AR	F
Familial deafness	AR	
Glycogen storage disease type III	AR	
Neurological syndrome simulating familial dysautonomia	AR	I
Partial albinism	XR	I
Radioulnar synostosis and craniosynostosis	AD	I
Tel Hashomer camptodactyly syndrome	AR	I

NORTH AFRICA (country not specified or mixed origin)
Celiac disease	M?	
Congenital adrenal hyperplasia	AR	
Congenital deafness and onychodystrophy	AR	I
Cystinosis	AR	
Familial Mediterranean fever	AR	
Glycogen storage disease type III	AR	
Hereditary deficiency of peroxidase and phospholipids in eosinophilic granulocytes	AR	NP
Hypouricemia, hypercalciuria, and decreased bone density	AR?	I
Leprechaunism	AR	F
Persistent mild hyperphenylalaninemia	AR	NP
Phenylketonuria	AR	F
Takayasu arteritis	U	F

TUNISIA
Blue sclerae and keratoconus	AR	F
Selective vitamin B$_{12}$ malabsorption	AR	

ALL THREE MAJOR ETHNIC GROUPS
Down syndrome	C	
Lactose intolerance	AR	
Left-handedness	M?	NP
Stub thumbs	AD	NP

OTHER

KARAITES
Hydrotic ectodermal dysplasia	AR	I
Werdnig-Hoffmann disease	AR	

SAMARITANS
Chronic airway disease in a Samaritan family	AD	

Note: All disorders discussed in this text are listed with the exception of those in Chapter 10, neoplasias, congenital malformations, and alcoholism. When a disorder involves more than one community it is listed more than once and is so designated by italics.

[a] AD = autosomal dominant; AR = autosomal recessive; C = chromosomal; M = multifactorial; NG = nongenetic; U = uncertain; XR = X-linked recessive.

[b] F = few families affected; I = isolate family affected; NP = nonpathological.

Genetic disorders classified according to major system(s) involved

Disorders by major system(s) involved	Mode of genetic transmission[a]	Country or ethnic group[b]	Special status[c]
BLOOD			
Acute hemolytic anemia with familial ultrastructural abnormality of the red-cell membrane	AD	Ashk.	I
Aldolase A deficiency	AR	Ashk.	I
Combined factor V and factor VIII deficiency	AR	Egypt	F
		Iraq	F
		Iran	F
		Syria	F
Familial neutropenia	AD	Yemen	NP
Glucose-6-phosphate dehydrogenase deficiency	XR	Kurdistan	
		Iraq	
		Iran	
Glanzmann thrombasthenia	AR	Iraq	
Hereditary deficiency of peroxidase and phospholipids in eosinophilic granulocytes	AR	North Africa	NP
		Yemen	
Polycythemia vera	M?	Ashk.	
PTA (plasma thromboplastin antecedent) deficiency	AR	Ashk.	
Thalassemia syndromes	AR	Oriental	
CARDIOVASCULAR			
Buerger disease	NG	Ashk.	
Coronary heart disease	M?	Ashk.	
Takayasu arteritis	U	India	F
		Seph.	F
Upper limb–cardiovascular syndrome type I	C	Ashk.	I
Upper limb–cardiovascular syndrome type II	U	Ashk.	I
CENTRAL NERVOUS SYSTEM			
Ataxia-telangiectasia	AR	Morocco	
Congenital ichthyosis with atrophy, mental retardation, dwarfism, and generalized aminoaciduria	AR	Iraq	I
Down syndrome	C	Ashk.	
		Seph.	
		Oriental	
Familial deafness	AR	Morocco	
Familial dysautonomia	AR	Ashk.	
Familial syndrome of central nervous system and ocular malformations	AR	Yemen	I
Gaucher disease type I	AR	Ashk.	

Disorders by major system(s) involved	Mode of genetic transmission[a]	Country or ethnic group[b]	Special status[c]
Gilles de la Tourette syndrome	U	Ashk.	
Left-handedness	M	Ashk.	NP
		Seph.	
		Oriental	
Meckel syndrome	AR	Iraq	
		Yemen	
Metachromatic leukodystrophy: Late infantile type			
among the Habbanites	AR	Habbanites	
Metachromatic leukodystrophy: A new variant	AR	Iran	I
Multiple sclerosis	NG	Ashk.	
Mucolipidosis type IV	AR	Ashk.	
Niemann-Pick disease	AR	Ashk.	
Neurological syndrome simulating familial			
dysautonomia	AR	Morocco	I
Phenylketonuria	AR	North Africa	
		Yemen	
Primary torsion dystonia	AR	Ashk.	
Spongy degeneration of the central nervous system	AR	Ashk.	
Tay-Sachs disease	AR	Ashk.	
Werdnig-Hoffmann disease	AR	Karaites	
CONNECTIVE TISSUE			
Blue sclerae and keratoconus	AR	Iraq	I
		Tunisia	F
Cleidocranial dysplasia (autosomal recessive type)	AR	Iraq	F
Familial Mediterranean fever	AR	Libya	
		North Africa	
		Iraq	
Werner syndrome	AR	Ashk.	F
Wrinkly skin syndrome	AR	Iran	F
		Iraq	
CHROMOSOMAL			
Down syndrome	C	Ashk.	
		Seph.	
		Oriental	
Upper limb–cardiovascular syndrome type I	C	Ashk.	I
EAR			
Congenital deafness and onychodystrophy	AR	Seph.	I
Deaf mutism with total albinism	AR	Morocco	I
Familial deafness	AR	Morocco	
Familial infantile renal tubular acidosis with			
congenital nerve deafness	AR	Iraq	I
Hairy ears	AD	Iraq	NP
	(Y-linked)	Iran	
Partial albinism and deaf mutism	XR	Morocco	I
EYE			
Blue sclerae and keratoconus	AR	Iraq	I
		Tunisia	F
Color blindness	XR	Ashk.	NP
Familial syndrome of central nervous system and			
ocular malformations	AR	Yemen	I
Ovoid pupils	AD	Ashk.	I+NP
X-linked recessive retinal dysplasia	XR	Iraq	I
GASTROINTESTINAL			
Abetalipoproteinemia	AR	Ashk.	
Celiac disease	M	North Africa	
		Yemen	

Disorders by major system(s) involved	Mode of genetic transmission[a]	Country or ethnic group[b]	Special status[c]
Congenital hepatic fibrosis and nephronophthisis	AR	Iraq	I
Dubin-Johnson syndrome	AR	Iran	
Lactose intolerance	AR	Ashk.	
		Seph.	
		Oriental	
Pyloric atresia	AR	Iraq	
Regional enteritis (Crohn disease)	M?	Ashk.	
Selective vitamin B₁₂ malabsorption	AR	Tunisia	F
Ulcerative colitis	M?	Ashk.	

MALFORMATION SYNDROMES

Acrocephalopolysyndactyly type IV: A new syndrome	AR	Iran	I
Camptodactyly with fibrous tissue hyperplasia and skeletal dysplasia	AR	Iran	I
Meckel syndrome	AR	Iraq	
		Yemen	
Radioulnar synostosis and craniosynostosis	AD	Morocco	I
Spondyloenchondrodysplasia	AR?	Iraq	I
Stub thumbs	AD	Ashk.	NP
		Seph.	
		Oriental	
Tel Hashomer camptodactyly syndrome	AR	Morocco	I

METABOLIC AND/OR ENDOCRINE

Abetalipoproteinemia	AR	Ashk.	
Aldolase A deficiency	AR	Ashk.	I
Bloom syndrome	AR	Ashk.	
Celiac disease	M	North Africa	
		Yemen	
Congenital adrenal hyperplasia	AR	North Africa	
Cystinosis	AR	North Africa	
Cystinuria	AR	Libya	
Essential pentosuria	AR	Ashk.	
Familial hyperglycinuria	U	Ashk.	I
Familial iminoglycinuria	AR	Ashk.	F
Familial Mediterranean fever	AR	Libya	
		North Africa	
		Iraq	
Gaucher disease type I	AR	Ashk.	
Gilles de la Tourette syndrome	U	Ashk.	
Glucose-6-phosphate dehydrogenase deficiency	XR	Kurdistan	
		Iraq	
		Iran	
Glycinuria associated with nephrolithiasis	AD	Ashk.	I
		North Africa	
Glycogen storage disease type III	AR	Morocco	
Glycoproteinuria, osteopetrosis, and dwarfism	AR?	Iraq	I
Hypouricemia, hypercalcemia, and decreased bone density	AR?	North Africa	I
Lactose intolerance	AR	Ashk.	
		Seph.	
		Oriental	
Leprechaunism	AR	North Africa	F
Metachromatic leukodystrophy in Habbanites	AR	Habbanites	
Metachromatic leukodystrophy: A new variant	AR	Iran	I
Mucolipidosis type IV	AR	Ashk.	
Niemann-Pick disease	AR	Ashk.	
Persistent mild hyperphenylalaninemia	AR	North Africa	NP
		Iran	
		Yemen	
Phenylketonuria	AR	North Africa	
		Yemen	

Disorders by major system(s) involved	Mode of genetic transmission[a]	Country or ethnic group[b]	Special status[c]
Pituitary dwarfism II (Laron type)	AR	Iran	
		Iraq	
		Yemen	
Pseudocholinesterase deficiency	AR	Iran	
		Iraq	
Selective hypoaldosteronism	AR	Iran	
Selective vitamin B$_{12}$ malabsorption	AR	Tunisia	F
Tay-Sachs disease	AR	Ashk.	
Tyrosinosis	AR	Ashk.	I
X-linked gout due to mutant feedback-resistant			
phosphoribosylpyrophosphate synthetase	XR	Ashk.	I
MUSCULOSKELETAL			
Acrocephalopolysyndactyly type IV: A new syndrome	AR	Iran	I
Camptodactyly with fibrous tissue hyperplasia and			
skeletal dysplasia	AR	Iran	I
Cleidocranial dysplasia (autosomal			
recessive type)	AR	Iraq	F
Glycoproteinuria, osteopetrosis and dwarfism	AR?	Iraq	I
Oculopharyngeal muscular dystrophy	AR	Ashk.	I
Spondyloenchondrodysplasia	AR?	Iraq	I
Tel Hashomer camptodactyly syndrome	AR	Morocco	I
RENAL			
Benign familial hematuria	AD	Iraq	NP
Congenital hepatic fibrosis and nephronophthisis	AR	Iraq	I
Cystinosis	AR	North Africa	
Cystinuria	AR	Libya	
Familial infantile renal tubular acidosis with			
congenital nerve deafness	AR	Iraq	I
Glycinuria associated with nephrolithiasis	AD?	Ashk.	I
X-linked gout due to mutant feedback-resistant			
phosphoribosylpyrophosphate synthetase	XR	Ashk.	I
RESPIRATORY			
Bronchial asthma	M	Iraq	
Chronic airway disease in a Samaritan family	AD	Samaritans	I
Cystic lung disease	M	Yemen	
SKIN			
Ataxia-telangiectasia	AR	Morocco	
Bloom syndrome	AR	Ashk.	
Congenital deafness and onychodystrophy	AR	Seph.	I
Congenital ichthyosis with atrophy, mental			
retardation, dwarfism and generalized			
aminoaciduria	AR	Iraq	I
Deaf mutism with total albinism	AR	Morocco	I
Hairy ears	AD	Iraq	NP
	(Y-linked)	Iran	
Hydrotic ectodermal dysplasia	AR	Karaites	I
Ichthyosis vulgaris (X-linked type)	XR	Iraq	
Ichthyosis vulgaris (autosomal dominant type)	AD	India	
Partial albinism	XR	Morocco	I
Wrinkly skin syndrome	AR	Iran	I
		Iraq	I

Note: All disorders discussed in this text are listed with the exception of those in Chapter 10, neoplasias, congenital malformations, and alcoholism. Because of difficulties in classifying these disorders, some are listed under more than one heading and are so designated by italics.

[a] AD = autosomal dominant; AR = autosomal recessive; C = chromosomal; M = multifactorial; NG = non-genetic; U = uncertain; XR = X-linked recessive.

[b] Ashk. = Ashkenazi; Seph. = Sephardi.

[c] F = few families affected; I = isolate family affected; NP = nonpathological.

Index

Abetalipoproteinemia: 68–73; basic defect in, 71; clinical features of, 69; diagnosis of, 69–70; genetics of, 71–72; historical note on, 68–69; prognosis and treatment of, 72

Achondroplasia, 38

Acidosis, familial infantile renal tubular, with congenital nerve deafness: 241–44; basic defect in, 243; clinical features and diagnosis of, 241–42; genetics of, 243; historical note on, 241; prognosis and treatment of, 243

Acrocephalopolysyndactyly type IV: 208–15; basic defect in, 213; clinical features and diagnosis of, 209–13; genetics of, 213–14; historical note on, 208–9; prenatal diagnosis of, 449; prognosis and treatment of, 214

Acromegaly, 404–5

Airway disease, chronic, 222

Albinism, partial, and deaf-mutism: 271–74; basic defect in, 273; clinical features of, 271–72; diagnosis of, 272–73; genetics of, 273; historical note on, 271; prognosis and treatment of, 273. *See also* Deaf-mutism, with total albinism

Albinism, total. *See* Deaf-mutism

Alcohol, tolerance to, 302

Alcoholism, 301–4

Aldolase A deficiency: 215–17; basic defect in, 216; clinical features of, 215–16; diagnosis of, 216; genetics of, 216; historical note on, 215; prognosis and treatment of, 216

Aliyah, 15

Alopecia, 48

Alpha-thalassemia. *See* Thalassemia

Amniocentesis, 448–50

Androgyny. *See* Hermaphroditism

Anemia, acute hemolytic, with familial ultrastructural abnormality of the red-cell membrane: 206–8; basic defect in, 207; clinical features of, 206–7; diagnosis of, 207; genetics of, 207; historical note on, 206; prognosis and treatment of, 208

Anosmia, 49. *See also* Kallmann syndrome

Anticipation, concept of, in autosomal dominant inheritance, 38–39

Anusim, 10

Arabian Jewry, history of, 6–8

Ashkenaz, 12

Ashkenazi Jewry: 12–16; early development of, 12–13; historical characteristics of, 6; migration of, to America, 15–16; migration of, to Israel, 15; persecution of, under Christian rule, 12–16; Polish-Lithuanian, 14; post–World War II, 16; rise of, in Poland, 13; in Russia, 15; in World War I, 16; in World War II, 16

Assimilation, 474–75

Asthma, 49–50. *See also* Bronchial asthma

Ataxia-telangiectasia: 124–31, 469; basic defect in, 127–28; clinical features of, 125–26; diagnosis of, 126–27; genetics of, 129–30; historical note on, 125; prenatal diagnosis of, 448; prognosis and treatment of, 130

Atherosclerosis, 43. *See also* Buerger disease; Coronary heart disease

Atresia, pyloric: 274–76; basic defect in, 274–75; clinical features of, 274; diagnosis of, 274; genetics of, 275; historical note on, 274; prognosis and treatment of, 275

Autosomal dominant inheritance: 37–39; anticipation theory of, 38; features of, 38; role of nonpenetrance in, 38; skipped generations in, 38

Autosomal recessive inheritance: 39–40; and homozygous state, 39; of inborn errors of metabolism, 39–40; of malformation syndromes, 40; pattern of

Specific disorders are listed according to ethnic group and system involvement in Appendixes 1 and 2.

485

Vitamin B$_{12}$ malabsorption, selective: 196–99, 468–69; basic defect in, 197–98; clinical features of, 197; diagnosis of, 197; genetics of, 198; historical note on, 196–97; prognosis and treatment of, 198, 452

Vitamin D–resistant rickets, 41

Werdnig-Hoffmann disease: 204–5; basic defect in, 204; clinical features of, 204; diagnosis of, 204; genetics of, 205; historical note on, 204; prognosis and treatment of, 205

Werner syndrome: 289–91; basic defect in, 290; diagnosis of, 290; genetics of, 291; historical note on, 289; prognosis and treatment of, 291

Wilson disease: 439–41; clinical features of, 439; ethnic distribution of, 440; genetic analysis of, 439, 440; treatment of, 452

Wisdom teeth, lack of, 388

Wolman disease: 441–45; basic defect in, 443; clinical features of, 442; diagnosis of, 442; genetics of, 443–44; historical note on, 441–42; prognosis and treatment of, 445

Wrinkly skin syndrome: 291–94; basic defect in, 293; clinical features of, 292–93; diagnosis of, 293; genetics of, 294; historical note on, 291; prognosis and treatment of, 294

X-linked inheritance: distinguishing features of, 40–42; of dominant disorders, 41; of recessive disorders, 41

Yiddish (Judeo-German), 4, 6, 11, 410
Y-linked inheritance. *See* Genetic transmission, modes of

Ziprkowski syndrome. *See* Albinism, partial, and deaf-mutism
Zomzom, 49

THE JOHNS HOPKINS UNIVERSITY PRESS

This book was composed in Linotype Times Roman text and Ludlow Times Roman display type by the Maryland Linotype Composition Co., Inc., from a design by Susan Bishop. It was printed on 70-lb. Paloma Coated Matte paper and bound in Holliston Roxite vellum cloth by Universal Lithographers, Inc.

Library of Congress Cataloging in Publication Data

Goodman, Richard Merle, 1932–
  Genetic disorders among the Jewish people.

  Includes index.
  1. Medical genetics. 2. Jews—Diseases. I. Title. [DNLM:
1. Hereditary diseases. 2. Genetics, Human—Jews. WB720 G653g]

RB155.G67   616′.042   78-21847
ISBN 0-8018-2120-7